MANUAL OF CLINICAL PROBLEMS IN GERIATRIC MEDICINE

WITH ANNOTATED KEY REFERENCES

MANUAL OF CLINICAL PROBLEMS IN GERIATRIC MEDICINE

WITH ANNOTATED KEY REFERENCES

EDITED BY
THOMAS M. WALSHE, M.D.
Assistant Professor of Neurology, Harvard Medical School, Boston; Associate Physician in Neurology, Brigham and Women's Hospital, Boston, and Associate Chief of Neurology, Brockton-West Roxbury Veterans Administration Medical Center, Brockton, Massachusetts

LITTLE, BROWN AND COMPANY
BOSTON/TORONTO

First Edition

Library of Congress Catalog Card No. 84-82147

ISBN 0-316-92077-0

Printed in the United States of America

HAL

CONTENTS

CONTRIBUTORS

DON BIENFANG, M.D.
Assistant Professor of Ophthalmology, Harvard Medical School; Surgeon, Brigham and Women's Hospital, Boston

ROBERT BROWN, M.D.
Assistant Professor of Medicine, Harvard Medical School, Boston; Chief, Pulmonary Section, Brockton-West Roxbury Veterans Administration Medical Center, West Roxbury, Massachusetts

EDWARD W. CAMPION, M.D.
Instructor in Medicine, Harvard Medical School; Chief, Geriatrics Unit, Massachusetts General Hospital, Boston

SANJIV CHOPRA, M.D.
Instructor in Medicine, Harvard Medical School, Boston; Associate Chief of Medicine, Brockton-West Roxbury Veterans Administration Medical Center, West Roxbury, Massachusetts, and Associate in Medicine, Brigham and Women's Hospital, Boston

RICHARD L. CURTIS, M.D.
Clinical Assistant Professor of Medicine, Tufts University School of Medicine, Boston; Attending Physician, Newton-Wellesley Hospital, Newton, Massachusetts

ANTHONY L. ESPOSITO, M.D.
Assistant Professor of Medicine, Boston University School of Medicine; Attending Physician in Medicine, University Hospital and Boston Veterans Administration Medical Center, Boston

LESLIE FANG, M.D.
Assistant Professor of Medicine, Harvard Medical School; Assistant in Medicine and Associate Director, Dialysis Unit, Massachusetts General Hospital, Boston

RALPH FREDIN, M.D.
Instructor in Social Medicine and Health Policy, Harvard Medical School, Boston; Staff Physician, Mount Auburn Hospital, Cambridge, Massachusetts

RICHARD A. GLECKMAN, M.D.
Professor of Medicine, University of Massachusetts Medical School; Director, Division of Infectious Disease, St. Vincent Hospital, Worcester, Massachusetts

SUSAN MAJOR HENDRICK, A.C.S.W., L.C.S.W.
Social Worker, Brockton-West Roxbury Veterans Administration Medical Center, West Roxbury, Massachusetts

ANDREW J. KEMPER, M.D.
Instructor in Medicine, Harvard Medical School, Boston; Director, Intensive Care Unit, Brockton-West Roxbury Veterans Administration Medical Center, Brockton, Massachusetts

KENNETH A. LABRESH, M.D.
Assistant Professor of Medicine, Brown University Program in Medicine; Director, Division of Cardiology, Roger Williams General Hospital, Providence, Rhode Island

CHERI LEONARD, PA-C
Assistant in Neurology, Brockton-West Roxbury Veterans Administration Medical Center, Brockton, Massachusetts

DANIEL A. PIETRO, M.D.
Instructor in Medicine, Harvard Medical School, Boston; Associate Chief of Cardiology, Brockton-West Roxbury Veterans Administration Medical Center, Brockton, Massachusetts

STEVEN M. SCHARF, M.D.
Senior Lecturer in Medicine, Faculty of Health Sciences, Ben-Gurion University; Director, Division of Lung Diseases, Soroka Medical Center, Beersheba, Israel

ARTHUR SKARIN, M.D.
Associate Professor of Medicine, Harvard Medical School; Associate Physican in Medicine, Dana-Farber Cancer Institute, Boston

DAVID M. SLOVIK, M.D.
Assistant Professor of Medicine, Harvard Medical School; Director of Endocrinology, Massachusetts Rehabilitation Hospital, and Associate in Medicine, Massachusetts General Hospital, Boston

LEWIS SUDARSKY, M.D.
Assistant Professor of Neurology, Harvard Medical School, Boston; Staff Neurologist, Beth Israel Hospital, Boston, and Brockton-West Roxbury Veterans Administration Medical Center, West Roxbury, Massachusetts

THOMAS M. WALSHE, M.D.
Assistant Professor of Neurology, Harvard Medical School, Boston; Associate Physician in Neurology, Brigham and Women's Hospital, Boston, and Associate Chief of Neurology, Brockton-West Roxbury Veterans Administration Medical Center, Brockton, Massachusetts

WILLIAM R. WILSON, M.D.
Professor of Surgery, George Washington University School of Medicine and Health Sciences; Chief, Division of Otolaryngology/Head and Neck Surgery, George Washington University Hospital, Washington, D.C.

ELAINE WOO, M.D.
Research Associate in Medicine, Harvard Medical School; Director of Clinical Pharmacology, Massachusetts Rehabilitation Hospital, Boston

PREFACE

All men wish to reach old age, yet they grumble when they have done so. The paradox suggests that aging is not merely a medical issue but an inevitable progression of social, emotional, and physiologic circumstances that changes the individual. Aging brings with it a withdrawal from career or other pursuits, reduced physical vigor, changes in the sensual pleasures, and an awareness of death unknown in youth. The total care of the geriatric patient must address each issue, but a physician is specifically trained to provide a basis for understanding the medical needs; the geriatrician provides a synthesis of medical and general skills that helps the individual confront the series of adjustments from youth to the senium. The geriatrician, therefore, tills a broader field than most others in medicine.

This book focuses on the medical issues that a physician or other health care provider may face in the care of the elderly patient. Social services are reviewed to enable the practitioner to associate the patient with the available resources. The medical topics covered reflect the interest and experience of the authors who, acting as subspecialist consultants, furnish information that can be added to the practicing geriatrician's broader background. The approach does not attempt to be all-encompassing but rather to present a point of view or attitude toward the problem.

There is no substitute for technical expertise even when the overall decision-making requires input from other areas. The diseases of the elderly are, for the most part, those confronted by internists and other specialists in the course of their practice. Modifications in the care of elderly patients are part of the expertise of specialists in their spheres and of geriatricians in general. The principles of good medical care underline the practice of geriatrics as they do any medical specialty; therefore, much of the information here is already imbedded in the literature of each specialty. This book, written by practicing physicians who treat adults of all ages, underlines the subtleties found in the elderly patient and attempts to point out methods helpful in the diagnosis and treatment of diseases of the elderly.

Each discussion is followed by a list of references chosen to reflect the geriatric aspects. Several general references are included to lead the reader to the more general works available. Topics that are special to geriatrics have more extensive bibliographies.

This book is the result of several years' preparation, false starts, and lengthy delays. I am grateful for the perseverance of the authors despite the delays. The publisher, patient in the face of a seemingly inviolate inertia, did not give up: for that, I am grateful. Thanks go also to our colleagues, who have continued to teach us and keep our thinking at least within some margin of reality. We also appreciate the help of Cecelia Shine, who typed the initial manuscript, and Ellie Shore, who typed the final manuscript.

T. M. W.

I. GENERAL MEDICAL ISSUES

NOTICE

The indications and dosages of all drugs in this book have been recommended in the medical literature and conform to the practices of the general medical community. The medications described do not necessarily have specific approval by the Food and Drug Administration for use in the diseases and dosages for which they are recommended. The package insert for each drug should be consulted for use and dosage as approved by the FDA. Because standards for usage change, it is advisable to keep abreast of revised recommendations, particularly those concerning new drugs.

1. AN APPROACH TO THE MEDICAL CARE OF THE AGED PATIENT

Ralph Freiden

The medical care of the elderly patient is a particularly challenging aspect of general medical practice. Elderly patients may have complex medical problems that require medical sophistication; in addition, the emotional and social aspects of their care are critical in allowing the patient to adjust to the illness and its treatment. Elderly patients do not always report symptoms, perhaps because they are afraid that serious illness may be diagnosed or because they merely accept serious problems as part of growing old. Often careful exploration of a seemingly trivial symptom will reveal a pathologic condition. The physician must keep a high level of awareness of subtle clues to the underlying problem, at the same time realizing that physical, emotional, or social stress may be the cause.

Most people age comfortably and in good health. They continue to yearn for and need the same gratifications and pleasures young people seek. In caring for elderly persons who seek medical care, however, it is necessary to understand the issues central to the experience of old age.

Among the **physical** problems that the elderly must face are arthritic diseases that affect locomotion; cardiovascular diseases that limit physical exertion; neurologic diseases that compromise intellectual function; pulmonary infections that lead to morbidity and mortality; and cancer that causes pain, dependency, and death. The **emotional** problems are no less serious and include depression and altered self-esteem. **Social stresses** such as retirement, dependency, death of family and friends, a changing neighborhood, and loss of economic security also confront the aging patient and complicate their medical care. Treatment of the elderly patient focuses on maximizing function and independence in a secure social and physically safe environment acceptable to the patient and his or her family.

The patient's social background provides the data needed to understand the relationships in his or her life. Integrating the background data into a general assessment of the patient improves patient-physician communication and compliance to therapy. The physician should try to view the present from the patient's historical perspective. For instance, an 80-year-old grew up at the turn of the century in an environment distinct from that of today. Asking about the patient's major accomplishments and disappointments, work history, and circumstances of retirement allows better assessment of complaints and better judgment for therapy. The patient's attitude about retirement and contact with previous work also may help clarify some unspoken needs. Knowledge of details of the patient's living arrangements, marriage, and previous relationships may facilitate the treatment plans. Relationship with the spouse may be crucial either in cause or treatment of complaints. If the spouse is not in good health, who provides for the spouse? If the patient is widowed, the time frame and adjustment may help to clarify the current complaint. Information about others who live with the patient and whether the patient lives in his or her "old neighborhood" may also provide useful background. Has the neighborhood changed? Does the patient feel safe walking outside? Knowing if the patient must use stairs inside and outside the house helps understand the limits of the environment. If the patient lives in special housing for the elderly or a nursing home, one needs to know when the move was necessary and for what reasons. Contact with siblings, children, grandchildren, or other family members provides important baseline information. Personal losses experienced by the patient, such as death of spouse, family, friends, or even pets, may explain new attitudes or problems. The ways that the patient spends time give insight into his or her range of function and abilities. The patient may have specific impairments that interfere with enjoyment of hobbies, social activities, or other personal interests. Collection of background data creates a better awareness of the impact of the illness and its management on the patient.

Older people seek medical care when a physical or psychological limitation becomes intolerable to either themselves or their families. Some elderly patients seek medical advice for complaints that do not add up and do not fit with their known disorders. Some of these hypochondriacal patients look for reassurance that they are still intact in the face of the increasing limitation of age. They realize they are more at risk because of their age and react by reporting all ailments. Other patients are depressed and somatize their depression. Direct inquiry is needed to identify the depression, so that appropriate therapy can be started. Many patients come to the physician for a measure of human contact not always available elsewhere. Such patients are benefited by frequent short visits that allow personal contact and advice.

Family and patient expect relief of symptoms and a return to previous level of function, rather than a cure. Like other patients, they fear fatal or progressive illness, but they also fear illness that reduces their independence.

Hospitalization or treatment that increases the patient's dependency may precipitate additional physical or psychological problems. Previous illnesses and experiences (personal, family, or friend) with health systems may influence a patient's judgment and must be explicitly discussed with the patient if they prevent acceptance of a treatment appearing to be advantageous.

A patient may believe that a particular behavior has led to disease or to a long life; an acute or chronic illness may be compounded by guilt. The physician's recommendations may, in some cases, run counter to the patient's own beliefs. The physician who understands the patient's background often can explain the facts in a way that allays the patient's concern. Depending on an individual's previous skills, a loss of one function may be more difficult to accept than another. For example, a lawyer who loses speech, a skilled mechanic who loses use of his hands, a homemaker who loses the stamina to shop and cook, are all equally disabled. Dependency and deterioration, more than death itself, is the specter of old age.

---

1. Abramson NS, et al: Adverse occurrences in intensive care units. *JAMA* 244:1582–1584, 1980.
   Age of the patient was not mentioned.
2. Anderson F: *Practical Management of the Elderly.* Oxford, Blackwell Scientific, 1976.
   A general text.
3. Anderson KE, Jensen O, Kvorning SA: Prevention of pressure sores by identifying patients at risk. *Br Med J* 284:1370–1371, 1982.
   Unconsciousness, dehydration, and paralysis were major risks. Lesser risk factors were age greater than 70 years, incontinence, emaciation, and restricted mobility.
4. Avorn J, Langer E: Induced disability in nursing home patients: A controlled trial. *J Am Geriatr Soc* 30:397–400, 1982.
   Excessive infantilization of residents, overly intrusive help in self-care and increased dependence were noted.
5. Besdine RW: The data base of geriatric medicine, in Rowe JW, Besdine RW (eds): *Health and Disease in Old Age.* Boston, Little, Brown, 1982, pp 1–14.
   A recent comprehensive text.
6. Blackburn GL, Bistrian BR, Maini BS, Schlamm HT, Smith MF: Nutritional and metabolic assessment of the hospitalized patient. *JPEN* 1:11–22, 1977.
   A compilation of the existing nutritional-metabolic assessment techniques. Contains the rationale, supporting dietary standards, and schemes for interpretation.
7. Brody JA: Life expectancy and the health of older persons. *J Am Geriatr Soc* 30:681–683, 1982.
   An editorial that emphasizes the need for research in chronic disease.
8. Caird FI, Judge TG: *Assessment of the Elderly Patient.* London, Pitman Medical Publishing, 1974.
   A general text.
9. Caranasos GJ, Stewart RB, Cluff LE: Drug induced illness leading to hospitalization. *JAMA* 228:713–717, 1974.
   Aspirin, digoxin, warfarin, hydrochlorothiazide, prednisone, vincristine, norethindrone, and furosemide produced one-third of the cases. Overall about 3% of patients had complications.
10. Davis NM, et al: *Medication Errors.* Philadelphia, George F. Stickley, 1981.
11. Flegel K, Oseasohn R: Adverse effects of diagnostic tests. A study of the quality of reporting. *Arch Intern Med* 142:883–887, 1982.
    This is a report of reports. The data in the literature are not adequate.
12. Freeman JT: *Clinical Features of the Older Patient.* Springfield, Thomas, 1965.
    Reviews the examination process.
13. Gilchrest BA: Age-associated changes in the skin. *J Am Geriatr Soc* 30:139–143, 1982.
    This article describes the common pathological lesions.

14. Gillick MR, Serrell NA, Gillick LS: Adverse consequences of hospitalization in the elderly. *Soc Sc Med* 16:1033–1038, 1982.
15. Hodkinson HM: *Biochemical Diagnosis of the Elderly.* New York, Wiley, 1977.
Puts the laboratory evaluation in perspective.
16. Kleh J: When to institutionalize the elderly. *Hosp Pract* 12:121–134, 1977.
Guidelines for choosing a nursing home as well as ideas for keeping the elderly at home longer are given.
17. Leaf A: Medicine and the aged. *N Engl J Med* 297:887–890, 1977.
An editorial that discusses the medical approach to elderly patients.
18. Munro HN: Nutrition and aging. *Br Med Bull* 37:83–88, 1981.
A review of the subject, including changes in body composition, tissue function, metabolism, known models of aging, and nutrient needs.

2. PHYSICAL CHANGES ASSOCIATED WITH AGING

Ralph Freiden and Thomas M. Walshe

The pathologic changes associated with aging have been known since Hippocrates listed them as "dyspnea, catarrh accompanied with cough, dysuria, pains in the joints, nephritis, vertigo, apoplexy, cachexia, pruritus of the whole body, insomlency, defluxions of the bowel, of the eyes, and of the nose, dimness of sight, cataract, glaucoma, and dullness of hearing." Besides the symptoms and signs of age-associated disease, however, the clinician must be aware—to avoid unnecessary, expensive, and sometimes dangerous testing—of the physical changes that accompany normal aging. Morphologic changes that occur as a part of aging may produce complaints, but only those changes that indicate a pathologic process need diagnostic evaluation. As in most of medicine, the foundation of good medical care of the elderly rests on a competent history and physical examination. By recognizing the changes expected with aging, the physician can avoid chasing phantom disease or neglecting important signs which indicate illness. Physical changes occur with aging in almost all organ systems. Most of them are easily identified as benign.

Physical Signs

Skin. As the skin ages, pigmentation increases, the epidermal sweat glands and hair follicles atrophy, and the supporting collagen and elastin degenerate. The subcutaneous fat also diminishes, and the blood vessels thicken. These morphologic changes result in the discolored, thin, wrinkled, dry, and fragile skin expected in older people. Elderly patients also develop senile purpura, senile keratosis, atrophic warts, and graying of the hair.

Unexpected dermatologic changes in older people include seborrheic keratoses, which appear in midlife on exposed or unexposed areas. They are irregularly round with a flat top. Initially they are light brown, but they may become heavily pigmented and must be distinguished from malignant melanoma. Aging skin can go through malignant degeneration to cause basal cell epithelioma, squamous cell carcinoma, or malignant melanoma. The physician should particularly search for these lesions in patients who have had outdoor occupations or excessive sun exposure. Any superficial lesion that changes its size, shape, or color should be considered suspicious. The malignant lesion appears to be firmly implanted in the skin, while the benign keratosis appears "stuck on" and has a waxy appearance. A close look shows keratin-filled follicle openings. The fragile skin of elderly patients is easily abraded and with steady pressure, "pressure sores" occur, allowing infection. The loss of sweat glands leads to dry, itchy skin, which is a particular problem in cold weather, when elderly patients tend to overheat and underhumidify their living quarters. The loss of subcutaneous fat also makes elderly patients less resistant to changes in ambient temperature. Thickened and curled toenails that cause chronic discomfort and interfere with walking sometimes become a problem for elderly patients.

Nose, Throat, and Tongue. Changes in the nose, throat, and tongue also accompany aging. Atrophy of the mucosa of the nose, throat, and tongue and neuronal degeneration of the taste buds are normal morphologic changes found later in life. The senses of taste and smell in older people are limited because of loss of primary neuronal centers. Most patients deal well with these changes; in some, however, problems of anorexia, weight loss, and malnutrition develop. Older patients are subject to food fads, which may lead to malnutrition, and anorectic patients may nibble at the same prepared food for several days, thus predisposing themselves to food poisoning.

Muscle and Skeleton. The muscle system atrophies with aging. Muscle bulk and physical strength decline in older people, but most remain able to carry out the activities of daily living. As the skeleton ages, osteoporosis occurs, especially when the rate of bone resorption exceeds that of new bone formation. The ligaments and cartilages of the joints lose resilience and elasticity. Cartilage also goes through degenerative changes as it ages. The combination of muscular weakness, stiff joints, and impaired sensory input reduces confidence in physical activity. The stooped posture of older people comes from the atrophy of supporting structures in the skeleton. Lost height in elderly patients is generally from a compression of the spinal column, first in the disks and then in the vertebral bodies themselves.

Teeth. Dental caries, gingival atrophy, atrophic changes in the jaw, and changes of the gastric and intestinal mucosa characterize the aging process of the gastrointestinal tract. Patients lose teeth and are less able to chew. Dentures are difficult to fit and maintain because of atrophy of the gums. Inability to chew, added to changes in gastric and intestinal function, produces a capricious appetite that sometimes leads to weight loss and malnutrition.

Kidneys. Renal function in the elderly is maintained, although there are definite changes associated with aging. The kidney mass is reduced by about one-third by age 85. The glomerular filtration rate is reduced by almost one-half between the ages of 20 and 90. Renal blood flow also decreases in the same age range. Despite the physiologic changes in renal function, most elderly patients maintain normal laboratory values except when under stress.

Heart. The aging aorta loses elasticity, dilates, and unfolds, so that occasionally it may obstruct venous return on the left side of the neck. Aortic aneurysm, particularly just below the renal arteries, is frequently encountered in older people and may be the cause of the poor arterial flow that produces clinical claudication, chronic abdominal pain or a lethal aortic dissection.

Heart valve cusps degenerate and calcify, a process that occasionally extends into the interventricular septum. Stiffened heart valves cause murmurs, particularly of aortic stenosis and mitral regurgitation. The calcific cusps make a good site for bacterial infection, and when the calcification extends to the interventricular septum, it causes electrocardiographic conduction defects (bundle branch blocks).

Laboratory Values

Second only to the history and physical examination in detection of illness, the routine laboratory evaluation aids the clinician in management of the elderly patient. The laboratory examination is particularly useful because of the high chance of multiple diseases, each looking clinically similar. Overuse of the laboratory, however, can cause the patient harm. Excessive blood sampling may lower the hematocrit, repeated fasting tests may provoke nutritional compromise, and extensive use of tests that require drugs may cause complications. As usual, the risk of the tests needs to be considered in light of the patient's clinical condition and the expected benefit.

Screening Tests. The subtlety of disease in the elderly is an argument for the use of screening tests such as the automated biochemical profiles now available almost everywhere. These test the function of each organ system, on the basis of which the clinician may order more specific tests. The most useful screening tests are those for electrolytes, blood urea nitrogen (BUN), creatinine, albumin, globulin, calcium, phosphate, alkaline phosphatase, thyroid hormone, fasting sugar, and bilirubin.

Meaning of Normal and Abnormal. The clinician must be able to recognize a laboratory value as pathologic or as a variant of normal. A "normal" lab value is the mathematic expression of a mean value, usually corrected for age. Of persons tested, generally 95% lie within the range of values cited as normal. A number of persons, however, have laboratory values outside the range of normal. The more separate tests obtained, the more chance there is to find a single value out of the normal range. Test value variation may be the result of aging, sex differences, or other individual idiosyncrasies. There is, of course, a range of values associated with disease, the majority (mean) of which are either higher or lower than the values in well patients. A small number of diseased patients, however, may have laboratory data that do not indicate the abnormality. The point is that the normal laboratory value is not absolute and must be evaluated in the context of the patient's clinical examination and the results of other tests.

Once the clinician understands the meaning of "normal" and "abnormal," he can deal with those values that are clearly abnormal. Some variations in laboratory tests come from error, but most laboratory errors are so blatant that they do not confuse the clinician. More difficult to interpret are the variations from the mean that are caused by circadian rhythm, level of hydration, level of nutrition, drugs, and complicating disorders.

Age-Altered Laboratory Values. The elderly patient is particularly susceptible to dehydration and renal dysfunction. When renal function is compromised, many laboratory values, for instance, phosphate and uric acid, have little significance as indicators of a primary pathologic condition. The hematocrit may also vary with the state of hydration.

The level of serum albumin is lower in elderly patients than in younger patients. When the albumin is very low, it usually indicates chronic disease rather than a specific disorder. Aging is accompanied by increased globulin, but the rise in globulin is less than the fall in albumin. The erythrocyte sedimentation rate is less useful in the elderly than in younger people, because it may be elevated in patients without overt disease. Albumin level is important because it binds calcium, so when albumin is low, calcium as usually measured may appear low. Magnesium, cortisol, free fatty acids, and bilirubin, also bound to albumin, may vary when albumin is low. Drugs are well known to alter lab values, especially in the elderly. Thiazides, by raising uric acid and blood sugar, may lead to a misunderstood set of laboratory values, unless the clinician is aware of the effects of the drug. The elderly patient often has more than one disease, so a test that screens for specific organ dysfunction may be less useful in the elderly. For example, in young persons elevated alkaline phosphatase indicates osteomalacia, but in an elderly patient it is usually from some other cause. Isoenzymes help to clear up the confusion.

Laboratory screening is very important in the detection of abnormal thyroid function, because the clinical features are easily missed. The T_3 uptake changes little with age, except that the value may be low when the patient is chronically ill from other disease. The T_4 uptake also changes little with advancing age, but in patients treated with L-dopa, digitalis, or other drugs it may be elevated.

Fasting blood sugar is elevated in the elderly, and the level of blood sugar following a glucose load may be increased by 8–12 mg/100 ml per decade of age.

Other laboratory tests are altered by age. Maximum breathing capacity declines, as does the timed vital capacity. Oxygen tension may also be reduced in the elderly without obvious illness. The cardiogram shows a shift of the QRS axis and changes in the S–T complex without known cardiac disease. The electroencephalogram is usually normal but may show generalized slowing.

The laboratory is critical to the management of the health needs of elderly patients, but laboratory data must be used with an understanding of their limitations and in concert with the findings from the history and physical examination.

---

1. Bailey AA: Changes with age in the spinal cord. *Arch Neurol* 70:299–309, 19 .
   After age 60, the changes become most obvious.
2. Besdine RW: Geriatric medicine: An overview. *Annu Rev Gerontol Geriatr* 1:135–153, 1980.
3. Besdine RW: The data base of geriatric medicine, in Rowe JW, Besdine RW (eds): *Health and Disease in Old Age*. Boston, Little, Brown, 1982, pp 1–14.
   A recent comprehensive text.
4. Freeman JT: *Clinical Features of the Older Patient*. Springfield, Thomas, 1965.
   Reviews the examination process.
5. Gilchrest BA: Age-associated changes in the skin. *J Am Geriatr Soc* 30:139–143, 1982.
   This article also describes the common pathological lesions.
6. Hodkinson HM: *Biochemical Diagnosis of the Elderly*. New York, Wiley, 1977.
   Puts the laboratory evaluation in perspective.
7. Brocklehurst JC: *Textbook of Geriatric Medicine and Gerontology*. Edinburgh and New York, Churchill Livingstone, 1978.
   This has been the standard English text in geriatrics.

8. Eckstein D: Common complaints of the elderly. *Hosp Pract* 11:67–74, 1976.
Symptoms direct the clinical examination.
9. Rossman I: *Clinical Geriatrics.* Philadelphia, Lippincott, 1979.
Basic text with clinical details.
10. Steel K, et al: Laboratory screening in the evaluation and placement of geriatric patients. *J Am Geriatr Soc* 22:538, 1974.
11. Samiy AM: Clinical manifestations of disease in the elderly. *Med Clin North Am* 67:333–344, 1983.
An excellent review in a volume devoted to clinical problems.

3. CHANGES IN THE NERVOUS SYSTEM WITH AGING

Thomas M. Walshe

The neurologic examination of an elderly person reflects both the aging process itself and the changes caused by disease. To interpret results properly, it is necessary to know what changes occur in elderly people who do not have underlying illness. Age-related changes in the gross, microscopic, and neurochemical structure of the nervous system produce the features that one associates with growing old.

The brain weight, which is about 1,400 gm at age 20, is reduced by about 11% between ages 45 and 85. There is no good evidence that brain weight is related to the loss of neuronal or other cellular material; it may be related to losses of extracellular fluid. There are, however, microscopic neuronal losses in many of the nuclei. Cell losses from aging alone have been shown in the superior temporal cerebral cortex, cerebellar Purkinje cells, putamen, substantia nigra, locus ceruleus, and anterior horn cells of the spinal cord. The brain weight varies with body size but does not reflect brain function. Ventricular size, as identified either at postmortem or by computerized tomography, increases in the normal aged patient without obvious clinical correlation.

Degenerative changes occur in neurons in elderly patients. The major changes are neurofibrillary degeneration, granulovacuolar degeneration, lipofuscin accumulation, and loss of dendritic processes. Aluminum concentration is also known to increase in aged neurons, but its significance remains unknown. The degree of change is mild in normal elderly persons.

The metabolic rate in the aging brain does not change. Oxygen consumption remains approximately the same throughout life, but there is more use of ketone in the aged brain, so that glucose consumption decreases. Glycolytic enzyme capacity also declines in the aged brain. Neurotransmitters change with aging but the details of the neurochemical changes are still being studied. Catecholamine synthesis decreases, and monamine oxidase activity increases. Gamma-aminobutyric acid (GABA) decreases during adulthood and increases in the senium. Acetylcholine decreases in the first 50 years of life and then remains stable.

Peripheral nerve conduction slows with advancing age, and central conduction of peripheral impulses probably also is altered. Somatosensory-evoked potential latencies and late responses are prolonged in patients older than 60 years. The latencies of F waves and somatosensory-evoked potentials vary with height, a factor that must be considered in analyzing differences in aged individuals.

The neurologic examination of the elderly is marked by many changes that one finds difficult to associate with an underlying pathologic state. The pupils are generally smaller in elderly patients, and the light reflex sluggish. There is progressive reduction in the movement of the eyes, with convergence. Upward gaze is limited in many normal elderly patients, usually because of degenerative changes in the elevator muscles. Wasting of the skeletal muscles is an expected finding, especially in advanced old age. The muscle wasting is usually symmetric, with only minimal focal weakness. Elderly patients without neurologic disease usually do not have muscle fibrillation, but fasciculation in the lower extremities occurs from aging and is not always a sign of serious disease. A rapid, low-amplitude, physiologic type tremor occurs in otherwise normal elderly patients. The sensory examination usually shows a decreased sensitivity for light touch and for pain. Lack of vibratory sense, particularly in the feet, is also quite common.

The deep tendon reflexes usually persist in old age, although in many cases ankle jerks are difficult to elicit. Knee jerks are almost always present in normal elderly patients. Superficial reflexes (cremasteric, abdominal) may disappear in the elderly. Abdominal reflexes disappear in some normal people shortly after middle age. Babinski signs are not found in elderly patients, unless there is a lesion in the spinal cord or brain.

Elderly persons have bradykinesia and slow reaction time, which may suggest Parkinson's disease, but the degree of deficit in normal aging is much less.

Changes in the spinal cord also occur but usually do not cause clinical signs. The major changes in the spinal cord after age 40 are thickening of the arteries and arterioles. There is also slight demyelination in the posterior portions of the fasciculus gracilis, with gliosis in some patients. Pigment atrophy (lipofuscin) and corpora amylacea is a constant feature also. After age 60 the arterial changes become more obvious.

1. Adams RD: Aging, involution, and senescence. *S Afr Med J* 43:1239–1244, 1969.
   A clinical neurologist's view.
2. Arnold KG: Cerebral blood flow in geriatrics—A review. *Age Ageing* 10:5–9, 1981.
   Brief discussion but many references.
3. Bailey AA: Changes with age in the spinal cord. *Arch Neurol* 70:299–309, 1953.
   After age 60 the changes become most obvious.
4. Bender, MB: The incidence and type of perceptual deficiencies in the aged, in Fields WS (ed): *Neurological and Sensory Disorders in the Elderly.* Chicago, Year Book, 1975, pp 15–32.
   The effects of aging are measurable but dementia causes more obvious and severe abnormalities.
5. Celesia GG, Daly RF: Effects of aging on visual evoked responses. *Arch Neurol* 34:403–407, 1977.
   Age increases the latencies.
6. Critchley M: The neurology of old age. *Lancet* 1:1119–1127, 1931.
   These are the well-known Goulstonian lectures.
7. Critchley M: Neurologic changes in the aged. *J Chronic Dis* 3:459–477, 1956.
   A definitive clinical discussion.
8. Dekaban AS: Changes in brain weights during the span of human life: Relation of brain weights to body heights and body weights. *Ann Neurol* 4:345–356, 1978.
   Brain weight is related to arm span and height.
9. Finch CE: Neuroendocrine and autonomic aspects of aging, in Finch CE, Hayflich L (eds): *Handbook of the Biology of Aging.* New York, Van Nostrand, 1977, chap 11.
   A survey of neurochemical changes.
10. Foley JM: Sensation and behavior, in Fields WS (ed): *Neurological and Sensory Disorders in the Elderly.* Chicago, Year Book, 1975, pp 1–14.
    A discussion of normal and abnormal changes.
11. Ford CV, Winter J: Computerized axial tomograms and dementia in elderly patients. *J Gerontol* 36:164–169, 1980.
    Enlarged ventricles and increased sulcal markings are related not to dementia but to age.
12. Howell TH: Neurological problems of the elderly. *Gerontol Clin* 8:77–94, 1966.
    Discusses normal changes and major pathologic problems.
13. Jacoby RJ, Levy R: Computed tomography in the elderly: II. Senile, dementia: Diagnosis and functional impairment. *Br J Psychiatry* 136:256–269, 1980.
    Compared with normals, demented patients had a greater tissue loss as measured by CT scans, but there was a large amount of overlap between abnormal and normal.
14. Klawans, HL, et al: Neurologic examination in an elderly population. *Dis Nervous System* 32:274–279, 1971.
    A survey of 3,141 patients between the ages of 65 and 74 years showed 972 without disease of the nervous system.
15. McGeer PL, McGeer EG, Suzuki JS: Aging and extrapyramidal function. *Arch Neurol* 34:33–35, 1977.
    Biochemical analysis shows reduced tyrosine hydroxylase in the striatum.

16. Morrison LR: The Effects of Advancing Age Upon the Human Spinal Cord. Cambridge, Mass, Harvard University Press, 1959.
A normative study of spinal cord morphology. Major changes occur after age 70.
17. Potvin AR, Syndulko K, Tourtellotte WW, Lemmon MS, Potvin JH: Human neurologic function and the aging process. *Am Geriatr Soc* 28:1–9, 1980.
Significant age-related linear decreases were found for almost all neurologic functions.
18. Squire LR: Remote memory as affected by aging. *Neuropsychologia* 12:429–435, 1974.
A decline in remote memory was noted in aged normals.
19. Wells CE, Duncan GW: Dangers of overreliance on computerized axial tomography. *Am J Psychiatry* 134:811–813, 1977.
There is no substitute for histories and physical exams.
20. Baron SA, Jacobs L, Kinkle WR: Changes in size of normal lateral ventricles during aging determined by computerized tomography. *Neurology* 26:1011–1013, 1976.
Data on 135 normals showed greatest enlargement in persons over 70 years.

4. IMMUNOLOGIC CHANGES WITH AGING

Anthony Esposito

Studies in man have demonstrated an attenuation in both the humoral and the cellular immune responses with advancing age. This decline in immunologic activity has been correlated with an increased incidence of infection, autoimmune disease, and malignancy in the elderly. It is not known, however, whether immunosenescence predisposes to these disorders or whether it is consequent to them; most immunopathologists favor the former concept.

The absolute number of circulating B lymphocytes remains stable with age. It is unknown, however, whether age-related shifts occur in the subpopulations of circulating B cells, or whether the number of B lymphocytes inhabiting the spleen and lymph nodes remains constant throughout life. B-cell responsiveness to stimulation by antigens that the host encounters for the first time (the *primary immune response*) declines with age. The attenuation of the primary immune response is dramatic if the antigen requires T-lymphocyte processing. The B-lymphocyte response to immunogens with which the host has previously been challenged (the *secondary immune response*) tends to remain intact; secondary responses are generally recognized as T cell–independent. Thus, abnormalities in T-lymphocyte function appear to play an important role in the age-associated decline in B-lymphocyte activity.

Data concerning age-related alterations in serum immunoglobulin levels remain contradictory. Most investigators report an increase in the total gamma-globulin levels between the third and seventh decades. This increase occurs in the IgG and IgA fractions; the IgM levels remain stable. By the eighth to ninth decades the concentration of IgG exceeds that of IgM, thereby reversing the immunoglobulin pattern of youth. Other investigators, however, have reported a maximum concentration of immunoglobulin in the third decade and a subsequent decline in the concentrations of all fractions with age.

When the levels of specific antibodies that are normally present in the sera of all healthy adults (natural antibodies) are evaluated, an age-associated decline is observed. For example, the concentrations of the blood group antibodies, natural anti-A and anti-B isohemagglutinins, decrease with age. Similarly, titers of naturally occurring, antibacterial, agglutinin antibodies decline in the elderly. The significance of these observations remains unknown.

Current evidence indicates that the decline in immune function associated with aging results primarily from alterations in the T-cell component of the immune system. The absolute number of circulating T lymphocytes appears to decline with age, but it is not known whether the quantity of circulating T cells reflects the total T-lymphocyte mass. The observed decrease in the number of peripheral T lymphocytes seems insufficient to explain the age-related attenuation in T-cell function, and most immunologists believe that aging results in qualitative T-lymphocyte changes. These qualitative changes likely occur as a consequence of the disappearance of functionally active T-lymphocyte subpopulations; in fact, surface marker analysis of T lymphocytes has revealed that while the absolute number of helper T lymphocytes remains stable throughout life, the number of suppressor T cells declines. Cortical atrophy of the thymus perhaps contributes to the alterations in T-cell populations by decreasing the number of thymic-dependent T-lymphocyte precursors or by impairing the differentiation of precursor cells into effector cells. Thymic involution begins at the time of sexual maturity, and by middle age the gland has lost 80–90% of its cellular mass. The serum concentrations of thymic hormones, which appear to contribute to the maturation of primitive T cells and to the regulation of T-cell function, are not detectable by the age of 60 years.

T lymphocytes from healthy elderly persons demonstrate in vitro an attenuation in their response to mitogen stimulation (e.g., phytohemagglutinin or concanavalin A) and a decrease in their cytolytic activity, when compared to cells from younger individuals. Moreover, the reduced in vitro responsiveness of T lymphocytes obtained from well elderly people is accentuated in cells garnered from aged persons with chronic disorders, such as diabetes mellitus and chronic renal failure. Finally, peripheral blood T lymphocytes from fit aged persons produce less T-cell growth factor (interleukin II) than do cells from younger adults. This recent observation has substantial implications since T-cell growth factor augments the response of lymphocytes to mitogens and promotes the proliferation of T-cell clones.

The ability of elderly persons to develop delayed cutaneous hypersensitivity to new antigens (e.g., dinitrochlorobenzene) appears to be impaired. Other in vivo functional studies of T cells have yielded conflicting results. In most series, skin testing for delayed cutaneous hypersensitivity to common antigens (e.g., mumps, *Candida*) has demonstrated a decreasing frequency of reactivity with increasing age. In other reports, however, investigators found no decrease in cutaneous responsiveness when the tested individuals were free from concomitant disease and when adequate antigenic challenge was presented; these investigators did note that the elderly seemed to be especially vulnerable to the transient attenuation in delayed cutaneous hypersensitivity that occurs in association with acute infections or changes in state of nutrition.

Immunocompetence appears to be a sensitive index of biologic age and an important marker for improved survival. For example, persons 80 years of age or older who maintain normal delayed cutaneous hypersensitivity to ubiquitous antigens have a significantly lower mortality than do clinically similar aged individuals who become hyporesponsive. Similarly, sequential measurements of serum immunoglobulin levels in patients older than 70 years reveal that individuals with a rising IgG fraction and a decreasing IgM fraction enjoy a longer survival than do persons who manifest the opposite changes. Indeed, these alterations in immunoglobulin concentrations appear more accurate than conventional parameters in predicting survival.

The absolute number of circulating neutrophils appears to remain stable with age and ranges from 4,100–6,200/μl. These data, however, result from cross-sectional population surveys; longitudinal investigations are not available. Information on polymorphonuclear leukocyte function in the elderly remains scant. Most investigations have been performed in adults with concomitant diseases such as diabetes mellitus or myeloproliferative disorders; in those individuals, derangements in neutrophil function have been demonstrated. However, the ability of neutrophils from healthy aged persons to migrate in response to chemotactic factors and to ingest and kill bacteria remains unimpaired. Thus, in well elderly individuals, polymorphonuclear function appears to be intact.

Healthy aged persons have been evaluated for abnormalities of the humoral elements that are important components of the host defense against infectious agents. The data are limited, but serum opsonic activity remains optimal, and the function of the classic and alternative pathways of complement activation persists unimpaired.

1. Gladstone JL, Recco R: Host factors and infectious diseases in the elderly. *Med Clin North Am* 60:1225, 1976.
2. Gardner ID: The effect of aging on susceptibility to infection. *Rev Infect Dis* 2:801, 1980.
3. Kay MB: An overview of immune aging. *Mech Ageing Dev* 9:39, 1979.

4. Lange CF: Immunology of aging. *Prog Clin Pathol* 7:119, 1978.
Readings 1–4 are extensive reviews.
5. Phair JP, et al: Host defenses in the aged: Evaluation of components of the inflammatory and immune responses. *J Infect Dis* 138:67, 1978.
Neutrophil function, complement activity, and other parameters of host defense in healthy aged persons were comparable to those observed in younger individuals.
6. Roberts-Thomson IC, et al: Aging, immune response and mortality. *Lancet* 2:368, 1974.
The mortality rate during the 2-year study period was significantly higher for elderly patients with fewer positive reactions to skin test antigens.
7. Buckley CS III, Buckley EG, Dorsey FC: Longitudinal changes in serum immunoglobulin levels in older humans. *Fed Proc* 33:2036, 1974.
Low or decreasing IgG levels identified a group of aged persons who subsequently died.
8. Jernigan JA, et al: Reference values for blood findings in relatively fit elderly persons. *J Am Geriatr Soc* 28:308, 1980.
The absolute number of polymorphonuclear leukocytes in the peripheral blood remains constant throughout life.
9. Gillis S, et al: Immunologic studies of aging: Decreased production of and response to T cell growth factor by lymphocytes from aged humans. *J Clin Invest* 67:937, 1981.
Cultured lymphocytes from aged persons produce and bind less interleukin II than do those from younger adults.
10. Nagel JE, et al: Human B-cell function in normal individuals of various ages. *In vitro* enumeration of pokeweed-induced peripheral blood lymphocyte immunoglobulin-synthesizing cells and the comparison of the results with numbers of peripheral B and T cells, mitogen responses and levels of serum immunoglobulins. *Clin Exp Immunol* 44:646, 1981.
Intrinsic defects in B-lymphocyte activity contribute to impaired immunoglobulin production in the elderly.
11. Goodwin JS, Messner RP: Sensitivity of lymphocytes to prostaglandin E_2 increases in subjects over age 70. *J Clin Invest* 64:434, 1979.
An increased sensitivity to prostaglandins results in a depression of effector T-lymphocyte activity in the aged.
12. Nagel JE, Chrest FJ, Adler WH: Enumeration of T-lymphocyte subsets by monoclonal antibodies in young and aged humans. *J Immunol* 127:2086, 1981.
While the total number of peripheral blood T lymphocytes remains unaltered in the elderly, the absolute number of suppressor-cytotoxic (OKT8) T cells declines.
13. Twomey JJ, Luchi RJ, Kouttab NM: Null cell senesence and its potential significance to the immunobiology of aging. *J Clin Invest* 70:201, 1982.
Bone marrows from aged persons contain substantially fewer T-lymphocyte precursors than do those from younger adults.

5. CHANGES IN RESPIRATORY PHYSIOLOGY IN THE ELDERLY

Robert Brown and Steven Scharf

Age-related changes in the respiratory system result in a predisposition to respiratory failure. What may be a relatively minor insult in a young patient may cause far more severe manifestations in an older one. In order to appreciate the reasons for this, it is essential to understand the effects of aging on the physiology of the respiratory system.

Airway development is complete in utero. During childhood, however, alveolar multiplication occurs and is largely responsible for lung growth. The age at which alveolar multiplication ceases is uncertain, but at some time it is replaced by alveolar enlargement. As aging continues, alveolar surface area diminishes, thereby reducing the area available for gas exchange. This, combined with age-related changes in the pulmonary capillary bed, is at least partly responsible for age-related diminution in pulmonary diffusing capacity and pulmonary capillary blood volume. Degeneration of alveolar-septal membranes occurs with aging. This results in hyperinflation (so-called senile emphysema) and is probably related to reported diminution in lung elasticity with age. Since parenchymal elastic forces act to hold airways open, loss of elasticity also results in airway narrowing. The combination of loss of alveolar surface area, diminished elastic recoil, and airway narrowing provides the basis for many of the age-related alterations in pulmonary mechanics.

After approximately age 20, the vital capacity diminishes by about 30 ml/year as a result of aging. The volume of gas in the lungs at the extremes of the vital capacity is influenced by the interaction of muscular strength, lung elastic recoil, and stiffness of the chest wall. The chest wall is much like a spring, which, when disturbed from its resting length, resists compression (deflation) and stretching (inflation). Functional residual capacity (FRC) (the volume in the lung at the end of tidal exhalation) is that volume at which the tendency of the lung to collapse (due to its elastic properties) is just balanced by an opposing tendency to expand on the part of the chest wall. With aging, lung elastic recoil diminishes more than chest wall recoil increases, and the result is in an increase in FRC. In young subjects without premature airway closure, residual volume is reached when the muscles of exhalation can no longer further deflate an increasingly stiff chest wall. In older subjects with airway narrowing due to loss of elastic recoil, however, as residual volume is approached, airway closure and gas trapping occur before exhalation is limited by chest wall stiffness, and residual volume is higher. Although the lung loses elastic recoil with age, and on that basis one might expect total lung capacity (TLC) to increase, in fact other forces predominate. The chest wall stiffens with age, presumably as a result of shape changes (kyphosis, scoliosis) and modifications in the joints of the thoracic skeleton. Also, just as progressive loss of strength occurs in other skeletal muscles with aging, so is there a diminution in the strength of the respiratory muscles after age 55. The net effect is that TLC diminishes and that there is an increase in the ratio of the residual volume to the total lung capacity.

In addition to the changes in static muscle strength already mentioned, changes in the endurance of the respiratory muscles affect the total lung capacity. When loads are greater than normal (e.g., intercurrent infection), diminished endurance may at times be a contributing factor in the onset of respiratory failure. The respiratory muscles of a young patient may be more capable of tolerating a given muscular load induced by respiratory disease. Endurance training of the respiratory muscles seems to be affected by exercise programs. Just as in the area of cardiovascular fitness, such programs may prove to be a useful form of conditioning for the elderly.

The flow of air from the lungs depends on the forces producing the flow (lung elastic recoil, chest wall recoil, and muscular effort) and on the airway resistance. Maximum expiratory flow from the lung demonstrates the phenomena of *flow limitation* and *effort independence*. Increasing exhalational effort will result in increasing flow, until a flow maximum is achieved. Subsequent further increases in effort fail to produce increases in flow. Although respiratory muscle strength wanes with age, it does not diminish sufficiently to prevent elderly subjects from producing enough effort to achieve flow limitation. Thus, loss of strength does not explain the fact that maximum exhalational flow at 50% and 25% of the vital capacity (VC) and maximum midexpiratory flow rate (MMFR) diminish with age. The answer lies in factors intrinsic to the lung itself. Once flow limitation is achieved, the force responsible for maximum flow is the elastic recoil of the lung. This force diminishes with age and may be partly responsible for decreases in maximum expiratory flows in the elderly. As well, large and small airways may become more compliant or "floppy" with age and may collapse during a forced exhalation, causing diminution in flow rates. Because flow limitation has not occurred during the early part of the forced expiratory maneuver, diminished muscle strength and changes in respiratory muscle force-velocity relationships may play a role in the progressive fall in FEV_1 with age.

Arterial oxygen tension (PaO_2) falls with age, but the arterial carbon dioxide tension does not change. These findings cannot be explained by age-related changes in diffusion capacity and probably are related to the phenomenon of airway closure. The *closing volume* is that lung volume at which regions of the lung cease to ventilate, presumably due to airway closure. As lung elastic recoil diminishes with aging, less negative pleural pressure is necessary to maintain a given absolute lung volume. The airways, which tend to be held open by the negative pleural pressure, will therefore narrow as elastic recoil di-

Table 5-1. Changes in pulmonary function with aging

Parameter	Direction of Change
TLC	↓
FRC	↑
VC	↓
RV	↑
DLCO	↓
FEV_1	↓
MMFR	↓
Static muscle strength	↓
PaO_2	↓
$PaCO_2$	—
Hypoxic response	↓
Hypercapneic response	↓

↓ = diminished; ↑ = augmented; TLC = total lung capacity; FRC = functional residual capacity; VC = vital capacity; DLCO = diffusion capacity of lung for carbon monoxide; FEV_1 = forced expiratory volume in 1 second; MMFR = maximum midexpiratory flow rate; PaO_2 = arterial oxygen tension; $PaCO_2$ = arterial carbon dioxide tension.

minishes. Furthermore, there is a normal gradient of pleural pressure from lung apex to base, such that pleural pressure is more negative at the apex than at the base, resulting in a progressive apex-to-base diminution in the tendency of the negative pleural pressure to hold the airways open. When there is loss of elastic recoil, this may cause airway closure, predominantly in dependent lung regions. In fact, closing volume increases with age, and airway closure may occur during the course of normal tidal breathing. This results in unventilated dependent lung regions where perfusion is greatest, low ventilation-perfusion ratios ("wasted perfusion"), and hypoxemia. The clinical significance of this should not be disregarded. If one examines the relationship between PaO_2 and percentage of saturation of hemoglobin (the latter is proportional to the oxygen content of arterial blood), it can be seen that in a patient with a PaO_2 of 95 mm Hg, a substantial diminution in PaO_2 can occur without great effect on hemoglobin saturation. On the other hand, if the PaO_2 is 70 mm Hg (commonly observed in subjects of about age 60 years and older), then a similar diminution in PaO_2 will be associated with considerably larger decreases in the oxygen content of arterial blood. Thus, with respect to oxygen delivery, the elderly patient is subject to greater risk from the same respiratory disorder than is a young subject.

The effects of aging on the respiratory system must consider not only the lung parenchyma, respiratory muscles, and chest wall, but also the neurologic apparatus responsible for coordinating and regulating ventilation. Hypoxic (carotid body receptors) and hypercapnic ("respiratory center") ventilatory responses provide a standardized method of studying the control of ventilation. Elderly subjects have been found to have a diminished ventilatory response to hypoxic or hypercapnic challenge. Once again, then, it would appear that the elderly patient is more vulnerable to respiratory diseases—in this case, those associated with hypoxia and hypercapnia.

In summary, then, age-related changes in the respiratory system cause a diminution in functional reserve of the lung parenchyma, respiratory muscles, and ventilatory control mechanisms, thereby predisposing the elderly patient to respiratory failure (Table 5-1). An awareness of this process should lead to close observation or prompt therapy of respiratory disorders that might otherwise be considered minor.

1. Anthonison NR, Ranson J, Robertson PC, Ross WRD: Airway closure as a function of age. *Respir Physiol* 8:58–65, 1969–1970.

2. Bates DV, Macklem PT, Christie RV: Maximal expiratory flow volume curve, in Bates DV (ed): *Respiratory Function in Disease*. Philadelphia, Saunders, 1971, pp 34–37.
3. Comroe JH: Mechanical factors in breathing, in Comroe JH: *Physiology of Respiration,* ed 2. Chicago, Year Book, 1974, pp 115–117.
4. Georges R, Saumon G, Loiseau A: The relationship of age to pulmonary membrane conductance and capillary blood volume. *Am Rev Respir Dis* 117:1069–1078, 1978.
5. Knudson RJ, et al: Effect of aging alone on mechanical properties of the normal adult human lung. *J Appl Physiol* 43:1054, 1977.
6. LeBlanc P, Ruff F, Milic-Emili J: Effects of age and body position on "airway closure" in man. *J Appl Physiol* 28:448–451, 1970.
7. Loew PG, Theus G: Die Altersabhangigkeit des Arteriellen Sauerstoffdruckes bei der Berufstatigen Bevolkerung. *Klin Wschr* 40:1093–1098, 1962.
8. Mead J, Turner TM, Macklem PT, Little JB: Significance of the relationship between lung recoil and maximum expiratory flow. *J Appl Physiol* 22:95–108, 1967.
9. Reid L: Embryology of the lung, in de Reuck AVS, Porter K (eds): *Symposium on Development of the Lung*. Boston, Little, Brown, 1967.
10. Sorbini CA, Gressi V, Solinas E, Muresan G: Arterial oxygen tension in relation to age in healthy subjects. *Respiration* 25:3–10, 1968.
11. Thurlbeck WM, Angus GE: Growth and aging of the normal human lung. *Chest* 67:35–75, 1975.
12. Turner JM, Mead J, Wohl ME: Elasticity of human lungs in relation to age. *J Appl Physiol* 25:664–671, 1968.

    Readings 1–12 provide information on the development of the lung and the effects of the aging process on respiratory system mechanics and gas exchange.
13. Black LF, Hyatt RE: Maximal respiratory pressures: Normal values and relationship to age and sex. *Am Rev Respir Dis* 99:969–702, 1969.
14. Goldman HI, Becklake MA: Respiratory function tests. *Am Rev Tuber* 79:457–467, 1959.
15. Grimby G, Soderholm B: Spirometric studies in normal subjects. *Acta Med Scand* 173:199–206, 1963.
16. Kory RC, Callahan R, Boven HG: I. Clinical spirometry in normal men. The Veteran's Administration–Army Cooperative Study of Pulmonary Function. *Am J Med* 30:243–258, 1961.
17. Leith DF, Mead J: Mechanisms determining residual volume of the lung in normal subjects. *J Appl Physiol* 23:221–227, 1967.
18. Morris JF, Koski A, Johnson LC: Spirometric standards for healthy non-smoking adults. *Am Rev Respir Dis* 103:57–67, 1971.
19. Schoenberg JB, Beck GJ, Bouhuys A: Growth and decay of pulmonary function in healthy blacks and whites. *Respir Physiol* 33:367–393, 1978.

    Readings 13–19 are standard references used to provide data for predicting normal pulmonary performance as a function of sex, height, weight, race, and age.
20. Leith DE, Bradley M: Ventilatory muscle strength and endurance training. *J Appl Physiol* 41(4):508–516, 1976.
21. Roussos CC, Macklem PT: Diaphragmatic fatigue in man. *J Appl Physiol* 43(2):189–197, 1977.

    These papers introduce the important new concept that respiratory muscle fatigue may sometimes be at least partly responsible for respiratory failure and speculate that respiratory muscle training may be a valuable prophylactic measure.
22. Kronenberg RS, Drage CW: Alteration of the ventilatory and heart rate responses to hypoxia and hypercapnia with aging in normal men. *J Clin Invest* 52:1812–1819, 1973.
23. Rebuck AS: Measurement of ventilatory response to CO_2 by rebreathing. *Chest* 70(Suppl):118–121, 1976.
24. Severinghaus J, Ozanne G, Massuda Y: Measurement of the ventilatory response to hypoxia. *Chest* 70(Suppl):121–124, 1976.

    Readings 20–24 provide evidence that the control of ventilation changes with aging.
25. Ferris BG, Pollard DS: Effect of deep and quiet breathing on pulmonary compliance in man. *J Clin Invest* 39:143–149, 1960.

    A good paper, which outlines the physiologic basis for the importance of periodic deep inflations of the lung.

6. FLUID AND ELECTROLYTE MANAGEMENT IN THE ELDERLY

Leslie Fang

The chronically hospitalized elderly patient, already impaired by a neurologic or other malady, easily falls prey to dehydration. The reason is at times as simple as inability to fetch liquid for him or herself, but in some cases an abnormality of fluid regulation in either the renal or the central mechanism is the cause. Careful fluid management of outpatients is possible but usually not necessary, except in renal disease.

Hydration

In acutely or chronically hospitalized patients, fluid balance becomes a serious issue. Routine chronic fluid management usually may be done by a competent nursing staff, but once an elderly patient becomes ill, he or she has a much greater risk of dehydration, so that careful measurement of losses and intake is necessary to prevent dehydration and its consequences.

To maintain a normal state of hydration, fluid requirements are anticipated and replaced daily. The insensible loss in an afebrile patient is generally 500–750 cc/day and is replaced daily with 5% dextrose in water. Insensible losses in a patient with a low-grade fever (a temperature $< 100.5°F$) are about 1,000 cc/day. Because of the increased salt loss with fever, replacement is with 700 cc of D_5W and 300 cc of normal saline (NS). The insensible loss in a patient with a high fever (temperature $> 100.5°F$) is about 2,000 cc. Fluid replacement for such patients is 1,400 cc of D_5W and 600 cc of NS. Of course, patients with cardiac failure and other complications must have the sodium adjusted according to their cardiac reserve.

To replace gastrointestinal losses, special electrolyte replacement is necessary. In general, gastrointestinal losses (vomiting and diarrhea) are measured and replaced as normal saline, to which is added potassium chloride, 20 mEq/liter.

Urinary losses are also replaced according to volume measured, using one-half normal saline with the addition of potassium chloride, 40 mEq/liter. In the case of dehydrated patients, additional fluid is added to the foregoing maintenance fluids, depending on the electrolyte balance and the patient's underlying condition.

Hypernatremia

Hypernatremia occurs frequently in the debilitated elderly patients and carries an exceedingly high morbidity and mortality. For patients with serum sodium in excess of 165 for more than 24 hours, the mortality has been reported as 50%. Elevated sodium levels are usually seen in elderly patients with excessive water losses and inadequate intake, often in the setting of severe neurologic disease. The reported high morbidity and mortality of such patients may reflect the nature of the underlying disease as well as the direct effect of the hypernatremia. Elderly patients may suffer dehydration even when their serum sodium is only slightly greater than normal. Patients will initially complain of thirst, but the usual presentation is one of altered mental status with drowsiness, lethargy, and at times seizures. Severely dehydrated and hypernatremic patients experience a confusional state leading to stupor and coma.

The clinical setting provides an important clue to the diagnosis. Elderly debilitated patients presenting with altered mental status, especially in hot and humid weather, should always have their serum sodium and osmolality determined. A history of fever, nausea, and vomiting or diarrhea in a patient with limited access to water should also heighten the clinician's suspicion. A careful physical examination may turn up evidence of infectious or other underlying etiologies that may lead to a deficit of free water. The laboratory, in addition to determining the electrolyte balance, may be of help in establishing the diagnosis of dehydration from data such as serum blood urea nitrogen (BUN), creatinine, blood sugar, calcium, and osmolality.

The management of hypernatremia is based on replacement of volume depletion. Prompt replacement with free water will prevent major complications. An estimate of the free water deficit can be calculated according to the formula

$$\text{Deficit in liters} = \frac{x - 140}{140} \times \frac{2}{3}\,(\text{BW})$$

where

x = observed serum sodium in mEq/liter

BW = body weight in kg

Using the formula, one can calculate that a 70-kg man with serum sodium of 169 mEq/liter has an estimated deficit of approximately 9 liters of free water. Half the estimated deficit should be replaced in the first 24 hours, with the remaining deficit corrected over the subsequent 48 hours. The replacement fluid should be D_5W, unless the patient presents with shock from severe volume depletion, in which case colloids and normal saline should be used. Serial determinations of serum electrolytes and blood sugar should be followed and appropriate adjustments made in the fluid therapy. With careful monitoring, hypokalemia or hyperglycemia can be prevented. Excessive fluid replacement is avoided with frequent assessment of the volume status.

Hyponatremia

Hyponatremia is somewhat less common in the elderly, although frequent use of diuretics and marginal cardiac function, characteristic of the elderly, make it a significant electrolyte problem when it does occur. Patients often have no symptoms, but some have mild anorexia, confusion, headache, or muscle cramps. Occasionally, moderate symptoms of nausea and vomiting with changes in personality are found. A few patients present with convulsions and coma subsequent to hyponatremia. The clinical presentation is not correlated with the degree of hyponatremia, although symptoms tend to occur more frequently after a rapid decrease in serum osmolality. Many diseases can lead to hyponatremia, and management is drastically different for each cause. It is therefore very important to assess the patient's underlying problems carefully, in order to arrive at an appropriate management plan. The history should include a careful review to evaluate the patient's cardiac, hepatic, renal, pulmonary, and neurologic function. A detailed history of drug use is also mandatory. A careful assessment of the volume status of the patient is crucial. Evidence of congestive heart failure and hepatic or renal disease should be sought. The laboratory examination must include determination of serum electrolytes, osmolality, BUN, creatinine, and blood sugar, in addition to urinary electrolytes and osmolality. At times, spurious hyponatremia may occur, particularly in elderly patients receiving intravenous fluids or those with hyperlipidemia or hyperproteinemia. Hyperglycemia is probably the most common cause of a spuriously low serum sodium. A rough estimate of the contribution of hyperglycemia to the lowering of serum sodium can be obtained by assuming a decrease of 1.6 mEq/liter in serum sodium for each 100 mg/dl of increase in blood sugar. Once the hyponatremia is established as real and not spurious, it will be found to fit in one of several groups, depending on the volume status of the patient and the urinary sodium.

Hyponatremic patients with clinical evidence of volume excess and a urinary sodium of less than 10 mEq/liter usually have ineffective renal perfusion from congestive heart failure with low cardiac output or from cirrhosis with hypoalbuminemia and a contracted plasma volume. The nephrotic syndrome with hypoalbuminemia is also a cause. In such cases, liver function studies and urinalysis should easily differentiate the three common etiologies.

Hyponatremia in patients who are clinically dehydrated and whose urinary sodium is high suggests a lesion in the renal or adrenal system. Diuretics causing renal salt-wasting, renal parenchymal diseases causing salt-wasting, or adrenal diseases causing excessive urinary sodium losses are most commonly at fault. Again, a careful history, clinical examination, and assessment of renal and adrenal function will clarify the etiologies.

Patients who are hypovolemic with low urinary sodium may have hyponatremia resulting from appropriate renal and adrenal responses to volume depletion. The hyponatremia is usually secondary to extrarenal losses, with replacement with hyponatremic solutions. The losses are often through the GI tract and at times through sweating. Hyponatremia in euvolemic patients with variable urinary sodium raises the possibility of the syndrome of inappropriate antidiuretic hormone, hypothyroidism, or "reset osmostat."

The syndrome of inappropriate antidiuretic hormone (SIADH) is an important diagnosis to make, since hyponatremia may be the only early warning of an associated underlying disease. The diagnosis of SIADH is made when the patient has normal cardiovascular, renal, thyroid, and adrenal functions. There is no peripheral edema, and there is decreased serum sodium, chloride, and osmolality. Urinary indices show a continued excretion of ingested sodium despite hyponatremia and a urine that is not appropriately dilute. SIADH is associated with a variety of tumors, pulmonary and central nervous system diseases, and a number of drugs.

Therapy for hyponatremia is determined by the underlying cause. For spurious hyponatremia, therapy is directed at correction of the underlying hyperglycemia, hyperlipidemia, or hypoproteinemia. Hypervolemic patients with low urinary sodium are treated by optimization of the cardiac output and plasma volume. Bed rest, appropriate salt and fluid restriction, and judicious use of digoxin (0.125–0.25 mg PO qd) are useful in managing such patients. Optimization of liver function, bed rest, salt and fluid restriction, and the use of spironolactone may be useful in the cirrhotic patient. Patients with a nephrotic syndrome should have a full renal evaluation to assess the etiology of the syndrome. Renal biopsy may be necessary for the delineation of the renal disease. The hypovolemic patient with a high urinary sodium is treated by stopping the diuretics, if they are determined as the cause. Patients with renal salt-wasting nephropathy need judicious salt replacement. Such patients may also have difficulty with salt excretion, and care should be taken to prevent excessive replacement. Urine volume and electrolyte measurements are important in maintaining the overall balance. Mineralocorticoid replacement is sometimes necessary. Hypovolemic patients with low urine sodium are treated by replacing the gastrointestinal or skin losses appropriately as delineated previously. Inappropriate ADH patients have their fluids restricted to 800–1,000 cc daily. If excessive fluid restriction is necessary, and the patient's thirst becomes a limiting factor, the use of doxycycline in doses of 300 mg PO qd is quite effective.

When severe hyponatremia causes neurologic symptoms, rapid reversal may be necessary. Furosemide in doses of 40-mg boluses may be used in combination with an infusion of 3% saline solution. Volume overload frequently complicates such therapy, especially in elderly patients. In all instances of SIADH, a search for the etiology may reveal an unsuspected occult malignancy or otherwise undetected pulmonary or neurologic disease.

Hyperkalemia

Patients with hyperkalemia usually have few prominent symptoms. The major clinical association is ventricular arrhythmia. The diagnosis is made by measuring the serum potassium; BUN, creatinine, and serum pH should also be determined. An electrocardiogram can provide an early clue to hyperkalemia. Early changes include shortening of the Q–T interval and peaking of the T wave. With increasing hyperkalemia, QRS prolongation and diminution of the P-wave amplitude occur. Sinus arrest, ventricular fibrillation, and asystole may supervene and cause death. The underlying cause of hyperkalemia needs to be determined in each case. In the case of a patient with compromised renal function, an increased intake of potassium may lead to lethal hyperkalemia. The common external sources of potassium are banked blood, low-sodium salt substitutes, and supplements given in conjunction with hypertension therapy. Another cause of hyperkalemia is potassium shifts, which occur in patients with acidosis. Increased catabolism also results in potassium shifts, as does loss of cellular membrane integrity in patients who have necrotic tissue. Decreased potassium excretion in acute renal failure, chronic renal failure, or mineralocorticoid deficiency is also an important determinant in potassium homeostasis.

Because of the cardiac risk with hyperkalemia, management requires acute adjustments of potassium balance. Glucose, insulin, and bicarbonate can be used to shift potassium from the extracellular to the intracellular compartment. One ampule of $D_{50}W$ with 10 units of regular insulin is given intravenously as a bolus. Its action begins within 30 minutes and lasts for 2–4 hours. Bicarbonate infusion (which is carried out over 20 min) has its onset of action within minutes and lasts for 30–60 minutes. Calcium gluconate can also be given as a direct antagonist of hyperkalemic depolarization blockage on the cardiac muscle. Its action starts within minutes but lasts only 30–60 minutes. For long-term therapy of hyperkalemia, a decreased potassium intake is necessary. In addition, exchange resins, for example, Kayexalate, can be given PO or per rectum. The starting dose is 15 gm PO and 50–100 cc of sorbitol. The onset of action for Kayexalate is 30–60 minutes, and the duration of action is 4–6 hours. Dialysis may be necessary in elderly patients with severe renal compromise and hyperkalemia.

Hypokalemia

Hypokalemia causes insidious and nonspecific symptoms. Muscle weakness, lethargy, easy fatigability, loss of libido, and depression are among the frequent complaints. A history of diuretic use or excessive GI losses is a clue to an underlying hypokalemia, and measurement of electrolytes, BUN, and creatinine generally defines the problem clearly. It is very unusual for decreased potassium intake to cause hypokalemia.

Gastrointestinal losses follow diarrhea, vomiting, or bowel fistulas. Excessive urinary potassium losses are usually caused by diuretic use, renal tubular acidosis, salt-losing nephropathy, hypercorticism, hyperaldosteronism, or pseudohyperaldosteronism from licorice ingestion; medications such as carbenicillin and other drugs with a large amount of poorly reabsorbable anions must be considered if there is no history of diuretic use.

The therapy of hypokalemia is aimed at the underlying endocrine disorder, if it is identified. The diuretic problem can be reversed with discontinuation of the drug, and potassium chloride may be needed orally or intravenously at times. Elderly patients who use diuretics usually require potassium supplement and frequent monitoring of potassium blood levels.

Hypernatremia

1. Ross EJ, Christie SBM: Hypernatremia. *Medicine* 48:441, 1969.
   Early paper on clinical manifestations and management of hypernatremia.
2. Arieff AI, Guisado R, Lazarowitz VC: Pathophysiology of hyperosmolar states, in Andreoli TE, Grantham JJ, Rector FC Jr (eds): *Disturbances in Body Fluid Osmolality.* Bethesda, Md, American Physiological Society, 1977, p 227.
   Excellent review of the pathophysiology of hyperosmolar states secondary to hypernatremia, hyperglycemia, and uremia.
3. Arieff AI, Guisado R: Effects on the central nervous system of hypernatremic and hyponatremic states. *Kidney Int* 10:104, 1976.
   Discusses effects of hypernatremia and hyponatremia on central nervous system, as well as the role of idiogenic osmols.
4. Loeb JN: The hyperosmolar state. *N Engl J Med* 290:1184, 1974.
   Develops the clinical manifestations of hyperosmolar states.
5. Berl T, Anderson RJ, McDonald KM, Schrier RW: Clinical disorders of water metabolism. *Kidney Int* 10:117, 1976.
   Discusses management of hyper- and hypoosmolar states.
6. Feig PV, McCurdy DK: The hypertonic state. *N Engl J Med* 297:1444, 1977.
   Deals with management of patients with hypertonicity due to hyperglycemia, hypernatremia, and uremia.

Hyponatremia

7. Berl T, Schrier RW: Water metabolism and the hypoosmolar syndromes. Sodium and water homeostasis, in Brenner BM, Stein JH (eds): *Contemporary issues in Nephrology.* New York, Churchill Livingston, 1978, vol. 1.
   Review of pathophysiology of hypoosmolar states.
8. Arieff AI, Llach F, Massry SG: Neurological manifestations and morbidity of hyponatremia: Correlation with brain water and electrolytes. *Medicine* 55:121, 1976.
   Neurologic manifestations of hyponatremia are related to rate of change of serum sodium.
9. Fichman MP, et al: Diuretic-induced hyponatremia. *Ann Intern Med* 75:853, 1971.
   Discusses pathophysiology of hyponatremia secondary to diuretics.
10. Moses AM, Miller M: Drug-induced dilutional hyponatremia. *N Engl J Med* 291:1234, 1974.
11. Leaf A: The clinical and physiologic significance of the serum sodium concentration. *N Engl J Med* 267:24, 77, 1962.
    Classic paper describing the clinical manifestations of hypernatremia and hyponatremia.
12. Bartter FC, Schwartz WB: The syndrome of inappropriate secretion of antidiuretic hormone. *Am J Med* 42:790, 1967.
    Describes the clinical manifestations of SIADH.

13. Cooke CR, Turin MD, Walker WG: The syndrome of inappropriate antidiuretic hormone secretion: Pathophysiologic mechanisms in solute and water regulation. *Medicine* 58:240, 1979.
Review of the pathophysiology of SIADH.
14. Hartman D, et al: Rapid correction of hyponatremia in the syndrome of inappropriate secretion of antidiuretic hormone. An alternative treatment of hypertonic saline. *Ann Intern Med* 78:870, 1973.
Deals with management of patients with severe hyponatremia using hypertonic saline and furosemide.
15. Bartter FC, Schwartz WB: The syndrome of inappropriate secretion of antidiuretic hormone. *Am J Med* 42:790, 1967.
Review of the pathophysiology of SIADH and a discussion of the clinical disorders commonly associated with this syndrome.
16. Miller M, Dalakos T, Moses AM: Recognition of partial defects in antidiuretic hormone secretion. *Annu Rev Med* 73:721, 1970.
Discusses identification of patients with partial defects in ADH secretion.

Hyperkalemia

17. Levinsky NG: Management of emergencies: VI. Hyperkalemia. *N Engl J Med* 274:1076, 1966.
Classic paper describing acute management of hyperkalemic patients.
18. Kliger AS, Hyslett JP: Disorders of potassium balance. *Contemp Issues Nephrol* 2:168, 1978.
Nice review of pathophysiology of hyperkalemia and hypokalemia.
19. Giebisch G, Stanton B: Potassium transport in the nephron. *Annu Rev Physiol* 41:241, 1979.
Review of potassium handling by the various segments of the nephron.
20. Surawicz B, Chlebus H, Mazzolini A: Hemodynamic and electrocardiographic effects of hyperpotassemia. Differences in response to slow and rapid increases in concentration of plasma potassium. *Am Heart J* 73:647, 1967.
Early paper indicating that acute hyperkalemia is associated with more significant hemodynamic and electrographic changes.
21. Cox M, Stearns RH, Singer I: The defense against hyperkalemia: The roles of insulin and aldosterone. *N Engl J Med* 299:525, 1978.
Hormonal control of potassium distribution in the various compartments of the body.
22. van Ypersele de Strihou C. Potassium homeostasis in renal failure. *Kidney Int* 11:491, 1977.
Review of the factors involved in potassium homeostasis in renal failure, including increases in renal tubular secretion of potassium and increased gastrointestinal losses of potassium.
23. Schambelan M, Sebastian A, Hulter HN: Mineralocorticoid excess and deficiency syndromes. *Contemp Issues Nephrol* 2:232, 1978.
Nice review of role of mineralocorticoids in potassium homeostasis.
24. Rosa RM, et al: Adrenergic modulation of extrarenal potassium disposal. *N Engl J Med* 302:431, 1980.
Epinephrine enhances the extrarenal disposal of an acute load of potassium. Propranolol impairs this disposal.
25. DeFronzo RA: Hyperkalemia and hyporeninemic hypoaldosteronism. *Kidney Int* 17:118, 1980.
Review of the syndrome of hyporeninemic hypoaldosteronism.

Hypokalemia

26. Cronin RE, Knochel JP: The consequences of potassium deficiency. *Contemp Issues Nephrol* 2:205, 1978.
Describes the clinical manifestations of hypokalemia.
27. Gennari FJ, Cohen JJ: Role of the kidney in potassium homeostasis: Lessons from acid-base disturbances. *Kidney Int* 8:1, 1975.
Discusses serum potassium changes with disturbances of acid-base balance.
28. Kassirer JP, Harrington JT: Diuretics and potassium metabolism: A reassessment of the need, effectiveness and safety of potassium therapy. *Kidney Int* 11:505, 1977.

Points out that potassium is not uniformly needed in patients on diuretic therapy and warns against indiscriminant use of potassium.

29. Kliger AS, Hayslett JP: Disorders of potassium balance. *Contemp Issues Nephrol* 2:168, 1978.
Excellent discussion of potassium handling and clinical disorders of potassium balance.
30. Lipner HI, et al: The behavior of carbenicillin as a non-reabsorbable anion. *J Lab Clin Med* 86:183, 1975.
Hypokalemic alkalosis as a consequence of carbenicillin therapy since carbenicillin acts as a non-reabsorbable anion.
31. Shapiro W, Taubert K: Hypokalemia and digoxin-induced arrhythmias. *Lancet* 2:604, 1975.
Hypokalemia worsened digoxin-induced arrhythmias.
32. Stearnes RH, Cox M, Feig PU, Singer I: Internal potassium balance and the control of the plasma potassium concentration. *Medicine* 60:339, 1981.
Review of the factors regulating the distribution of potassium between the intracellular and extracellular space.
33. Adrogue HJ, Madias NE: Changes in plasma potassium concentration during acute acid-base disturbances. *Am J Med* 71:456, 1981.
Review of the changes in potassium level during acute acid-base disturbances.
34. Wright FS, Giebisch G: Renal potassium transport: Contributions of individual nephron segments and populations. *J Physiol* 235:F515, 1978.
Review of renal handling of potassium, particularly with reference to the heterogeneity of the different segments of the nephrons.

7. DRUG TREATMENT OF THE ELDERLY

Elaine Woo

Although it is becoming increasingly clear that good geriatric medicine requires multiple therapeutic modalities, drugs continue to be the mainstay of therapy. Drug treatment of older patients is complicated by several factors. Geriatric patients require more medication and medical attention because of concomitant chronic diseases. Although the elderly make up about 10% of the total population in the United States, they spend annually 25% of the total national expenditure for drugs. Unfortunately, drug treatment of the elderly includes medications that are inappropriately prescribed by the physician and inappropriately used by the patient. Adverse drug reactions in hospitalized patients over 65 years of age occur three times more often than in patients younger than 50. Thus it is evident that drug therapy may not always solve a geriatric medical problem but may create another problem in itself.

It often appears that the elderly are more "sensitive" to drug effects and toxicity. There are certain ways in which the elderly are unique in their response to drugs. Awareness of these differences can allow practitioners to optimize therapeutic benefits while decreasing undesired drug effects in the elderly population.

Sources of Altered Drug Effects in the Elderly

Pharmacokinetics. Altered drug effects in the elderly have several sources. One is pharmacokinetics, which describes the processes by which the body absorbs, metabolizes, stores, and excretes a drug and the rate at which these processes occur. The endpoint of interest is the drug's tissue concentration, which governs the resultant drug effect and toxicity. If the tissue concentration is excessive, there may be drug toxicity; if the tissue concentration is too low, the therapeutic effects are inadequate. Available pharmacokinetic data on most drugs is derived from young, healthy volunteers, but it is becoming evident that there are significant age-related changes in pharmacokinetics that cause excessive tissue drug levels and exaggerated or unexpected drug effects.

Absorption. The absorption of a drug is the first determinant of its tissue level. Most medications are administered orally, and changes in gastric function may alter absorption. Among the physiologic alterations in the gastrointestinal tract associated with increasing age are increased gastric pH, decreased gastric motility, and decreased mesenteric blood flow (by 40–50%). Although these changes theoretically can impede or alter the rate of oral drug absorption, in fact there is little or no significant change in oral absorption in the elderly. Drugs absorbed from the gastrointestinal tract pass initially through the liver before reaching the systemic circulation. Some drugs are inactivated significantly during the initial pass through the liver. In the elderly, liver metabolic functions can be sufficiently compromised so that the expected inactivation of a drug via the first pass effect is less, and the apparent bioavailability of a single dose of the drug is increased. Propranolol is an example: serum levels are as much as four times greater in elderly patients than in young patients at all time points after an identical oral dose. Other drugs with increased bioavailability after the first pass effect are acetaminophen, aspirin, diphenhydramine, guanethidine, hydralazine, lidocaine, meperidine, methyldopa, morphine, pentazocine, phenothiazines, propoxyphene, reserpine, and tricyclic antidepressants.

Distribution. The distribution of a drug in the body is governed by its molecular size, pKa, lipid solubility, the presence and integrity of active transport systems, and its affinity to binding proteins. In elderly patients there is a decrease in total body water (61–53%) and an increase in total body lipids (14–30%). Although theoretically there might be significant differences in the extent and manner in which drugs are distributed in the elderly, in fact, alterations do not occur in a predictable fashion. Protein binding of drugs to serum proteins also can reduce the pharmacologically active unbound fraction in many cases. For example, phenytoin, warfarin, salicylates, sulfonamides and benzodiazepines are all more than 90% bound to serum proteins. A decrease in serum protein binding of these drugs can occur either because of a decrease in the binding proteins or because of interference in protein binding by other substances. This can cause a substantial relative increase in the unbound fraction and produce an excessive drug effect with the same total serum drug level. In the elderly, there is no evidence that affinity of drugs to proteins is altered; however, elderly patients have reduced protein binding of drugs associated with depressed serum albumin concentration.

Elimination. Removal of drugs from the body occurs principally by two routes: (1) **metabolism** in the liver to less active, more water-soluble compounds, and (2) **excretion** of drugs and their metabolites by the kidney. The time needed to eliminate half the drug in the body is called the *elimination half-life*. The action of some drugs is terminated primarily by metabolism to inactive compounds (examples: lidocaine, propranolol, and morphine). Impaired liver function or impaired delivery of the drug to the liver would result in prolongation of the elimination half-life and accumulation of the drug at higher and possibly toxic levels. Many other drugs are eliminated by renal excretion (examples: digoxin, procainamide, disopyramide, and most antibiotics). Even in healthy individuals, the glomerular filtration rate declines by 1%/year after the age of 40, with comparable deterioration in tubular function as well. Thus, underlying renal dysfunction is the cause of altered elimination of many drugs in the elderly.

Concurrent Disease. Concurrent diseases, such as chronic malnutrition or organic heart disease with congestive heart failure and decreased organ perfusion, can be expected to exacerbate these deficiencies even further.

It appears that the aging process results in (1) prolongation of drug elimination half-life, (2) reduction in total drug clearance, (3) unpredictable changes in volume of distribution, and (4) no inherent changes in binding of drugs to serum proteins.

Types of Altered Drug Responses

Before the advent of techniques to measure blood and tissue drug concentrations, it was assumed that the elderly were unique in their sensitivity to drug effects. Demonstrable pharmacokinetic alterations now indicate that, in many cases, increased drug sensitivity in the aged is actually an appropriate clinical response to excessive tissue drug levels. Nonetheless, true age-related alterations in drug responsiveness are known and include decreased clinical response, increased clinical response, abnormal response, and altered homeostasis.

In healthy elderly patients, beta-active agents such as propranolol and isoproterenol appear to have less clinical activity than the same dosages in younger patients. This is attributed to the decreased number of beta-receptors in the elderly. It must be borne in mind, however, that most elderly patients would be predisposed to toxicity from these agents because of the increased incidence of concomitant heart disease.

As yet, there are surprisingly few well-documented examples of increased clinical response. The elderly are more sensitive than the young to benzodiazepines, even when serum drug levels are comparable. The mechanism for this sensitivity is unknown. The elderly also seem to be more sensitive to warfarin. At high concentrations of warfarin, there is decreased serum protein binding, producing higher concentrations of unbound drug. However, at therapeutic levels, there is also a greater inhibition of synthesis of vitamin K–dependent clotting factors, suggesting an intrinsic receptor sensitivity to the effects of warfarin.

The development of agitation and confusion with administration of sedative agents to the elderly is one of the best-known abnormal clinical responses to medicine. The elderly are also vulnerable to undesired side effects even at therapeutic drug concentrations. Often, nonspecific side effects such as a depressed affect, confusion, or poor appetite may be missed by even the most alert clinician.

Age-related deficits in homeostasis can cause undesired or excessive drug effects. For example, an elderly patient is more sensitive to antihypertensive agents because (1) cerebral blood flow autoregulation may be abnormal and require a higher blood pressure for adequate perfusion, (2) postural mechanisms for maintaining blood pressure are deficient, and (3) underlying cardiac disease causes greater susceptibility to the fluid retention seen with virtually all nondiuretic antihypertensive agents.

Compliance is a major issue in geriatric treatment, as it is in all medicine. Studies employing objective measures of compliance suggest that elderly patients are no more likely to commit errors in medication than a younger cohort. This does not mean that compliance is not a problem in the elderly, however, but, rather, that it is a significant universal problem! The incidence of noncompliance is high, and up to 60% of chronically ill, hospitalized elderly patients make one or more medication errors, of which over one-fourth are potentially serious. The most common medication error is omission of a medication. Up to 50% of outpatients do not take their prescribed medications at all.

The objective studies of patient compliance deal with compliance to only a single drug of interest. Elderly patients generally use many more medications than young patients, and rate of compliance with several pills and multiple daily doses might be quite different from compliance with a single one-a-day tablet. The elderly patient often has several disorders being treated simultaneously. Subtherapeutic or toxic drug levels can early decompensate the interdependent diseases.

Complications of Commonly Used Medications

The following drugs, given commonly to the elderly, illustrate problems of particular importance in geriatric therapeutics.

Digitalis. Although there is no evidence of inherent sensitivity to digitalis in the elderly, digitalis intoxication is one of the most frequent adverse drug reactions in this group of patients. This frequency is partly explained by the fact that digoxin and its congeners are among the drugs most commonly prescribed for the elderly. Moreover, these medications have a low therapeutic ratio, so that the margin of reserve between the therapeutic and toxic concentrations is small. In addition, digoxin clearance falls with the age-related decrease in creatinine clearance; hence, digoxin will accumulate to higher levels in the elderly, even when appropriate corrections are made for body weight. Digoxin clearance is decreased further when the patient is dehydrated or has intercurrent renal disease. Serum levels of digoxin are not always indicative of the level of treatment. For example, congestive heart failure causes a lower volume of distribution of digoxin, so that serum levels will be higher for a given total body load of drug. Digitalis toxicity also can be precipitated by abnormalities in electrolytes (potassium, calcium, and magnesium), even at acceptable serum drug concentrations. Dietary deficiencies and the use of diuretics increase the likelihood of electrolyte abnormalities in the elderly.

Antihypertensives. Antihypertensive drugs may cause several problems. Adequate cerebral perfusion in elderly patients with carotid or other large vessel stenosis requires higher blood pressure than in younger patients. Clinicians should not attempt to lower blood pressure in the elderly to levels "acceptable" for younger patients. Impaired baroreceptor responses and poor peripheral vascular tone also contribute to symptomatic postural hypotension in the elderly. The bioavailability of some of the antihypertensive agents increases because of a decreased first pass effect, and the clinical effect of the drug thus is enhanced. Toxicity can be hard to recognize in the elderly. Nonspecific symptoms such as lethargy, confusion, and dizziness result both from excessive drug effect, causing low blood pressure, and from direct central nervous system activity of the drugs at therapeutic levels.

Diuretics. Diuretics are the mainstay of therapy for both congestive heart failure and hypertension. Although the complications of diuretics—volume depletion, abnormalities of electrolyte and uric acid excretion, and glucose intolerance—are not unique to the elderly, their sequelae can cause serious effects to patients whose homeostatic mechanisms are deficient. Diuretics can create major problems in patients with potassium deficiency from poor diet or overall oral intake. Patients who take digoxin, or who have diseases such as adult-onset diabetes mellitus, gout, or borderline renal function, are at high risk for complications of diuretic therapy. Elderly patients, even off diuretics, are at risk for dehydration; with diuretic use they may become severely dehydrated.

Anticoagulants. Several factors must be considered in giving anticoagulants to elderly patients. Alterations in receptor sensitivity and pharmacokinetics seem to cause increased sensitivity to warfarin in the elderly. Increased capillary fragility predisposes older persons to bruising, even when anticoagulation therapy is carefully controlled. Instability of gait means an increased chance of trauma and hemorrhage. The concurrent self-administration of aspirin or compounds containing aspirin, which potentiates risk of bleeding, is a constant worry in treatment of the elderly. Older patients find it difficult to come to the hospital or clinic for adequate follow-up of their anticoagulation. Visiting nurses can help to solve this problem in some cases. Dementia may complicate compliance, when frequent changes are necessary in warfarin dosage.

Sedatives. Drugs acting on the central nervous system may create complications, even when blood levels are acceptable. Among the major offenders are the sedative, hypnotic, and anxiolytic agents. In the elderly, paradoxical response to these agents may range from mild restlessness to frank psychosis and may be confused with irreversible nervous system dysfunction. When drug activity is prolonged because of pharmacokinetic alterations, the excessive sedation can render the patient dependent and institutionalized. The benzodiazepines, Valium and Librium, have long elimination half-lives and are metabolized to a series of active metabolites with even longer elimination half-lives. Accumulation of clinically active compounds can cause stupor or confusion when the drugs are used chronically.

Antidepressants. The greatest problem with the antidepressants may be their inappropriate use in the elderly. Patients who have chronic aches and pains, physical illness, and losses of job, family, and friends sometimes become depressed; and when the depression is clearly diagnosed, the antidepressants are of use. Clinicians should be extremely vigilant for side effects, which can be especially severe and devastating in the elderly. Orthostatic hypotension, aggravation of cardiac arrhythmias, urinary retention, aggravation of glaucoma, and confusional states are the most usual adverse effects in elderly patients treated with tricyclics.

Antipsychotic Drugs. Antipsychotic drugs cause parkinsonism (extrapyramidal symptoms) in the elderly. Choreiform movement disorders are five times more frequent in the elderly than in the young and are not always reversible when the medication is stopped. Other movement disorders, such as tardive dyskinesia and akathisia, are also common in the elderly. Such iatrogenic symptoms are indeed tragic, if the diagnosis of psychosis was in error and an undiagnosed medical illness such as thyroid dysfunction, glucose abnormalities, or hyponatremia was the cause of the altered mental state.

Guidelines to Successful Drug Therapy

The cornerstones of any successful therapeutic program can be summarized by four concepts: parsimony, vigilance, education, and compliance.

Use the fewest drugs possible. Not every patient complaint needs a prescription; and drugs should be given only for a specific diagnosis that has been well documented. Use the lowest dose and the least number of daily doses. Elderly patients may require less medication to reach a desired clinical effect. Moreover, longer elimination half-lives may mean that drugs can be taken much less frequently than by younger patients. Choose the least toxic drugs possible and, when there are equivalent medications, try to provide the lowest-costing one.

Take repeated and frequent drug histories. Keep in mind that patients have access to many sources of drugs besides the ones you prescribe and may avail themselves of these sources at any time. Nonprescription, over-the-counter medications are easily available from well-meaning friends or family. A trip to the local walk-in clinic or emergency room for an acute complaint can also result in an unrecorded addition to the patient's drug inventory. Evaluate the patient often for the desired clinical or laboratory effect, so that the dosage can be reduced, where possible, or discontinued if there is no demonstrable benefit. It is necessary to reevaluate the need of a medication, since patients receiving it chronically often tolerate a reduction or discontinuation of the drug without ill effects. When there is a change in the medical findings, even in the subtlest ways, consider first the effect and potential complications of the drugs being used.

Before prescribing any drug, know its contraindications, adverse effects, and, when possible, pharmacokinetics, so that you can anticipate problems in drug disposition or response. Educate the patient by frequent verbal and written explanations of the expected effects and possible side effects of the drugs.

A patient who understands his or her own disease and medications can be a valuable addition to the therapeutic team, willingly compliant and vigilant for adverse effects. It helps to establish a medication diary or calendar for the patient, consisting of a booklet with a sample pill on the front with its name, its dosage, and a brief statement of its intended action. Make sure containers are labeled clearly. Large print or color codes may be helpful for patients with decreased vision. Instructions in a specific foreign language may be needed for a non–English-speaking patient. Consider use of standard container lids, child-proof lids may also be elderly-proof and may prevent the patient from opening the box. Choose convenient dosing regimens: When possible, reduce the number of times per day the patient needs to take a medication, administer agents with sedative side effects at night and diuretic agents during the day, and consider prescribing an elixir if the patient has trouble swallowing pills.

---

1. Crooks J, Stevenson IH (eds): *Drugs and the Elderly.* Baltimore, University Park Press, 1979.
Proceedings of symposium held in University of Dundee, Great Britain, September 1977. This is a comprehensive review of the field to 1977 describing the aging process at the cellular and biochemical level.
2. Jarvik LF, Greenblatt DJ, Harman D (eds): *Clinical Pharmacology and the Aged Patient,* no. 16, Aging Series. New York, Raven Press, 1981.
This is the most recent textbook to date that provides a brief but complete review of the general problems of drug treatment in the elderly, followed by an organ-specific approach by particular drug categories.
3. Ouslander JG: Drug therapy in the elderly. *Ann Intern Med* 95:711–722, 1981.
Briefly describes problems unique in the aged, such as compliancy and polyphamacy, and pharmacokinetic differences. Contains 146 references.
4. Richey DP, Bender AD: Pharmacokinetic consequences of aging. *Annu Rev Pharmacol Toxicol* 17:49–65, 1977.
Includes a detailed table listing comparative pharmacokinetic data accumulated up to 1977.
5. Salzman C: A primer on geriatric psychopharmacology. *Am J Psychiatry* 139:67–74, 1982.
Discusses problems of therapy in the aged for (a) disordered behavior and psychosis, (b) depression, (c) anxiety, (d) memory and cognitive disturbance, and (e) sleep disorder.
6. Vestal RE: Drug use in the elderly: A review of problems and special considerations. *Drugs* 16:358–382, 1978.
This article is the predecessor to the Ouslander article and to the author's own review article in 1982.
7. Vestal RE: Pharmacology and aging. *J Am Geriatr Soc* 30(3):191–200, 1982.
This is a briefer, up-dated version of the author's more extensive earlier review.
8. Vestal RE: Report of the technical group on use of medicaments by the elderly (World Health Organization). *Drugs* 48:279–294, 1981.
Defines indications for use of drugs in the elderly, describes problems of inappropriate use, and provides information on the most useful drugs for use in the elderly.

8. ANTIBIOTIC-RELATED ADVERSE REACTIONS

Anthony Esposito and Richard Gleckman

Geriatric patients experience a higher incidence and a greater severity of antibiotic-related adverse events than do younger individuals; for example, gentamicin-induced untoward reactions occur three times more frequently in the aged. The adverse effects of antibiotics commonly administered to seriously ill elderly patients are reviewed in this section and are outlined in Appendix A, together with recommendations for monitoring patients during therapy. Important drug–antibiotic interactions are delineated in Appendix A.

Penicillin G

Aqueous penicillin G continues to be widely prescribed for a diverse group of serious infections that include bacteremia, pneumonia, meningitis, and endocarditis. When administered in doses that exceed 14–16 million units/day, or when prescribed for azotemic patients, aqueous penicillin G has the potential for producing serious metabolic, hematologic, renal, and neurologic toxicities. The infusion of large doses of potassium penicillin G to patients with renal insufficiency can induce life-threatening hyperkalemia, because each million units of this penicillin salt contains approximately 1.7 mEq of potassium. Geriatric patients often have congestive heart failure or renal insufficiency; when challenged with sodium penicillin G, such patients may have rapid expansion of the extracellular fluid volume and pulmonary edema. Further, like carbenicillin and ticarcillin, sodium penicillin can induce hypokalemic alkalosis, which may precipitate cardiac arrhythmias. Finally, excessive serum concentrations that result from massive doses of penicillin G (14–40 million units/day) can evoke hemolysis, acute tubular necrosis, and neurotoxicity. The neurotoxic events include myoclonic jerks and focal or generalized seizures. Failure to identify these reactions as manifestations of drug toxicity and to discontinue therapy can result in the patient's demise.

Carbenicillin and Ticarcillin

These semisynthetic penicillin analogues have become an essential part of the antibiotic treatment of choice for life-threatening *Pseudomonas aeruginosa* infections in patients with burns and hematologic malignancies. More recently, indications for these antibiotics have been extended to include treatment of serious anaerobic infections, empiric therapy for febrile patients with cancer and granulocytopenia, and prevention of posthysterectomy infections. Carbenicillin and ticarcillin possess a sodium content that exceeds 4.7 mEq/gm. The recommended daily doses for patients with life-threatening infections are 30–40 gm of carbenicillin and 18–24 gm of ticarcillin. Administration of these compounds in doses of this magnitude, as with infusion of large parenteral doses of aqueous penicillin G, can precipitate or exacerbate pulmonary edema and can produce generalized muscular twitching and focal or generalized seizures.

Therapeutic doses of carbenicillin have induced profound hypokalemia associated with serious cardiac arrhythmias. Elderly patients who receive digitalis preparations and diuretics or who have sustained potassium depletion through gastrointestinal fluid losses appear to be particularly susceptible to the hypokalemia resulting from carbenicillin administration. When elderly patients are given therapeutic doses of carbenicillin for serious infections, serial determinations of the serum potassium concentration and frequent electrocardiographic monitoring should be performed to detect carbenicillin-induced hypokalemia.

Carbenicillin increases plasma antithrombin III activity, interferes with platelet aggregation, and impedes conversion of fibrinogen to fibrin. Severe spontaneous bleeding resulting from the administration of carbenicillin has developed postoperatively. Elderly individuals seem to be particularly vulnerable to hemorrhage, especially when they are uremic or receive drugs that alter platelet function (e.g., aspirin) or produce anticoagulation (e.g., warfarin). Ticarcillin can also impair platelet function and has been associated with clinically significant hemorrhage.

Azlocillin, mezlocillin, and piperacillin are new acylamino penicillins that expand the antibacterial spectrum of carbenicillin and ticarcillin. These drugs possess less than half the sodium content of carbenicillin and ticarcillin and, therefore, they decrease the risk of hypokalemia or volume overload. Reversible neutropenia and prolongation of bleeding times have been observed in patients given the newer penicillins, however, and it appears that the side effects of these drugs are similar to those observed with other broad-spectrum penicillins that are administered in high doses.

Tetracyclines

Tetracyclines are rarely the antibiotics of first selection for bacterial infections prevalent in the elderly. These antibiotics are extensively prescribed, however, because they possess broad-spectrum activity and have proved effective for the treatment of pulmonary, biliary, and urinary tract infections in penicillin-allergic patients. Tetracyclines should be avoided for elderly patients with renal impairment: These antimicrobials can directly exacerbate preexisting abnormal renal function and can produce a catabolic state leading to azotemia, acidosis, and death. For the patient with impaired renal function who requires a tetracycline, doxycycline can be administered, since this antibiotic will not exacerbate renal dysfunction.

Minocycline has been extensively prescribed for geriatric patients because, compared to tetracycline, it possesses a wider spectrum of activity for both aerobic and anaerobic bacteria, demonstrates enhanced tissue penetration, requires less frequent dosing, and fails to cause phototoxicity. Minocycline, however, evokes a significant incidence of vestibular side effects that include nausea, vomiting, dizziness, vertigo, and ataxia. These symptoms usually appear within 72 hours of drug administration and, although reversible, represent such a major threat of injury that compelling reasons should exist before this medication is prescribed to the elderly.

Cephalosporins

The cephalosporins have proved to be highly effective therapy for a wide range of life-threatening infectious diseases and have accumulated an exceptional record of safety. Parenteral administration of these compounds, however, has produced pain on intramuscular injection and chemical phlebitis following intravenous infusion.

Cephalothin enhances aminoglycoside-related nephrotoxicity and, on rare occasions, has precipitated acute tubular necrosis. Cephalothin has emerged as an attractive alternative for the treatment of the penicillin-allergic patient. Elderly patients hypersensitive to penicillin, however, have experienced anaphylaxis when exposed to cephalothin. Individuals with a history of immediate or accelerated hypersensitivity to penicillin, including giant urticaria, laryngeal spasm, and anaphylaxis, should not receive cephalothin or any other cephalosporin antibiotic.

Two unique untoward reactions have been described for a number of the newer cephalosporins, including cefamandole, cefoperazone, and moxalactam. These antibiotics appear to inhibit a vitamin K–dependent step in the synthesis of clotting factors, resulting in hypoprothrombinemia and an enhanced tendency to bleed. These drugs are also capable of producing disulfiramlike reactions, including nausea, vomiting, and cardiovascular instability, in patients who consume alcohol or alcohol-containing preparations, such as cough syrups and elixirs, while receiving the antibiotic.

Aminoglycosides

Aminoglycosides, such as gentamicin, tobramycin, and amikacin, exhibit a narrow therapeutic-toxic ratio. Consequently, aged patients who receive these antibiotics must be monitored frequently for evidence of nephrotoxicity and ototoxicity (App. A). Aminoglycoside-associated nephrotoxicity can be prolonged, result in acute tubular necrosis, or, rarely, be irreversible. An enhanced potential for renal toxicity exists in aged patients who simultaneously receive cephalothin sodium, methoxyflurane, or other nephrotoxic drugs such as vancomycin or *cis*-dichlorodiaminoplatinum (*cis*-platinum). Aminoglycoside-induced ototoxicity includes irreversible vestibular injury and bilateral permanent hearing loss in the conversational range. Ototoxicity has been attributed to a number of factors, including the impaired renal function that accompanies aging, the inability of critically ill elderly patients to communicate, concomitant therapy with loop diuretics, and inappropriate dosage or duration of therapy.

The invaluable information provided by serum antibiotic assays reduces the potential for aminoglycoside-related nephrotoxicity and ototoxicity. Sequential monitoring of both peak and trough aminoglycoside serum concentrations is essential (App. A). If aminoglycoside assays are not available, the dosing intervals should be guided by determinations of the creatinine clearance (App. A). Because the serum creatinine may not accurately reflect renal function in the aged, formulas and nomograms that are solely based on that serum value should be avoided.

Clindamycin

Antibiotic-associated pseudomembranous colitis caused by clindamycin affects the elderly especially. This toxicity follows either oral or parenteral administration of the drug and can develop during therapy or weeks after discontinuation of the antibiotic. Manifestations of pseudomembranous colitis include fever, crampy abdominal pain, watery diarrhea, and, at the extreme, acute toxic colon. This syndrome constitutes a potentially lethal disorder, and deaths have resulted from colonic perforation, rectal hemorrhage, and intractable fluid and electrolyte depletion. The majority of these fatalities have been elderly patients. The *sine qua non* for the diagnosis of antibiotic-related pseudomembranous colitis consists of the detection of plaques by sigmoidoscopy or biopsy. Enterotoxigenic strains of *Clostridium difficile* contribute to the pathogenesis of this disorder, and the isolation of the *Cl. difficile* toxin from the stool appears sufficient to establish a diagnosis. Therapy of clindamycin-associated colitis consists of immediate cessation of the antibiotic and vigorous supportive treatment. Oral vancomycin administration (250–500 mg qid) is recommended for patients with severe disease.

Chloramphenicol

Chloramphenicol-induced bone marrow suppression and aplastic anemia occur more frequently in older patients. Bone marrow suppression produced by chloramphenicol is a dose-related phenomenon, characterized by anemia with or without leukopenia or thrombocytopenia. Dose-related marrow suppression tends to occur more commonly in elderly, malnourished patients, often follows infusions of large doses, and is reversible with discontinuation of the antibiotic. In contrast, aplastic anemia results from an idiosyncratic reaction, usually occurs weeks to months after cessation of therapy, and is almost invariably fatal. Chloramphenicol can also produce neuropsychiatric abnormalities that include nightmares, lethargy, hallucinations, and confusion. These symptoms resolve when therapy is terminated.

Chloramphenicol should be restricted to the therapy of serious infections for which acceptable alternatives are not available. Chloramphenicol remains an invaluable antibiotic for the treatment of invasive salmonellosis, life-threatening infections caused by *Hemophilus influenzae,* rickettsial diseases, and central nervous system infections.

Trimethoprim-Sulfamethoxazole

Hematologic toxicity attributable to trimethoprim-sulfamethoxazole has occurred rarely. Elderly patients with borderline folate stores resulting from drugs, malnutrition, malabsorption, or chronic alcoholism, however, are particularly susceptible to trimethoprim-sulfamethoxazole–induced blood dyscrasias. In addition, hypersensitivity events culminating in death have developed in aged individuals with severe renal dysfunction who received this drug in conventional doses.

Erythromycin

Erythromycin remains an antibiotic with relatively few toxicities. The most serious adverse reaction associated with the drug is cholestatic hepatitis. Hepatotoxicity most frequently occurs following the parenteral use of the estolate form but also can result from the ethyl succinate preparation. Aged patients with renal failure who receive high intravenous doses of erythromycin are at risk to experience sensorineural hearing loss. Fortunately, unlike the deafness associated with aminoglycosides, erythromycin ototoxicity is reversible on discontinuation of the drug.

1. Gleckman RA, Esposito AL: Antibiotics in the elderly: Skating on therapeutic thin ice. *Geriatrics* 35:26, 1980.
2. Bennett WM, et al: Drug therapy in renal failure: Dosing guidelines for adults. *Ann Intern Med* 93:62, 1980.
Comprehensive reviews with extensive bibliographies.

II. SOCIAL SERVICES

9. SOCIAL SERVICES FOR THE ELDERLY

Susan Hendrick

The experienced physician generally acknowledges that a major part of caring for elderly patients involves dealing with financial and social problems. "Quality of life," a goal often stated, very often depends more on the social than on the medical resources available to the patient. The long-term effect of an acute illness on an elderly patient and his or her family often requires a major reorganization of daily life. The patient may have to change jobs, alter the home, or otherwise change the routine. Such an adjustment is not easy at any age but, because of multiple medical and social constraints, elderly patients find it particularly difficult.

Even without medical illness, the changes of age and retirement alone may precipitate the need for social services, and some elderly patients may present with medical complaints that are signals of social, rather than physiologic, distress. In any case, in addition to medical care, the physician should attempt to provide guidance, so that the patient can maintain the best possible lifestyle. When physical dysfunction is minimal, usually minimal social services are required. When the residual problems of disease involve motor or mental function, the needs grow exponentially. Elderly patients who are disabled by financial and social problems may require intensive social work intervention, even when illness is minimal. Loss of a spouse, loss of income, and limited mobility require greater dependency of the elderly on family and community sources. The physician may not have the time and expertise required to associate the needy patient with the available resources but can refer the patient to a social worker.

Social programs exist on a federal, state, and community level (see App. 9-1) and vary depending on funding and locality. The utilization of social welfare has become difficult because of its fragmentation and duplication. Moreover, lack of common planning, uniformity, and goal-setting make the system unwieldy. The traditional bureaucratic process often causes delay, but an experienced social work professional can usually channel a client to the right service. Most clinics have social workers who are aware of the resources available in the community and the prerequisites for eligibility. Social services for the elderly may be used to assist them through a crisis or to improve the overall quality of life. Even patients with a firm financial footing may need some social services when advancing age or other disability creates dependency. The major needs remain, however, in the elderly patients with limited resources.

The following outline gives a broad view of social services that are generally available to elderly patients. The details of eligibility and application vary from community to community, but with diligent searching most patients can receive much of what they need.

Services Related to Health Care

The local health department in most communities provides free screening for hypertension, diabetes, glaucoma, cataracts, and hearing problems. Immunizations, chest x-rays, eyeglass prescriptions, dietary guidance, and general health counseling are also available locally from the health department.

"Service-connected" and some "non–service-connected" veterans can receive free health care from the Veterans Administration. The local VA office, VA medical center, or VA Central Office* will provide details of eligibility and help with entering the system. Inpatient and outpatient care is available in many areas. Mental health services, long-term care, and alcohol and drug treatment are also available in the VA. The VA can also provide eligible veterans with discharge planning and placement, hospital-based home care services, and prostheses, as well as medical equipment and supplies.

Availability of mental health services depends on the patient's economic or insurance status. Local mental health clinics are usually available on a prorated fee basis. Psychiatric, psychological, or social work professional organizations can help with referrals. The local state hospital usually can accommodate patients who have no financial resources.

Long-term care is a most difficult resource to obtain, since few beds are available. Chronic disease hospitals, nursing homes, and some VA medical centers provide most long-term and custodial care.

*Washington, D.C. 20420.

Hospice Care. Hospice associations can be found in many communities by calling the local hospital. These associations provide many services for terminally ill patients and their families, including those of a physician, nurse, clergyman, social worker, psychologist, and psychiatrist. Some of these services are covered by third-party payers. After the patient's death, the hospice association can also provide bereavement follow-up. There are a few private hospice units in the country that provide medical care and pain relief in an atmosphere that is as homelike as possible.

Services for Special Groups. The local Social Security office can help refer special groups such as American Indians, miners, merchant mariners, and fishermen to the appropriate government agencies for medical care.

Home Health Care Services. Home health care is available locally from the Visiting Nurse Association and the local public health department. RNs, LPNs, and home health aides (who provide personal care) are available to some patients. Homemaker services for child care, light housekeeping, laundry, food preparation, and errands often allow the patient to live outside an institution. Transportation, escort services, and companion services are also available in some communities. In-home medical supplies and equipment, as well as physical, occupational, and speech therapies and the services of a social worker may also be obtained from the Visiting Nurse Association.

Services for Patients with a Specific Illness. Direct services, counseling, support, and advocacy can be obtained from the relevant local voluntary health association (e.g., the American Cancer Society and American Heart Association). These groups are usually listed in the phone book or can be contacted through the local hospital.

Hospital-Sponsored or Hospital-Based Home Care. Large general hospitals and some VA medical centers offer services in the home after hospital discharge. The services of a physician, nurse, physical or occupational therapist, dietitian, and social worker may be provided when necessary. The hospital from which the patient is being discharged can give details of available services.

Paying for Health Care

Medicare. Medicare is a federal health insurance program primarily for, but not limited to, people 65 years old or older. The Medicare program has two components. Medicare, Part A, which is free to all eligible persons, helps to pay for medically necessary inhospital care, medically necessary care in a skilled nursing facility, and home health care after a hospital discharge. Medicare, Part B, is based on voluntary enrollment, and the cost, currently about $15 per month, changes each year. Medicare B helps to pay for physicians' services and some services provided by chiropractors, podiatrists, optometrists, dentists, and oral surgeons. Part B pays for outpatient hospital and emergency room services, for some surgical procedures performed in walk-in surgical centers or in a doctor's office, and for rehabilitation services in an approved outpatient rehabilitation center. It also pays for blood (after the first three units), x-rays and clinical laboratory services, physical and speech therapies, certain ambulance services, and home health services. Purchase or rental of durable medical equipment (e.g., beds, braces) and supplies, and the cost and administration of drugs that cannot be self-administered, as well as of pneumococcal vaccine, are also covered. The Medicare program can be rather intricate. A publication called *Your Medicare Handbook* (SSA Publication No. 05-10050) is an excellent source of more detailed information regarding eligibility rules, covered services, definitions of medical necessity, reasonable charges, and reserve days. The local Social Security office or the fiscal intermediary responsible for administering the Medicare program in a given geographic area can also give more information.

Medicaid. The Medicaid assistance program covers patients who are below certain income levels or have high medical bills in relation to their income. Medicaid also covers patients who are receiving cash benefits from the Supplemental Security Income (SSI) program because of age, disability, or blindness. Low-income individuals who are eligible for both can supplement Medicare with Medicaid. Medicaid coverage includes the following (varying according to state): inpatient and outpatient hospital services, outpatient x-ray and clinical laboratory services, rural health clinics, skilled nursing services, home health services, physicians' services, prescription drugs, prosthetic devices, dental services, optometrists and eyeglasses, podiatrists and chiropractors, emergency room services, ambulance services, private duty nursing, physical therapy, intermediate care facilities, and, in some cases, residential care facilities. The state welfare or social services office can give the details for entry into the Medicaid system.

Private Insurance. Private insurance plans may be single or comprehensive policies. Private plans are used by the over-65 population primarily as a supplement to the gaps left by the government programs. Those forms of insurance designed to supplement government programs are most important for the older age groups. The Medex I, II, and III plans (with Medex III being the most comprehensive) are offered by most Blue Cross and Blue Shield plans around the country. Different insurance companies call their supplemental programs by different names. The private plans reimburse the policyholder or, more commonly, the provider of services for the components not paid because of deductible(s) or co-insurance (co-payment) in the Medicare program. The state insurance department or the state consumer protection agency can give details about cost and coverage. In general, most private insurance policies **do not** pay for the following services: private duty nursing, personal services (telephone and television while in a hospital or skilled nursing facility and the cost of a private room), custodial nursing care, homemaker services, routine medical checkups, routine immunizations, dental care and dentures, routine examinations for eyeglasses and hearing aids, orthopedic shoes and routine foot care, acupuncture, most chiropractic services, and elective cosmetic surgery.

Services That Provide Chronic Care

Nursing Homes. Nursing homes are the most widely used form of chronic care for elderly patients who can no longer live alone in the community. There are several types of nursing homes. A *skilled nursing facility* (SNF) provides skilled nursing care and rehabilitative services. Short-term, convalescent, and rehabilitative care are emphasized. This type of environment is referred to as *level I* care. Another type of care, *level II,* may also be available in the SNF. Level II is usually indicated for total bed patients who can do very little for themselves and who need very prolonged or lifelong care. An *intermediate care facility* (ICF) provides nursing supervision primarily for medications, some personal care services, room and board, and social and recreational services. An individual would have to function fairly independently to be accepted. This type of care is usually referred to as *level III* and, at times, is provided in the same facility as levels I and II. A *residential care facility* (RCF) provides room and board, a protective environment, limited supervision, and a basic social program for the individual who cannot live alone at home. This is usually referred to as *level IV* care, or a rest home. Level IV care can be found in a nursing home that provides multiple levels of care or in a separate level IV facility.

Financing is often the most important limit on obtaining a nursing home bed. Persons financially able to pay the cost must pay the rate that is set by the facility. Medicare will pay for only 100 days of level I care upon hospital discharge. Medicare payment is 100% for all covered services in the first 20 days and all charges, less a deductible per day, for all covered services for the next 80 days. The deductible amount is subject to change each year. Medicaid payment is different from Medicare. With Medicaid the individual signs over his or her government benefit check(s) to the nursing home each month. The individual then receives a check for $35 to cover personal expenses. Medicaid pays the balance of the cost, or the reimbursement rate set by the state, directly to the nursing home facility. Persons not eligible for Medicaid because of excess income, savings, or personal property must reduce their assets to a certain amount before they become eligible. Private insurance usually pays only a stated amount per day for skilled nursing care received in an SNF.

The Veterans Administration is a source of chronic care for certain patients. If the veteran is "non–service-connected," the VA usually will pay the total cost of care for the first 6 months in a VA contract nursing home. After 6 months the veteran's income and Medicaid are expected to pay the cost. If a veteran is "service-connected" and needs nursing home care for a service-related illness, the VA will pay for the entire cost of care in a VA contract nursing home for the length of time required. Some VA medical centers have their own nursing home care units.

There are a number of sources of information about nursing home **placement.** The social work or continuing care department at the hospital will assist in placement of hospitalized persons and in applying for financial assistance. The patient who has returned home from a nursing home but is again in need of placement may contact the social work or continuing care department that assisted originally. Service-connected veterans can be placed by most VA medical centers directly from home into a nursing home. Direct placement is not possible for non–service-connected veterans. They must be placed after discharge from a VA medical center.

The patient and family who select a nursing home should consider several factors. The patient, family, and physician should discuss the patient's individual needs in order to determine the type of facility and level of care required. It is important to consider the location of the nursing home in relation to family, friends, hospital, and physician, and the facility's financial policy as to accepting Medicare and Medicaid. A visit to the nursing home for a discussion with the administrator and a tour of the facility should be an integral part of the selection process. Others who can assist the family include clergy, family counseling agencies, the local board of health, the local Social Security office, senior citizens' organizations, the state office for the elderly, and welfare and social services offices. Some private agencies in a few states offer a nursing home placement service. They are reimbursed for this service by the nursing home or the patient. In many communities there are social workers in independent practice who receive a fee for such a service. The feelings of the patient and family toward nursing home placement must be considered. Counseling and support may be necessary to make the transition as smooth as possible for both patient and family.

Services That Maintain Income. The retired person's income usually is from a company or private pension plan and/or Social Security retirement insurance. Social Security can begin at age 62, at a reduced rate, or at age 65 at the full amount. A worker's dependents and survivors might also be eligible for benefits.

The Veterans Administration also provides pensions for non–service-connected veterans 65 years of age or older, depending on their income level. A service-connected veteran continues to receive the monetary compensation benefit awarded to him or her on discharge from the service for illness or injury sustained as a result of military service. A service-connected veteran at retirement could elect to receive a pension, if that option could result in an income higher than his disability payment. If a patient's spouse or children served in the armed forces, the patient also should investigate his or her eligibility for benefits.

Massachusetts is the only state that sponsors a program for veterans in each town or city hall. The program provides temporary funds to a veteran who is without a source of income until a VA or Social Security pension is awarded, or who is in a financial crisis. The veterans' agent at each town or city hall has the information needed.

Supplemental Security Income (SSI) is an income source for persons who are aged, blind, or disabled and have very little or no income. The local Social Security office is the point of entry for this program.

Housing Services. Low- and moderate-income housing for the elderly is available on a limited basis, depending on the community. Special housing developments for the elderly have a few units especially equipped for the handicapped. Unfortunately, long waiting lists limit the accessibility to such housing. The town housing authority or manager of the specific housing development is the source of information. Moderate-income housing is sometimes sponsored by churches and other private, nonprofit organizations.

Retirement centers or communities are complexes of apartments and/or homes, sometimes with an infirmary and a nursing home. Some old hotels have been converted into retirement hotels. The retirement centers usually have a main dining room with central meal service, planned activities, and indoor and outdoor recreational space as special features. There is usually space for religious activities, facilities for therapy, and proximity to shopping centers and hospitals. The local senior citizens' group or council on aging can give information as to what is available in a specific area.

Congregate or cooperative housing or shared living arrangements are another form of special housing for the elderly. These units consist of various sizes of apartments or bedrooms, each with full or partial bathroom facilities, in a communal, cooperative setting. The bathrooms and kitchens are shared, or there are central kitchens and dining rooms. There are activity and meeting rooms. The rent is usually limited to a percentage of the person's income. The local senior citizens' group or council on aging will provide the details.

Housing for veterans is available on a limited basis. Level IV patients self-sufficient in daily living are eligible for foster homes. Soldiers' and airmen's homes provide several levels of care. Domiciliary care provides medical and personal care services in a residential, dormitory-type setting for veterans not requiring hospitalization. The local VA office or VA medical center will provide details. Some local housing authorities give preference to veterans for housing in subsidized housing complexes.

"Sheltered" housing for the elderly and physically impaired adult consists of medically oriented, barrier-free facilities near or attached to a hospital. Special services, such as a nurse on duty at all times and physical and occupational therapy, are available. Congregate dining and recreational activities provide social opportunities for the residents. The local senior citizens' center or council on aging can provide information about local programs.

Halfway houses, group homes, and residential treatment programs provide a sheltered environment and treatment within a community for people with similar problems or disabilities. Many of these facilities have an age limit of 65. For referral, contact the local hospital's social work or continuing care department.

Services That Maintain Nutrition. Hot meal programs are provided in some communities for ambulatory elderly. Nutritionally balanced hot lunches are served on weekdays and sometimes on nights and weekends at designated sites (school cafeterias, churches, public housing, and senior citizens' centers). Some programs provide escort and transportation to the site. Recreation, education, volunteer opportunities, information, referral, and counseling are also available at the centers.

For the home-restricted elderly person, the "meals on wheels" type programs deliver nutritionally balanced hot lunches on weekdays. If a homebound patient needs, in addition to meals, someone to check on him or her regularly, this program may serve both purposes. The hot lunch programs ask for a small voluntary donation, charge a minimal fee, or charge according to ability to pay. The local home care corporation, council on aging, senior citizens' center, or Visiting Nurse Association usually has information on the hot meal programs available in the community.

The Food Stamp program is for low-income individuals. Food stamps can be used to purchase food in grocery stores and to pay for the hot lunch program. For information, contact the local welfare or social services office.

In some areas there are also "mobile markets," which bring a full range of groceries, at supermarket prices, to designated neighborhood sites. For information, contact the town or city hall. Food cooperatives in some towns provide groceries at lower prices, and they can be found through a senior citizen center.

Miscellaneous Support Services. Adult day care centers provide medical monitoring, meals, transportation (in some centers), and recreational activities for individuals in need of supervision during the day while family members work, or when the family needs relief from the stress of constant care-giving. Some VA medical centers also provide day care programs. The local Visiting Nurse Association or the council on aging will have information.

Many communities provide a handyman service or volunteers who do home repairs. Some localities sponsor subsidy programs for the elderly to help pay for home repairs, painting, or heavy housework and yardwork. Contact the town or city hall for details. The Community Action Agency may assist in preparing a home for winter and in paying fuel bills.

Most transit authorities, as well as some taxicab companies, offer reduced rates for the elderly. Many organizations and church groups provide free transportation for medical appointments, shopping, and various other activities. Some public transportation systems provide barrier-free transportation for the handicapped. For information, contact the local transit authority and council on aging.

"Telephone reassurance" and "friendly visitor" programs are available that check on a patient every day. Contact the local council on aging for details.

There are programs to assist the low-income, elderly individual who needs direct legal assistance, protective services, advice about wills, or advocacy services. The Legal Aid Society, Bar Association, or local law school can usually arrange the services. Some senior citizen centers have paralegal assistance available at a reduced rate. Some consumer councils and the Better Business Bureau could also be of assistance.

For the widow or widower who needs support and/or counseling following the death of a spouse, some communities have supportive groups and programs. Local churches or the local council on aging can help locate the programs.

Information and referral agencies exist in most communities to assist the elderly in finding the appropriate resources for their needs. Shortly after referral, the agency should contact the individual to see if he or she was referred properly and received the needed service. Contact the state and area agencies on aging.

Services That Provide Activities. Employment and volunteer programs help retired people fill their time and use their skills. These programs usually pay the minimum wage for part-time work, or a minimum salary. The local ACTION agency can give information about the Foster Grandparents Program, Senior Companion Program, Volunteers in Service to America (VISTA), and Peace Corps. The local senior citizens' center or town hall may have programs such as Green Thumb, Green Light, Older American, Service Employment, Senior Aides, and the Senior Community Service Project. Many senior citizens' centers have an employment service or job registry, as does the local Office of Employment Security. "Mature Temps" is a recently formed private employment agency that provides older workers for temporary jobs throughout the business community.

Volunteer opportunities include the Service Corps of Retired Executives (contact the Better Business Bureau) and the Retired Senior Volunteers Program (contact the local ACTION agency). Other volunteer opportunities can be found in outreach programs for the elderly and in schools, courts, hospitals, United Way agencies, and Red Cross chapters.

Elderly patients wishing to extend their education can enroll in community and junior colleges, technical institutes, and universities, which offer special programs and regular courses for the elderly at little or no tuition. The local board of education or school committee offers educational programs for the non–English-speaking elderly.

Recreational and cultural programs offered at reduced rates may be of great interest to some elderly patients. Public libraries often have senior citizen activities. Also, the Department of Parks and Recreation, local cinemas and community theaters, concert halls, museums, and galleries offer reduced rates to the elderly. Senior citizens' centers also have a variety of leisure activities, ranging from card games to group trips.

Services Available on the Death of a Spouse. Social Security provides a death payment (if the decreased had been covered by Social Security) to an eligible surviving widow, widower, or entitled child. Dependents and survivors of the deceased also could be eligible for monthly Social Security benefits. The VA provides eligible veterans and their families with the following benefits: a Spanish-American War death pension, a death pension for families of non–service-connected veterans, dependency and indemnity compensation or death compensation for families of service-connected veterans, and reimbursement of some burial expenses. The government also provides eligible veterans with free burial in a national cemetery, an American flag, a headstone or grave marker, and a Presidential Memorial Certificate. The local VA office and the local funeral director can give information about these services.

Other sources of financial assistance might be found through union and employers' pension funds, fraternal organizations, and professional groups. If death is employment-related, Workmen's Compensation may provide some financial benefits.

Appendix 9-1. Some National Agencies and Organizations for the Elderly

American Association of Retired Persons
1909 K Street, N.W.
Washington, D.C. 20006

Gray Panthers
6342 Greene Street
Philadelphia, Pennsylvania 19144

National Caucus on the Black Aged
1730 M Street, N.W.
Washington, D.C. 20036

National Council of Senior Citizens
1511 K Street, N.W.
Room 202
Washington, D.C. 20005

Administration on Aging
Office of Human Development
Department of Health and Human Services
Washington, D.C. 20201

National Council on Aging
1828 L Street, N.W.
Washington, D.C. 20036

The Gerontological Society
1 Dupont Circle, N.W.
Washington, D.C. 20036
The American Geriatrics Society
10 Columbus Circle
New York, New York 10023
The Urban Elderly Coalition
250 Broadway
New York, New York 10007

III. SYMPTOMS AND SIGNS

10. CONSTIPATION

Sanjiv Chopra and Richard L. Curtis

Constipation may be defined as infrequent defecation, insufficient defecation, feeling of incomplete evacuation, or increased hardness of stools. Volvulus of the sigmoid may be seen more frequently in patients with chronic and severe constipation.

Constipation of recent onset is usually a symptom of a significant pathologic condition and justifies a meticulous clinical evaluation. After drug-related and other toxic causes have been excluded, it is mandatory to perform a proctosigmoidoscopy and barium enema examination to identify more serious causes such as volvulus or colonic carcinoma. Films of the abdomen reveal feces in the colon, and findings depend on the site of the impaction. Less specific roentgenographic changes include small bowel air-fluid levels and dilatation proximal to the site of impaction. Barium enema should not be performed in the setting of impaction, since concretions of barium may occur in the distended atonic colon.

Paradoxical diarrhea is especially noted in the elderly. The patient will complain of a long period of constipation preceding the diarrhea, and will be expelling frequent loose, watery movements past a hard, incompletely obstructing fecal mass (fecaloma or stercoroma). Physical examination may reveal a mass in the right lower quadrant. Treatment includes digital disimpaction and enemas containing 20% water-soluble x-ray contrast agents. In extreme cases, intestinal obstruction and bleeding or perforation from stercoraceous ulcers may necessitate a surgical procedure.

Laxative abuse also may contribute to constipation. An abnormal brown or black pigment in the colonic mucosa (melanosis coli) may be seen on sigmoidoscopy in patients who have taken anthracene cathartics for several months. Microscopic examination of a rectal biopsy specimen shows striking pigmentation of the mucosa.

The presentation of constipation is sometimes misleading, as it may appear as an acute confusional state with disorientation or agitation. Furthermore, the associated signs may mimic a more severe disorder such as volvulus or intestinal perforation. Such signs may include hypotension, tachycardia, abdominal distention and rigidity, nausea and vomiting.

The etiology of chronic constipation in the elderly may be local or systemic. In the first category, diverticular disease and carcinoma predominate, although constipation may be a presenting manifestation of stricture, volvulus, or anal fissure. Conditions that cause nervous system dysfunction are also associated with constipation. Multiple sclerosis, Parkinson's disease, pseudoobstruction, and paraplegia are examples. Constipation from a systemic etiology is usually a result of drug ingestion. Major offenders are analgesics, aluminum-containing antacids, anticholinergics, hematinics (iron), psychotherapeutics, and laxatives. Metabolic disorders such as diabetes, uremia, and hypothyroidism may also produce constipation.

Treatment of constipation is aimed at finding reversible causes. Prevention—encouraging fluid intake and prescribing stool softeners or bulk laxatives—helps geriatric patients. Lactulose syrup, 10–50 mg as a bedtime dose, often is enough to prevent problems.

1. Connell AM, Hilton C, Irvin G: Variations in bowel habit in two population samples. *Br Med J* 2:1095, 1965.
   No correlation was noted between advancing age and bowel habits.
2. Gurll N, Steer M: Diagnostic and therapeutic considerations for fecal impaction. *Dis Colon Rectum* 18:509, 1975.
   The authors emphasize that patients with fecal impaction may present with symptoms and signs of acute intestinal obstruction.

11. ABDOMINAL PAIN IN THE ELDERLY

Sanjiv Chopra and Richard L. Curtis

The evaluation of abdominal pain in the elderly patient poses a formidable diagnostic and therapeutic challenge to the physician. Precise historical information regarding the site, radiation, intensity, duration, and aggravating or relieving factors is often unobtainable. The pain may be chronic with exacerbations, or it may be acute. The presence of an acute abdomen demands accurate, astute decisions on the part of the physician. Elderly patients with acute abdominal pain require surgery more often than younger patients. As many as 33% of patients over age 65 have been reported to require immediate operation, as contrasted with only 16% of patients less than 65 years of age. Moreover, the mortality for patients over age 65 is 8.4% compared with 0.9% for patients less than 65 years old.

Pain preceding vomiting as a general rule signifies a surgical condition. The speed and character of the onset of pain are helpful clues, with **sudden** onset of pain suggesting a perforated viscus or an abdominal vascular accident. Pain of **rapid** onset (developing over an hour or so) suggests obstruction of a hollow viscus or an inflammatory process. Pain that is **gradual** in onset, peaking in 12–24 hours, may be a manifestation of the acute surgical conditions or signify pancreatitis, appendicitis, neoplasm, inflammatory bowel disease, or urinary retention. The slower onset should **not** mislead the physician into thinking that there is no urgency in establishing a diagnosis. The development of severe abdominal pain and shock suggests a perforated viscus, strangulated obstruction, or ruptured aortic aneurysm.

Patients with acute abdominal pain may be divided into three groups. The first are those with intraabdominal lesions requiring urgent surgical intervention, for example, incarcerated hernias or perforated viscus. The second group are those with intraabdominal conditions usually **not** requiring immediate surgical interaction, e.g., acute pancreatitis and inflammatory bowel disease. The last group are those with medical conditions simulating the acute abdomen. Myocardial infarction, pneumonia, diabetic ketoacidosis, Addisonian crises, congestion of the liver, and viral hepatitis have been found to underlie abdominal pain.

Causes of chronic abdominal pain in elderly patients include neoplasms, biliary tract disorders, diverticular disease, peptic ulcer, and abdominal angina. Abdominal pain may be absent in the elderly with an acute abdomen. Symptoms may consist only of restlessness, altered mental status, respiratory distress, obstipation, sepsis, or fever. Morbidity and mortality increase in direct proportion to the delay in surgical management of a ruptured viscus or necrotic bowel. Therefore, when in doubt, it is useful to remember that the consequences of failing to operate on a patient requiring prompt intervention are more dire than those of performing a diagnostic laparotomy.

Acute appendicitis has its peak incidence in the second and third decades. About 7% of patients with acute appendicitis, however, are over 60 years of age. The older patients often seek medical attention late, with as many as half seeking help 3 days or longer after onset. Acute appendicitis is often not considered as a diagnostic possibility in elderly patients with abdominal pain, since other disorders are more common. The symptoms of right lower quadrant pain, nausea, and vomiting occur in one-third of cases. In many elderly patients the pain is minimal and the abdominal tenderness is deceptively mild. The shift of the pain, from the epigastric area or periumbilical region to the right lower quadrant, often happens late in elderly patients and may not happen at all in about half of cases, and the temperature may be normal or only minimally elevated.

Despite these deceptively reassuring findings, life-threatening gangrene, perforation, abscess formation, and peritonitis are encountered more frequently in elderly patients. In addition, carcinoma of the cecum or appendix may cause acute appendicitis. Not infrequently the underlying carcinoma is not recognized at the time of surgical procedure. The increased **virulence** of the disease process, together with the delay in diagnosis and treatment of this condition, and the presence of concomitant medical illnesses contributes to the high morbidity and mortality of acute appendicitis in elderly patients. Mortality is as high as 15% or at least 10 times higher than that of younger age groups.

1. Albano WA, Zielinski CM, Organ CH: Is appendicitis in the aged really different? *Geriatrics* 30:81, 1975.
Of the patients studied, 61% experienced major or minor postoperative complications.
2. Brewer RJ, et al: Abdominal pain. *Am J Surg* 131:219, 1976.
Retrospective study of 1000 consecutive cases of abdominal pain. Elderly patients required immediate operation more often than patients under the age of 65 years and had a much higher in-hospital mortality. The authors stress the need for careful evaluation and reevaluation in elderly patients with abdominal pain.

3. Fabr PJ, Carey LC: Cecal carcinoma presenting as acute appendicitis: A reappraisal. *J Clin Gastroenterol* 12:173, 1980.
A high index of suspicion in patients with atypical presentations or unusual operative findings might provide for an earlier diagnosis of associated carcinoma.
4. Peltokallio P, Jauhianen K: Acute appendicitis in the aged patient: Study of 300 cases after the age of 60. *Arch Surg* 100:140, 1970.
Perforated appendix was present in 32% of the aged patients as opposed to 6% of the younger patients. The mortality in the group of aged patients was 7 times that of the entire group.
5. Steinheber FM: Interpretation of gastrointestinal symptoms in the elderly. *Med Clin North Am* 60:1141, 1976.
Excellent review article in an issue devoted to geriatric medicine.
6. Thorbjarnarson B, Loehr WJ: Acute appendicitis in patients over the age of sixty. *Surg Gynecol Obstet* 125:1277, 1967.
In this series of 195 patients, over 70% had perforations.
7. Williams JS, Hale HW: Acute appendicitis in the elderly: Review of 83 cases. *Ann Surg* 162:208, 1965.
While all patients had abdominal pain and tenderness, associated symptoms and signs were minimal. Of the patients, 50% presented with symptoms after 72 hours. A mortality rate of 14% was attributed to delay in diagnosis, infection, and high incidence of associated diseases.

12. HYPOTHERMIA

Thomas M. Walshe

Accidental hypothermia occurs when the body temperature falls below 95°F. It usually is provoked by exposure to cold weather or immersion in cold water. Elderly persons, however, are known to develop low core body temperature without clear exposure to excessive cold. In fact, hypothermia has been found in certain elderly patients living where the temperature is as high as 60°F. Most of our information about hypothermia, however, comes from studies of persons who have been seriously exposed to a cold environment. There is very little data regarding elderly persons who develop hypothermia occultly without toxic or environmental provocation. Although the susceptibility of the elderly to hypothermia is unexplained, elderly patients are known to have varying degrees of vasoconstriction, so that, when cooled under experimental control, they do not always adapt normally. Moreover, elderly persons maintain lower resting temperatures, perhaps because of reduced activity, poor diet, or as-yet-undocumented anterior hypothalamic-preoptic area central nervous system dysfunction. The elderly also shiver less, so they produce less heat when cooled.

Hypoglycemia and hypothyroidism cause low body temperatures but account for very few cases of hypothermia in the elderly. Drugs that interfere with temperature regulation provoke hypothermia in the elderly, as they do in others. Chlorpromazine (and other phenothiazines), barbiturates, and other sedatives are clearly associated with hypothermia. Alcohol is perhaps the most common predisposing factor in hypothermia, but less so in elderly patients.

The incidence of hypothermia in the elderly is not clearly established, but British studies suggest that almost 4% of patients older than 65 years admitted to hospital are hypothermic. Hypothermia may be missed when temperature is measured by the usual clinical thermometer, which reads only from 94°F. To identify hypothermia more reliably, one must use a low-reading thermometer, which allows temperatures to be recorded from 84°F.

The clinical findings in hypothermia are not specific. Patients with mild hypothermia complain of being cool, but once their temperature drops below 95°F, they usually do not remark about feeling chilly. The family or friends may note that the patient is less alert and has become less able to manage routine activities. As the temperature falls further, the patient passes into stupor and then to coma. There are usually no focal neurologic signs, unless the patient has had a prior neurologic lesion. As with other systemic illness, a patient who has a previous neurologic disorder and develops hypothermia may show the signs of the old lesion. Hypothermia on its own seldom causes focal neurologic deficits. Seizures may occur, especially if there is previous cerebral injury. Patients shiver when body temperature is above 95°F, but in hypothermic patients with lower temperature, shivering is absent. Rigidity of the limbs may appear in the older patient with hypothermia, suggesting a parkinsonian syndrome. The reflexes are usually normal. The patient feels cool to the touch, even on the trunk, which is usually warm. An erythematous, generalized, purpuric rash appears in some cases, and the face may become puffy. Heart rate falls to a sinus bradycardia; blood pressure drops, to the point of shock in some cases. Atrial fibrillation, atrial flutter, and later idioventricular rhythms become major problems in the hypothermic patient. Death from ventricular fibrillation or asystole may occur at any time while the patient is hypothermic, although ventricular fibrillation is usually encountered during rewarming. The left ventricular electrocardiogram leads show a depression in the QRS–ST junction (called *J waves*) in about 30% of hypothermic patients. When present, the left J waves are indicative of hypothermia. Urine output remains normal until tubular function becomes impaired, usually at temperatures lower than 81°F (27°C). Hypovolemia and hemoconcentration occur because of the shift in intravascular volume. Thrombocytopenia is another complication that should be monitored. Metabolic acidosis and spuriously elevated PCO_2 and PO_2 are other features that accompany hypothermia.

Severe hypothermia strikes patients who are already ill from neurologic or medical disease, but some generally well elderly persons also develop the syndrome. The spontaneous cases are usually less severe than those associated with illness, intoxication, or exposure. The diagnosis is not always obvious in the mild cases, and unexplained cognitive or physical deficits may be the only clues. Dehydration is a common companion to accidental hypothermia. Laboratory tests in hypothermic patients usually show signs of dehydration or may show another underlying metabolic abnormality. Signs of hemoconcentration and hypernatremia occur, and the blood urea nitrogen (BUN) may be elevated. Blood glucose is frequently elevated in patients with hypothermia. Hypoglycemic patients also develop mild hypothermia, but the hypothermia is only a by-product of the underlying hypoglycemia. When blood sugar is low, therefore, one should suspect a problem with glucose metabolism rather than a primary problem with temperature regulation.

Once the diagnosis of accidental hypothermia is clear and complications are identified, gradual rewarming will correct the condition. The mildly hypothermic patient can be put into a warm room with appropriate cardiac monitoring and allowed to rewarm over several hours. As long as the core temperature rises by at least 1°F/hr, the spontaneous method is satisfactory. Careful attention to correct dehydration and other metabolic problems prevents further complications. Many hypothermic patients have atelectasis or pneumonia, and most should be given antibiotics prophylactically. Cultures of blood and urine are needed before starting antibiotics. When hypothermia is severe, external heat may need to be applied for more rapid rewarming. The patient should be in an intensive care unit with cardiac and blood pressure monitors. Immersion in warm water (105–113°F) or use of a heating blanket will allow the temperature to rise by 1°F/hr. Rapid rewarming may precipitate hypotension or cause cardiac arrhythmia. These complications should be treated with pressors and antiarrhythmic management. Some of the atrial arrhythmias, however, will convert spontaneously as the temperature rises.

The prognosis in hypothermia depends on the degree of the hypothermia and the underlying condition of the patient. In mild hypothermia (temperature $>$ 90°F), recovery is good if complications are managed. When the temperature falls below 90°F, many patients will not recover fully, and many will die. Hypothermic patients with underlying diseases have a worse prognosis than those who are otherwise healthy.

1. Anderson WF: Accidental hypothermia, in Anderson WF: *Practical Management of the Elderly.* Oxford, Blackwell, 1976, chap 19, pp 354–357.
A review in a book with many other useful topics.
2. Besdine RW: Accidental hypothermia: The body's energy crisis. *Geriatrics* 34:51–59, 1979.
A good general review with practical sugggestions.

3. Bini G, et al: Thermoregulatory and rhythm-generating mechanisms governing the sudomotor and vasoconstrictor outflow in human cutaneous nerves. *J Physiol* 306:537, 1980.
The rhythm is probably produced by the central nervous system.
4. Collins KJ: *Hypothermia: The Facts.* Oxford, Oxford University Press, 1983.
General review of the subject.
5. Collins KJ, et al: Accidental hypothermia and impaired temperature homeostatis in the elderly. *Br Med J* 1:353–358, 1977.
A 4-year follow-up study shows that thermoregulation decreased with age.
6. Collins KJ, Easton JC, Exton-Smith AN: Shivering thermogenesis and vasomotor responses with convective cooling in the elderly. *J Physiol* 320:280, 1981.
The character of the shivering response is different in the elderly.
7. Collins KJ, Exton-Smith AN: Thermal homeostasis in old age. *J Am Geriatr Soc* 31:519–524, 1983.
Neurohumoral control of body temperature, drugs, and stressful changes in environmental temperature play a role.
8. Collins KJ, Exton-Smith AN, Dore C: Urban hypothermia: Preferred temperature and thermal perception in old age. *Br Med J* 282:175–177, 1981.
Elderly subjects were less able than young subjects to control the temperature and maintain comfort in a controlled-environment room. This suggests behavioral aspects responsible for susceptibility to hypothermia.
9. DaVee TS, Reineberg EJ: Extreme hypothermia and ventricular fibrillation. *Ann Emerg Med* 9:100–102, 1980.
A case report on a 31-year-old man.
10. Foster KG, et al: Sweat responses in the aged. *Age Ageing* 5:91–101, 1981.
Addresses susceptibility of the elderly to excessive heat but discusses thermoregulation.
11. Fox RH, MacGibbon R, Davies L, Woodward P: Problems of the old and the cold. *Br Med J* 1:21–24, 1973.
Elderly persons have lower body temperatures.
12. Fox RH, et al: Body temperatures in the elderly: A national study of physiological, social, and environmental conditions. *Br Med J* 1:200–206, 1973.
States the problem and analyzes data on 1,000 elderly subjects.
13. Horvath SM, et al: Metabolic responses of old people to a cold environment. *J Appl Physiol* 8:145, 1965.
Shivering is less effective in raising body temperature in the elderly.
14. Horvath SM, Rochelle RD: Hypothermia in the aged. *Environ Health Perspect* 20:127–130, 1977.
A good review of basic issues.
15. Ledingham I MacA, Mone JG: Treatment of accidental hypothermia: A prospective clinical study. *Br Med J* 26:1102–1105, 1980.
A 15-year study showed that surface rewarming of the torso was the simplest effective method.
16. Levy LA: Severe hypophosphatemia as a complication of the treatment of hypothermia. *Arch Intern Med* 140:128–129, 1980.
A 72-year-old woman developed low phosphate during rewarming.
17. Lewin S, Brettman LR, Holzman RS: Infections in hypothermic patients. *Arch Intern Med* 141:920–925, 1981.
Prompt empiric antibiotic therapy is needed.
18. MacLean D, Emslie-Smith D: *Accidental Hypothermia.* Oxford, Blackwell, 1977, p 286.
General review of large experience.
19. O'Keeffe KM: Accidental hypothermia: A review of 62 cases. *J Am Coll Emerg Physicians* 6:491–496, 1977.
The age range was from 14 to 87 years. Most cases were from outdoor exposure, but the indoor cases had an average age of 72.
20. Reuler JB: Hypothermia: Pathophysiology, clinical settings, and management. *Ann Intern Med* 89:519–527, 1978.
The best recent review.
21. Southwick FS, Dalglish PH: Recovery after prolonged asystolic cardiac arrest in pro-

found hypothermia. *JAMA* 243:1250–1253, 1980.
Vigorous cardiopulmonary resuscitation over 2½ hours left the patient with no neurologic deficits.
22. Watts AJ: Hypothermia in the aged: A study of the role of cold sensitivity. *Environ Res* 5:118, 1972.
In patients aged 74–86 years, a few were unable to regulate the temperature of the room appropriately.
23. Weyman AE, Greenbaum DE, Grace WJ: Accidental hypothermia in an alcoholic population. *Am J Med* 56:13–21, 1974.
Mortality depended on existence of underlying disease.

13. HEADACHE IN THE ELDERLY

Thomas M. Walshe

Headache is usually benign and is commonly encountered in young and middle-aged adults, but also occurs in the elderly. When headache occurs in elderly patients without a prior history, there is a higher risk of a serious underlying disorder. As in most neurologic disorders, a careful history and thorough examination will separate the benign from the serious disorders.

Vascular headache is a major cause of head pain, even in the elderly, although it is more often seen in the younger age groups. Careful questioning to obtain a past history of migraine during early or middle adult life may help establish the diagnosis. Most people "outgrow" their migraine syndromes, but headache or other migrainous features may recur as isolated instances after many asymptomatic years. Migraine occurs often, but not always, with visual phenomena. The headache may not be the same as it was in the past. Migraine is often unilateral, but no generalization can summarize the type, severity, or duration of the headache. Patients are often nauseated, may vomit, and experience scalp tenderness and photophobia. The headaches usually have their onset over several minutes to an hour and then last for several hours. Most patients find it necessary to lie quietly and take analgesics. The headaches are intermittent and not constant, do not cause loss of consciousness, and usually cause no permanent neurologic findings. There are occasional patients who experience transient neurologic signs and symptoms with migraine. The signs are usually, but not invariably, associated with headache and often include scotoma, scintillations, hemianopsia, or other visual phenomena. Patients usually have a past history of migraine and are middle-aged rather than elderly. It is not wise to attribute transient neurologic findings in elderly patients to migraine except after other possibilities are excluded.

So-called tension headache and headache of depression are unusual in elderly patients, but should be considered, since they require specific treatment. The headaches are usually moderate or mild in severity, bilateral, and not associated with other neurologic complaints. Depression, often overlooked in elderly patients, produces headache that is moderately severe and unrelenting and that devastates the ability to do almost everything. Patients often are tearful, but not always; most feel depressed, but some do not admit feeling sad. The chronicity, lack of neurologic signs, and the melancholy help to identify the nature of the headache.

Patients who complain of sinus headache almost always have some other type. Sinus infection causes pain and tenderness over the affected sinus. There may be purulent drainage, and the sinus cannot be transilluminated. Signs of infection, fever, malaise, elevated white cell count, and sedimentation rate are usually found. Roentgenograms of the sinuses show opacification of the air spaces.

Dangerous Headaches

The serious headaches, some of which may become lethal, are almost always associated with other neurologic signs. The causes of dangerous headache that present diagnostic problems in the elderly are subarachnoid hemorrhage, stroke, temporal arteritis, meningitis, cervical spondylosis, tumor, and glaucoma.

Headache is an invariable symptom in subarachnoid hemorrhage from ruptured aneurysm. Although the peak age for ruptured aneurysm is between ages 50 and 60, it may occur later, but is unusual after age 80. The headache is severe and dramatic, usually causing the patient to seek emergency aid. The patient generally loses consciousness at onset but may not have any residual neurologic signs after the initial bleed. When the headache is dramatically severe and the patient has little or no previous headache history, subarachnoid hemorrhage can be confirmed by spinal fluid examination. All patients with a ruptured aneurysm have grossly bloody spinal fluid. The noncontrast computed tomography (CT) scan sometimes shows blood in the subarachnoid space or may show a hematoma; however, the scan is normal in up to 20% of patients with subarachnoid hemorrhage. A helpful diagnostic sign on physical examination is a subhyloid retinal hemorrhage, which is very suggestive of ruptured aneurysm but is seen also in intraparenchymal hemorrhage. When the aneurysm bleeds into the brain parenchyma, causing a hematoma, there are usually fixed neurologic signs. Patients with a posterior communicating artery aneurysm may develop diplopia from a third nerve palsy after an initial bleed or if the aneurysm is large enough to compress the nerve.

Stroke also causes headache, but the headache is usually a minor part of the clinical picture. Carotid artery dissection presents with a subjective bruit (the patient hears it), headache, and a small pupil on the same side as the dissection. Some patients have a hemiparesis associated with occlusion of the artery. Others have transient ischemic attacks. The diagnosis is made by angiography, which shows a very thin line of contrast in the carotid *(string sign)*. With time the carotid may reopen, and later films may show a normally patent carotid artery.

Thrombotic occlusion of the internal carotid artery produces a mild or moderate frontoorbital headache on the side of the vascular lesion or bilaterally. Occlusion of the basilar artery produces mild to moderate headache in the back of the neck, around the head, or in the parietotemporocervical region on one side. Most ischemic strokes have little or no associated headache. Headache alone is almost never a sign of stroke or transient ischemic attack. A hypertensive hemorrhage may cause headache, especially if the hemorrhage is in the cerebellum.

Headache from glaucoma occurs late, and before the headache becomes a problem, the patient complains of blurred vision and halos around lights. The headache of glaucoma is generally in and around the eye but may spread to include the forehead. Patients with chronic glaucoma may develop headache after prolonged use of the eyes in poor light, because the pupillary dilatation increases the intraocular pressure.

Intracranial infections cause headache, but there are always other symptoms and signs to point to the correct diagnosis. Brain tumor may present with headache alone, but on neurologic examination there is usually some focal sign to suggest a lesion. Pain in the neck from cervical arthritis may radiate into the occipital region and cause an occipital head pain. There may be associated signs of cervical spondylosis and degenerative changes on films of the cervical spine. Giant cell arteritis (GCA) is a major concern when an elderly patient complains of headache of recent onset.

The evaluation of headache depends on the history and the clinical findings. All elderly patients with headache should be evaluated for giant cell arteritis with a sedimentation rate and hematocrit. As long as the neurologic examination is normal, and there is no history of transient neurologic spells, a CT scan or other tests are not needed in elderly patients with headache. Follow-up examinations in 3 or 4 months will identify evolving signs of serious neurologic disease. If the pain persists or other signs develop, the patient must be evaluated and treated more vigorously.

Treatment

Treatment of a headache that has no clear etiology is aimed at relief of the pain. When the headache is mild, aspirin (600 mg qid) or acetaminophen (600 mg qid) is often enough and is the best first drug to use if the patient has not been treated. Combinations of analgesics and barbiturate (Fiorinal) are very effective when used as needed for nonspecific (tension) headache. Propranolol (80–320 mg qd) or amitriptyline (25–100 mg qhs) is useful in migraine. Sansert (methysergide) (2 mg bid or qid) is useful when the other two drugs fail. Ergotamine is generally not given to elderly patients because of its vasoconstrictor effects. Amitriptyline in higher doses (75–250 mg) is helpful for depression headaches. Other antidepressants are also useful. Many patients improve when assured that the headache has no serious cause. Patients often worry that their headaches are caused by a brain tumor and feel great relief at learning that there is no tumor. Patients with headache should be followed monthly while being treated actively, but once the headache is under control, follow-up once or twice a year is usually enough. The headaches may "break through" the treatment or reappear after a period off medication. Changing the medication, increasing the dose, or restarting a previously successful drug often relieves the problem. When a new headache appears, the clinician must be wary lest he miss a lesion not present before. A repeat evaluation is then needed.

---

1. Austen FK, Carmichael MW, Adams RD: Neurologic manifestations of chronic pulmonary insufficiency. *N Engl J Med* 1957:579–590, 257.
   Chronic pulmonary insufficiency with congestive heart failure was associated with headache, papilledema, impairment of consciousness and asterixis in 4 patients.
2. Fisher CM: Headache in cerebrovascular disease, in Vinkin PJ, Bruyn GW (eds.): *Headache and Cranial Neuralgias, Handbook of Clinical Neurology.* New York, Wiley, 1968, vol 5, pp 124–156.
   A detailed description of headache in stroke. The volume is a review of all aspects of headache.
3. Fisher CM, Ojemann RG, Roberson GH: Spontaneous dissection of cervicocerebral arteries. *Can J Neurol Sci* 5:9–19, 1978.
   The 16 patients had headache, facial pain, subjective bruit, oculosympathetic palsy, and monocular blindness.
4. Hunt WE, Hess RM: Surgical risk as related to time of intervention in the repair of intracranial aneurysms. *J Neurosurg* 28:14–19, 1968.
   The risk is greatest in patients with the most severe deficit. Early surgery is safe in patients with minimal deficit.
5. Huston KA, Hunder GG: Giant cell (cranial) arteritis: A clinical review. *Am Heart J* 100:99–105, 1980.
   Of 60 patients, 18 had headache as the initial complaint.
6. Huston KA, Hunder GG: Giant cell (cranial) arteritis: A clinical review. *Am Heart J* 100:99–107, 1980.
   A comprehensive clinical review with 79 references.
7. Locksley HB: Natural history of subarachnoid hemorrhage, intracranial aneurysms, and arteriovenous malformations. *J Neurosurg* 25:219–235, 1966.
   A detailed review of 6,368 cases.
8. Raskin N: Headaches associated with organic diseases of the nervous system. *Med Clin North Am* 62:459–466, 1978.
   This book contains a number of monographs on headache.
9. Ropper AH, Davis KR: Lobar cerebral hemorrhages: Acute. *Ann Neurol* 8:141–147, 1980.
   Headache was a prevalent symptom and hypertension was unusual.
10. Stewart MR, Samson D, Diehl J, Hinton RC, Ditmore QM: Unruptured cerebral aneurysms presenting as recurrent transient neurologic deficits. *Neurology* 30:47–51, 1980.
    Focal signs lasting less than 30 minutes were present in 4 patients.
11. Sundt TM, Whisnant JP: Subarachnoid hemorrhage from intracranial aneurysms: Surgical management and natural history of disease. *N Engl J Med* 299:116–122, 1978.
    In 310 patients severe initial bleeding, rebleeding usually within two weeks, and delayed ischemia were the major preoperative problems. Operative mortality was 1.6% in patients without neurologic signs and 35% in patients with severe deficits.
12. Twomey C: Brain tumors in the elderly. *Age Ageing* 7:138–145, 1978.
    Mental impairment with motor signs was the most common finding in patients with malignant tumors. Headache was common in the benign cases.
13. Weisberg LA: Computed tomography in aneurysmal subarachnoid hemorrhage. *Neurology* 29:802–808, 1979.
    Computed tomography identified bleeding in 28 of 50 patients. The CT scan may not identify all cases of SAH, but lumbar puncture will.

14. DIZZINESS IN THE ELDERLY

Thomas M. Walshe

Dizziness is a nonspecific description used by patients and physicians to indicate a variety of discomforts. The first step in the evaluation of dizziness is to understand the exact nature of the complaint. The feeling of dizziness usually involves the loss of normal spatial perception. In some patients it may appear as a sensation of moving or whirling, in others as a feeling of unsteadiness in gait or station, and in others as an uncomfortable, vague head sensation without a sense of motion. Blurred vision, faint feeling, and nausea also may be described as dizziness. Because of its multiple meanings, "dizziness" is not a helpful clinical description unless its meaning is made clear. Once the quality of the discomfort is defined, the clinician will be able to emphasize a cardiac or neurologic evaluation.

Dizziness, even in elderly patients, is usually not associated with dangerous neurologic illness. About 70% of patients referred for dizziness have a labyrinthine or other benign cause; 12% or 13% have multiple sensory loss; 4% or 5% have cardiovascular causes, and about 12% have central nervous system disease. In elderly patients, the multiple sensory causes are slightly more prevalent. Dizziness without other signs may warn of serious disease outside the nervous system, but the neurologic syndromes causing dizziness can usually be recognized by signs found on neurologic examination. The disorders outside the nervous system that cause dizziness are usually labyrinthine or cardiovascular. In some cases no clear disorder is diagnosable.

Differentiation of Central and Peripheral Vertigo

Both central nervous system and labyrinthine disorders produce *vertigo,* the sensation of spinning or whirling. The sensation of movement may be mild or severe and is associated in some cases with nausea, vomiting, diaphoresis, and unsteadiness of gait. The sensation of falling or moving while being supine is also a form of vertigo. Vertigo provoked by changes in position is commonly found in patients with labyrinthine disorders.

Focal Signs. Patients with labyrinthine vertigo usually do not have other complaints. Indeed, vertigo alone is seldom caused by a central nervous system lesion. Both neurologic and labyrinthine disorders, however, produce *nystagmus,* a rhythmic jerking of the eyes. Although it is not fully valid to generalize, most patients with labyrinthine disease have nystagmus with the fast component beating in a single horizontal direction away from the affected ear. Nystagmus caused by lesions of the brain often changes its direction, so that the fast component beats toward the direction of gaze. When the nystagmus beats upward or downward, the lesion is almost always in the brainstem. Nystagmus caused by brainstem lesions can occur when there is no vertigo, but labyrinthine nystagmus is almost always present only while the patient is vertiginous. When the complaint is vertigo, an underlying neurologic disorder can often be recognized through associated signs such as diplopia, facial numbness or weakness, Horner's syndrome, and motor deficits.

Transient Ischemia. When a patient has transient episodes of severe or moderate vertigo, one must search for clues to a cerebrovascular or other neurologic disorder. Vertigo may be a prominent symptom in transient brainstem ischemia, cerebellar ischemia, lateral medullary infarction, or seizure disorder. There are almost always clues in addition to vertigo that localize the dysfunction to the brain. Patients with transient ischemia have diplopia, facial numbness or weakness, and sometimes transient motor or sensory complaints in the extremities. The lateral medullary stroke causes a fixed (or progressing) deficit which adds ataxia, Horner's syndrome, and a sensory deficit to the vertigo. Cerebellar ischemia or infarction almost always produces such ataxia that the patient cannot walk.

Seizure. Temporal lobe seizures are difficult to separate, but the vertigo is usually less severe and of shorter duration than that seen in labyrinthine disorders. The seizure may produce a nonvertiginous feeling that resembles the complaints found in hypotension. The EEG is often abnormal, and the symptoms disappear or diminish with anticonvulsant treatment.

Hearing Loss. Hearing loss is found in patients having inner ear lesions, but the rare patient with occlusion of the anterior inferior cerebellar artery (AICA) may present with vertigo and hearing loss. There are, however, always other findings of cranial nerve dysfunction in such strokes.

Patients with Ménière's disease, a disorder of the labyrinth and cochlea, complain of decreased hearing, tinnitus, fullness in the ear, and dizziness that may or may not be vertigo. Audiometry can help separate Ménière's disease from lesions of the eighth nerve, which also cause hearing loss. Speech discrimination is good in Ménière's disease but poor in lesions of the eighth nerve. Recruitment and short increment sensitivity are preserved in Ménière's disease but become poor with nerve lesions. Tone decay occurs with nerve lesions but not with cochlear lesions.

Hearing loss usually occurs without vertigo in tumors of the eighth nerve (acoustic neurinoma). Some patients with acoustic neurinoma lose their corneal reflex on the side of the deafness, and the "dizziness" in acoustic neurinomas is usually an unsteadiness of gait described as stumbling or imbalance. Computed tomography (CT) scan with contrast can show the tumor in most cases.

Cardiac Syndromes. Elderly patients who suffer dizziness, diaphoresis, blackout spells, and a feeling of faintness sometimes have seizures but more often suffer from cardiac arrhythmia, hypotension, or other cardiovascular dysfunction. Elderly patients with dizziness need a thorough cardiac evaluation, and when the history sounds like arrhythmia, cardiac monitoring sometimes can confirm it.

Other Syndromes. Elderly patients also complain of a less specific syndrome thought to be associated with the aging changes of the labyrinth and vestibular system. Severe vertiginous episodes that follow certain head positions are sometimes caused by *cupulolithiasis,* an abnormality of the semicircular canal. The vertigo is usually of short duration, but in a few patients it persists. A few cases studied pathologically have shown deposits of an insoluble material in the posterior semicircular canal. Clinical evidence for the syndrome is inferential, and patients should be evaluated thoroughly for other causes. Other syndromes of vertigo with head movement, so-called *dysequilibrium syndromes,* have been postulated, but no pathologic verification has been produced. Hearing is often spared in these cases, and no cardiac or neurologic findings explain the vertigo.

Another large group of elderly patients complain of a nonspecific, less discrete discomfort that is not easily associated with a clear etiology. The patient usually describes an unsteadiness, lightheadedness, feeling of about to fall, or other nonvertiginous complaint. Occasional vertigo may be superimposed on the other discomfort. The patients have reduced sensory (visual, hearing, proprioception) input, and it is thought that the lack of sensory feedback produces part of the syndrome. An abnormality of the vestibular apparatus may also be involved.

Tests

Elderly patients who come to the neurologist because of dizziness do not always have a diagnosable condition. It is crucial that each patient be carefully examined, although most have nonspecific syndromes that can be treated symptomatically. If the patient has no other neurologic symptoms or signs, it is usually correct to assume the problem is labyrinthine or one of the nonspecific syndromes.

Provocative tests that precipitate the symptoms often help to identify the cause. Measurement of the orthostatic variation in blood pressure and use of the Valsalva maneuver may explain symptoms in some patients. Hyperventilation reproduces the symptoms in patients who suffer from that cause of dizziness. Positional testing—having the patient move quickly from the seated to the supine position with the head rotated 90 degrees—produces vertigo and nystagmus in patients with positional vertigo. Electronystagmography, by quantitating the nystagmus and other parameters, is sometimes helpful in establishing the site of the lesion. Audiometry may confirm a suspected hearing loss and thus point to a peripheral localization.

Patients should be observed serially to ensure that there are no evolving neurologic signs, since some patients with brainstem stroke may have vertigo alone and develop telltale neurologic signs 12–24 hours later. Elderly patients with severe or moderate vertigo usually should be observed in the hospital.

Treatment

Treatment of labyrinthine vertigo consists of reassuring the patient that the condition is not serious and relieving the symptoms. Elderly patients with acute labyrinthine vertigo should be hospitalized and watched closely, because they become dehydrated and ill from the vomiting. Mild sedation with phenergan (25–50 mg tid) helps relieve the discomfort. Time and rest are the major therapies, however. Patients with milder, chronic vertigo can also be given phenergan or meclizine (25 mg bid or tid). Mild sedatives such as oxazepam or lorazepam in low doses reduce the vertigo in some cases.

Elderly patients who have no clear neurologic or labyrinthine etiology may benefit from increased sensory input to help them feel less dizzy. The physician can ensure that the patient has the proper glasses, and a hearing aid if needed. Some patients find that a cane helps them to sense their position.

1. Facer GW, Maragos NE: The dizzy patient. *Postgrad Med* 57:73–77, 1975.
   A short description.
2. Alford B: Ménière's disease: Criteria for diagnosis and evaluation of therapy for reporting. *Trans Am Acad Ophthalmol Otolaryngol* 76:1462, 1972.
   No references.
3. Drachman DA, Hart CW: An approach to the dizzy patient. *Neurology* 22:323–334, 1972.
   A diagnosis was made in 91% of patients, but only 12% had central nervous system lesions.
4. Fisher CM: Vertigo in cerebrovascular disease. *Arch Otolaryngol* 85:529–534, 1967.
   Dizziness without other findings is seldom a sign of stroke. This article describes the specific syndromes that have dizziness as a major component.
5. Frederic MW: Central vertigo. *Otolaryngol Clin North Am* 6:267–285, 1973.
   Discusses the vertiginous syndromes caused by stroke and other neurologic disorders.
6. Morgenstein K, Seung H: Vestibular neuronitis. *Laryngoscope* 81:131–139, 1971.
   Covers what little is known about labyrinthine disorders.
7. Schuknecht HF: *Pathology of the Ear.* Cambridge, Mass, Harvard University Press, 1974.
   A comprehensive description.
8. Smith BH: Vestibular disturbances in epilepsy. *Neurology* 10:465–469, 1960.
   Describes patients with symptoms that resemble labyrinthine or vestibular lesions, but who have seizure disorder.
9. Wolfson RJ (ed): Symposium on vertigo. *Otolaryngol Clin North Am* 6:1, 1973.
   A group of monographs that covers the subject in detail.
10. Jonas S, Klein I, Dimant J: Importance of Holter monitoring in patients with periodic cerebral symptoms. *Ann Neurol* 1:470–474, 1977.
    Arrythmia does not cause focal signs or symptoms but may cause dizziness, lightheadedness, and blackout spells.
11. Overstall PW, Hazell JWP, Johnson AL: Vertigo in the elderly. *Age Ageing 10:105–109, 1981.*
    Half the patients seen in this group had a central vestibular lesion; the details of the criteria were not stated.
12. Stuart WH: Geriatric neurology for the otolaryngologist. *Otolaryngol Clin North Am* 15:329–350, 1982.
    Among other topics this article covers dizziness in the elderly.

15. TREMOR IN THE ELDERLY

Thomas M. Walshe

Tremor, a neurologic sign commonly found in elderly patients, is a spontaneous, involuntary, rhythmic movement of a body part about a joint. The tremor may be fast or slow, have a large or small excursion, and be constant or intermittent. The clinical details of the tremor and its electrophysiologic parameters help to separate the three main types of tremor: *action tremor, cerebellar tremor,* and *extrapyramidal tremor.*

Action Tremors

Action tremor is most obvious during voluntary activity and may be present but less noticeable at rest. The EMG recordings of action tremor show that the agonist muscles and antagonist muscles across a joint contract synchronously, and the movement results from the imbalance between the two competing muscle groups. With careful electrophysiologic recording, everyone can be shown to have a fine clinically undetectable action tremor. Such physiologic action tremors are asymptomatic. The involuntary movement is usually rapid (8–12 times/sec), and the excursion small (a fine, fast tremor). Physiologic tremor may become enhanced with anxiety, following exercise, or following other stresses. The tremor usually disappears when the stress abates.

Alcohol withdrawal causes an enhanced physiologic tremor that has a slightly larger amplitude than other physiologic tremors. Lithium, tricyclic antidepressants, and xanthines enhance the physiologic tremor. When the tremor is from medication, stopping the drug usually stops the tremor. Drug-induced action tremors often abate spontaneously after a few months on the drug or with reduction in dose. Other physiologic tremors may respond to antianxiety medicines such as oxazepam, but when the tremor is minimal, no treatment is needed. Patients with action tremor should be evaluated for hyperthyroidism and hypoglycemia, which cause an enhanced physiologic tremor.

Essential, familial, and senile tremors are action tremors that each have approximately the same physiology and clinical significance. Essential tremor may appear to be similar to enhanced physiologic tremor but is slower (4–8 times/sec) and seems to depend on central nervous system rather than myoneural mechanisms. Postural tone activates the tremor, so that it seems to disappear at rest and increase with action. Since even slight postural tone will produce it, some patients have essential tremor when apparently resting.

Essential tremor occurs usually in the hands and arms and sometimes in the legs. The head, jaw, and tongue are involved in many patients, and when the voice is tremulous, essential tremor is a likelier diagnosis than enhanced physiologic tremor. Essential tremor is benign, except that it may disfigure the patient and, when severe, cause difficulty with the activities of daily living. Essential tremors are usually not indicative of dangerous progressive neurologic disease, although the patient may be quite uncomfortable and inconvenienced.

The action tremor manifested by some patients with chronic hereditary neuropathy (Charcot-Marie-Tooth disease) resembles essential tremor clinically but has different physiological findings.

Treatment of benign, essential, or familial tremor in elderly patients depends on the severity of the tremor and the presence of concomitant disease that would make drug therapy unwise. Alcohol in moderate doses will abolish essential tremor, and patients who drink usually notice the benefit of alcohol on their tremor. Because treatment with alcohol may lead to addiction, it is not a useful method for control of tremor.

Propranolol is the most effective drug in many patients (about three-fourths) with essential tremor. The dose should be increased slowly, starting with 10–20 mg tid and going up to 60–80 mg qid. The effect is usually apparent within a week of treatment. The tremor may improve but not disappear completely. Another useful drug is diazepam, in doses of 5–10 mg tid or qid. Although relief of anxiety reduces tremor, diazepam probably works for other reasons. When propranolol alone fails, the addition of diazepam is sometimes effective. Other beta-blockers are not as effective as propranolol in most patients. It is best to start with lower doses of diazepam (2 mg) in elderly patients and to keep the dose constant for at least a week before increasing it, to avoid excess sedation. Other sedatives also may be useful in low doses, especially when used before a social function or other stressful event. Primidone (250 mg bid) has been helpful in some patients when other drugs fail. Phenothiazines and butyrophenones make essential tremor worse. Alcohol and propranolol are specific for essential tremor and do not improve enhanced physiological tremor or the tremor that accompanies neuropathy.

Cerebellar Ataxia

Abnormality of the cerebellum or its connections in the brainstem causes a type of action tremor. Cerebellar ataxia calls for thorough evaluation of the patient for serious neurologic disease. The cerebellar, or *ataxic,* tremor (really a failure to control movement rather than a tremor in the strict sense) is coarse and is much worse at the end of a movement. A patient moves an extremity toward a target adroitly, but, as it approaches the target, the extremity develops a coarse tremor and fails to hit the target accurately. A lesion involving the cerebellar outflow tracts produces a proximal, coarse (2–4 times/sec), and sometimes violent action tremor, which disappears at rest and begins with the onset of movement. Such tremors are usually quite violent and often unilateral, so they are easily distinguished from benign essential tremor. Patients with cerebellar lesions usually have other neurologic findings in addition to tremor. Many patients have abnormalities of balance and gait, findings not seen in essential tremor. The tremor and ataxia caused by cerebellar lesions improve only as the lesion improves. There is no symptomatic treatment for cerebellar tremor, and management depends on diagnosis of the underlying cerebellar disease.

Extrapyramidal Tremor

The tremor of basal ganglial disease (of which Parkinson's disease is most common) differs from the tremors described. This extrapyramidal tremor diminishes during movement and is not enhanced with precise, goal-directed movement. It is most obvious when the patient is in a resting position. The tremor is provoked by anxiety, as are almost all movement disorders, and is a coarse (3–7 times/sec), rhythmic movement that is usually more obvious in the hands but often involves the lower extremities. The head and trunk are involved in the minority of cases. There is a tendency for extrapyramidal tremor to involve the mouth and lips, but it does not interfere with speech or swallowing. The EMG shows an alternating agonist-antagonist muscle activity, which produces the abnormal movement. The tremor is of greater amplitude and slower than that seen in benign essential tremor. The diagnosis of an extrapyramidal disorder usually becomes obvious when other neurologic signs exist along with tremor, whereas the benign tremor exists alone. The extrapyramidal tremor produced by neuroleptic drugs is the same as that seen in Parkinson's disease. Very rarely, a stroke or tumor in the basal ganglia causes an extrapyramidal tremor. (Treatment is discussed in Chap. 95, Parkinson's Disease.)

Benign essential tremor frequently occurs in patients with Parkinson's disease and is the source of the "cogwheel" phenomenon. Essential tremor can be differentiated from the tremor of Parkinson's disease, because it is faster (6.5 times/sec) and continues during action.

---

1. Brumlik J, et al: A critical analysis of the effects of trihexyphenidyl (Artane) on the components of the parkinsonian syndrome. *J Nerv Ment Dis* 138:424–431, 1964.
   Evaluation of the drug's efficacy on individual disabilities based on a breakdown of symptoms of parkinsonism.
2. Calzetti S, et al: Effect of a single oral dose of propranolol on essential tremor: A double-blind controlled study. *Ann Neurol* 13:165–171, 1983.
   Double-blind placebo study in 26 patients showed a reduction of essential tremor after a single oral dose of 120 mg.
3. Calzetti S, Findley LJ, Perucca E, Richens A: The response of essential tremor to propranolol: Evaluation of clinical variables governing its efficacy on prolonged administration. *JNNP* 46:393–398, 1983.
   Double-blind crossover placebo-controlled study in 16 patients showed propranolol was better than placebo only in doses of 240 mg qd.
4. Chakrabarti A, Pearce JMS: Essential tremor: Response to primidone. *JNNP* 44:650, 1981.
   A letter describes 5 patients who improved within a few days.
5. Critchley E: Clinical manifestations of essential tremor. *JNNP* 35:365–372, 1972.
   In a study of 42 patients, the tremor affected the upper extremities in 41 patients, the head in 25, the lower limbs in 15, and the trunk in 2.
6. Dupont E, Hansen HJ, Dalby MA: Treatment of benign essential tremor with propranolol. *Acta Neurol Scand* 49:75–84, 1973.
   Propranolol is the best drug for essential tremor but more effective in younger patients.
7. Fahn S: Differential diagnosis of tremors. *Med Clin North Am* 56:1363–1375, 1972.
   A general review.
8. Fann WE, Whelan JC: Therapeutic principles in the management of movement disorders in elderly patients, in Ruge W (ed): *Interdisciplinary Topics in Gerontology.* Basal, Karger, 1979, vol 15, pp 194–210.
   Discusses tardive dyskinesia, Huntington disease, and Parkinson's disease.
9. Gresty MA, Findley LJ: Tremors in Parkinson's disease, in Rose FC, Capildeo R (eds): *Research Progress in Parkinson's Disease.* Turnbridge Wells, Kent, Pitman Medical, 1981, chap 11.

10. Hoehn MM, Yahr MD: Parkinsonism: Onset, progression, and mortality. *Neurology* 17:427–442, 1967.
Describes 856 patients who were diagnosed as having paralysis agitans, Parkinson's disease, or parkinsonism.
11. Jankovic J, Fahn S: Physiologic and pathologic tremors. *Ann Intern Med* 93:460–465, 1980.
Reviews "basic mechanisms and clinical features" of tremors with a concentration on current advances in pathophysiology and management.
12. Manyam BV: Amantidine in essential tremor. *Ann Neurol* 9:198–199, 1981.
A letter describes improvement in 15 of 26 patients.
13. O'Brien MD, et al: Benign familial tremor treated with primidone. *Br Med J* 282:178–180, 1981.
In 20 patients with essential tremor, 12 improved and 6 had nausea and vertigo that prevented treatment.
14. Shahani BT, Young RR: Physiological and pharmacological aids in the differential diagnosis of tremor. *J Neurol Neurosurg Psychiatry* 39:772–783, 1976.
An excellent description of the physiologic characteristics of the various tremors.
15. Stern M, et al: The parkinsonian tremor in sleep. *J Nerv Ment Dis* 147:202–210, 1968.
Reviews the relationship of sleep and tremor. The effect of trihexyphenidyl (Artane) on nocturnal tremor was not clear.
16. Sweet RD, Blumberg J, Lee JE, McDowell F: Propranolol treatment of essential tremor. *Neurology* 24:64–67, 1974.
Authors had limited success using doses of up to 320 mg qid.
17. Teychenne PF, et al: Bromocriptine: Low-dose therapy in parkinson's disease. *Neurology* 32:577–583, 1982.
Double-blind placebo study in 29 patients showed improvement using bromocriptine in doses between 3 to 4 mg daily.
18. Winkler GF, Young RR: Efficacy of chronic propranolol therapy in action tremors of the familial, senile or essential varieties. *N Engl J Med* 290:984–988, 1974.
Double-blind crossover study in 24 patients showed improvement using propranolol in doses of 60 to 160 mg qid.
19. Young RR, et al: Beta-adrenergic mechanisms in action tremor. *N Engl J Med* 293:950–953, 1975.
Function of peripheral beta-adrenergic tremorogenic receptors is not necessary for production of essential tremor, and the efficacy of chronic propranolol therapy in the suppression of essential tremor is not mediated via its peripheral blocking action.
20. Zetusky WJ, et al: Clinical categorization of parkinsonian patients. *Neurology* 33 (suppl 2):61–62, 1983.
Abstract describes two subgroups, one characterized by "rigidity, bradykinesia, postural instability, and gait difficulty" and the other by tremor alone.

16. TREATMENT OF TARDIVE DYSKINESIA

Thomas M. Walshe

Mechanism

Current teaching holds that tardive dyskinesia results from chronic high-dose neuroleptic drugs that interfere postsynaptically with dopamine neurotransmission. Clinical analogues are Huntington's disease and, more closely, L-dopa–induced dyskinesia. The opposite clinical condition is Parkinson's disease. Drugs (amphetamine, L-dopa) or conditions that increase dopamine transmission in the striatum (caudate, globus pallidus, putamen) cause dyskinesia or make chorea worse. Drugs (neuroleptics) or conditions (Parkinson's disease) that decrease dopamine transmission improve chorea. The neurochemical mechanism is most likely postsynaptic, i.e., an alteration in number or sensitivity of the dopamine receptors. In Huntington's disease, it is suspected that there are abnormal striatal cells that are overly activated by the normal levels of striatal dopamine. Likewise, in L-dopa–induced dyskinesia, excess dopamine stimulation is one explanation for the abnormal movements. In Parkinson's disease the effect is the opposite—striatal dopamine concentration is decreased. In tardive dyskinesia, chronic blockage of the dopamine receptor by neuroleptics creates hypersensitive receptors (or some other membrane abnormality), which produce the dyskinesia that confronts the clinician.

Dopamine transmission excess appears to be the major factor in tardive dyskinesia, but cholinergic striatal interneurons also play an important role. For instance, in Huntington's disease, a disorder that causes movements somewhat similar to those in some cases of tardive dyskinesia, increased acetylcholine activity improves chorea but anticholinergic drugs worsen it. The reverse is true for Parkinson's disease. In tardive dyskinesia, increased acetylcholine activity reduces the movements, but the anticholinergics make them worse. Using simplified generalizations, based on incomplete understanding of the physiology, clinicians attempt to predict the efficacy of certain classes of drugs in tardive dyskinesia.

Prevention

Tardive dyskinesia is a iatrogenic problem caused by the use of drugs that act as dopamine-receptor blockers. The drugs are used mostly for the treatment of psychosis and include several generic types. As a group they are known as *neuroleptics* because of their primary effect on the nervous system. Phenothiazines, butyrophenones, and the other major tranquilizers are among the most widely used neuroleptics. The physician who uses such a drug must be sure that there is a clear need for it and that no other drugs will suffice. For serious psychoses and a few other indications, neuroleptics are valuable drugs. They should not be used, however, when another, less toxic drug will do. Simple prevention is the most effective way to reduce the morbidity of tardive dyskinesia.

When a neuroleptic drug is needed, the lowest dose for the shortest duration should be administered, as tardive dyskinesia usually occurs after months or years of chronic neuroleptic treatment. In elderly, demented, and other brain-damaged persons, the incidence of tardive dyskinesia seems to be greater than in others. Patients with senile dementia of the Alzheimer type develop particularly vigorous movement disorders at relatively low doses of neuroleptics. Although behavioral problems are one of the major targets for management in demented patients, high doses of neuroleptics for long periods are seldom necessary. The short-acting benzodiazepines often successfully control unwanted behavior, and when they fail, low doses of neuroleptic for a short time will minimize the risk of tardive dyskinesia.

The routine use of anticholinergic drugs with the neuroleptics seems to promote the onset of tardive dyskinesia. Anticholinergics are useful, indeed, for neuroleptic-induced parkinsonism, but should not be given until the parkinsonian syndrome appears, and only when it becomes bothersome to the patient. A short course (2 mo) of anticholinergics will usually reverse the parkinsonian syndrome, and after the anticholinergic drug is removed, the parkinsonian syndrome may not return.

When possible, it is best to use the neuroleptic drugs intermittently, giving the patient as long a period off the drug as his or her condition safely permits. Low dose and short duration seem the best preventive methods for patients who need neuroleptics.

The final principle in primary prevention of tardive dyskinesia is to be **watchful** for the **earliest** signs (usually minimal buccolingual dyskinesia), so that the neuroleptic can be reduced or stopped. Tardive dyskinesia is a progresive syndrome, and the longer the dyskinesia remains, the more likely it is to be permanent.

Treatment

Many patients, despite careful neuroleptic management, develop persistent, disfiguring dyskinesias. When the dyskinesia is mild, sedatives, short-acting benzodiazepines or barbiturates may reduce the movements enough to satisfy the patient. Only when the dyskinesia is severe enough to disrupt the patient's life does one need to treat vigorously. The first step in management of even mild tardive dyskinesia is discontinuation, or at least reduction, of the neuroleptic drug. When the drug is discontinued, the movement disorder increases or first becomes noticeable. If the patient happens to develop the restlessness called *akathisia,* those taking care of him may erroneously interpret the excess movement as a psychiatric symptom and reinstitute treatment. The increase in neuroleptic will mask the movement but only increase the later risk of an unmanageable disorder. Some patients with dementia develop so vigorous a withdrawal dyskinesia that the neuroleptic must be restarted. The dyskinesia that occurs following reduction in neuroleptic dose or after discontinuation of a neuroleptic can sometimes be handled by a very slow reduction in the dose plus concomitant treatment with reserpine. Tapering the dose by about 10% every 2 weeks helps to reduce the movement disorder.

The best drug for established tardive dyskinesia is reserpine, which depletes presynaptic amines and thus reduces the amount of dopamine released at the synapse. The effective dose of reserpine is usually 6–8 mg in tardive dyskinesia. The major side effects of reserpine are mild parkinsonism, hypotension, and bradycardia. The side effects of reserpine are usually well tolerated, and the hypotension, when symptomatic, can be improved with a mineralocorticoid (Florinef). Reserpine can increase or cause depression and should not be given to depressed patients. Drowsiness is the most commonly encountered side effect, but it usually disappears with time.

When reserpine alone fails to control the dyskinesia, the addition of alpha-methyltyrosine may be effective. Alpha-methyltyrosine competitively inhibits tyrosine hydroxylase, which catalyzes the rate-limiting step in the conversion of L-tyrosine to L-dopa. The drug reduces the amine concentration available at the synapse. Alpha-methyltyrosine is sometimes effective used alone in doses of 250–1,500 mg/day. Experience with the drug is limited, since it is used almost exclusively in patients with pheochromocytoma. Sedation, the major side effect, begins in about 24 hours and usually diminishes in several days. Extrapyramidal signs are mild and occur infrequently. When added to reserpine, alpha-methyltyrosine is very effective. The dose may be as low as 250 mg every other day for some patients, but most require 500–750 mg daily in addition to 6 mg of reserpine. Careful titration of the dose is necessary to achieve the best effect at the lowest dose. Sedation, parkinsonism, bradycardia, and hypotension are almost always caused by the combination of reserpine and alpha-methyltyrosine but are not usually severe enough to prevent therapy. Careful monitoring is needed throughout the treatment.

Other drugs are seldom effective in tardive dyskinesia. Deanol (acetamidobenzoate, thought to be an acetylcholine precursor) can be used in doses of 200–2,000 mg with almost no risk of adverse reaction but is rarely effective. Lecithin helps some patients but seems less convincingly successful the more it is tried. The dose of lecithin is about 10–40 gm/day, depending on the purity of the product. Weight gain is the only known side effect.

Neuroleptic-induced movements, such as rabbit mouth (rhythmic pursing of the lips), acute dystonic reactions, and akathisias, are not tardive movements but are associated with ongoing treatment. These movements can sometimes be treated with the anticholinergic drugs such as benztropine mesylate (Cogentin) in doses of 2–4 mg bid or tid. The major side effects are associated with the anticholinergic action on the bladder and on vision.

---

1. Baldessarini RJ, Lipinski JF: Risks versus benefits of antipsychotic drugs. *N Engl J Med* 289:427–428, 1973.
There is a substantial misuse of antipsychotic drugs for the "chronically malfunctioning psychiatric patient."
2. Casey DE: Managing tardive dyskinesia. *J Clin Psychiatry* 39:748–753, 1978.
Prevention is more successful than drug treatment.
3. Dovoisin RC: Reserpine for tardive dyskinesia. *N Engl J Med* 286:611, 1972.
This letter suggests that reserpine is "symptomatically effective even in relatively severe cases of tardive dyskinesia."
4. Fahn S: Treatment of tardive dyskinesia with combined reserpine and alpha-methyltyrosine. *Trans Am Neurol Assoc* 103:100–103, 1978.
The combination was effective in 7 patients.
5. Growden JH, Gelenberg AJ, Doller J, et al: Lecithin can suppress tardive dyskinesia. *N Engl J Med* 298:1029–1030, 1978.
A letter that is more optimistic than current experience supports.
6. Growden JH, Hirsch MJ, Wurtman RJ, Wiener W: Oral choline administration to patients with tardive dyskinesia. *N Engl J Med* 297:524–527, 1977.
Choline is rarely used today.
7. Huang C, Wang RIH, Hasagawa A, Alverno L: Evaluation of reserpine and alpha methyldopa in treatment of tardive dyskinesia. *Psychopharmacol Bull* 16:41–43, 1980.
Compared to placebo, neither drug caused improvement in 30 inpatients.

8. Jus A, Jus K, Fontaine P: Long-term treatment of tardive dyskinesia. *J Clin Psychiatry* 40:72–77, 1979.
A study of 62 patients who were followed and treated for 4 years. The best results were in young patients.
9. Kazamatsuri H, Chien CP, Cole JO: Treatment of tardive dyskinesia: I. Clinical efficacy of a dopamine depleting agent, tetrabenazine. *Arch Gen Psychiatry* 27:95–99, 1972.
Of 400 ambulatory long-term patients with tardive dyskinesia, 24 improved with tetrabenazine.
10. Klawans HL: Therapeutic approaches to neuroleptic-induced tardive dyskinesias, in Yahr MD (ed): *The Basal Ganglia.* New York, Raven Press, 1976, pp 447–457.
An authoritative review.
11. Klawans HL, Rubovits R: Effect of cholinergic and anticholinergic agents on tardive dyskinesia. *J Neurol Neurosurg Psychiatry* 37:941–947, 1974.
Anticholinergic therapy in patients capable of developing tardive dyskinesia lowers the threshold for the "appearance of these movements" and consequently may increase the occurrence of abnormal movements.
12. Klett JC, Caffey E: Evaluating the long-term need for antiparkinson drugs by chronic schizophrenics. *Arch Gen Psychiatry* 26:374–379, 1972.
Antiparkinson medication was replaced by placebo in chronic schizophrenic males who were taking both antipsychotic and antiparkinson medication. Improvement occurred in 82% of subjects, while 11% became worse and 7% withdrew from the study.
13. Kobayashi RM: Drug therapy of tardive dyskinesia. *N Engl J Med* 296:257–259, 1977.
A brief, accessible review.
14. Linnoila M, Vivkari M, Hietala O: Effect of sodium valproate on tardive dyskinesia. *Br J Psychiatry* 129:114–119, 1976.
In 32 chronic psychiatric patients, sodium valproate had no effect on dyskinesia or on psychiatric symptoms.
15. Sedman G: Clonnazepam in treatment of tardive oral dyskinesia. *Br Med J* 2:583, 1976.
16. Sato S, Daly R, Peters H: Reserpine therapy of phenothiazine induced dyskinesia. *Dis Nerv Syst* 32:680–685, 1971.
A significant improvement followed large doses of reserpine in 5 patients.
17. Jenke MA: Tardive dyskinesia: Special risk in the elderly. *J Am Geriatr Soc* 31:71–73, 1983.
Neuroleptics should be avoided except when necessary. This is a short literature review.
18. Johnson GFS, Hunt GE, Rey JM: Incidence and severity of tardive dyskinesia with age. *Arch Gen Psychiatry* 39:486, 1982.
This letter reports that 66 psychiatric outpatients evaluated with the Abnormal Involuntary Movement Scale showed that the severity of tardive dyskinesia was greater with older age.
19. Hunter R, et al: Neuropathological finding in 3 cases of persistent dyskinesias following phenothiazine medication. *J Neurol Sci* 7:763, 1968.
20. Christensen E, Moller JE, Faurbye A: Neuropathological investigation of 28 brains from patients with dyskinesias. *Acta Psychiatr Scand* 46:14–23, 1970.
Comparison between oral dyskinesia and a control group without dyskinesia showed that cell degeneration in the substantia nigra was more marked in the dyskinesia group.
21. Smith JM, Baldessarini RJ: Changes in prevalence, severity and recovery in tardive dyskinesia with age. *Arch Gen Psychiatry* 37:1368–1373, 1980.
The severity of tardive dyskinesia increases with age, and there is an inverse relationship between age and remission.
22. Carroll BJ, Curtis GC, Kokmen E: Paradoxical response to dopamine agonists in tardive dyskinesia. *Am J Psychiatry* 134:785–789, 1977.
Dimethyaminoethanol, dozapine, and thioridazine failed to modify dyskinesia.
23. Baldessarini RJ: Tardive dyskinesia: An evaluation of the etiologic association with neuroleptic therapy. *Can Psychiatry Assoc J* 19:551–554, 1974.
A review of the problem, its prevalence, and its etiology.

24. Casey DE, Gerlach J: Oxiperomide in tardive dyskinesia. *J Neurol Neurosurg Psychiatry* 43:264–267, 1980.
The drug suppressed dyskinesia, but symptoms returned when the drug was stopped.
25. Nasrallah HA, Pappas NJ, Crowe RR: Oculogyric dystonia in tardive dyskinesia. *Am J Psychiatry* 137:850–851, 1980.
An unusual side effect.
26. Christensen E, Møller JE, Faurbye A: Neuropathological investigation of 28 brains from patients with dyskinesia. *Acta Psychiatr Scand* 46:14–23, 1970.
"Cell degeneration" was found in substanta nigra in 27 of 28 cases.

17. GAIT DISORDERS IN THE ELDERLY

Lewis Sudarsky

Gait disorders are common among nursing home patients, some of whom are admitted because their walking fails and they can no longer carry on their daily activities independently. The causes of falls among the elderly are often not understood. As the population grows older, the incidence of injury related to gait instability and fall can be expected to rise. According to U.S. National Health Survey statistics, one-half of all impairments among persons 65 and older are due to injury, of which falls account for nearly half. This actuarial analysis of the morbidity of aging understates a common clinical teaching: Old people are often unsteady in their walking and are increasingly likely to fall and sustain injuries.

An older literature describes the "senile gait disorder" but opinion differs as to whether it is in fact a single entity. Elderly people characteristically move slowly and cautiously, being uncertain in foot placement and step. They use a widened stance and have a tendency to be displaced easily, especially backwards. The underlying causes of such gait disorders are not understood, but evidence suggests a loss of postural supporting reflexes, and the release of grasping and other subcortical functions may account for some of the problem. Subcortical systems are important in organizing ambulation. Certain automatic stepping movements are elicited from the human neonate prior to myelination of the corticospinal tract. Walking movements can be elicited from the decerebrate cat by the systemic administration of clonidine, an alpha-adrenergic agonist, or L-dopa. Presumably some encephalization occurs in the primate bipedal gait; in primates, the subthalamic nucleus and mid-brain tegmentum function as locomotor control centers from which stimulation evokes controlled walking. Certainly our lack of knowledge about the basic motor program for walking, the anatomic and physiologic substrate for the performance, has been a major stumbling block to advancing our understanding of normal and abnormal gaits.

Data on marathon runners suggest that a decline in motor performance occurs with age. The capacity for running a marathon begins to deteriorate at age 35, and this loss progresses linearly until age 70, after which there is a more dramatic and accelerated decline. A variety of factors contribute to this incapacity. Alterations in metabolism and respiration and changes in skeleton, joints, and muscle fibers occur with age. It is likely that the changes in the central and peripheral nervous system are important at the geriatric end of the spectrum.

Causes

Patients with gait disorders seen in clinical practice are not a homogenous group but suffer from a variety of disorders, all of which affect ambulation. In our experience, a single etiologic diagnosis can be made in slightly more than half of the cases of gait disorders; the others usually have several causes. About one-fourth of elderly patients with gait disorders have a treatable condition. Gait failure in the elderly is most frequently caused by disorders affecting the motor system, such as myelopathy, stroke, Parkinson's disease, cerebellar atrophy, and hydrocephalus. Sensory disorders such as neuropathy and labrynthine disorders may also compromise stance and gait, in addition to causing subjective dizziness. Essential gait disorders—disorders without obvious neurologic cause—affect about 15% of patients.

Myelopathy. The most common cause of myelopathy in the elderly is cervical spondylosis. Foraminal osteophytes and cervical bars are frequently found on spine films of elderly patients. Autopsy studies of patients over 70 often show changes in the spinal cord caused by compression from spondylotic bars. Patients with myelopathy have spasticity in the legs, proprioceptive deficits (positive Romberg test), and correlated findings on laboratory tests (spine films, myelograms, or Schilling tests). Urinary frequency and urgency are also common. Not all such patients have limitation of neck movement, pain, atrophy in the arms, or other signs of nerve root irritation.

Stroke. Walking difficulty is at times related to a series of nonparalyzing strokes. The diagnosis of multiple cerebral infarcts can be made when patients, referred for undiagnosed gait disorder, have clear evidence of cerebral infarcts by computed tomography (CT) scan with or without a clinical history of previous stroke. Episodes of nonparalyzing stroke occur in outpatients and may go undiagnosed.

Parkinson's Disease. The prevalence of Parkinson's disease is estimated at 0.5–1.5% of the population over 65. The cardinal clinical features are bradykinesia, rigidity, and a 3–5 Hz resting tremor, often distal (see Chap. 15). A constellation of secondary features is common and assists in diagnosis: dysarthria, dysphonia, drooling, micrographia, seborrhea, and a tendency toward flexion in posture. Depression occurs in patients with early disease, and dementia is also common in advanced disease. Parkinson's disease must be differentiated from an akinetic-rigid state induced by the phenothiazines and from degenerative neurologic disease involving the striatum and pallidum. Alzheimer's disease and lacunar state are often associated with akinesia and rigidity, but the "pill-rolling" tremor at rest is not seen in Alzheimer's disease (unless the patient has been treated with neuroleptics).

The normal elderly tend to have parkinsonian features without the disease. A slightly flexed attitude, a paucity of facial expression, a positive glabellar response, and a mild uniform increase in tone often are seen in elderly patients. Elderly gait disorders may be akin to Parkinson's disease, and, indeed, dopamine systems in the forebrain are known to be differentially affected by aging. The clinical experience with L-dopa, however, in treating the elderly gait disorders has been disappointing. Only patients with bona fide Parkinson's disease benefit from L-dopa. For patients with Parkinson's disease, amantadine and anticholinergics are usually the first drugs tried.

Hydrocephalus. The pathogenesis of the gait disorder associated with adult hydrocephalus is not well understood. Frontal lobe centers for the integrative control of locomotion are thought to be compromised by the anterolateral expansion of the ventricles. Normal pressure hydrocephalus presents as a slowly progressive frontal gait disorder in association with dementia and incontinence. Pressures are often in the high normal range of 150–180 cm H_2O, although prolonged monitoring may reveal sustained pressure waves. There is at present little agreement about the cause of the hydrocephalus in this syndrome or about the criteria to follow in selecting patients for shunting. Ventricular enlargement is relatively common in patients with undiagnosed gait disorder. Formal determinations of cerebrospinal fluid (CSF) dynamics and conductance to outflow of spinal fluid are the most useful measures of actual dynamic hydrocephalus.

Cerebellar Ataxia. Cerebellar atrophy as seen by CT scan is a common incidental finding in asymptomatic elderly patients. The presence of a wide-based ataxic gait along with CT scan evidence of cerebellar atrophy should suggest chronic alcoholism or the presence of a systems degeneration involving the cerebellum.

Other Causes. *Multiple sensory deficits* is the term used to characterize a subgroup of patients, often diabetic, often elderly, whose unsteadiness is attributable to their sensory disorders. These patients illustrate the deafferentation hypothesis for gait problems: failure due to loss of input from visual, vestibular, and proprioceptive systems. The peripheral neuropathy seen so commonly in elderly patients with gait disorders may be of clinical importance. A loss of proprioceptive information from IA afferents, muscle spindles, and joint receptors might compromise the fine control of postural support. Vestibular disorders and visual changes (common in aging) may also be important in this regard. The acute visual change that follows a cataract surgical procedure may be particularly destabilizing for elderly people.

A variety of other diagnosable illnesses occur infrequently but may present as undiagnosed gait disturbances. Orthostatic hypotension must be considered, particularly in the case of diabetics and patients on antihypertensive medications. A small number of patients who complain of gait disorders will have skeletal muscle disease, metabolic encephalopathy, intracranial tumor, or other important treatable disorders. Treatment with the phenothiazines is a frequent cause of gait disorders in institutionalized patients. Drug-induced parkinsonism, akathisia, or axial tardive dyskinesia may cause bizarre stereotypic gaits. Depression can also affect motor performance and gait.

Arthritis. Arthritis causes gait disorders; fifty or sixty percent of the geriatric population will be found to have joint swelling, limited range of movement, crepitance, or skeletal changes on x-ray films. Many patients who complain of gait disorder are taking aspirin or antiarthritic drugs. In some patients the gait disorder is due to a major deformity at the hip, knee, or ankle. Some patients will have a analgic gait related to painful arthritic involvement of their joints. Despite the high incidence of arthritic findings in the elderly, however, many gait abnormalities are incorrectly attributed to arthritis, because neurologic deficits are overlooked.

Idiopathic Disorder. An *essential (idiopathic) gait disorder* is one with no clear cause. Patients generally exhibit the nonspecific features observed in any gait disorder: short steps, a wide base, and a tendency to be easily displaced backward. It is not clear whether patients represent a single entity or a collection of patients with undiagnosed diseases.

Treatment

As mentioned, a treatable illness contributes to the gait problem in almost one-fourth of gait disorders. Parkinson's disease often responds to antiparkinsonian therapy. Orthostatic hypotension responds to a readjustment in the patient's medical regimen. Refractory cases can be treated with mineralocorticoids, and/or elastic stockings. Patients with communicating hydrocephalus or frontal tumor are often amenable to primary neurosurgical treatment. Other disorders, such as metabolic encephalopathy and depression, also respond to therapy. It is not always possible to reverse peripheral neuropathy; patients in whom B-vitamin deficiencies can be documented respond to supplemental vitamin therapy. Improved diabetic control may make a difference in the severity of neuropathy in diabetics; the issue remains controversial.

Many patients with undiagnosed gait disorders have increased ventricular size as revealed by CT scan. Patients with gait disorder often have a ventricular diameter across the frontal horns in excess of 12.0 mm, as measured on the CT scan hard copy at the level of the caudate nucleus (38–40 mm actual size). This degree of ventricular enlargement is unusual in age-matched controls, but it remains unclear whether ventricular enlargement contributes to gait disorders.

Physical therapy is often helpful for elderly patients with gait disorders. Sessions with the therapist emphasize practical training in ambulatory skills. Physical therapists universally point to patient motivation as the major predictor of outcome.

When no treatable disorder is found, the gait disorder tends to progress. Such patients often lose independence and may require nursing home care.

---

1. Sabin T: Biologic aspects of falls and mobility limitations in the elderly. *J Am Geriatr Soc* 30:51–58, 1982.
A nice review of the subject, with a discussion of the neuropathy of aging and deafferentation hypothesis.
2. Grillner S, Zanger P: On the central generation of locomotion in the low spinal cat. *Exp Brain Res* 34:241–261, 1979.
Data on automatic walking elicited from the decerebrate cat. Brainstem and spinal centers may be capable of autonomous execution of the motor program.
3. Eidelberg E, et al: Locomotor control in the macaque monkey. *Brain* 104:647–663, 1981.
Failure to elicit spinal automatic walking in the primate.
4. Fries JF: Aging, natural death, and the compression of morbidity. *N Engl J Med* 303:130–132, 1980.
Discussion of health and disease in the geriatric population.
5. Brownwell B, Hughes JT: Necropsy observations on the damage to the nervous system in degenerative disease of the cervical spine. *Proc Fifth Int Congress Neuropathol* 39:551–554, 1975.
The autopsy study that documents prevalence of spondylitic myelopathy.

6. Beasley B, Ford D: Aging and the extrapyrimidal system. *Med Clin North Am* 60:1315–1323, 1976.
Parkinsonian features occur in normal elderly persons.
7. Adams RD, et al: Symptomatic occult hydrocephalus with "normal" cerebrospinal fluid pressure. *N Engl J Med* 273:117, 1965.
A description of the characteristic clinical features of the syndrome.
8. Fisher CM: Hydrocephalus in walking problems of the elderly. *Trans Am Neurol Assn* 105:29–33, 1980.
Computed tomography data suggest ventricular enlargement is frequent in elderly patients with gait disorders.
9. Koller W, et al: Cerebellar atrophy. *Neurology* 31:1486–1489, 1981.
Cerebellar atrophy is seen on CT scan in asymptomatic elderly patients.
10. Drachman D, Hart C: An approach to the dizzy patient. *Neurology* 22:323–324, 1972.
Characterizes a group of patients with sensory disorders.
11. Sudarsky L, Ronthal M: Gait disorders among elderly patients. *Arch Neurol* 40:740–743, 1983.
Survey study concentrating on the etiology of gait disorders in 50 patients.

18. EPILEPSY IN THE ELDERLY

Thomas M. Walshe

Epilepsy, or recurrent seizures, is most often encountered in children or young adults, but in elderly patients who suffer from neuropsychiatric disease, recurrent seizures are also a clinical concern. The incidence of seizure disorder with late-life onset varies with the population but may be as high as 6% in high-risk elderly patients. When a seizure disorder first begins in late adult life, it almost always indicates a pathologic lesion involving the cerebral cortex; therefore, proper management of a new seizure disorder in an elderly patient requires a search for an underlying cause.

Causes

Among the several pathologic processes that occur in late-life epilepsy, the most feared, but not the most common, is brain tumor. Patients with brain tumor almost always have a progressive onset of signs and symptoms, in addition to onset of the seizure disorder. Tumor, in fact, accounts for only 10–12% of late-life onset seizure disorders in patients who are older than 50.

On the basis of postmortem findings the most common diagnosis in late-life epilepsy is cerebrovascular disease. Acute stroke rarely causes seizure, although seizures occasionally may occur at the onset of cerebral embolism. Elderly patients who suffer small (at times undiagnosed) cerebral infarcts over their lifetime may develop a seizure disorder with little history of a known stroke. Most patients with cerebrovascular disease-related seizure disorder, however, have a clear past history of at least one stroke from which they have recovered. The seizure disorder usually begins during the first year after the stroke, but in some cases the seizures develop later on. Although vascular disease is a common underlying condition in seizure disorder, the majority of patients with stroke never develop seizures. It is, therefore, not necessary to treat stroke patients prophylactically with anticonvulsants.

Other, less common, neurologic problems that cause late-life seizures are head trauma, neurosyphilis, brain abscess, subdural hematoma, and certain degenerative diseases. Patients having advanced Alzheimer's disease develop seizures. Myoclonus is also common in advanced Alzheimer's cases and may at times be confused with a seizure disorder.

Diagnosis

Seizure itself, in elderly patients, is not always obvious, since the seizure is not always a convulsive fit. Episodic sensory or motor phenomena must always provoke the suspicion of an underlying seizure focus, even when there is not clear loss of consciousness or a convulsion. Usually there is a history of previous stroke affecting nearly the same location as the paroxysmal symptoms. In such cases the EEG is often abnormal and may help in making the diagnosis.

A few elderly patients have seizures that cause vertigo or a vague sense of discomfort, which they describe as dizziness. Such patients may have a history of stroke or a temporal lobe lesion of some other type. Other paroxysmal features help identify the problem as a seizure, or there may be a major motor seizure that follows the vertiginous episode.

The seizures caused by reversible medical disorders, such as hyponatremia and alcohol withdrawal, are usually not recurrent. Elderly patients with underlying subclinical lesions, however, may have seizures brought on by minor metabolic perturbations, yet remain seizure-free at other times. It is necessary, therefore, when an elderly patient has a seizure, to evaluate the blood chemistry in an effort to identify an easily treatable metabolic cause of seizure.

Evaluation

Evaluation of the elderly patient with a seizure disorder of new onset begins with a careful history and review of past medical history. Specific questions regarding alcohol or other toxins may lead to the diagnosis immediately. A general medical and thorough neurologic examination will usually eliminate most systemic disorders or point to a specific neurologic condition. A general metabolic screen will identify electrolyte abnormalities, hypoglycemia, hypocalcemia, uremia, or liver disease. When a patient has a clear-cut seizure, an electroencephalogram is not needed to verify it. An abnormal EEG, however, adds credence to the clinical history, especially when the seizure itself is not typical. The EEG further helps to lateralize and sometime localize the electrical focus and identify an electrical abnormality that does not cause clinical signs. The most helpful test in the differential diagnosis of a late-life seizure disorder is the computed tomography (CT) scan of the head. The CT scan will identify tumor, abscess, areas of infarction, subdural hematoma, and other structural lesions.

A lumbar puncture is needed if neurosyphilis or other infection is suspected. When blood serologic findings are negative, however, there is little chance that central nervous system syphilis is the cause of a seizure.

Treatment

Despite thorough medical and neurologic evaluation, many patients have no clear-cut cause of seizure disorder. Obvious cerebrovascular disease is found in about one-third of cases, and the other etiologies in a few instances. When the underlying disorder can be corrected, therapy is aimed at it. Patients who have undiagnosable or irreversible lesions are given anticonvulsants to prevent the recurrence of seizures.

The treatment of a single or several isolated seizures is not an emergency, and even when the seizures are particularly vigorous, rapid treatment with oral medicines is usually sufficient. A 1000-mg loading dose of phenytoin can be given orally (or intravenously) to establish seizure control in hours. Phenytoin is not used intramuscularly, because it crystallizes in the tissue and is erratically absorbed.

Most patients can be treated with oral drugs, since the seizures occur infrequently, and as long as the patient is aware of the possibility of a seizure, he or she can avoid situations that would be dangerous. Trauma is the major risk to elderly persons who fall with seizures. Adequate blood levels of the drug can be achieved safely in a few days or a week in most cases, avoiding the side effects associated with rapid treatment.

Single-Drug Therapy. Phenytoin or carbamazepine is the usual drug of first choice, and it is effective in most idiopathic and vascular cases. The effective daily dose of phenytoin or other anticonvulsant varies among patients. The dose is adjusted in the elderly, just as it is in younger patients. When elderly patients have frequent seizures (daily or weekly), the daily dose of anticonvulsant that stops the symptoms without toxicity is the dose to be used, regardless of the serum drug level. When seizures are infrequent (monthly or less often), it is usually best to administer enough anticonvulsant to establish mild to high therapeutic blood levels, and follow the patient for several months to assess efficacy.

Increasing the Dosage. If a patient has a seizure while on a single anticonvulsant, and the serum level is well into the therapeutic range, one must consider adding another drug. On the other hand, when a seizure occurs in a patient with a low serum anticonvulsant level, the best approach is to increase the dose. The usual starting dose of phenytoin is 200 mg qd, for older individuals, but most will need 300–500 mg to achieve therapeutic success or adequate serum levels. In patients with seizure disorder from degenerative disorders such as Alzheimer's disease, lower doses of phenytoin (100–200 mg qd) are usually adequate to prevent seizures. Carbamazepine in the form of 200-mg tablets is given in increasing doses up to 1,200 mg qd.

It is very important to increase the dose of anticonvulsants slowly, because the steady state is not reached for several days. At the onset of phenytoin therapy (unless a 1,000-mg loading dose is given), it takes about 7 days for the given dose to reach the maximum steady state level. We prefer to start elderly patients on 200 mg of phenytoin orally and increase it by 100 mg each week, unless success, toxicity, or therapeutic blood levels are reached. Some patients' seizures are controlled on serum drug levels that are not in the therapeutic range; therefore, the criterion of success is not blood level but abolition of the seizure. At times, the major motor or convulsive seizures are stopped, but the patient continues to have smaller paroxysmal phenomena that represent partial seizures. The drug can be increased until all the seizure phenomena are stopped, unless toxicity prevents further increases. At the maximum dose tolerated, an additional drug is started, if the seizure phenomena continue to interfere with the patient's life.

Side Effects. The side effects of phenytoin are usually mild and are not much of a problem when low doses are used. Patients may develop nystagmus at midtherapeutic levels and almost always have it when serum levels are in the toxic range. Intoxication by phenytoin produces involuntary movements, ataxia, and dysarthria. Somnolence and coma are unusual but occur especially in older, phenytoin-intoxicated patients. Falls caused by ataxia can be a major threat in the elderly, but gingival hyperplasia, teratogenecy, and hirsutism are not problems in elderly patients. Although calcium metabolism and folate metabolism are altered in phenytoin treatment, it is rarely necessary to treat the patient with supplements. Patients who are on phenytoin treatment for many years may develop a mild peripheral neuropathy, which may require supplemental folate. Folate sometimes reduces the efficacy of the drug, however, so the patient may start to have seizures again.

Using More than One Drug. When phenytoin alone fails to control seizures, another drug may be added. The next choice is usually phenobarbital in oral doses of 30–90 mg qhs. When the second drug is added, serum levels of both drugs can be measured to assure compliance and to assure maintenance of therapeutic levels. In general, each drug is given until success or side effects intervene. If two drugs fail, a third is added. It is rare that more than two drugs are needed for elderly patients. If phenytoin-induced ataxia or other side effects appear at a serum level too low to control the seizures, phenobarbital can be added, to allow both drugs to be used in doses lower than are usually successful. In some patients, especially those with cerebellar degeneration, even a small dose of phenytoin can cause disabling ataxia. Such patients are best treated with phenobarbital alone.

Handling Toxicity. When a patient develops toxicity from phenytoin or phenobarbital, the medication must not be stopped completely. Toxicity is usually not life-threatening, and, if the medicine is stopped abruptly, seizures will recur and status epilepticus may appear. When phenytoin is used alone and the patient becomes toxic, it is usually adequate to skip one day's dosage and then to reduce the dose by 100 mg or more. The patient will remain symptomatic from the toxicity for several days but will not run the risk of status epilepticus. Toxicity with phenobarbital is treated similarly by skipping one day's dosage and then reducing subsequent doses.

Carbamazepine and Sodium Valproate. Other first-line drugs in the treatment of adult seizure disorders are carbamazepine and sodium valproate. Both are very effective and, in some instances, may be used before phenytoin or phenobarbital. Generalizations are not adequate to guide therapy when several drugs are used, but the principle of using each drug at its highest tolerated dose before adding another usually holds. The clinical situation dictates the exact choice of drug and the dose used in each case.

Follow-Up. Patients who are on anticonvulsants should be evaluated frequently at the beginning of therapy to ascertain efficacy. After it is clear that the seizures have been stopped, follow-up every 3–4 months for several visits is usually enough. When the seizure disorder is stable, and the patient is tolerating the medication, yearly follow-ups are usually adequate. When phenytoin and phenobarbital are used, blood counts and liver function studies can be done yearly or even less often. Patients treated with carbamazepine require more frequent metabolic and hematologic surveillance, although complications are exceedingly rare. Serum levels of the drug are needed only when treatment fails to prevent seizure, or if the patient has so few seizures that the drug's efficacy cannot be monitored clinically.

Status Epilepticus. Treatment of major motor seizures that recur repeatedly within minutes (status epilepticus) is not the same as treatment of an established seizure disorder.

When the patient is under treatment already, it is best to add phenobarbital intravenously (100–250 mg) to stop an acute flurry of seizures. Elderly patients may remain drowsy for 12–24 hours following large doses of phenobarbital. Acute administration of intravenous phenytoin in doses of 500–1,000 mg is effective for patients who have not received chronic anticonvulsant treatment. There is little risk of serious cardiac or respiratory complication with phenytoin, and, once given, the drug is continued as the maintenance medication. Intravenous diazepam is the most popular remedy for recurrent seizures. It is effective in small doses of 2–5 mg intravenously in status epilepticus. It is dangerous, however, to give diazepam to patients treated with phenobarbital because of the risk of respiratory arrest. When small doses of diazepam are used, the risk is small, but when doses of 10–30 mg are given, respiratory problems arise. Moreover, the drug causes more sedation than phenobarbital, and its efficacy in seizure control is brief. Phenobarbital and phenytoin take slightly longer to act but are perhaps better in most instances. When diazepam treatment controls the seizures in a patient with status epilepticus, but the patient continues to have single isolated seizures, it is best to start the maintenance medications rather than repeat the doses of diazepam.

While the seizures are being treated, infection and other causes of the status epilepticus should be sought and corrected. Single seizures, or even a flurry of two or three seizures with an interval between, do not require emergency anticonvulsant treatment but do require emergency medical evaluation and identification of a cause. In established seizure patients, status epilepticus is frequently caused by withdrawal of anticonvulsants or by an infection.

1. Graham K, Williams BO, Rowe MJ: Idiopathic hypoparathyroidism: A cause of fits in the elderly. *Br Med J* 1:1460–1461, 1979.
   Case reports.
2. Roberts MA, Godfrey JW, Caird FI: Epileptic seizures in the elderly: I. Aetiology and type of seizure, II. Diagnostic problems. *Age Aging* 11:24–34, 1982.
   Two-part review noting that 44% of patients had cerebrovascular disease, 12% had tumor, 11% had disease outside the brain, and 16% had unknown cause. No pathology was done.
3. Dodge PR, Richardson EP, Victor M, Recurrent convulsive seizures as a sequel to cerebral infarction: A clinical and pathological study. *Brain* 77:610–638, 1954.
   Establishes stroke as a major cause of late-life epilepsy.
4. Easton JD: Diphenylhydantoin and epilepsy management. *Ann Intern Med* 77:421–423, 1972.
   Brief review of how to use phenytoin.
5. Penry JK, Newmark ME: The use of antiepileptic drugs. *Ann Intern Med* 90:207–218, 1979.
   Reviews the principles of management based on pharmacokinetics and other pharmacologic data.
6. Pinder RM, et al: *Drugs* 13:81, 1977.
   Valproic acid is effective for generalized motor seizures.
7. Richardson EP: Late life epilepsy. *Med Clin North Am* March:349–359, 1958.
   Review of the pathology found in late-life onset seizure disorders.
8. Sjögren H: Cerebral seizures in the presenile-senile period of life: A study of 77 patients. *Acta Psychiatr Scand* 40:265–274, 1964.
   This somewhat opaque paper reviews a large experience and shows that late-onset seizures occur in about 6 percent of geriatric patients with neuropsychiatric disorders.
9. Stuteville P, Welch K: Subdural hematoma in the elderly person. *JAMA* 168:1445–1449, 1958.
   None of the 75 patients had seizures.
10. Troupin, et al: Carbamazepine—a double-blind comparison with phenytoin. *Neurology* 27:511–519, 1977.

Carbamazepine treatment is recommended for partial seizures and major motor seizures.

11. Wallis W, Kutt, H, McDowell F: Intravenous diphenylhydantoin in treatment of acute repetitive seizures. *Neurology* 18:513–525, 1968.
The basis for using a loading dose for Dilantin.
12. Otomo E: Convulsion in the Aged. *Folia Psychiatr Neurol Jpn* 35:295–300, 1981.
In 2,625 cases the incidence of recurrent seizure was 0.076%. Among stroke patients, the incidence was 26.4%.
13. Shigemoto T: Epilepsy in middle or advanced age. *Folia Psychiatr Neurol Jpn* 35:287–294, 1981.
Older patients had complex partial seizures more often than younger patients.

IV. CANCER

19. CANCER IN THE ELDERLY

Arthur Skarin

The incidence of malignancies increases with age. Among persons 85–89 years old, 3,000 in 100,000 men and 1,650 in 100,000 women have cancer. The overall incidence rates decline after age 85–89. The **current** probability of developing cancer within 5 years for a male rises from 1 in 700 at age 25 to 1 in 14 at age 65. Incidental microscopic invasive cancers of the prostate (stage A) are found in 15–50% of autopsies, which is 100 times the clinical incidence. Other asymptomatic tumors are found at autopsy in 43% of males between ages 76 and 85 and 34% of men over age 85.

In men over age 75, the most common malignancies are cancer of the digestive tract (colon and rectum, pancreas, and stomach) and prostate. These account for 25% of total cases and 35% of cases between ages 85 and 89. Respiratory malignancies are third in frequency but decrease from 20% of all cancers between ages 70 and 74 to about 5% of cancers for patients in their late 90s. In contrast, men under age 74 develop lung cancer as the most common tumor (22% of cases). In the same age group, digestive tract cancer accounts for about 17% of cases and prostate cancer for 16%.

In women between ages 75 and 79, the digestive tract accounts for about 40% of cancer cases, and the incidence rises until age 90 and then decreases. Breast cancer accounts for 20%, then plateaus at menopause, with a slight decrease eventually after age 89. The incidence of respiratory cancer is 5% and is fairly constant throughout ages 75–99. In women under age 74, breast cancer is the most common malignancy (26%), followed by colorectal cancer (15%), uterine cancer (14%), lung cancer (7%), and ovarian cancer (5%).

About 350,000 persons die of cancer each year, representing almost one-fifth of all deaths in the United States. More than 60% of cancer deaths are caused by a few common malignancies, while the remainder are caused by more than 100 uncommon cancers. Death rates from all forms of cancer increase with age until 85–89 years, then decrease in both sexes for most cancers. Exceptions are cancer of the buccal cavity, pharynx, bone, and connective tissue, all of which are more common in younger patients. Lung cancer is the leading cause of cancer death in men of all ages, with a death rate 18 times that recorded 40 years ago. In women, lung cancer ranks third among deaths caused by tumor but has increased sixfold compared to 40 years ago. It is expected to be as common as breast cancer in women within 10 years.

Several models have been proposed to account for the increasing incidence of cancer in old age. One acceptable hypothesis states that each cell has several genes that independently restrain it from becoming malignant. After successive mutations that inactivate the genes, a cancer will develop. The probability of gene inactivation increases directly with age. As an example, when the logarithm of the death rate from colon cancer is plotted against the logarithm of age, a linear relationship is seen. The slope of the line suggests that five mutations are required to create the cancer. Another theory postulates an age-related breakdown of the immunosurveillance system, which allows for unrestrained malignant growth. The immunosurveillance system involves a complex interrelationship of various lymphocyte subsets that normally destroy or reject foreign agents (viruses) or damaged (altered) cells.

From examination of the cancer experience of successive cohorts of patients (a group of individuals born in the same year) as they grow older, it seems that the increase in some cancers (e.g., lung and breast cancer) between cohorts is not from age per se but from exogenous factors. Some of the factors identified in carcinogenesis are environmental mutagens (chemical or physical), spontaneous errors in DNA replication, heredity, hormones, and the influences of hormones or viruses.

In breast cancer, the cohort effect suggests that recent generations, which have an increased incidence of cancer, have been exposed more to causal factors than past generations.

1. Hodgkinson HM: Cancer in the aged, in Brocklehurst J (ed): *Textbook of Geriatric Medicine and Gerontology,* Edinburgh, New York, Churchill Livingstone, 1978, pp 646–650. *Brief review of epidemiology, screening, clinical evaluation, and general principles of cancer management in the elderly.*

2. Howell TR: Multiple primary neoplasms in the elderly. *J Am Geriatr Soc* 28:65–67, 1980.
A brief review of multiple primary cancers occurring in geriatric patients, which vary considerably (0.6–36%) in incidence.
3. Kent S: What is the relationship of cancer to aging? *Geriatrics* 32:105–108, 1977.
Brief review of carcinogens and other factors implicated in the etiology of cancer.
4. Harris CC: Individual differences in cancer susceptibility. *Ann Intern Med* 92:809–825, 1980.
A comprehensive review of the interactions of environmental carcinogens and predisposing host factors in cancer susceptibility.

20. THERAPEUTIC PLAN FOR ELDERLY CANCER PATIENTS

Arthur Skarin

The treatment plan for a cancer patient must be specific for the patient, the type of tumor, and the extent or stage of disease. Several general considerations enter into treatment planning. The goal of treatment may be to cure or to palliate. Several factors help to determine which is appropriate. The possibility of cure should be balanced against maintenance of patient function, comfort, and self-esteem. Furthermore the cost of treatment in both financial and human terms becomes increasingly important for geriatric patients, for whom cure may not be possible because of concurrent diseases.

Goals of Treatment

The cure rate depends on type of malignancy, stage of disease, advances in surgical techniques, radiotherapy technology, and available chemotherapeutic armamentarium. If cure is not possible or is achieved only with marked morbidity, then palliation of symptoms becomes the primary goal. Much can be done to benefit the incurable patient. Among the management modalities, appropriate analgesics are most important to making life bearable for many patients with chronic pain. Limited surgery may be useful for spinal cord compression or other local problems that would otherwise limit mobility or comfort. Local irradiation for refractory bone pain is useful for some tumors and reduces the need for analgesic drugs that have adverse side effects. Chemotherapy may reduce soft tissue masses in responsive tumors such as metastatic breast cancer, giving needed relief.

A clinical measure of the performance status can help to predict outcome of tumor treatment. The performance status is defined as follows:

STATUS	DESCRIPTION
0	Carries on normal activities without symptoms
1	Ambulatory, but symptoms present
2	Bedridden less than 50% of the day
3	Bedridden more than 50% of the day
4	Completely bedridden and requires assistance for daily maintenance

The patients with the lowest performance status have the best chance of a good therapeutic result, and patients with a performance status of 3 or 4 benefit least from any major treatment modality. The performance status may be improved in some patients by hyperalimentation, either intravenously or with a 10 Fr. nasogastric feeding tube.

To justify treatment of patients with a poor performance status, **quality** of survival rather than survival itself must be considered. The prognosis of malignant tumors in older patients must be compared to the relatively short life expectancy of patients in the same age group without cancer. The average life expectancy at age 80 is about 5 years for men and 6 years for women. At age 85 the life expectancy is 4 years, and at age 90, 3 years. Most treatment successes in cancer are reported as 5-year survivals, making them of little value in the treatment of elderly patients. In elderly patients disease other than cancer commonly determines the prognosis. For instance, 75% of breast cancer patients older than 75 years die from vascular disease, and only 15% from the malignancy. Many older patients die **with** cancer rather than **from** cancer, a fact that must enter into the overall therapeutic plan. Several complications limit the therapeutic approach to older patients. Motor difficulties caused by aging or nervous system disease, forgetfulness, and other central nervous system problems common to the elderly interfere with compliance with the therapeutic program.

Special Concerns in Elderly Patients

Enlistment of family, friends, and social workers aids in ensuring proper compliance with treatment of elderly patients. When neurologic impairment is severe, the aim of treatment is the patient's comfort. Elderly patients often have coronary artery disease and chronic congestive heart failure; and even in the healthy, cardiac output is lower than in youth. Therefore orthostatic hypotension as a side effect of drugs is more common, and anthracycline drugs, for example, adriamycin, may produce excessive cardiac side effects in the elderly. Corticosteroids may increase the muscle atrophy and weakness that occurs in elderly patients without disease. Osteoporosis is exacerbated also by corticosteroids in the elderly. Arthritis interferes with endoscopy, endotracheal anesthesia, and surgical procedures, because it causes difficulty in positioning the patient. Renal and liver changes in elderly patients alter drug clearance and metabolism and may prolong the half-life of chemotherapeutic drugs. Changes in lungs, GI tract, and bone marrow give the elderly patient less reserve and increase his or her susceptibility to drug and radiation complications. Excessive use of laxatives may interfere with absorption of chemotherapeutic agents. Achlorhydria, well known in elderly patients, appears to decrease absorption of phenylalanine mustard (L-PAM). Respiratory depression occurs with lower doses of analgesics or sedatives in elderly patients. Autoimmune phenomena also become more common with age and may interfere with chemotherapy.

In treating elderly patients with chemotherapy, lean body weight should be estimated before surface area is calculated to guide drug doses, because body composition changes with aging. Total body water decreases, but extracellular water increases in elderly patients. Loss of muscle mass and loss of body fat also occur, but fat may replace muscle mass. Older patients are not usually as big when measured as they appear at first. Serum albumin is lower in the elderly, so drugs that bind to protein produce more unbound drug, causing toxicity at a lower dose. Moreover, competitive binding in drug combinations may cause variable and unpredictable drug levels. Finally, the clinical picture may not reflect the extent of disease, since the elderly often have less prominent symptoms with tumor than younger patients.

The major treatment modalities—surgery, radiotherapy, and chemotherapy—are adjusted to compensate for the age and performance status of the patient. For example, fever, a poor prognostic sign in patients with lymphoma, may be absent in the elderly, even with extensive disease. Pain may be less severe even with large bone lesions, and the usual leukocytosis seen with infection may be absent in the elderly. Elderly patients often present with advanced cancer, because they deny warning signs and symptoms or attribute them to "old age." Symptoms and signs may also be attributed to already diagnosed disease, or may be misdiagnosed when caused by paraneoplastic syndromes.

Surgical Treatment

For good-risk patients, the mortality rate from a present-day surgical procedure is only 8% for those 71–80 years old and 10% for those over 80 years. Mortality from surgical procedures (including thoracenteses) in patients with advanced or metastatic cancer increases to 15–20% but is not much greater than in younger age groups with similar disease. Mortality can be reduced in the elderly by careful postoperative care and anesthesia. Preoperative management reduces mortality, also. Preoperative planning to ensure proper hydration, nutrition, and adequate hematocrit improves the chances of survival through the postoperative period.

After the operation, geriatric patients recover more slowly than younger patients and have a higher morbidity. The choice of surgical procedures for cancer resection must be individualized, depending on the decision to palliate or cure. Some tumors tend to be slow growing and localized in the elderly, and standard curative resection should be carried out whenever possible. Palliative procedures such as segmental bowel resection, simple mastectomy, or biliary diversion may provide enough local control for the remaining lives of some patients. Electrocoagulation for small rectal cancers may be especially appropriate in the aged. The patient's optimal performance status, the presence or absence of irreversible coexisting disease, and the general life expectancy also dictate the extent and aim of the surgical procedure.

Radiotherapy

As a rule, megavoltage irradiation (high-energy electrons in the 1–25 million electron volt range) is better than orthovoltage, because it generates doses of better depth with more efficient tumor treatment. There is also less side-scatter and therefore less radiation sickness, and more uniform dosage is possible with no differential bone absorption. Megavoltage also has a skin-sparing effect, with less radiation dermatitis. The goal of cure or palliation needs to be defined in each case, according to type of tumor and results of staging procedures, just as in surgical therapy. In the case of poor surgical risks, radiotherapy may be curative. Early bladder or prostate cancer in patients with severe heart disease may be cured by radiotherapy. Palliative **surgical intervention,** however, may be preferable sometimes to palliative radiotherapy. As an example, subtotal or simple mastectomy is better for a patient with a large lesion who is unable to tolerate daily radiation treatments over a 3- to 4-week period. The goals of radiotherapy apply **equally** to young and elderly patients. The planned doses and time course should be identical in both groups. Mucositis and other side effects take longer to occur in geriatric patients, however. Some delay in radiation doses may be necessary in the elderly.

Chemotherapy

Chemotherapy cures are associated with a few tumors that occur for the most part in young patients. Pediatric cancers, Hodgkin's disease, Burkitt's lymphoma, diffuse histiocytic lymphoma, testicular cancer, choriocarcinoma, and osteosarcoma in an adjuvant setting are often curable with chemotherapy. Cancers in which chemotherapy has resulted in **survival improvement** but not cure occur in middle-aged as well as in elderly patients. The major malignancies in this group are breast, ovarian and adrenocortical carcinomas, malignant insulinoma, small cell undifferentiated lung cancer, acute myelogenous leukemia, and multiple myeloma. The more common cancers show a variable response rate to chemotherapy, but improvement in survival with chemotherapy has not been conclusively demonstrated. Patients who show objective disease regression with treatment occasionally survive longer than nonresponders. Responders include patients with tumors of the GI tract, head and neck, lung, soft tissue, liver, bladder, prostate, and endometrium, as well as malignant melanoma.

The usual objective of cancer chemotherapy in geriatric patients, therefore, is palliation of various symptoms by shrinkage of the tumor. Prolongation of survival is a secondary goal, since there is often no objective disease regression. The **quality of life** is the major guide, since the effects of treatment must not be worse than the disease itself. Rigorous chemotherapy is dangerous to geriatric patients because of decrease in bone marrow reserve as well as impaired function of other organs and a higher incidence of significant coexisting morbid disease.

Patients aged 65–75 years with a performance status of 0 or 1 may tolerate some combination chemotherapy programs, but the **starting dose of each drug should be decreased by 50%.** The dose can be escalated gradually if weekly blood counts do not show cumulative or severe myelosuppression. Single agents may be employed, but also with initial dose reduction by 50%. Use of **adjuvant chemotherapy** after operation or radiotherapy in geriatric patients at risk of relapse must be decided according to performance status. Except as part of a properly designed research trial, such treatment is not recommended.

Supportive Measures

Wise supportive care is often as important to the total care of the patient as the primary treatment modalities. Nutritional therapy should not be used to prolong life when no effective antitumor therapy is available but, in carefully selected cases of malnourished patients who have a responsive malignancy with a potential for increase in survival, hyperalimentation may facilitate adequate treatment. The signs of nutritional depletion usually include unintentional loss of 10% or more of body weight, serum albumin of less than 3–4 gm/100 ml, and anergy to a series of skin test antigens. Oral nutrition through a small-bore nasogastric feeding tube may help patients who have severe, persistent anorexia or nausea, or malabsorption. Also, a feeding tube can safely bypass a fistula and allow continuous slow feeding of a dietary formula. Intravenous hyperalimentation is indicated during management of bowel obstruction or for bowel or pancreatic fistulas. It can also be helpful in radiation or drug enteritis or stomatitis and when persistent emesis interferes in nutrition (e.g., during prolonged chemotherapy or radiotherapy). Short-term intravenous hyperalimentation is used at times following an extensive surgical procedure. The usual course of hyperalimentation varies from 1–4 weeks and may be repeated periodically if the patient benefits. Standard oncology textbooks should be consulted for the technique.

Nausea and vomiting sometimes follow chemotherapy and radiotherapy and may require treatment. Nausea usually responds to prochlorperazine (Compazine), 10 mg IM or PO q3–6h, but extrapyramidal reactions (dyskinesia) are likely to develop in geriatric patients. The latter reactions usually subside with diphenhydramine hydrochloride (Benadryl), 150 mg PO or IM. Thiethylperazine maleate (Torecan), trimethobenzamide hydrochloride (Tigan), or continuous IV infusion of perphenazine (Trilafon) are also useful in controlling nausea and vomiting. Hypnotics and opiates employed with antiemetic drugs can potentiate serious respiratory depression, if not used carefully.

Pain occurs frequently in cancer patients and is a major target of therapy. Unpredictable side effects of analgesics in geriatric patients dictate a sequential steplike approach to drug use. It is best to start with aspirin or acetaminophen, 650 mg q3–4h. Often the major part of the pain is relieved with aspirin alone, so the patient can tolerate his disease. Codeine sulfate, 30–60 mg q3–4h, can be added if needed. If there is a dysphoric reaction to codeine, an aspirin or acetaminophen-oxycodone combination (Percodan or Tylox) may be effective, 1–2 tabs q3–4h PO. For more refractory pain, hydromorphone hydrochloride (Dilaudid), 5–10 mg q4h IM, may help. For severe chronic pain in terminal cancer, Brompton's Mixture (10 mg cocaine, 5–20 mg morphine sulfate, 2.5 ml 95% grain alcohol, flavor, and chloroform water for a total of 20 ml/dose) is given q4–6h. Methadon (5–10 q8h PO), economical and well tolerated, provides stronger and longer analgesia than other PO narcotics.

Narcotic analgesics, particularly codeine, cause constipation, which in geriatric patients can lead to obstipation. One useful preventative of constipation with narcotics is dioctyl sodium sulfosuccinate (Colace), 100 mg tid, with a senna preparation (Senokot) at bedtime. Cancer pain is usually chronic. Good management requires that medication be given in adequate amounts and often enough to "get ahead" of the pain, rather than always tagging behind. Tolerance frequently develops, and drugs must be increased or switched for effectiveness. There is no value in denying a patient with cancer pain adequate narcotic analgesia when needed.

Blood product transfusion may relieve symptoms of anemia but, before use of this supportive modality, the overall prognosis must be seriously considered, so that life is not needlessly or unmercifully prolonged. Appropriate transfusions are indicated for good-risk elderly patients with temporary life-threatening myelosuppression from therapy or underlying disease. Packed red blood cells (usually 2 units at a time) can now be safely administered for symptomatic anemia. With acute hemorrhage, fresh whole blood is usually given. Platelet transfusions are readily available in most hospitals and should be given for thrombocytopenia causing acute bleeding. Platelets may be prophylactically administered, if the count is under 10,000–20,000/mm^3, especially if mucous membrane hemorrhages are present. White blood cell (WBC) transfusions are administered for patients with fever and severe acute granulocytopenia (polymorphonuclear luekocytes usually $< 1{,}000/\text{mm}^3$), but only under supervision by experts, because of serious reactions. WBC transfusions may reduce infection and mortality. Combination antibiotics are also generally administered, with the choice depending on the most likely infection, until results of cultures are available.

1. Albano WA: Should elderly patients undergo surgery for cancer? *Geriatrics* 32:105–108, 1977.
Various mortality rates for surgical procedures in common cancers are listed and briefly discussed.
2. Copeland EM III: Intravenous hyperalimentation as an adjunct to cancer patient management. *CA* 28:322–330, 1978.
Good review of indications, techniques, and results of IV hyperalimentation. Nutrition-

ally healthy patients appear to tolerate treatment (and have a better prognosis) than malnourished patients.
3. Kalchthaler T, Rigor Tan ME: Anemia in institutionalized elderly patients. *J Am Geriatr Soc* 28:108–113, 1980.
Anemia in geriatric patients is most commonly due to iron deficiency and responds to iron replacement. Diagnostic studies and other etiologies are discussed.
4. Lamy PP, Vestal RE: Drug prescribing for the elderly. *Hosp Pract* 11:111–118, 1976.
Good review of the altered physiology and pharmacology that occur in the elderly.
5. Lee PV: Drug therapy in the elderly: The clinical pharmacology of aging. *Clin Exp Res* 2:39–42, 1978.
Basic review of multiple factors associated with aging that must be considered before prescribing drugs to geriatric patients.
6. Reichel W: Multiple problems in the elderly. *Hosp Pract* 11:103–108, 1976.
A discussion of the approach to disease in the elderly based upon a problem list.
7. Shimm DS, Logue GL, Maltbie AA, Dugan S: Medical management of chronic cancer pain. *JAMA* 241:2408–2412, 1979.
Thorough review of analgesics, antiemetics, antidepressants, and stimulants useful in the management of patients with chronic cancer.
8. Ouslander JG: Drug therapy in the elderly. *Ann Intern Med* 95:711–722, 1981.
Comprehensive review of age-related biologic and physiologic changes in the elderly, including important considerations for the prescription of medications.

21. SKIN CANCER

Arthur Skarin

Skin cancer, the most common of all cancers, has the best cure rate, except in the case of malignant melanoma. Its high tendency to remain localized, with early detection because of location, explains the favorable prognosis for skin tumors. All types of skin cancer increase with age and are partly related to sun exposure. It is estimated that 40–50% of all people will have had at least one type of skin cancer by age 65. If a person has had a cancer of any other site, there is a 50–60% chance that he or she will later have skin cancer.

Premalignant lesions such as senile and actinic keratoses, Bowen's disease, and radiation dermatitis, if untreated, may progress to invasive cancers. Basal cell carcinoma usually appears on the forehead, eyelids, cheek, nose, and lips (T zone). The lesion is hard and red gray, with a pearly appearance. It may have a rolled border and marked central ulceration. Squamous cell carcinoma occurs usually in sun-exposed areas as a scaly, keratotic lesion with an irregular border. It is elevated and may be ulcerated or have scabs that will not heal. Surgical and radiotherapeutic treatments of geriatric patients offer comparably high cure rates (90–95% for basal cell and 75–80% for squamous cell). Excisional biopsy with 0.5- to 1.0-cm margins is curative therapy for lesions smaller than 2 cm across; however, regional node dissections are sometimes indicated for squamous carcinoma. Irradiation is preferable for small facial lesions, where cosmetic reconstruction is a problem, or for lesions with a poor surgical margin. In the case of more advanced lesions that invade bone, cartilage, or regional lymph nodes, a surgical procedure combined with radiotherapy may be successful.

Malignant (cutaneous) melanoma, when metastatic, has a poor prognosis, but lesions detected early and properly treated have a reasonably good prognosis, with 70–90% cure rates. Tumors of the extremities carry a better prognosis than those of the head, neck, and trunk. Overall management of geriatric patients with good performance status does not differ from that of other age groups. Treatment for primary melanoma begins with wide local excision (2- to 5-cm margins) that includes underlying fat and usually requires a skin graft. For small lesions the present trend is toward a less radical removal of surrounding skin. Careful pathologic evaluation is mandatory, since prognosis is related to the following levels of skin invasion:

LEVEL	DESCRIPTION
I	In situ (entirely within epidermis); 100% cure
II	Invasion of papillary dermis and/or <0.75 mm in thickness; 95% cure
III	Invasion to papillary-reticular dermis and/or 0.75–1.5 mm in thickness; 60–90% cure*
IV	Invasion into reticular dermis and/or 1.51–3.0 mm in thickness; 25–80% cure*
V	Invasion into subcutaneous fat and/or >3.0 mm in thickness; 0–15% cure

If regional lymph nodes are **not** palpable, "prophylactic" node dissection is generally **not** indicated. If regional lymph nodes are palpably enlarged but not fixed, removal avoids problems caused by local tumor progression but does not usually increase survival. Considerable morbidity from lymphedema may result from node dissection in the inguinal regions. Regional nodes that are fixed to adjacent tissue should not be resected. Treatment of metastatic melanoma is rarely successful. The prognosis is poor, but the erratic behavior of malignant melanoma includes spontaneous remissions in rare instances. Chemotherapy with dacarbazine (DTIC) results in temporary disease regression in 10–20% of patients. Women improve more frequently than men, especially with soft tissue lesions; however, the risk-benefit ratio must be seriously considered in the case of geriatric patients. All patients should not receive chemotherapy, and combination chemotherapy programs have no advantage over DTIC alone. Local immunotherapy by injection is experimental but may reduce the size of cutaneous metastases. Hyperthermia (especially in organs perfused with antitumor agents) and new drugs are under investigation but are usually not appropriate for geriatric patients. Several randomized studies are being evaluated in which adjuvant chemotherapy, immunotherapy, or chemoimmunotherapy has been tried on patients with histologic levels III, IV, and V, and on patients classified as having "no-evident-disease" after resection of nodes or localized metastases. The results are equivocal, and unless an elderly patient with a good performance status is entered into a clinical study, adjuvant treatment is not indicated.

1. Chanda JJ, Callen JP, Stawiski MA: Malignant melanoma and its therapy: A review. *Cutis* 23:759–783, 1979.
   Has 103 references.
2. Emmett AJJ, O'Rourke MGE (eds): *Malignant Skin Tumors.* Edinburgh, New York, Churchill Livingstone, 1982.
   A detailed monograph covering the Australian experience.
3. Epstein E, et al: Curability of melanoma: A 25-year retrospective study. *Cancer* 46(4):818–821, 1980.
   Discusses the prognosis and treatment plan.
4. Gilchrest BA, Blog FB, Szabo G: Effects of aging and chronic sun exposure on melanocytes in human skin. *J Invest Dermatol* 73:141–143, 1979.
   Melanocyte density declines by 6–8% per decade.
5. Griffel M: Survival of cutaneous malignant melanoma patients at University of Iowa hospitals. *Cancer* 47:176–183, 1981.
   Age at diagnosis was greater than 60 years in 39% of patients.
6. Hall JH, Lupton ES: Office management of malignant melanoma: A report of 132 patients. *Cutis* 24:453–456, 1979.
   Describes a method to follow and treat patients without hospitalization.
7. Helm F: *Cancer Dermatology.* Philadelphia, Lea & Febiger, 1979.
   A comprehensive textbook covering all aspects of the subject.
8. MacDonald EJ, Bubendorf E: Some epidemiologic aspects of skin cancer. In University of Texas, M.D. Anderson Hospital, *Tumors of the Skin.* Chicago, Year Book 1964, pp 23–66.
   Excludes melanoma and shows high incidence of skin cancer in elderly patients. This reference has many other articles of use.

*Percentage is lower if regional nodes are involved.

9. Robinson JK, Roenigk HH: The big three of skin cancer. *Postgrad Med* 67:92–107, 1980.
Surveys the types of skin cancer and their treatment.
10. Shaw HM, McGovern VJ, Milton GW, Farago GA, McCarthy WH: Malignant melanoma: Influence of site of lesion and age of patient in the female superiority in survival. *Cancer* 46:2731–2735, 1980.
More women than men are under 50 years when diagnosed. Tumor thickness was most important.

22. GUIDELINES FOR MANAGEMENT OF COMMON MALIGNANCIES

Arthur Skarin

Extensive staging procedures, including multiple organ scans, are generally not performed on geriatric patients once the diagnosis of a specific tumor is made. Management decisions are rarely affected by multiple investigative studies, which are time-consuming, expensive, and often unsafe for the elderly. Such evaluations are unjustified unless they may effect a cure or manage a crisis.

Lung Cancer

Localized (stage I or II) lung malignancies that are not of the small cell type (adenocarcinoma and squamous cell and large cell undifferentiated malignancies) are best managed by surgical resection, when possible. Postoperative "adjuvant" radiotherapy or chemotherapy is still experimental and is not indicated for geriatric patients. Primary radiation therapy may be given to patients who are poor operative risks, but the cure rate is low in most studies. Palliative irradiation is effective in relieving obstruction of the superior vena cava or bronchial obstruction with atelectasis. Painful bone metastases, hoarseness, and brain metastases may respond to palliative radiotherapy. Recent chemotherapy programs for metastatic lung cancer (e.g., cyclophosphamide, adriamycin, and *cis*-platinum) have shown response rates of 30–50%, with a suggestion of increase in median survival, but are rarely indicated for patients over age 75 because of significant side effects. Small cell (oat cell) lung cancers present with early dissemination of disease in the majority of patients. Surgical procedure is not indicated except for the rare localized "coin lesion." Bone, liver, and brain scans show metastases in a high percentage of asymptomatic patients. Radiation therapy is of value in palliation of local disease. Several chemotherapy regimens are effective in causing regression of disease. The large doses of drugs necessary to obtain a meaningful remission cause myelosuppression and are dangerous in the elderly. Median survival in small cell lung tumors is usually 2–3 months but may increase to 9–12 months in patients responding to therapy.

Colonic and Rectal Cancer

Screening and early detection of colonic and rectal cancer help detect treatable lesions. Periodic sampling of stool for occult blood may prove to be a cost-effective method of cancer detection. Rectal examination, of course, should be a part of every physical examination in elderly patients. Annual sigmoidoscopy can no longer be strongly recommended except for high-risk patients (previous polyp or colonic cancer, strong family history). Preoperative carcinoembryonic antigen (CEA) may predict the risk of relapse. Patients with CEA levels greater than 6 ng/ml have higher relapse rates than those with levels under 6 ng/ml.

The prognosis for colorectal cancer depends on the findings at operation. Lesions of mucosa and submucosa only (Duke's A) carry a 70–90% chance of 5-years' survival. Lesions invading the bowel wall but not the regional nodes (Duke's B) denote a 50–70% 5-years' survival rate. Lesions involving regional nodes (Duke's C) portend a 20–50% chance of 5-years' survival. With metastases beyond the regional nodes (Duke's D), 0–10% of patients survive for 5 years.

Patients who present with metastatic disease may benefit symptomatically from a bypass procedure or colostomy, if bowel obstruction is present. Curative resection of invasive rectal lesions usually requires a permanent colostomy. Some geriatric patients with a poor performance status but with low rectal lesions may not tolerate a colostomy. In addition, psychological factors may be an obstacle to acceptance of the colostomy. Electrocoagulation or other local measures should be attempted in early disease, if possible, in order to avoid the colostomy, especially in cases of coexisting disease.

Preoperative radiotherapy renders some rectal lesions more resectable and reduces the incidence of local recurrence, but overall survival is minimally affected. Postoperative radiotherapy may benefit selected patients with Duke's B or C lesions. Standard bowel resection (e.g., hemicolectomy) is indicated in nonrectal invasive cancers, if the patient can tolerate it medically. Adjuvant chemotherapy after resection of colon cancer has so far not prolonged survival in Duke's B or C cases. This treatment is under investigation in a number of large studies. Unless a patient is assigned to such a study or protocol, use of adjuvant chemotherapy in geriatric patients is not indicated. Chemotherapy of metastatic colorectal cancer is marginally successful. The most active drug, 5-fluorouracil, may cause partial response in 15–20% of patients and in some cases gives beneficial palliation of symptoms. New drug combinations, however, may be too toxic for geriatric patients. Treatment should be considered only when the patient potentially will benefit, is fully able to comprehend the dose schedule, and can tolerate the various side effects of the antitumor agents.

Breast Cancer

Primary surgical treatment for breast cancer remains controversial, but preference for modified radical mastectomy over the standard radical procedure is growing. Survival is similar, and morbidity (arm edema) is reduced with the less radical procedures. Primary radiotherapy after lumpectomy has been successful for early lesions and can be considered for geriatric patients. Adjuvant chemotherapy (e.g., methotrexate, 5-fluorouracil, and cyclophosphamide [CMF]) in patients with positive axillary nodes (stage II) decreases the relapse rate and increases survival in premenopausal women. Recent data show that postmenopausal patients may benefit if 85% or more of the standard drug doses are given; however, adequate chemotherapy may be too toxic for geriatric patients, so adjuvant chemotherapy is not generally recommended. Postoperative radiotherapy decreases local recurrence in stage II disease but does not improve survival. In geriatric cases it may be best to use local radiotherapy when needed rather than routinely postoperatively.

With the availability of estrogen receptor protein (ERP) assays, the endocrine (hormonal) treatment of metastatic breast cancer has become more rational and predictable. When ERP levels are very low or absent, the probability of response to any hormonal manipulation is less than 5%. High ERP values indicate that 40–75% of patients will benefit. A recently introduced synthetic nonsteroidal antiestrogen, tamoxifen citrate (Nolvadex), has proved effective with minimal side effects in metastatic breast cancer. Standard estrogen compounds carry a high incidence of nausea, vomiting, fluid retention, and cardiovascular complications, all of which are prominent in geriatric patients. When hormonal treatment fails, or in combination with hormonal treatment, chemotherapy should be considered. Overall, 50–75% of ERP-negative patients will respond, and 10–20% of these will have complete remission. Active agents include cyclophosphamide (C), adriamycin (A), 5-fluorouracil (F), vincristine (V), methotrexate (M), and prednisone (P). Effective regimens are CMF, CAF, AV, and CMFVP. These chemotherapeutic programs offer palliation, with remissions lasting 6–12 months or more. Geriatric patients are given half the usual drug dosages to start, with gradual increases if blood counts permit. Chemotherapy should be used cautiously in patients over 75–80 years, with close monitoring for side effects. In most cases chemotherapy is effective regardless of the patient's ERP status.

Prostate Cancer

Treatment of prostate cancer depends on the extent or stage of disease. The incidence increases with age. In asymptomatic patients (stage A disease) the diagnosis is made during prostatectomy for hypertrophy and requires no further treatment in most cases. Treatment of stage B disease, a palpable tumor confined to prostate, is more controversial. Radical prostatectomy and irradiation (6,500 rads) each give similar 10-year survival rates (50–60%). Patients must be treated individually according to operative risk, coexisting disease, and consideration of complications from each modality. Treatment of tumors with contiguous spread beyond the capsule, which may extend to the pelvic side wall (stage C), usually consists of radiotherapy, although a surgical procedure may be considered. Treatment of metastatic disease (stage D) depends on the patient's symptoms. Since therapy does not cure metastatic disease, some asymptomatic patients may require only periodic evaluation. Orchiectomy or use of estrogens will palliate pain or other symptoms in about 80% of symptomatic patients. About 50% will have objective evidence of tumor regression for 6–12 months.

In prostate cancer, chemotherapeutic agents (cyclophosphamide, 5-fluorouracil, and adriamycin) may alleviate symptoms and cause objective disease regression when hormonal manipulation has failed. Toxicity is considerably greater than with hormonal treatment. Palliation of bone pain can be achieved in the majority of cases by local irradiation. The most useful guide to disease status is the serum acid phosphatase level. Minimal elevation can now be detected by the newer methods of radioimmunoassay. Improved survival through the use of hormones or chemotherapy has not been conclusively demonstrated for any stage of prostate cancer. With large doses of estrogens or diethylstilbesterol (DES), survival may actually decrease because of cardiovascular complications. The dose of DES should be limited to 1–3 mg daily.

Gastric Cancer

Stomach cancer is rarely localized when first diagnosed, but removal of the primary lesion with correction of obstruction offers palliative treatment to most patients. Operation is indicated if the patient is a surgical candidate without widespread metastases. A combination of chemotherapeutic agents (5-fluorouracil, adriamycin, and mitomycin-C) causes regression of metastatic disease in 40% of patients, who survive longer (up to 8–12 mo) than nonresponders (4- to 6-month survival). This drug regimen causes predictable, severe myelosuppression and is not recommended for most geriatric patients.

Hematologic Malignancies

Acute Leukemia. Acute leukemia in elderly patients is more often the myeloblastic than the lymphoblastic type. New combination chemotherapy programs employing adriamycin and cytosine arabinoside achieve beneficial remissions in the elderly, although the complete remission rate is less than in younger patients. Intensive chemotherapy is recommended in good-risk patients, younger than 70 years, who fully understand the side effects, costs, and benefits involved. Less intense chemotherapy to reduce the WBC does not improve survival. Chronic leukemia is most likely to be of the mature lymphocyte type and does not require therapy in most instances. Occasionally palliation with alkylating agents (chlorambucil) can be offered to geriatric patients who suffer from massive lymphadenopathy, organomegaly, or a WBC of over 100,000/mm^3. Corticosteroids may alleviate Coomb's-positive hemolytic anemia, which occurs in 10–20% of cases. Patients with early chronic myelogenous leukemia may not require therapy. Busulfan or hydroxyurea may relieve hypermetabolic symptoms, organomegaly, or rapidly increasing WBC when the patient is symptomatic.

Lymphomas. Non-Hodgkin's lymphomas are classified histologically as having a favorable or an unfavorable prognosis. The prognosis is favorable for nodular, well-differentiated lymphocytic; nodular poorly differentiated lymphocytic; nodular mixed; and diffuse, well differentiated lymphocytic disease. The prognosis is unfavorable for diffuse undifferentiated; diffuse histiocytic; diffuse mixed; diffuse, poorly differentiated lymphocytic; and nodular histiocytic lymphomas. In the elderly, staging procedures should be limited to bone marrow biopsy, chest roentgenograms and abdominal ultrasound or CT scan. Patients with a favorable histologic prognosis may not require any treatment. If lymph node masses or organomegaly become symptomatic, single alkylating agents or localized radiotherapy can be employed. Corticosteroids and vincristine can also be used but have an added toxicity for geriatric patients. Elderly patients with unfavorable histologic findings have a poor prognosis, since intensive chemotherapy is not justified because of the excessive risk of toxicity. Active drugs include adriamycin (A), cyclophosphamide (C), oncovin (O) (vincristine), bleomycin (B), and prednisone (P). Standard combination chemotherapy programs are COP, ACOP, and BACOP. Use of lower doses of drugs may cause temporary clinical improvement in some cases. Palliative radiotherapy can be employed to treat bone pain, skin lesions, spinal cord compression, or the superior vena cava syndrome.

Hodgkin's disease in good-risk elderly patients should be approached as in younger patients. Staging laparotomy should not be carried out indiscriminately because of increased complications. Early nodal disease (stages I and II) can be cured by modern radiotherapy. A significant number of elderly patients have more advanced (stages III and IV) disease, with abdominal and bone marrow involvement, but achieve prolonged remissions after MOPP (mechlorethamine hydrochloride [*M*ustargen], *O*ncovin, *P*rocarbazine, *P*rednisone) chemotherapy. Blood counts should be carefully monitored for serious myelosuppression.

Multiple Myeloma. Multiple myeloma in geriatric patients should be treated only when significant symptoms occur. Symptomatic anemia improves with transfusion of packed red blood cells. Bone pain usually responds to palliative radiation therapy or analgesics. Specific chemotherapy may improve progressive disease, especially with Bence-Jones proteinuria and/or massive hyperproteinemia. L-PAM (phenylalanine mustard) with or without prednisone is a standard, effective regimen in multiple myeloma. The drugs may be administered continuously (in low doses) or intermittently (in moderate doses).

1. Harviel JD, McNamara JJ, Straehley CJ: Surgical treatment of lung cancer in patients over the age of 70 years. *J Thorac Cardiovasc Surg* 75:802–805, 1978.
Surgery still offers the best chance for cure in early lesions, but patients must be carefully selected owing to an operative mortality of 18%.
2. Peterson BA, Kennedy BJ: Aging and cancer management: I. Clinical observations. *CA* 29:322–340, 1979.
A general review of various problems encountered in geriatric patients with cancer. Specific types of cancers are briefly discussed.
3. Ouslander JG: Durg therapy in the elderly. *Ann Intern Med* 95:711–722, 1981.
Comprehensive review of age-related biologic and physiologic changes in the elderly, including important considerations in prescribing medications.
4. Boyd JB, Bradford B Jr, Watne AL: Operative risk factors of colon resection in the elderly. *Ann Surg* 92:743–746, 1980.
Mortality from colon resection increases with the number of preexisting medical problems but not with age per se.
5. Tomita M, et al: Surgical treatment for the elderly patient with lung cancer. *Nippon Kyobu Rinsho* 39:779–786, 1980.
Postoperative pulmonary complications are significant in the immediate postoperative period and therefore must be anticipated and dealt with accordingly. Some data is presented that show a slower growth rate for lung cancer compared to younger age groups.

23. APPROACH TO OCCULT PRIMARY MALIGNANCIES

Arthur Skarin

Some patients with a solitary metastasis may not initially develop a readily apparent primary tumor. Survival may be related more to complications of other nonmalignant disease than to the lone metastasis or occult primary tumor; further metastases usually develop with passage of time, however.

In cases of multiple metastases without an identified primary, the overall prognosis is poor, with a median survival of about 3 months; therefore, a rigorous diagnostic evaluation offering a low yield of useful information does not necessarily help the elderly patient. A comprehensive pathologic evaluation of the metastasis itself may be the most important predictor of survival. Lymphatic, breast, prostatic, ovarian, or uterine cancer may be identified and treated successfully in selected good-risk patients, but standard therapy of malignancies at other sites is disappointing. In general, therefore, the chance of finding useful information must be balanced against the costs of searching for an occult tumor.

Laboratory Techniques

It is not always possible to identify the primary tumor from a biopsy of the metastatic lesion, using routine histopathologic methods, but special laboratory techniques increase the chances of success. In adenocarcinoma, positive mucicarmine stains usually indicate a gastrointestinal tract or lung primary tumor. Mucin, however, may occasionally be present in breast, ovarian, and other adenocarcinomas. Glycogen stains are especially positive in adenocarcinoma of the kidney. Estrogen receptor protein (ERP), if present at high levels, usually indicates a breast origin. In tumors of the ovary, uterus, and GI tract, and in malignant melanomas, ERP also may be slightly positive. Histopathologic findings in metastatic squamous cell carcinoma usually indicate lung or head and neck as the primary site. The source of an undifferentiated metastatic carcinoma may be identified in some cases as malignant melanoma, if the Fontana argentaffin stain is positive.

Electron microscopy (EM) may identify specific ultrastructures, such as dense-core rootlets in microvilli, which are seen mainly in colon adenocarcinomas. Electron microscopy is also helpful in making the diagnosis of rhabdomyosarcoma, malignant fibrous histiocytoma, leiomyosarcoma, epithelial tumors, malignant melanoma, malignant lymphoma, carcinoid, oat cell carcinoma, and hepatoma, all of which are undifferentiated morphologically by light microscopy but have a specific EM ultrastructure.

Surface-marker studies showing the presence of immunoglobulin or T-cell markers are diagnostic of B-cell or T-cell malignant lymphomas. Moreover, histochemical stains such as peroxidase and esterase on tissue touch preparations or fixed tissue section are diagnostic of myeloblastoma, an extramedullary manifestation of acute myelogenous leukemia. Finally, recent immunologic research utilizing immunoperoxidase has allowed the specific identification of the B subunit of human chorionic gonadotropin (HCG) alphafetoprotein (AFP), and other markers in trophoblastic, testicular, and other carcinomas, which may present as undifferentiated metastatic carcinoma.

Likely Sources

Although laboratory techniques are most helpful in identification of the primary tumor, knowledge of common presenting metastatic sites for primary tumors helps to narrow the choice. Malignant cervical adenopathy in the upper neck often is the first site of metastases from squamous cell carcinoma, lymphoepithelioma, or lymphoma of the oral cavity, nasopharynx or pharynx (head and neck primaries). A detailed ear, nose, and throat evaluation begins the search in such cases. If no primary lesions are seen, several blind biopsies by a specialist may reveal the primary occult tumor. Adenopathy of the lower neck less frequently arises from head and neck primaries, so that lung, GI tract, and thyroid tumors and malignant lymphoma must also be considered. In about 30% of patients with cervical adenopathy, the primary tumor will not be determined, and surgical excision may be adequate, especially in geriatric patients. Regional irradiation may be indicated for patients with a high probability of head and neck primary tumors.

The most likely tumor in axillary adenopathy in a woman is occult breast cancer. Other possibilities are lymphoma, melanoma, and lung, GI, and ovarian tumors. In cases of malignant axillary adenopathy, even when xeroradiograms are negative, resection of the outer upper quadrant of the breast (or simple mastectomy) will reveal an occult primary tumor in a significant number of cases. The majority of patients, however, have no obvious primary tumor, and only 15–20% will survive for 5 years after initial node dissection. Local irradiation is employed in some cases.

Inguinal adenopathy in women is associated with cancer of the cervix, uterus, or ovary. In men, the prostate is the most common primary site when inguinal nodes are found. In both sexes, occult malignant melanoma, especially of the extremities, must be sought also. A history of a small, "benign" lesion that "regressed spontaneously" or a skin "lesion" resected many years previously is a helpful clue. Other occult tumors with inguinal nodes include anal, rectal, and urinary tract carcinoma and malignant lymphoma. Management must be individualized for each set of circumstances. If no primary is detected, then surgical resection of the involved nodes is indicated in most cases. Local radiation therapy in the inguinal region may lead to refractory peripheral lymphedema, so radiation must be used discriminately.

A solitary coin lesion on a chest film from an elderly patient may not require an extensive evaluation for eventual resection, because morbidity from other illnesses usually precludes thoracotomy. Growth rate in primary lung cancer is usually slow; therefore, periodic follow-up is suitable for patients who are poor operative or radiotherapy risks. However, since 50–60% of patients with stage I primary lung cancer can be cured by surgical procedures, thoracotomy is recommended in suitable cases. Other primary tumors that occasionally present with a solitary lung metastasis are cancers of the breast, GU tract, and GI tract and melanomas. Multiple lung metastases are much more usual and, because of the poor prognosis, seldom require extensive diagnostic studies. Primary lung adenocarcinoma may present with this pattern, as may several other primary lung tumors.

Liver metastases arise from occult primary tumors in the GI tract, lung, kidney, and breast and from melanomas. Extensive GI work-up in the absence of symptoms, anemia, or blood in the stool rarely identifies the tumor so is not cost-effective. Selected patients may benefit from regional hepatic perfusion with 5-fluorouracil or hepatic irradiation, but these treatment modalities are not often useful for the elderly.

Malignant osteolytic lesions can arise from primary tumors of the lung, head and neck, breast, and genitourinary tract. Multiple myeloma may also present with lytic bone lesions, but examination of bone marrow usually identifies myeloma. Multiple osteoblastic lesions usually originate from breast, prostate, stomach, or thyroid tumors. Management of bone metastases includes local radiotherapy for pain, if analgesics are unsuccessful. Prophylactic orthopedic pinning can prevent future disability from fracture if more than half of a major weight-bearing bone (e.g., femur) is destroyed. If breast or prostate cancer is the likely diagnosis, hormonal therapy may result in bone recalcification.

Metastases to the brain may originate from tumors of the breast, lung, skin (melanoma), kidney, head and neck, stomach, colon, or other sites. Metastatic brain tumors are initially treated with dexamethasone (Decadron), 4–6 mg qid, which often provides dramatic symptomatic improvement. The dose is tapered during or after irradiation to avoid the adverse effects of steroids, which are especially common in the elderly. In the majority of cases, 3,000 rads total brain irradiation with local coned-down rads to the lesion offers good palliation for 6–12 months. Surgical resection of a brain metastasis is rarely indicated, except when a solitary, easily accessible lesion arises from a previous malignancy with a long free interval (3 yr or more). In a patient without evidence of a primary cancer, the morbidity from biopsy of an accessible brain metastasis must be carefully weighed against the use of steroids and radiotherapy without a tissue diagnosis. Chemotherapy is unsatisfactory in brain metastasis. Only rare responses from nitrosourea drugs are reported.

1. Krementz ET, Cersie EJ, Foster DP: Metastatic cancer of undetermined source. *Curr Probl Cancer* 4:1–37, 1979.
Thorough review of the differential diagnosis, pathology, natural history, and therapy of metastatic malignancy from an unknown primary site.
2. Stewart JF, Tattersall MHN, Woods RL, Fox RM: Unknown primary adenocarcinoma: Incidence of over-investigation and natural history. *Br Med J* 1:1530–1533, 1979.
Presentation of data showing that the majority of patients are over-investigated with no effect on survival.
3. Osteen RT, Kopf F, Wilson RE: In pursuit of the unknown primary. *Am J Surg* 135:494–498, 1978.

24. CHEMOTHERAPEUTIC AGENTS IN GERIATRIC PATIENTS

Arthur Skarin

The goal of chemotherapy in geriatric patients is mainly palliation of symptoms for a reasonable period of time with minimal or acceptable side effects. Most patients have the types of malignancies that are rarely cured by drugs. Survival may be increased in patients who show either partial or, less commonly, complete disappearance of tumor. Increase in useful life, usually measured in months, and not prolongation of agony, is the only worthwhile goal. Considerable judgment is necessary in choosing elderly patients for a chemotherapy program.

Because of variability in body fat and water content, doses of chemotherapeutic agents are based on body surface area (m^2), which is calculated from a standard nomogram. Surface area calculations minimize the diversity of total dose among various patients. If the drug dosage is listed in mg/kg, multiplication by 40 will convert the dose to mg/m^2 with reasonable accuracy. Risk of toxicity is increased in elderly patients. Age older than 65, prior radiotherapy to the axial skeleton or pelvis, prior chemotherapy, significant renal or liver disease, and weight loss equal to 10% or more of total body weight are all associated with increased toxic side effects.

In general, geriatric patients are started on 50% of the usual dose of chemotherapeutic agents in order to avoid unpredictable toxicity. With subsequent courses, the dose can be increased by 50% increments, if serial blood counts (generally weekly) do not show serious myelosuppression, and if other side effects are minor. Before each chemotherapy course, the leukocyte and platelet count should be rising (from the previous course), with the white count above 4,000/mm^3 and platelet count above 125,000/mm^3.

Common Chemotherapeutic Agents

The following summarizes the most commonly used cancer chemotherapeutic drugs. Dosages apply to use as a single agent. When combined with myelosuppressive drugs, dosage is reduced by 50%.

Alkylating Agents.

Busulfan (Myleran). The mechanism of action is cell cycle nonspecific with interference in DNA, RNA, and protein function. The dosage is 2–4 mg/m^2/day PO for 1–2 weeks, followed by maintenance doses of 1–2 mg/m^2 depending on CBC. The major side effect is myelosuppression, which may be delayed and prolonged. Irreversible pulmonary fibrosis after prolonged therapy, occasional hyperpigmentation, and adrenocortical insufficiency–like syndrome have been seen. Among the indications for use are chronic myelogenous leukemia, selected cases of essential thrombocythemia, and polycythemia vera. Special precautions in the case of elderly patients include monitoring CBC and platelet counts weekly and watching for myelosuppression.

Carmustine or bis-*Chloroethyl Nitrosourea (BCNU) (BiCNU).* The mechanism of action is cell cycle–nonspecific, with alkylation of DNA, inhibition of DNA repair by isocyanate carbamylation, and protein modification. The dosage is 75–100 mg/m^2 diluted in 250 cc of 5% dextrose in water, administered IV bid, every 6–8 weeks. Major side effects are nausea and emesis about 2 hours after injection. Myelosuppression is delayed, with the platelet nadir at day 30 and WBC nadir at day 34. The solution contains 3 ml of absolute alcohol, which may cause dizziness and vein irritation. Indications for use include malignant gliomas, Hodgkin's disease, and multiple myeloma. Precautions needed for elderly patients are related to delayed and prolonged myelosuppression. Rarely, renal and liver toxicity is a problem.

Chlorambucil (Leukeran). The mechanism of action is cell cycle–nonspecific, with alkylation of DNA. The dosage is 0.03–0.1 mg/kg/day PO. Side effects include gradual modest myelosuppression (prolonged therapy may cause marrow failure). Major indications for use are chronic lymphatic leukemia, Waldenström's macroglobulinemia, mycosis fungoides, and breast and ovarian cancer. In the elderly, rare dermatitis and hepatotoxicity may occur rarely.

Cis-*Diamminedichloroplatinum or DDP (Platinol, Cisplatin).* The mechanism of action is cell cycle–nonspecific, with inhibition of DNA synthesis by binding to DNA, RNA, and transfer RNA. The dosage is 60–75 mg/m^2 IV every 3–4 weeks or, alternatively, 20 mg/m^2 IV daily $\times$ 5, repeated every 3 weeks. Pretreatment hydration should be carried out, plus furosemide or mannitol diuresis. Common side effects are nausea and emesis for 1–12 hours after infusion. Reversible myelosuppression occurs in only 20–30% of patients. Renal toxicity may appear if hydration is inadequate. Tinnitus and hearing loss, which may be reversible, have also occurred. Indications for use are testicular carcinoma and ovarian, bladder, prostate, head and neck, and lung cancer. The drug is usually combined, in doses of 40–50 mg/m^2, with other chemotherapeutic agents. Special precautions to ensure proper hydration in elderly patients will help prevent renal failure.

Cyclophosphamide (Cytoxan). The mechanism of action is cell cycle–S phase specific and nonspecific with inhibition of DNA synthesis and reaction with sulfhydryl, phosphate, and amine groups, resulting in multiple lesions in dividing and nondividing cells. The dosage for oral maintenance therapy is 1.5–3.0 mg/kg/day PO; for pulse dose therapy, 0.5–1.0 gm/m^2 IV every 3 weeks. Side effects are reversible myelosuppression (leukopenia more often than thrombocytopenia); nausea and vomiting after a single large IV dose; hemorrhagic cystitis, especially after large doses; chronic cystitis with bladder fibrosis; and alopecia. Indications for use are lymphomas, multiple myeloma, and carcinomas of the breast, lung, ovary, and prostate. The elderly require adequate fluid intake (2,000 ml/day) when large doses are given IV.

Dacarbazine or Dimethyl-Triazeno-Imidazole-Carboxamide (DTIC) (Dome). The mechanism of action is cell cycle–nonspecific. Major effects are alkylation of nucleic acids and purine antagonism. The drug may interact with sulfhydryl groups. The dosage is 250 mg/m^2/day IV $\times$ 5 every 3–4 weeks. Alternatively, 750 mg/m^2 IV every 3–4 weeks can be used. Myelosuppression is an uncommon side effect and may be delayed (10–15 days); nausea and emesis are prominent but subside with successive daily doses. A flulike illness and hepatic toxicity have been encountered. The indications for use (in combination with other chemotherapeutic drugs) are malignant melanoma, Hodgkin's disease, and soft tissue sarcomas. In the elderly, liberal use of antiemetics helps to prevent dehydration.

Lomustine or Chloroethyl-Cyclohexyl-Nitrosurea (CCNU) (CeeNU). The mechanism of action is the same as for other alkylating agents, but it may also inhibit enzymatic processes leading to DNA synthesis. The dosage is 100–130 mg/m^2 PO every 6–8 weeks. Major side effects are nausea and emesis, which may be delayed 4–6 hours and persist for 24 hours. Myelosuppression is delayed, with platelet nadir at 4 weeks and WBC nadir at 5–6 weeks. Indications for use are central nervous system malignancies, Hodgkin's disease, multiple myeloma, and gastrointestinal tumors. The dosage should be reduced for elderly patients, especially those with compromised marrow function.

Methchlorethamine Hydrochloride or Nitrogen Mustard (HN_2) (Mustargen). The mechanism of action is cell cycle–nonspecific, with interference in DNA replication function. The dosage is 0.2 mg/kg IV for 2 days. The dose with other chemotherapeutic agents is 6 mg/m^2 IV on days 1 and 8 once monthly. Side effects are nausea and vomiting, alopecia, and myelosuppression. Extravasation outside a vein causes tissue necrosis. When extravasation occurs, the area should be infiltrated by isotonic sodium thiosulfate. The major indication is Hodgkin's disease. The drug is rarely indicated for the elderly, except with MOPP chemotherapy in Hodgkin's disease (Mustargen, Oncovin, procarbazine, prednisone).

Melphalan or L-*Phenylalanine Mustard* (L-*PAM) (Alkeran).* The mechanism of action is the same as for nitrogen mustard (preceding paragraph). Intermittent dosage is 0.15–0.20 mg/kg PO daily for 5 days, repeated every 4–6 weeks. Continuous dosage is 0.1 mg/kg/day PO for 2–3 weeks, followed by maintenance with 2–4 mg/day (total) when the bone marrow has recovered. Delayed myelosuppression that may persist for weeks is a side-effect. Indications for use are multiple myeloma and breast and ovarian cancer.

Antimetabolites.

5-Fluorouracil (5-FU). The mechanism of action is cell cycle–specific for S phase, with inhibition of thymidylate synthetase. For weekly treatment the dose is 10–15 mg/kg IV. The intermittent treatment dosage is 500 mg/m^2 IV for 5 consecutive days, repeated every 4–5 weeks. Mixed with glucose solution (e.g., Glucola) in the same doses, the drug can be given orally. Absorption is variable, and oral treatment is not generally recommended. Side effects are nausea, emesis, and alopecia, which are mild. Myelosuppression and mucositis are dose-dependent. Hyperpigmentation occurs, and reversible cerebellar ataxia is seen in 1% of patients. Indications for use are colon, breast, gastric, and pancreatic cancers. In the elderly, dose-related mucositis and neurotoxicity are more likely to occur.

Methotrexate (MTX). The mechanism of action is cell cycle–specific for S phase. Inhibition of dihydrofolate reductase leads to decreased synthesis of thymidylic acid (DNA) and inosinic acid (part of RNA synthesis). The weekly dose is 20–40 mg/m^2 IV; daily dosage is 15–30 mg total PO or IM for 5 consecutive days, repeated every 2–3 weeks. Intermittent dosage is 30–50 mg/m^2 IV on days 1 and 8 every 2–4 weeks, in combination with other chemotherapeutic drugs. Side effects are mucositis, myelosuppression, hepatotoxicity with chronic use, allergic pneumonitis, and nephrotoxicity with large doses. The drug has increased efficacy when used with other chemotherapeutic agents. Major indications are breast, lung, head and neck, and cervical cancers and acute leukemia. High-dose MTX with leucovorin factor rescue is experimental in osteosarcoma, lymphoma, breast, and lung cancers. In the elderly, the drug is used with caution because of reduced renal function.

Natural Products—Plant Alkaloids.

Vinblastine Sulfate (Velban). The mechanism of action is cell cycle–specific for M phase, causing inhibition of mitosis. The dosage is 4–6 mg/m^2 IV every 3–4 weeks. Mild nausea and vomiting, myelosuppression, alopecia, local phlebitis, neurotoxicity (parasthesias and jaw pain), constipation, and abdominal pain are the major side effects. Indications are Hodgkin's disease and testicular and breast carcinoma. Myelosuppression and neurotoxicity are more common in the elderly. The drug is usually combined with other chemotherapeutic agents.

Vincristine Sulfate (Oncovin). The mechanism of action is cell cycle–specific for M phase, with metaphase arrest. Dosage is 0.5–1.0 mg/m² IV weekly (not to exceed a total weekly dose of 2.0 mg). Side effects include neuropathy (paresthesias, loss of deep tendon reflexes, extreme weakness, cranial nerve palsies); gastrointestinal effects (constipation and adynamic ileus); and inappropriate ADH release with hyponatremia and orthostatic hypotension. The drug is useful when combined with other agents in acute leukemia and lymphomas and in breast and lung (oat cell) cancer. In the elderly, the use of stool softeners helps to reduce gastrointestinal complications.

Antitumor Antibiotics.

Bleomycin Sulfate (Blenoxane). The mechanism of action is cell cycle–specific for G_2 and M phases with scission of double-stranded DNA. The dosage is 10–20 units/m² IM or IV weekly or twice weekly (cumulative dose limitation, 400 mg). A febrile reaction occurs in about 10–25% of patients, usually 4–6 hours after administration. An anaphylactic reaction (fever, wheezing, urticaria, and shock) is seen rarely (1%), usually in patients with lymphoma. A 1-mg test dose is recommended for lymphoma patients. Skin toxicity (inflammation, ulcers, and hyperpigmentation) occurs in 45% of patients and is usually dose-related. Pulmonary fibrosis occurs in 5–10% of patients and is also dose-related but may be fatal. Indications for use are lymphomas and testicular cancer (in combination chemotherapy) and squamous cell carcinoma of the head, neck, and cervix. Precautions should be taken in the elderly because of lung toxicity.

Doxorubicin or Hydroxydaunomycin Hydrochloride (Adriamycin). The mechanism of action is cell cycle–specific for the S phase. It binds to DNA by intercalation with base pairs and also inhibits RNA synthesis by steric obstruction and template disordering. When it is given as a single agent, the dosage is 60–75 mg/m² IV every 3 weeks. When it is combined with other myelosuppressive agents, its dosage is 30–45 mg/m² IV every 3 weeks. If the bilirubin is increased to 3.0 mg/100 ml, 50% of the usual dose should be given; if over 3.0 mg/100 ml, 25% of the dose should be used. Nausea and vomiting develops in 50% of patients; myelosuppression with leukopenia greater than thrombocytopenia is dose-related. Local tissue necrosis occurs if the drug is extravasated outside the vein. Other side effects are red urine (no clinical significance); hyperpigmentation of skin, mucous membranes, nail beds, palms, and soles (especially in black patients); and transient ECG changes. Dose-related cardiotoxicity occurs and irreversible congestive heart failure increases significantly with total doses exceeding 450 mg/m². Cardiotoxicity is potentiated by mediastinal irradiation or concomitant cyclophosphamide. Indications for use are acute leukemia; lymphomas; soft tissue sarcomas; and breast, bladder, lung, ovarian, gastric, prostate, thyroid, pancreatic, and hepatocellular cancers. In the elderly, myelosuppression and cardiac toxicity require close monitoring. Use with caution.

Mitomycin-C. The mechanism of action is cell cycle–nonspecific but also active in early (G_1) and (S) phases. The drug causes cross-linking of DNA chains and may also inhibit RNA and protein synthesis. Dosage when used as a single agent is 10–20 mg/m² IV, every 6–8 weeks. Side effects include myelosuppression (delayed and unpredictable); severe tissue necrosis if extravasated; renal and hepatic toxicity; and pulmonary fibrosis. Indications for use (generally in combination with other agents) are gastrointestinal, breast, and head and neck cancer. Serious myelosuppression limits use in the elderly and in patients with compromised marrow.

Miscellaneous Chemotherapeutic Agents.

Mithramycin. The mechanism of action is probably cell cycle–specific for S phase by complexing with DNA. Also, it directly affects osteoclasts that block bone resorption. Its dosage as an antitumor drug is 0.025–0.050 mg/kg IV, daily or every other day for 5–10 doses, until toxicity occurs. The courses are repeated every 4 weeks. For hypercalcemia the dose is 0.025 mg/kg IV as a single daily dose, which can be increased up to 3 times. Side effects are nausea and vomiting, myelosuppression (mainly thrombocytopenia), hemorrhagic diathesis (5–10% of cases), facial flushing, fever, skin lesions, and hepatic and renal toxicity. Indications for use are testicular embryonal cell carcinoma (occasionally) and hypercalcemia due to bone metastases. In the elderly, the risk of a hemorrhagic disorder and thrombocytopenia limits usefulness.

Mitotane or o,p'-*DDD (Lysodren).* The mechanism of action is direct suppression of adrenocortical cell growth. Dosage is 6–10 gm PO daily given in 3 or 4 divided doses. The major side effects are nausea and vomiting, which occur in over 80% of patients; lethargy, somnolence, visual disturbances, dermatitis, and adrenal insufficiency are also common. The drug is indicated in carcinoma of the adrenal cortex. In the elderly, begin with a low dose (1–2 gm) and gradually increase. Supplemental use of corticosteroids, larger than normal replacement, is essential.

Procarbazine or Methylhydrazine (Matulane). The mechanism of action is cell cycle–specific for (S) phase. Complex actions inhibit DNA, RNA, and protein synthesis. Dosage is 100 mg/m^2 PO daily for 14 days of each 28-day cycle (MOPP). Side effects are nausea and vomiting (70% of patients), myelosuppression, neuropathy and depression or stupor, and dermatitis. There may be significant interaction with other drugs (especially ethyl alcohol) due to monoamine-oxidase inhibiting properties. The drug is useful in lymphomas and is employed occasionally in brain and lung cancers.

Hormonal Agents.

Estrogens. The mechanism of action is not completely known but may involve a dual effect: pituitary suppression and a direct effect on the stroma of the tissue or malignant cell. The dosage of diethylstilbestrol (DES) is 5 mg tid PO for breast cancer or 1–3 mg/day PO for prostatic cancer. Side effects are anorexia, nausea and vomiting, fluid retention, vaginal discharge, urinary urgency, breast tenderness, gynecomastia, and skin changes. Indications are breast cancer (mainly ERP-positive) and prostatic cancer. A temporary flare-up in breast cancer with bone pain and hypercalcemia may threaten the elderly patient. Analgesics, fluids, and mithramycin may be required during this temporary phase. Cardiovascular complications in men also occur with doses of DES above 3–5 mg/day.

Antiestrogens. The mechanism of action is not completely known but involves interference in DNA, RNA, and protein functions. The dosage of tamoxifen (Nolvadex) is 10 mg bid PO. Side effects are nausea, dermatitis (dry skin), and occasional mild myelosuppression (thrombocytopenia). Indication for use is breast cancer (mainly ERP-positive). Temporary flare-up may occur (see Estrogens), but the incidence is much less than with estrogens.

Androgens. The mechanism of action is not completely known but involves interference in DNA, RNA, and protein functions. The dosage of testosterone propionate is 100 mg 3 times weekly. Fluoxymesterone (Halotestin) is given at 10 mg tid PO. Indication for use is breast cancer (ERP-positive). Side effects are fluid retention, virilization, and hepatic toxicity. Temporary disease flare-up and hypercalcemia (see Estrogens) may occur.

Progestins. The mechanism of action is not completely known. Dosage of megestrol (Megace) is 100 mg tid PO in uterine and kidney cancer; less for breast cancer. Medroxyprogesterone acetate (Provera) is given at 1 gm IM weekly for uterine and kidney cancer, less for breast cancer. A major side effect is fluid retention at high doses. Indications for use are adenocarcinoma of the uterus (well-differentiated), and occasionally breast and renal cell cancer. Fluid retention in elderly patients with cardiovascular disease may be intolerable.

---

1. Pratt WB, Ruddon RW: *The Anticancer Drugs—The Antimetabolites.* New York, Oxford University Press, 1979, chap 6, pp 118–119.
   Handbook with concise review of cancer chemotherapeutic agents, including brief discussion of choice of drugs for specific malignancies.
2. Kiely JM: Series on pharmacology in practice. *Mayo Clin Proc* 56:384–392, 1981.
   Excellent updated review of chemotherapy and hormonal agents, including numerous tables of drug classes, indications, and side effects.
3. Begg CD, Cohen JL, Ellerton J: Are the elderly predisposed to toxicity from cancer chemotherapy? *Cancer Clin Trials* 3:369–374, 1980.
   Elderly patients with metastatic breast, lung, and colon cancer did not experience increased toxicity during chemotherapy when compared to younger patients receiving the same regimens.
4. Harris CC: Individual differences in cancer susceptibility. *Ann Intern Med* 92:809–825, 1980.
   A comprehensive review of the interactions of environmental carcinogens and predisposing host factors in cancer susceptibility.

V. INFECTIOUS DISEASES

25. INFLUENZA

Anthony L. Esposito and Richard A. Gleckman

Primarily an infection of respiratory tract epithelium, influenza is a viral disease transmitted from man to man by the inhalation of infected, aerosolized droplets. The incubation period appears to be 18–36 hours.

Clinical Course

Prodromal symptoms, such as malaise and chilliness, occur in some cases, but the onset of the illness is characteristically abrupt. Severe headache, diffuse myalgias, fever, and marked prostration represent typical early manifestations. Cough and chest pain usually appear as the systemic manifestations begin to subside. In most adults, the illness resolves within 5–7 days of onset and recovery is prompt; in the elderly, the course of the infection can be protracted. In addition, the elderly appear to be especially vulnerable to severe debilitation following influenza infection, and their convalescence can require weeks. Pneumonia, caused either by the influenza virus itself or by bacterial superinfection, represents the primary complication of the disease and the leading cause of death. *Streptococcus pneumoniae* and *Staphylococcus aureus* are the two organisms most frequently isolated from patients with secondary bacterial infection. Eighty percent of deaths attributable to influenza are of persons 65 years of age or older; the majority of deaths involve persons with preexisting cardiac or pulmonary disease.

Virus Types

Influenza viruses are typed (A, B, or C) on the basis of their core nucleoprotein antigen. Type A viruses are responsible for most cases and remain the only strains isolated during pandemics; the B and C influenza viruses can cause isolated outbreaks and sporadic epidemics. The surface proteins of the influenza A virus, hemagglutinin and neuraminidase, confer infectivity; they are also antigenic and elicit protective antibody formation. New strains of the influenza A virus emerge every 10–15 years and result from a spontaneous alteration in the surface proteins. These antigenically novel viruses are unaffected by antibodies to earlier strains and therefore have the potential to produce epidemics or pandemics.

Vaccination

Immunity to influenza is conferred by antibodies to the viral surface antigens. Immunity reduces susceptibility to influenza and mitigates the severity of the illness in persons who contract the disease. As a result, efforts have been made in the United States to prevent or control influenza through vaccination. Because the aged represent those at greatest risk for serious illness and death, large-scale immunization programs have been aimed primarily at this group. Clinical trials of immunization with inactivated influenza vaccines have yielded inconsistent results. In some reports, persons 65 years of age or older exhibited antibody responses to vaccination similar to those of younger adults. In other investigations, significant increments in antibody titers were not noted in the aged. It has also been reported, however, that even though vaccination may produce a blunted humoral response, elderly persons who receive influenza vaccine experience a substantially reduced incidence of bronchopneumonia and enjoy a significantly lowered mortality than aged individuals not vaccinated who contract the disease.

The formulation of the influenza vaccine is periodically reviewed by the U. S. Public Health Service to ensure that the antigenic composition of the vaccine provides immunity against the most currently prevalent viruses. Information on the specific composition of the vaccine and recommendations for immunization are published annually by the Public Health Service Advisory Committee on Immunization Practices. In general, vaccination is recommended for all persons 65 years of age or older. The vaccine should be administered in a single dose 1–2 months before an expected epidemic; in the presence of a major antigenic shift, a second dose of vaccine should be given. Pain and tenderness at the injection site occur commonly but are usually transient and clinically insignificant. Occasionally, systemic symptoms, such as fever, chills, and malaise, appear 6–24 hours after vaccination; these symptoms are rarely disabling.

Use of Amantadine Hydrochloride

Amantadine hydrochloride is a drug of established value for the prophylaxis and therapy of influenza A infections. When administered prophylactically, it results in a significant reduction in both rate of infection and duration of illness produced by influenza A strains. Amantadine has been shown to be effective against all strains of influenza A, but it demonstrates no action against other viruses. Its prophylactic effect ceases abruptly with its discontinuation. The use of amantadine after the clinical onset of influenza reduces the duration of fever and other symptoms and accelerates the resolution of pulmonary function abnormalities associated with uncomplicated disease. The efficacy of the drug in treating primary influenzal pneumonia or in preventing bacterial superinfection remains to be demonstrated.

Because amantadine hydrochloride exhibits no prophylactic or therapeutic action in viral infections other than those caused by influenza A, its use requires accurate detection of influenza A infection in the community. Once an outbreak has been identified, amantadine can be prescribed for persons over 65 years of age who have not been protected by appropriate vaccines. Thus, amantadine should be employed when adequate supplies of appropriate vaccines are not available, or during the first 2 weeks after vaccination, before the protective effect has been achieved. In addition, because the combined use of vaccine and amantadine augments the protection conferred by either alone, and because amantadine does not interfere with the immunologic response elicited by the vaccine, some authorities recommend the routine employment of both in the elderly. The prophylactic dose of amantadine is 100 mg twice daily and must be adminstered for the entire duration of the outbreak. The therapeutic dosage is identical to the prophylactic; administration should begin within 24 hours of the onset of influenza and should be continued for 24–48 hours after the disappearance of symptoms.

Adverse effects of amantadine occur most commonly in elderly patients, particularly those with impaired renal function. Central nervous system dysfunction, manifested by agitation, confusion, or depression, represents the most frequently observed toxicity; these symptoms are dose-related, usually appear within the first 48 hours of therapy, and are reversible with discontinuation of the drug. Toxic psychosis, seizures, and coma have also been reported.

---

1. Seneca H: Influenza: Epidemiology, etiology, immunization and management. *J Am Geriatr Soc* 28:241, 1980.
   A concise review in which the efficacy and safety of influenza vaccine are discussed.
2. Mather U, Bentley DW, Hall CB: Concurrent respiratory syncytial virus and influenza A infections in the institutionalized elderly and chronically ill. *Ann Intern Med* 93:49, 1980.
   Respiratory syncytial virus appears to be an important pulmonary pathogen in the debilitated aged and produces illness clinically similar to that caused by influenza A.
3. Horadam VW, et al: Pharmakokinetics of amantadine hydrochloride in subjects with normal and impaired renal function. *Ann Intern Med* 94:454, 1981.
   Guidelines are presented for the use of amantadine in patients with impaired renal function.
4. Goodman RA, et al: Impact of influenza A in a nursing home. *JAMA* 247:1451, 1982.
5. Hall WN, et al: An outbreak of influenza B in an elderly population. *J Infect Dis* 144:297, 1981.
   Outbreaks of influenza A or B may occur in nursing home patients. Among the debilitated geriatric patients in these two studies, the viral illnesses produced high attack rates (25–40%) and excessive case fatality rates (10–30%).

26. URINARY TRACT INFECTION

Anthony L. Esposito and Richard A. Gleckman

Community-acquired Urinary Tract Infections

The diagnosis of a urinary tract infection is readily apparent when the patient experiences an acute onset of fever, flank pain, suprapubic discomfort, urinary frequency, and dysuria. However, aged patients with this infection can also present with incontinence, confusion, vague abdominal pain, anorexia, nausea, vomiting, progressive azotemia, or uncontrolled diabetes mellitus. Elderly catheterized patients typically experience no symptoms localized to the urinary tract.

Urinalysis of specimens from patients with symptomatic infection usually reveals pyuria (5 WBC/high power field) and, occasionally, white blood cell casts; the presence of casts lends considerable support to a presumptive diagnosis of urinary tract infection. Gram stain of the unspun urine demonstrates organisms in 85% of cases of symptomatic infection. The urine colony count is the accepted method of establishing the diagnosis of a bacterial urinary tract infection, and a clean-voided urine specimen containing 100,000 or more colonies/ml confirms the diagnosis. However, because factors such as state of hydration, frequency of micturation, and presence of obstruction or of an antimicrobial agent influence the urine colony counts, the diagnosis of infection is not necessarily excluded when counts of less than 100,000/ml are obtained.

Polymicrobic bacteriuria usually reflects contamination; however, the clinical significance of multiple isolates must not be underestimated in the presence of a suprapubic tube, indwelling urethral catheter, neurogenic bladder, or structural abnormality of the bladder, such as a stone, tumor, or diverticulum. To ensure the validity of culture results, elderly patients should be assisted in urine collection. When warranted, urine can be obtained by bladder catheterization or aspiration.

An initial episode of community-acquired urinary tract infection is usually caused by *Escherichia coli, Proteus mirabilis,* and *Klebsiella* species that are predictably susceptible to a large number of antibiotics, and a prompt clinical and microbiologic response to therapy is the rule. Recurrent urinary tract infections are caused by a wider spectrum of organisms that have less predictable susceptibility patterns; these infections are often complicated by structural abnormalities, and, in general, are notoriously recalcitrant to antimicrobial therapy.

The diagnostic and therapeutic approach to the aged patient with community-acquired urinary tract infection is dependent on the patient's clinical appearance. If the patient does not appear to be toxic, a midstream, clean-voided urine specimen should be submitted for colony count, culture, and susceptibility, and a Gram stain of unspun urine should be made. Initial antibiotic therapy will be guided by the results of the Gram stain of the urine; if gram-negative bacilli are present, and if the patient has not recently received antibiotics, has no history of penicillin allergy, and is not known to harbor an *Enterobacter, Serratia,* or *Pseudomonas* species, cephalexin (500 mg q6h PO) can be administered. For the patient with significant penicillin allergy, trimethoprim-sulfamethoxazole (2 tabs bid) can be prescribed. If gram-positive cocci in chains are noted on the Gram stain of the unspun urine, and the patient is not penicillin-allergic, ampicillin (500 mg q6h PO) is the antibiotic of choice; in the case of a penicillin-hypersensitive patient, erythromycin (500 mg q6h PO) can be administered while disc susceptibility testing is being performed. Therapy for acute urinary tract infection should be continued for 2–4 weeks. Males who are experiencing an initial episode of infection should undergo radiologic evaluation because of the high incidence of structural abnormalities in infected males.

The elderly patient with a urinary tract infection who appears toxic, or who has concomitant illness, such as uncontrolled diabetes mellitus, should be hospitalized. In addition to a Gram stain of unspun urine, a colony count, and culture and susceptibility testing of a clean-voided specimen, the physician must obtain three sets of blood cultures. Initial antimicrobial therapy is guided by the results of the Gram stain: If gram-negative bacilli are seen, and if the patient has no history of penicillin hypersensitivity and is not known to harbor *Enterobacter, Serratia,* or *Pseudomonas aeruginosa* in the urine, cefoxitin (1.5 gm q4h IV) or a cephalosporin (App. A) is acceptable therapy. If an aged patient is seriously ill and has a significant penicillin allergy, or a history of recurrent episodes of urinary tract infection, or known recent exposure to antimicrobials, an aminoglycoside (App. A) should be administered while results of urine culture and susceptibility testing are awaited. Therapy should be continued for a minimum of 2 weeks. The patient who is receiving appropriate antimicrobial therapy, as determined by repeat in vitro susceptibility testing of the offending pathogen, and who fails to demonstrate a prompt clinical and bacteriologic response (e.g., persistent bacteremia or bacteriuria) should undergo thorough investigation of the genitourinary tract with excretory urography and ultrasonography, so that obstruction or intrarenal or perinephric abscess may be detected.

In the treatment of an aged patient with a community-acquired urinary tract infection, a number of practical aspects of therapy should be considered. A bactericidal drug is no more effective than a bacteriostatic agent in eradicating this infection. An unselected combination of multiple antibiotics produces a cure rate no greater than that achieved by an effective single member of the combination. Bacterial cystitis in the female responds adequately to a 1- to 3-day course of therapy; bacterial pyelonephritis probably requires weeks of treatment. Cure of the urinary tract infection is achieved when the organism has been completely eradicated and the urine remains sterile for at least 6 weeks after cessation of therapy. Forcing fluids does not improve the therapeutic results when an appropriate antimicrobial has been administered. Bacteriuria that persists 1–2 days after therapy has been initiated suggests an incorrect selection of antibiotics or the presence of polymicrobic bacteriuria, a significant reduction in the glomerular filtration rate, or an anatomic abnormality, such as staghorn calculus or obstruction.

Hospital-acquired Urinary Tract Infections

Symptomatic urinary tract infections that develop in hospitalized elderly patients invariably follow urethral catheterization or urologic instrumentation. These infections represent the most common hospital-acquired infectious disease and the most frequent source of nosocomial gram-negative bacteremia. Most hospital-acquired urinary tract infections are caused by *E. coli*; however, other gram-negative bacilli, such as *Enterobacter, Klebsiella, Proteus, Pseudomonas,* and *Serratia* contribute to these nosocomial infections.

Fifteen percent of elderly patients in a community hospital have indwelling catheters; these catheters predispose to local infections that are manifested primarily by bacteriuria. However, catheter-related infections can produce pyelonephritis and often serve as a source of metastatic infections that involve surgical wounds, hip prostheses, and cardiac valves. Elderly, critically ill females who remain catheterized for prolonged periods appear to be at greatest risk to develop bacteriuria. The risk of infection is augmented in both sexes in proportion to the number of breaks that occur in the closed catheter drainage system.

The closed sterile drainage system has become the preferred method of preventing catheter-associated urinary tract infections. This system is not infallible but is effective for short-term prophylaxis. Continuous antibiotic irrigation with neomycin or polymycin through a triple-lumen indwelling catheter is not more effective than the closed sterile drainage system in preventing infection, and antibiotic irrigation does not enhance the prophylactic benefit of a closed system. Administration of systemic antimicrobial prophylaxis is not indicated.

Bacteriologic evaluation of catheterized patients can be performed by aspiration of urine from the catheter, using a sterile syringe with a 21-gauge needle. Patients with indwelling catheters inevitably develop bacteriuria. Asymptomatic bacteriuric patients require no chemotherapy, because the ultimate outcome will be recolonization with drug-resistant organisms. Antimicrobial therapy is reserved for those catheterized patients who develop symptomatic infection, with or without concomitant bacteremia. Specific antimicrobial therapy is predicated on identification of the offending pathogen and determination of its antimicrobial susceptibility. Initial antibiotic therapy should be guided by the Gram stain of the urine, the results of previous urine cultures, and a knowledge of the susceptibility patterns prevalent in the hospital. In addition to specific antimicrobial therapy, patients with symptomatic infection associated with indwelling catheters should have those catheters removed, if possible. When catheter removal is not possible, patency of the device and free urine flow must be assured.

Nursing personnel and physicians often become unduly concerned about the appearance of bladder catheters and tend to remove them when concretions form. As long as the catheter functions well, however, it should be left in place, regardless of its appearance.

It is not necessary to detect or treat asymptomatic bacteriuria in geriatric patients, except in those subjected to urologic surgical procedures; rather, the goal of therapy is a reduction in the incidence and magnitude of bacteremia and its complications (e.g., vertebral osteomyelitis and endocarditis). Some authorities have recommended treatment of asymptomatic bacteriuria if the patient has a neurogenic bladder or obstructed flow of urine, however, the high recurrence rate and the significant potential for antibiotic toxicity argue against this approach.

1. Kay D: Urinary tract infections in the elderly. *Ball NY Acad Med* 56:209, 1980.
2. Lye M: Defining and treating urinary infections. *Geriatrics* 14:71, 1978.

Concise reviews on the diagnosis and management of infections of the urinary tract in the aged.

3. Sourander LB, Kasanen A: A 5-year follow-up of bacteriuria in the aged. *Gerontol Clin* 14:274, 1972.
Bacteriuria was detected in 10% of elderly men and 20% of elderly women living at home; 20 and 25%, respectively, of geriatric male and female patients in extended care facilities; and 35% of aged men and 40% of aged women in long-stay hospitals.
4. Brocklehurst JC, et al: Bacteriuria in geriatric hospital patients: Its correlates and management. *Age Aging* 6:240, 1977.
In long-stay, aged patients, bacteriuria is a fluctuating condition that is closely associated with dementia and incontinence of feces and urine.
5. Dontas AS, et al: Bacteriuria and survival in old age. *N Eng J Med* 304:939, 1981.
Among clinically similar residents of a home for the aged, bacteriuria was associated with a 30–50% reduction in survival.
6. Stamey TA, Condy M, Mihara G: Prophylactic efficacy of nitrofurantoin macrocrystals and trimethoprim-sulfamethoxazole in urinary infection. *N Engl J Med* 296:780, 1977.
Elderly patients with frequent, symptomatic reinfection may benefit from long-term chemoprophylaxis with trimethoprim-sulfamethoxazole (one-half tablet) or nitrofurantoin (100 mg) nightly.
7. Holmberg L, et al: Adverse reactions to nitrofurantoin. *Am J Med* 69:733, 1980.
The risk for acute and chronic pulmonary reactions, allergic phenomena, and liver damage in patients receiving prolonged treatment with low doses of nitrofurantoin increases significantly with age.
8. Harding GK, et al: Prophylaxis of recurrent urinary tract infection in female patients. *JAMA* 242:1975, 1979.
Thrice-weekly trimethoprim-sulfamethoxazole therapy (one-half tablet) was effective for prophylaxis of recurrent, symptomatic urinary tract infections and did not predispose to colonization or infection with trimethoprim-resistant Enterobacteriaceae.
9. Gleckman RA, et al: Community-acquired bacteremic urosepsis in elderly patients: A prospective study of 34 consecutive episodes. *J Urol* 128:79, 1982.
Deaths in aged patients with community-acquired urosepsis are infrequent if appropriate antibiotic therapy is administered.
10. Gleckman RA, et al: Symptomatic pyelonephritis in elderly men. *J Am Geriatr Soc* 30:690, 1982.
Noncatheterized elderly men who require hospitalization for acute bacterial pyelonephritis often have bacteremia and usually have anatomic abnormalities of the urinary tract.
11. Gleckman RA, et al: Catheter-related urosepsis in the elderly: A prospective study of community-derived infections. *J Am Geriatr Soc* 30:255, 1982.
Geriatric patients with catheter-related urosepsis typically experience a traumatic catheter-associated event preceding the acute illness; they usually have polymicrobic bateriuria with pathogens resistant to antimicrobial agents commonly given for community-acquired urinary tract infection.
12. Nicolle LE, et al: Bacteriuria in elderly institutionalized men. *N Engl J Med* 309:1420, 1983.
The therapy of asymptomatic bacteriuria in elderly institutionalized men does not reduce either infectious morbidity or long-term survival.

27. INFECTIVE ENDOCARDITIS

Anthony L. Esposito and Richard A. Gleckman

Although the peak incidence of infective endocarditis is in younger adults, 20–30% of patients with this disorder are 60 years of age or older, and its incidence in the aged is increasing. Nevertheless, physicians appear to have difficulty in establishing a diagnosis in the elderly. The interval between onset of symptoms and diagnosis increases dramatically with age, and in a remarkable number of cases—estimated to be up to 50%—geriatric patients remain undiagnosed during life.

Symptoms

Elderly patients with either acute or subacute bacterial endocarditis usually present with primarily constitutional symptoms, such as weakness, anorexia, and fatigue. Patients with acute bacterial endocarditis (ABE) tend to seek medical attention because of a nonspecific illness of recent onset; the abrupt appearance of fever, rigors, prostration, myalgias, or arthralgias; or the development of symptoms produced by metastatic infection, such as meningitis, pneumonia, and brain abscess. Aged individuals with subacute bacterial endocarditis (SBE) typically experience a chronic illness of insidious onset that is characterized by anorexia, inanition, and malaise; these vague and debilitating symptoms are often attributed to the aging process itself or to occult malignancy. Backache, peripheral vascular occlusion, congestive heart failure, renal insufficiency, and central nervous system disease—such as confusion, sterile meningitis, stroke, and coma—are manifestations of SBE that often precipitate hospitalization and evaluation.

Over 90% of aged patients with infective endocarditis exhibit fever; in both ABE and SBE, however, the temperature elevation is often mild and intermittent and frequently goes undetected by the patient and family. The physical examination reveals a cardiac murmur in 70–80% of elderly patients with infective endocarditis. These murmurs have often been present for years and rarely demonstrate clinically recognizable changes over time. In the absence of any cardiac murmur, the diagnosis of bacterial endocarditis is invariably delayed until postmortem examination. Osler's nodes and Janeway's lesions are rarely observed, but splenomegaly, splinter hemorrhages, and retinal abnormalities appear to occur as frequently in elderly patients as they do in younger individuals.

Laboratory Findings

Routine laboratory investigation typically reveals anemia and an elevated erythrocyte sedimentation rate (ESR). The polymorphonuclear leukocyte count can be normal or elevated; extreme leukocytosis has been associated with ABE and a high mortality. Microscopic hematuria is observed in the majority of elderly patients with bacterial endocarditis. Blood cultures will detect the offending pathogen in 80–90% of these cases, if three sets of aerobic and anaerobic cultures are obtained on the first and second hospital days. Prior antimicrobial administration represents the most frequent explanation for sterile blood cultures; other factors that can impede the isolation of the offending pathogen include infection involving the tricuspid valve, the presence of organisms that possess unusual growth requirements, such as thiol-dependent streptococci, and inadequate bacteriologic techniques, such as failure to perform blind subcultures or to observe the culture bottles for a minimum of 2 weeks. In the case of an elderly patient with suspected bacterial endocarditis and sterile blood cultures, isolation of the organism can occasionally be facilitated if hyperosmolar media are employed or bone marrow aspirates cultured. Rheumatoid factor appears in approximately 50% of patients with untreated endocarditis of 6 or more weeks' duration, but this serologic finding is also present in 30% of healthy persons 65 years of age or older. In untreated patients with infective endocarditis, the rheumatoid factor titer rises rapidly, but in the healthy aged person, it remains stable for years; thus, serial determinations must be performed for meaningful interpretation. The detection of cryoglobulins, teichoic acid antibodies, intraleukocyte bacteria in the peripheral blood, phagocytic reticuloendothelial cells in blood from an earlobe, or valvular vegetations by M-mode or cross-sectional echocardiography can lend considerable support to a presumptive diagnosis of bacterial endocarditis.

Pathophysiology

Isolated aortic valve endocarditis occurs twice as commonly in elderly patients as in younger individuals and accounts for 30–40% of the cases of infective endocarditis in the aged. Isolated mitral valve endocarditis (30–40%) and combined aortic and mitral valve infection (20–30%) are common. Endocarditis restricted to the pulmonic or tricuspid valve, and infection involving one of these valves plus an aortic or mitral valve, are rare. Valvular abnormalities that might predispose to infection are observed less frequently in the elderly; the most commonly detected valvular lesions include fibrocalcific changes in a bicuspid or tricuspid aortic valve and rheumatic fibrosis of the mitral valve. In 30–40%

of aged patients with infective endocarditis examined at autopsy, no underlying valvular abnormality is found. The history of an event that might have induced bacteremia and initiated endocarditis is elicited from only 20–30% of elderly patients with this infection; tooth extractions, genitourinary manipulation, abdominal surgical procedures, and intravenous catheters represent the most frequently identifiable precipitating causes. *Streptococcus viridans* and *Staphylococcus aureus* are the organisms most commonly isolated; other streptococcal strains, *Staph. epidermidis, Escherichia coli,* and *Pseudomonas aeruginosa* occasionally produce infective endocarditis in the aged. In the absence of a cardiac prosthesis, fungal endocarditis remains uncommon.

Treatment

Treatment of elderly patients with infective endocarditis consists of the parenteral administration of a bactericidal antibiotic for 4–6 weeks without interruption. The selection of appropriate antimicrobials is determined by the isolated pathogen's antibiotic susceptibility pattern; Appendix A outlines the usual therapy for specific isolates. Antimicrobial therapy of infective endocarditis is initiated on the basis of the results of routine disc susceptibility testing, but it is best monitored by determinations of the minimal bactericidal concentration (MBC) and the serum-bactericidal activity. The measurement of the MBC ensures that the selected antimicrobial is bactericidal against the offending pathogen at drug concentrations attainable by conventional dosing regimens. The serum-bactericidal test employs the patient's serum, obtained 1–2 hours after antibiotic administration. Through a series of twofold tube dilutions, the highest titer at which the serum remains bactericidal against the infecting organism is determined; a titer of at least 1 : 8 appears to be important to eradicate infection in patients with endocarditis. Because the antimicrobials employed in the therapy of bacterial endocarditis are administered in maximum doses and for prolonged periods, careful surveillance for toxicity must be performed (App. A).

Patients who remain bacteremic while receiving antibiotic therapy require prompt investigation. The serum-bactericidal activity and MBC for the antibiotics being given must be ascertained for the patient's blood isolate. The physician must review the drug orders to ensure that adequate doses of the antibiotic are being administered by the appropriate route and that other drugs that have the potential to interfere with the action of the antimicrobial are not being given concomitantly. The possibility of metastatic or myocardial abscess should be considered. Finally, antibiotic combinations that demonstrate synergistic activity should be sought, if the evaluation does not reveal a specific reason for persistent bacteremia. Persistent or recurrent fever in the aged patient receiving antibiotics can be consequent to drug reaction, metastatic infection, phlebitis, thromboembolic events, or inadequate antimicrobial therapy. Surgical intervention should be considered for the management of intractable congestive heart failure caused by valvular damage or ruptured chordae, or for the eradication of continuous bacteremia produced by persistent valvular infection or by myocardial or metastatic abscess.

When the diagnosis of infective endocarditis appears likely, but blood cultures remain sterile, a therapeutic trial of antibiotics must be considered. The abacteremic patient should be given an aminoglycoside plus ampicillin or, in the presence of significant penicillin allergy, an aminoglycoside plus vancomycin (App. A). Patients who are given a therapeutic trial of antimicrobials usually experience a resolution of fever and an amelioration of systemic symptoms within 2 weeks, if bacterial endocarditis is present.

1. Petersdorf RG, Goldman PL: Changes in the natural history of bacterial endocarditis. *J Chronic Dis* 32:287, 1979.
   The incidence of endocarditis in the aged is increasing because most persons with rheumatic valvular heart disease are reaching maturity, calcific valvular lesions represent a potential nidus for infection, and an increasing population of hospitalized elderly patients are at risk for nosocomial endocarditis.
2. Hartman TL, Myers WK: Occurrence of bacterial endocarditis in older individuals. *Geriatrics* 14:374, 1959.
   Aged patients usually respond to antibiotic therapy, as do younger individuals with infective endocarditis.
3. Wallach JB, et al: Bacterial endocarditis in the aged. *Ann Intern Med* 42:1206, 1955.
   A presentation of autopsied cases with an extensive review of a previous series of infective endocarditis in the elderly.

4. Anderson HJ, Stafforth JS: Subacute bacterial endocarditis in the elderly. *Lancet* 2:1055, 1955.
The average interval from the time of apparent onset to diagnosis was found to be 2.6 months in patients 40–49 years of age, 2.9 months in patients 50–59 years, 5.6 months in those 60–69 years, and 10 months in patients 70–79 years of age.
5. Watanakunakoin C, Tan JS: Diagnostic difficulties of staphylococcal endocarditis in geriatric patients. *Geriatrics* 28:168, 1973.
Endocarditis should be suspected when S. aureus *bacteremia is detected in the aged patient with anorexia, nausea, vomiting, and mental deterioration.*
6. Habte-Gabr E, January LE, Smith IM: Bacterial endocarditis. The need for early diagnosis. *Geriatrics* 29:164, 1973.
In one third of the elderly patients, the diagnosis was made either late in the course of the infection or at postmortem examination.
7. Thell R, Martin FH, Edwards JE: Bacterial endocarditis in subjects 60 years of age and older. *Circulation* 51:174, 1975.
In the absence of a cardiac murmur, the diagnosis of infective endocarditis is rarely considered in the elderly patient with fever.
8. Rubin RH, Fallon JT: Case records of the Massachusetts General Hospital. *N Engl J Med* 303:627, 1980.
Pacemakers as well as prosthetic valves may become infected and produce bacterial endocarditis.
9. Ziment I: Nervous system complications in bacterial endocarditis. *Am J Med* 47:593, 1969.
A comprehensive review.
10. Churchill MS, Geraci JE, Hunter GG: Musculoskeletal manifestations of bacterial endocarditis. *Ann Intern Med* 87:754, 1977.
Arthralgias, arthritis, low back pain, or myalgias may represent the first or only symptoms of infective endocarditis.
11. Sande MA, Scheld WM: Combination antibiotic therapy of bacterial endocarditis. *Ann Intern Med* 92:390, 1980.
A review of synergistic antibiotic treatment of infective endocarditis caused by Streptococcus faecalis *and other bacteria.*
12. Cannady PB, Sanford JP: Negative blood cultures in infective endocarditis. *S Med J* 69:1420, 1976.
13. Gleckman RA: Culture negative endocarditis: Confirming the diagnosis. *Am Heart J* 94:125, 1977.
Reviews on the approach to patients with suspected endocarditis but negative blood cultures.
14. Everett, ED, Hirschmann JV: Transient bacteremia and endocarditis prophylaxis. *Medicine* 56:61, 1977.
A comprehensive review of the indications for antibiotic prophylaxis for bacterial endocarditis.
15. Bayer, AS, et al: Use of circulating immune complex levels in the serodifferentiation of enterocarditic and nonenterocarditic septicemias. *Am J Med* 66:58, 1979.
Discusses the role of circulating immune complexes as an adjunctive diagnostic test.
16. Applefeld MM, Hornich RB: Infective endocarditis in patients over age 60. *Am Heart J* 88:90, 1974.
17. Cummings V, et al: Subacute bacterial endocarditis in the older age group. *JAMA* 172:137, 1960.
The case fatality rate for geriatric patients was greater than 70% in these two series. This grave prognosis was attributed to difficulties in establishing a diagnosis, delays in initiating therapy, and the presence of serious associated illness.
18. Tan JS, et al: *Streptococcus viridans* endocarditis: Favorable prognosis in geriatric patients. *Geriatrics* 28:68, 1973.
In this report, the case fatality rate was identical in aged and younger patients.

28. PULMONARY TUBERCULOSIS

Anthony L. Esposito and Richard A. Gleckman

During the past three decades, the number of newly diagnosed cases of active tuberculosis in the United States has steadily declined. Concomitantly, the incidence of a positive delayed cutaneous hypersensitivity response to purified protein derivative (PPD) has diminished in young persons. Tuberculosis in the elderly remains a significant problem, however. Epidemiologic data demonstrate that the incidence of PPD reactivity increases dramatically with age: In the United States, the reactor rate appears to be five or six times greater for persons 60 years of age or older than for individuals 20–30 years of age. Because a positive PPD identifies persons with arrested infection with *Mycobacterium tuberculosis* and, more significantly, those individuals at highest risk for developing active tuberculosis, it is apparent that the major reservoir for this disease resides in the elderly. Indeed, the peak tuberculosis case rate in the United States occurs in patients 65 years of age or older.

Pathogenesis

Infection with *M. tuberculosis* invariably results from the inhalation of infectious aerosolized droplets of minute size produced by the cough of a patient with pulmonary tuberculosis. The person not previously exposed to the tubercle bacillus has immunologic defenses that are initially inadequate to prevent multiplication of the organism in the lungs. Lymphatics transport the tubercle bacilli from the pulmonary parenchyma to regional lymph nodes, and vascular dissemination subsequently occurs. The upper lung zones, kidneys, meninges, and epiphyses provide unusually favorable environments for bacterial multiplication. On occasion, local pulmonary host defenses become overwhelmed, and extensive lung disease results. Approximately 1 month after the initial infection, immunity develops and bacterial multiplication becomes arrested; however, not all mycobacteria are destroyed. Many viable organisms remain dormant for decades; these mycobacteria represent a perpetual threat of subsequent active infection.

Detection of Infection

The intracutaneous injection of Tween-stabilized purified protein derivative (PPD-S) is the most reliable technique available for detecting infection with *M. tuberculosis*. A *positive* response is indicated by the development of 10 mm or more of induration to the injection of 0.1 cc of intermediate-strength (5 TU) PPD-S. Lesser degrees of induration are designated as *doubtful* (5–9 mm) or *negative* (0–4 mm); doubtful reactions can result from infection with either *M. tuberculosis* or atypical mycobacteria, and individuals demonstrating such a reaction should be retested with PPD-S. Induration produced by second-strength (250 TU) PPD-S must be interpreted with caution, since such responses can result from cross-sensitization to atypical mycobacteria or as a nonspecific reaction to the antigen. Conversely, a negative response to second-strength PPD-S in the nonanergic aged person usually excludes the diagnosis of active tuberculosis. The delayed cutaneous hypersensitivity response can transiently diminish in magnitude or disappear entirely in the presence of malnutrition, fever, viral infection, immunosuppressive drugs, or overwhelming tuberculosis. Patients over the age of 55 years who demonstrate a doubtful or negative response to initial testing with intermediate-strength PPD-S may exhibit a typically positive reaction upon retesting; this is referred to as the *booster phenomenon*. In this circumstance, a positive response to PPD-S does not represent recent primary infection (i.e., conversion), but simply reflects a diminished antigenic responsiveness that occurs secondary to an age-associated attenuation in immunologic function and that can be overcome by repeated antigenic challenge.

Active Tuberculosis

Reactivation of dormant tubercle bacilli accounts for 90% of newly diagnosed cases of active tuberculosis in the elderly. The risk of developing active disease is greatest in the first year after primary infection and has been estimated to be 3–4%. Although the subsequent yearly risk is considerably smaller, that risk is cumulative; thus, 4–6% of patients with a positive reaction to PPD will develop active tuberculosis during their lifetime. Moreover, the chance of active disease evolving increases substantially for all years after the primary infection, when roentgenographic evidence of healed tuberculosis exists. Factors that augment the probability of reactivation include alcoholism, diabetes mellitus, lymphoreticular malignancies, cancer, and immunosuppressive drugs. How much age-associated alterations in immune competency may predispose to reactivation is speculative.

Active tuberculosis can occur in any of the organs that were infiltrated with *M. tuberculosis* during the primary infection. The lungs, lymph nodes, kidneys, bones, and meninges represent the most common sites of postprimary infection in the elderly. Occasionally a geriatric patient can present with disseminated infection. In general, the signs and symptoms of active tuberculosis in the elderly tend to be less prominent than those exhibited by younger persons, regardless of the site of reactivation.

Prophylaxis

Active tuberculosis can be prevented by treating patients who manifest a positive response to PPD with isoniazid (INH). However, enthusiasm for widespread prophylaxis is tempered by the recognition that INH can produce hepatitis, liver failure, and death. The risk of developing INH hepatitis increases with age. The frequency of this complication is 2.3% in patients 55 years of age or older, against 0.3% for persons 24–34 years of age and 1.2% for individuals 35–49 years of age. Thus, when chemoprophylaxis is considered for an aged person, the projected risks of INH hepatitis must be weighed against the probability of active tuberculosis.

The following recommendation is adapted from the Guidelines on Tuberculosis Chemoprophylaxis established by the American Thoracic Society, the medical section of the American Lung Association. One year of INH (300 mg daily as a single dose, without interruption) should be considered for patients 65 years of age or older who exhibit a positive response to PPD **and** who demonstrate radiographic evidence of nonprogressive pulmonary infection, who have recently been infected, who have been exposed to household members or close associates with active pulmonary tuberculosis, or who appear to be at high risk of developing active infection because of corticosteroid or immunosuppressive therapy, leukemia or lymphoma, gastrectomy, diabetes mellitus, or silicosis. Many authorities believe, however, that the risk of INH-induced hepatotoxicity constitutes an absolute contraindication to chemoprophylaxis for geriatric patients. They emphasize the difficulty of distinguishing between a recent tuberculin conversion and a booster phenomenon, and they argue that once an aged patient is identified as PPD-reactive, careful clinical, bacteriologic, and radiographic monitoring will allow detection of active infection. Finally, these authorities stress the fact that tuberculosis remains a disease eminently responsive to antimicrobials. Regardless of whether or not the physician caring for an aged person with a positive PPD elects to administer a year of INH chemoprophylaxis, efforts must be made to ensure that active infection is not already present. If the chest roentgenogram demonstrates fibrocalcific changes of the apices, or if urinalysis reveals unexplained hematuria or pyuria, sputum and urine should be obtained for acid-fast staining and culture. Appendix A outlines recommendations for the surveillance of patients receiving INH.

Diagnosis

Fever, weight loss, malaise, and productive cough are the usual symptoms associated with active pulmonary tuberculosis in the elderly. The significance of these symptoms is not always apparent to the aged person and family, however. The chest roentgenogram of elderly patients with active pulmonary tuberculosis frequently fails to reveal the presence of a discrete new infiltrate, but it almost invariably demonstrates apical fibrosis or pleural or parenchymal calcifications; the significance of these latter abnormalities is often overlooked, because they are assumed to represent "inactive" or "old" granulomatous disease. On occasion, an aged person presents with endobronchial tuberculosis and a normal-appearing chest roentgenogram or nonspecific nodule. Among elderly patients with pulmonary tuberculosis, 80–85% will demonstrate a positive response to PPD-S; those patients who fail to respond often have malnutrition, extreme debility, or overwhelming infection and usually exhibit anergy to most common antigens. Aged patients in whom the diagnosis of tuberculosis is strongly considered should be retested with second-strength PPD-S (250 TU), if the intermediate-strength challenge (5 TU) elicits a negative or doubtful reaction; a negative response to second-strength PPD-S does not completely eliminate the possibility of tuberculosis, but other diagnostic considerations should be pursued, especially when the patient is not anergic.

The diagnosis of pulmonary tuberculosis is established by the identification of acid-fast bacilli in pulmonary secretions and by the isolation of *M. tuberculosis* in culture. When the diagnosis of pulmonary tuberculosis is considered, multiple collections of pulmonary secretions should be performed; sputum should be induced or obtained by transtracheal aspiration from those aged persons who cannot spontaneously produce secretions. Occasionally the organism can be isolated from early morning gastric aspirates of a patient whose sputum examination is negative.

When considered, the diagnosis of pulmonary tuberculosis usually can be established or excluded quickly. In the occasional case of an elderly patient whose chest roentgenogram is suggestive but whose evaluation remains unproductive, however, confirmation of the diagnosis may be prolonged. When the patient manifests progressive deterioration, therapy should be initiated while appropriate investigative procedures are being performed.

Therapy

Isoniazid remains the cornerstone of antituberculous therapy and shoud be included in all initial treatment regimens. Elderly patients with active pulmonary tuberculosis should be given INH, 300 mg daily, plus ethambutol, 15 mg/kg daily, for 2 years without interruption. Alternatively, such patients may be treated with two bactericidal drugs (INH and rifampin) daily for 9 months. Patients seriously ill with extensive disease probably should receive an additional antimicrobial, such as streptomycin (0.5–1.0 gm daily IM) or rifampin (600 mg daily PO), for 2–3 months. The toxicities and surveillance recommendations for these antituberculous medications are outlined in Appendix A.

Elderly patients with pulmonary tuberculosis who appear clinically well, experience minimal cough, and are reliable can be discharged 14–21 days after initiation of antituberculous therapy; these patients are not highly infectious, even though sputum smears and cultures remain positive. Nursing home residents, severely debilitated individuals, and patients who are noncompliant or who have difficulty controlling their pulmonary secretions require more prolonged hospitalization. The initial follow-up evaluation occurs within 1 month of discharge and should include a repeat chest roentgenogram as well as sputum smears and cultures. Subsequent evaluations should be conducted approximately every 4–6 weeks for 6 months, then every 3–4 months for the duration of the antituberculous therapy. Elderly patients must be instructed repeatedly on the importance of drug compliance and the necessity of promptly reporting any symptoms suggestive of INH hepatitis; these include unexplained fever, weakness, fatigue, anorexia, nausea, or vomiting.

Cases of active pulmonary tuberculosis must be reported to the local public health authorities. Notification ensures that close contacts of the infected patient receive appropriate screening and adequate prophylaxis for tuberculosis.

---

1. Stead WW: Pathogenesis of the sporadic case of tuberculosis. *N Engl J Med* 277:1008, 1967.
2. Kasik JE, Schaldt S: Why tuberculosis is still a health problem in the aged. *Geriatrics* 25:63, 1977.
3. Glassroth J, Robbins AG, Snider EE Jr: Tuberculosis in the 1980's. *N Engl J Med* 302:1441, 1980.

   Readings 1-3 discuss the epidemiology and the magnitude of the problem of tuberculosis in the aged.
4. Dubrow EL: Reactivation of tuberculosis: A problem of aging. *J Am Geriatr Soc* 24:481, 1976.
5. Geboes K, Bossaert H: Reactivation of tuberculosis in old age. *J Am Geriatr Soc* 25:318, 1977.

   These reports illustrate that reactivation of pulmonary tuberculosis may occur 20–50 years after the initial diagnosis in patients who receive inadequate chemotherapy.
6. Stead WW: Tuberculosis among elderly persons: An outbreak in a nursing home. *Ann Intern Med* 94:606, 1981.

   An epidemic of tuberculosis in a nursing home resulted in many tuberculin conver-

sions, clinical tuberculosis, and even death in both residents and employees. Atypical clinical and roentgenographic manifestations contributed to the spread of infection.

7. Novick A, et al: Tuberculin skin testing in a chronically sick aged population. *J Am Geriatr Soc* 20:455, 1972.
   The significance of a negative reaction to even very large doses of PPD should be viewed in the context of the overall clinical picture when dealing with debilitated patients.
8. Thompson NJ, et al: The booster phenomenon in serial tuberculin testing. *Am Rev Respir Dis* 119:587, 1979.
   The booster phenomenon was observed most often in the elderly. Persons in chronic care facilities should have a second tuberculin test administered 1 week after the first before they are designated as tuberculin negative.
9. Comstock GW, Edwards PQ: The competing risks of tuberculosis and hepatitis for adult tuberculin reactors. *Am Rev Respir Dis* 111:573, 1975.
   A salient review of the data on isoniazid (INH) chemoprophylaxis.
10. Johnston RF, Wildrick KH: The impact of chemotherapy on the care of patients with tuberculosis. *Am Rev Respir Dis* 109:636, 1974.
    An extensive review of the diagnosis and contemporary management of patients with tuberculosis.
11. Stead WW, Datt AK: What's new in tuberculosis? *Am J Med* 71:1, 1981.
    Includes a discussion of short-course chemotherapy regimens.
12. Alexander WJ, et al: Simple primary tuberculosis in an elderly woman. *J Am Geriatr Soc* 27:123, 1979.
    The presence of an infiltrate and enlarged hilar lymph nodes on chest radiography suggests the possibility of primary tuberculosis.

29. EXTRAPULMONARY TUBERCULOSIS

Anthony L. Esposito and Richard A. Gleckman

Osteoarticular Tuberculosis

A common manifestation of extrapulmonary infection, osteoarticular tuberculosis is invariably caused by the reactivation of a previously dormant focus that resulted from hematogenous dissemination during the primary infection. Younger adults with osteoarticular infection often have concomitant active pulmonary or renal tuberculosis or display roentgenographic evidence of prior pulmonary infection; the most frequently involved sites in these adults include the vertebral bodies, hip, and knee. Elderly patients with osteoarticular tuberculosis less commonly manifest roentgenographic evidence of prior infection, rarely experience concomitant active renal or pulmonary disease, and often demonstrate unusual sites of infection such as the humerus, ribs, and sternoclavicular joint.

The pathologic lesion consists of a combination of osteomyelitis and contiguous arthritis. Destruction of articular cartilage results from a pannus of granulation tissue but proceeds slowly; consequently, the joint space tends to be preserved. In advanced disease, paraosseous abscesses (cold abscesses) and sinus tracts can form.

Diagnosis. The insidious onset and subtle manifestations of osteoarticular tuberculosis in the elderly frequently result in delays in diagnosis. Often months or years pass, and advanced joint destruction and severe functional disability supervene, before a correct diagnosis becomes established. Most aged patients complain of joint or bone pain and deny constitutional symptoms. The physical examination usually reveals localized tenderness and swelling over the involved bone or joint. Weight-bearing joints often demonstrate a limited range of motion and synovial thickening or effusion. Chronic draining sinuses can be present. Roentgenographic findings include soft tissue swelling, localized areas of subchondral osteoporosis, and relative preservation of the joint space. Multiple skeletal areas can be involved simultaneously, and the patient can present with multiple osteolytic lesions.

Patients with osteoarticular tuberculosis uniformly demonstrate a positive response to either intermediate-strength (5 TU) or second-strength (250 TU) PPD-S. In the elderly, nonanergic patient, a negative tuberculin skin test should alert the physician to the possibility of an alternative diagnosis, such as primary or metastatic carcinoma, multiple myeloma, or disseminated fungal infection. Confirmation of the diagnosis usually requires culture and acid-fast smears of synovial fluid, drainage from open sinuses, or aspirates of "cold abscesses." On occasion, bone or synovial biopsy must be performed to isolate the organism.

Therapy. If clinical manifestations and histologic examination of biopsy material are consistent with the diagnosis of tuberculosis, therapy should be administered while confirmatory culture results are awaited. Antimicrobial treatment is identical to that for pulmonary tuberculosis. Surgical intervention is reserved for the prevention of deformity, the improvement of function, and the eradication of infection that has not responded to antibiotics.

Renal Tuberculosis

Tuberculosis of the urinary tract usually results from the breakdown of foci acquired by hematogenous dissemination during the primary infection. Elderly patients with this disorder typically present with signs or symptoms of urinary tract disease, such as dysuria, hematuria, or flank pain; systemic complaints of fever, anorexia, or weight loss are usually not prominent. Some individuals with renal tuberculosis experience no symptoms and undergo evaluation because of abnormalities noted on a routine urinalysis.

Diagnosis. The chest roentgenogram demonstrates lesions consistent with inactive tuberculosis in 60–70% of elderly patients with active renal tuberculosis; typical roentgenographic findings include apical fibrosis and pleural or parenchymal calcification. More than 90% of patients with renal tuberculosis will have either pyuria (5 WBC/high power field) or hematuria (5 RBC/high power field) or both on routine urinalysis. Excretory urography frequently reveals nondiagnostic abnormalities, such as calyceal dilatation, papillary necrosis, cortical scarring, or parenchymal calcifications; renal cavitation, urethral strictures, or multiple deformities of the upper and lower urinary tract are less commonly observed but represent extremely valuable clues to the presence of tuberculosis. Virtually all patients with this infection exhibit a positive tuberculin reaction to either intermediate-strength (5 TU) or second-strength (250 TU) PPD-S.

The diagnosis of renal tuberculosis will be confirmed in 90% of patients with the disease, if 3 first-morning-urine specimens are cultured for *Mycobacterium tuberculosis;* 24-hour urine collections are reserved for those patients with suspected renal tuberculosis in whom first-morning-urine cultures are negative.

Therapy. The antimicrobial therapy for this disease is identical to that for pulmonary infection. The role of surgical intervention remains controversial; in general, nephrectomy should be reserved for the treatment of patients with advanced unilateral renal tuberculosis complicated by hemorrhage, intractable pain, severe hypertension of recent onset, bacterial superinfection recalcitrant to antimicrobial therapy, and persistent tuberculous infection unresponsive to chemotherapy. In addition to periodic evaluation for signs of drug toxicity (App. A), elderly patients should have repeat urine cultures to ensure that eradication of the infection has occurred, as well as periodic intravenous pyelograms to detect the appearance of urethral strictures that can develop during or following therapy.

Miliary Tuberculosis

Disseminated tuberculosis in the elderly results from the recrudescence of a previously established focus, usually a lymph node. Originating from this lesion, massive numbers of tubercle bacilli invade the bloodstream, embolize to the capillary beds of many organs, and form granulomas. The peak incidence of miliary tuberculosis is found at a younger age than 65 years; nevertheless, elderly patients with this disease experience more prolonged delays in diagnosis and a greater mortality than do younger individuals.

Symptoms. Geriatric patients with miliary tuberculosis usually present with nonspecific constitutional symptoms, such as weakness, fatigue, anorexia, or weight loss. These symptoms are often insidious in onset and tend to be present weeks before the patient seeks medical attention. Intermittent, low-grade fever occurs in most elderly patients with disseminated tuberculosis, and fever of unknown origin (FUO) represents a common reason for hospitalization and investigation. Localized symptoms, such as headache and abdominal pain, and suggestive physical findings, such as choroidal tubercles, lymphadenopathy, and signs of meningitis or peritonitis, are noted infrequently in the aged.

Laboratory Findings. Routine laboratory investigation typically reveals an anemia, neutropenia, or monocytosis; pancytopenia and leukemoid reactions rarely occur. Elevation of the erythrocyte sedimentation rate and of serum alkaline phosphatase is frequently observed. Although a miliary pattern will be present on the initial or subsequent chest roentgenograms of virtually all younger adults with disseminated tuberculosis, similar roentgenographic evidence of the infection may never appear in aged patients; these elderly individuals with "cryptic" dissemination usually remain undiagnosed during life. Sixty to seventy-five percent of elderly patients with miliary tuberculosis, including those patients with "cryptic" disease, will exhibit a positive response to either intermediate- (5 TU) or second-strength (250 TU) PPD on initial testing; eventually 80–90% of these patients will demonstrate a positive tuberculin reaction.

Confirmation of the diagnosis of disseminated tuberculosis requires isolation of *M. tuberculosis*. Sputum, gastric washings, and urine represent accessible specimens that should be obtained for smear and culture. In the presence of meningeal signs or an abnormal neurologic examination, cerebrospinal fluid should be stained by a concentration technique and cultured for *M. tuberculosis;* similarly, when pleural effusions or ascites is detected, pleural and peritoneal biopsy material, as well as fluid, should be secured for analysis and culture. Percutaneous liver biopsy represents the single most helpful diagnostic procedure to confirm the diagnosis of miliary tuberculosis; in approximately 90% of patients with the infection, the liver biopsy will yield noncaseating granulomas, even in the absence of significant hepatomegaly or abnormalities in liver function tests. However, because other disorders such as brucellosis, sarcoidosis, lymphoma, infectious mononucleosis, and drug reactions can be associated with hepatic granulomas; and because in most cases of miliary tuberculosis, acid-fast bacilli cannot be identified histologically in tissue section and, on occasion, *M. tuberculosis* cannot be grown in culture; the results of the liver biopsy must be interpreted in conjunction with the entire clinical picture. In some cases the diagnosis of miliary tuberculosis will be established by histologic examination and culture of tissue obtained by bone marrow, lymph node, pleural, peritoneal, or transbronchial lung biopsy. Bone marrow biopsy is the diagnostic procedure of choice when a patient's abnormalities of hemostasis prohibit liver biopsy; this test should be performed by trephine biopsy to ensure that an adequate specimen for histologic and microbiologic evaluation is secured.

Therapy. If the diagnosis of miliary tuberculosis appears likely, chemotherapy should be initiated while diagnostic procedures are being performed and before extreme cachexia, respiratory failure, or neurologic dysfunction supervenes. Treatment of this disease consists of the continuous administration for 2 years of INH (300 mg/day PO) plus either ethambutol (15–25 mg/kg/day in a single dose) or rifampin (600 mg/day in a single dose); like INH, these latter two antimicrobials penetrate most tissues and fluids, including the cerebrospinal fluid, in therapeutic concentrations. In addition, a third antituberculous drug, such as streptomycin (10–15 mg/kg/day in a single IM dose), should be added for the initial 2–3 months of chemotherapy. The role of corticosteroids remains controversial; in general, corticosteroids appear to be effective in reducing cerebral edema and in preventing cerebral herniation but should be employed only when other drugs, such as mannitol or urea, fail to effect an appropriate response. Because elderly patients with miliary tuberculosis so frequently have inanition, vigorous attempts, including total parenteral nutrition, should be made to improve their nutritional state. In addition, attention must be directed toward detecting subtle signs or symptoms suggestive of drug toxicity in these debilitated and often depressed patients (App. A). The guidelines outlined for the follow-up care of elderly patients with active pulmonary tuberculosis apply also to aged persons with miliary disease.

---

1. Hunt DD: Problems in diagnosing osteoarticular tuberculosis. *JAMA* 190:95, 1964.
Unusual sites of involvement, the lack of detectable pulmonary involvement, secondary pyogenic infections, and the absence of classical roentgenographic signs resulted in delays in diagnosis.
2. Davidson PT, Horowitz Z: Skeletal tuberculosis: A review with patient presentations and discussion. *Am J Med* 48:77, 1970.

A previous history of tuberculosis or exposure should be sought, and tuberculin testing should be performed in elderly patients with destructive monoarticular arthritis.

3. Wallace R, Cohen AS: Tuberculosis arthritis. *Am J Med* 61:277, 1976.
Of patients with tuberculosis arthritis 20% will have a positive synovial fluid acid-fast smear for tubercle bacilli, 80% will have positive synovial fluid cultures, and greater than 90% will have synovial biopsy specimens that are diagnostic.
4. Meade RH, Hyslop NE Jr, Putschar WG: Case records of the Massachusetts General Hospital. *N Engl J Med* 294:267, 1976.
Discusses an elderly man with tuberculous osteomyelitis of the femur, arthritis of the hip, and tuberculous otitis media.
5. Simon HB, et al: Genitourinary tuberculosis. *Am J Med* 63:410, 1977.
Male genital tuberculosis often presents as a mass in the epididymis, testicle, or prostate, and female infection can be manifested by pelvic pain or abnormal vaginal bleeding.
6. Schulze K, Warner HA, Murray D: Intestinal tuberculosis. *Am J Med* 63:735, 1977.
The diagnosis of intestinal tuberculosis should be considered in an aged patient with recent onset of inflammatory bowel disease.
7. Foster GS, Badger TL, Galdabihi JJ: Case records of the Massachusetts General Hospital. *N Engl J Med* 303:445, 1980.
An elderly patient with ileocecal tuberculosis carried the incorrect diagnosis of Crohn's disease for 51 years.
8. Munt PW: Miliary tuberculosis in the chemotherapy era: With a clinical review in 69 American adults. *Medicine* 51:139, 1971.
9. Sahn S, Neff TA: Miliary tuberculosis. *Am J Med* 56:495, 1974.
Readings 8 and 9 are comprehensive reviews.
10. Proudfoot AT, et al: Miliary tuberculosis in adults. *Br Med J* 2:273, 1976.
Miliary mottling on chest roentgenograph may be absent in aged patients with disseminated tuberculosis.
11. Peel AL: Peripheral tuberculous lymphadenitis in the elderly. *Br J Surg* 59:568, 1972.
Tuberculous adenitis in the aged can occur in the absence of acute infection elsewhere, usually involves cervical nodes, and may require lymph node excision for cure.

30. COMMUNITY-ACQUIRED BACTERIAL PNEUMONIA

Anthony L. Esposito and Richard A. Gleckman

Etiology

Clinicians have traditionally assumed that *Streptococcus pneumoniae,* the pneumococcus, causes virtually all community-acquired bacterial pneumonia in the elderly. Recent epidemiologic and bacteriologic observations do not support that assumption, however. *Haemophilus influenzae* has emerged as a significant etiologic agent in the elderly and represents the second most commonly isolated bacterium from patients 60 years of age or older with community-acquired pneumonia. Although infection with *H. influenzae* can occur in previously healthy aged persons, the majority of patients with this disorder have chronic underlying disorders, such as lung cancer, obstructive pulmonary disease, and alcoholism. The mortality from *H. influenzae* pneumonia has been correlated with age, presence of bacteremia, serious associated disease, and inappropriate antibiotic selection.

Community-acquired aspiration pneumonia is an infection usually produced by anaerobic bacteria. Aspiration pneumonitis occurs primarily in geriatric patients with dysphagia or an altered state of consciousness. The organisms most frequently isolated from patients with community-acquired aspiration pneumonia include *Bacteroides melaninogenicus, Fusobacterium nucleatum,* and various species of *Peptostreptococcus* and *Peptococcus.* The clinical and roentgenographic manifestations of *H. influenzae* and anaerobic pneumonitis are indistinguishable from those of pneumococcal pneumonia. Nursing home residents requiring hospitalization for bacterial pneumonia, especially those individuals who have previously received antibiotics, are frequently infected by *Klebsiella pneumoniae* or *Staphylococcus aureus*. Thus, although *Strep. pneumoniae* remains the pathogen most commonly isolated from aged patients with community-acquired infection, a number of other organisms contribute significantly to this disease.

Antibiotic Therapy

Gram stain and culture of sputum traditionally guide initial selection of antibiotics. Many elderly patients, however, are incapable of expectorating lower respiratory tract secretions. In addition, meaningful interpretation of expectorated sputum is hindered by the inevitable contamination of the sputum specimen by oropharyngeal flora; thus, the value of the stained and cultured specimen appears to be limited. Transtracheal aspiration eliminates the upper respiratory tract contamination but remains a procedure that is not widely employed. The diagnostic evaluation of the aged patient with community-acquired pneumonia must also include cultures of blood and pleural fluid and smears of sputum or acid-fast bacteria; additionally, acute phase sera should be secured and frozen for possible subsequent immunologic testing.

The initial selection of antibiotics for the aged patient with community-acquired pneumonia will be guided by a knowledge of the patient's environment prior to hospitalization, the presence of underlying disease and the results of the Gram stain of quality sputum. When adequate sputum is not available, or when the establishment of a definitive microbiologic diagnosis appears unlikely, cefamandole, and not penicillin or erythromycin, should be considered standard treatment for the non–penicillin-sensitive patient. This new cephalosporin derivative has an enhanced spectrum of activity as compared to cephalothin sodium or cefazolin and appears to have retained the safety that characterizes the cephalosporin family of drugs. Cefamandole is bactericidal for *Strep. pneumoniae, Staph. aureus, H. influenzae,* including most beta-lactamase–producing strains that are resistant to ampicillin, *Klebsiella species,* and those anaerobic bacteria implicated in community-acquired aspiration pneumonia. It should be administered parenterally in doses of 1–2 gm q4h for patients with life-threatening infections, such as staphylococcal and *Klebsiella* pneumonia, and at a dose of 1 gm q6h for less threatening situations, such as presumed pneumococcal or aspiration anaerobic pneumonia. Cefamandole should not be administered to patients known to be allergic to penicillin.

When the diagnosis of pneumococcal pneumonia appears certain, penicillin remains the antibiotic of choice. Patients with uncomplicated pneumococcal pneumonia should be treated with penicillin G, 600,000 units q6–8h IV; erythromycin (500 mg q6h IV) can be given to patients who are penicillin-sensitive. Elderly patients with adequate clinical and microbiologic evidence to substantiate the diagnosis of aspiration pneumonia should also be treated with penicillin G (10–12 million units daily IV); clindamycin (300–600 mg q6h IV) can be substituted for penicillin in the case of patients with penicillin allergy. Finally, aged patients with documented gram-negative bacillary pneumonia (e.g., *K. pneumoniae, E. coli, P. mirabilis*) should be treated with an aminoglycoside plus either a cephalosporin or a newer semisynthetic penicillin (azlocillin, mezlocillin, or piperacillin) to which the isolate is sensitive.

Supportive Measures. The treatment of bacterial pneumonia requires supportive measures in addition to specific antimicrobials. Adequate hydration and nutrition appear to be essential. Metabolic derangements, such as hyperglycemia, azotemia, and alkalosis, should be corrected promptly. Hypoxemia or conditions that interfere with tissue oxygenation, such as congestive heart failure, must be reversed. Serial determinations of arterial blood gases are invaluable for evaluating patients with respiratory insufficiency and for monitoring the response to supplemental oxygen administration; arterial oxygen tensions should be maintained at greater than 65 mm Hg. Chest physiotherapy and intermittent positive-pressure breathing do not appear to accelerate the rate of resolution of the infection but can be considered as ancillary treatment.

Differential Diagnosis

When elderly patients do not respond to antibiotic therapy and supportive measures, alternative diagnosis should be considered. The entities that can simulate community-acquired acute bacterial pneumonia in the elderly include influenza pneumonia, tuberculosis, Legionnaires' disease, and pulmonary embolism.

Pneumococcal Vaccination

In the era preceding the advent of antibiotics, polyvalent antiserums were administered for the therapy of pneumococcal infections, and vaccines were given to prevent pneumococcal disease. The efficacy of polyvalent vaccines in preventing infection caused by *Strep. pneumoniae* was clearly demonstrated in young adults, the chronically ill, and the elderly. With the introduction in the 1940s of sulfonamides and penicillin, enthusiasm for immunization quickly waned. Recently, a resurgence of interest in pneumococcal vaccination has occurred and has resulted in the release of a new polyvalent vaccine approved for use by the Food and Drug Administration.

The commercially available dodecavalent vaccine, pneumococcal polyvalent vaccine (Pneumovax), contains capsular polysaccharide antigens from pneumococcal serotypes 1, 3, 4, 6, 7, 8, 9, 12, 14, 18, 19, and 23; these serotypes account for 80% of the pneumococcal disease in the United States. Included in the vaccine are antigens from approximately two-thirds of those serotypes associated with pneumonia in the elderly. When administered to healthy aged persons, the vaccine elicits significant rises in antibody titers and induces few systemic or local reactions. However, the efficacy of the new vaccine in preventing pneumococcal infection in the chronically ill and debilitated elderly remains to be demonstrated.

Pneumovax has been recommended for elderly patients who reside in chronic care facilities or who have cardiopulmonary disease or other chronic illnesses, such as renal failure and diabetes mellitus. Some authorities suggest that all persons 50 years of age and older be vaccinated. The vaccine should be administered subcutaneously or intramuscularly as a single 0.5-ml dose; revaccination should not be performed because of a marked increase in adverse reactions associated with reinjection of the vaccine in adults.

---

1. Garb JL, et al: Differences in etiology of pneumonias in nursing home and community patients. *JAMA* 240:2169, 1978.
   Klebsiella pneumoniae, Hemophilus influenzae, *and* Staphylococcus aureus *are prominent pathogens in elderly patients with nursing home–acquired pneumonia.*
2. Ebright JR, Rytel MW: Bacterial pneumonia in the elderly. *J Am Geriatr Soc* 27:220, 1980.
   Gram-negative bacillary pneumonia occurred in 21% of aged patients with community-acquired infection and produced a 70% mortality.
3. Lavala DC: The threat of aspiration pneumonia in the aged. *Geriatrics* 3:46, 1977.
   A review of the pathogenesis, clinical manifestations, and management of aspiration pneumonitis.
4. Schwartz P: Asylyum pneumonitis. *Gerontol Clin* 15:281, 1973.
   On postmortem examination, 30% of chronically institutionalized elderly patients were found to have asylyum pneumonitis, a condition resulting from the aspiration of cooked vegetables.
5. Hirschmann JV, Lipsky BA: Pneumococcal vaccine in the United States. *JAMA* 246:1428, 1981.
   A critical review of the efficacy of the vaccine in aged patients.
6. Advisory Committee on Immunization Practices: Recommendation for pneumococcal vaccine. *MMWR* 30:411, 1981.
   The current Public Health Service recommendations are presented.
7. Everett ED, et al: *Haemophilus influenzae* pneumonia in adults. *JAMA* 238:319, 1977.
8. Berk SL, et al: Nontypable *Hemophilus influenzae* in the elderly. *Arch Intern Med* 142:537, 1982.
9. Musher DM, et al: Pneumonia and acute febrile tracheobronchitis due to *Haemophilus influenzae. Ann Intern Med* 99:444, 1983.
   Type B and nontypable strains of H. influenzae *are capable of producing lower respiratory tract infection in the elderly. Since both strains can produce beta-lactamases, all isolates should be routinely tested for ampicillin susceptibility.*
10. Ninane G, et al: Bronchopulmonary infection due to *Branhamella catarrhalis:* 11 cases assessed by transtracheal puncture. *Br Med J* 1:276, 1978.
11. West M, et al: *Branhamella catarrhalis* pneumonia. *South Med J* 75:1021, 1982.
    B. catarrhalis *is becoming recognized as an important cause of lower respiratory tract*

infection. Many strains produce beta-lactamases and consequently are resistant to penicillin, ampicillin, amoxicillin, and methicillin.

12. Esposito AL: Community-acquired bacteremic pneumococcal pneumonia. Effect of age on manifestations and outcome. *Arch Intern Med* 144:945, 1984.
In contrast to previous reports, this prospective study did not detect substantial differences in the presenting features, clinical course, or outcome between aged and younger patients.

31. HOSPITAL-ACQUIRED BACTERIAL PNEUMONIA

Anthony L. Esposito and Richard A. Gleckman

Elderly patients who are hospitalized and seriously ill rapidly undergo an alteration in their oropharyngeal flora and soon become colonized with gram-negative aerobic bacilli. The pathophysiology of colonization remains incompletely understood, but impairment of pharyngeal clearance mechanisms and local bactericidal activity appear to play important roles. Because bacterial pneumonias usually result from the inapparent aspiration of oropharyngeal contents, the significance of colonization is apparent. Clinically, gram-negative aerobic bacilli such as *Klebsiella, Pseudomonas aeruginosa, Escherichia coli,* and *Proteus* are frequently isolated from elderly patients with nosocomial pneumonias. Gram-negative aerobic bacteria are not, however, the sole pathogens responsible for hospital-acquired pneumonia; anaerobes, combinations of gram-negative bacilli and anaerobes, and gram-positive cocci such as *Staphylococcus aureus* and *Streptococcus pneumoniae* can cause nosocomial infection. *Legionella pneumophila* also produces hospital-associated bacterial pneumonia in geriatric patients.

Identification of Etiologic Agent

Earnest attempts must be made to isolate the etiologic bacterial agent from elderly patients with nosocomial pneumonia. An empiric selection of antibiotics for patients with this infection is difficult because of the complexity of the infecting flora and the unpredictability of organism susceptibility. Many hospital-acquired bacterial pneumonias occur in patients with a compromised level of consciousness; these patients include individuals who have sustained a cerebrovascular accident or who have developed stupor or coma because of metabolic disorders. Elderly patients with a depressed state of consciousness often cannot expectorate a "quality" specimen of respiratory secretions for Gram stain analysis and culture; in such cases it may be necessary to perform transtracheal aspiration or nasotracheal suctioning in order to establish definitively the bacterial etiology of the pulmonary infection. Transtracheal aspiration provides a means of obtaining lower respiratory secretions that are devoid of oropharyngeal contamination. If the patient refuses transtracheal aspiration, or if there exist contraindications to the procedure, such as a bleeding diathesis, excessive coughing, or patient uncooperativeness, initial therapy should consist of an aminoglycoside plus a cephalosporin, clindamycin, or an acylamino penicillin (piperacillin, mezlocillin, or azlocillin). Blood and pleural fluid must be cultured before antimicrobials are administered; the isolation of a pathogen from these sources will allow the selection of specific antimicrobial therapy.

Differential Diagnosis

Hospital-acquired bacterial pneumonia should be quickly differentiated from gastric aspiration and pulmonary embolism. These disorders are all characterized by the acute onset of dyspnea, tachypnea, tachycardia, fever, abnormal blood gas values, and pulmonary infiltrates and can be clinically indistinguishable. Bacterial pneumonia and pulmonary emboli frequently occur in patients with similar predisposing conditions, such as immobility and congestive heart failure; moreover, these entities cannot be differentiated by pulmonary perfusion scanning alone. The documentation of pulmonary embolism can require selective pulmonary angiography. The diagnosis of chemical pneumonitis secondary to the aspiration of gastric contents is often difficult to establish, because the aspiration usually occurs unwitnessed and the neutralization of the gastric acid content proceeds rapidly. Patients strongly suspected of having experienced gastric aspiration should be treated primarily with supplemental oxygen, if hypoxemia is present; antibiotics and corticosteroids have no role in the therapy of chemical pneumonitis.

Antibiotic Therapy

Patients with hospital-acquired pneumonia caused by *Staph. aureus* should receive oxacillin or nafcillin, 20–25 mg/kg q4h IV; the penicillin-sensitive but cephalosporin-tolerant patient should receive cephalothin, 30 mg/kg q4h. Individuals with serious reactions to penicillins and cephalosporins can be treated with vancomycin or clindamycin (App. A). Finally, patients known to be colonized with methicillin-resistant staphylococci should be given vancomycin pending results of susceptibility tests.

When gram-negative aerobic bacilli are the etiologic organisms, an aminoglycoside antibiotic should be administered, pending identification of the pathogen and susceptibility testing; the initial selection of an aminoglycoside (gentamicin, tobramycin, or amikacin) is best guided by the patterns of resistance that prevail in each hospital. The initial dose of amikacin is 7.5 mg/kg IV; and that of gentamicin and tobramycin, 1.5–1.75 mg/kg IV; subsequent administration is best monitored by assays of the peak and trough serum aminoglycoside concentrations (App. A) or, if unavailable, by determinations of the patient's creatinine clearance (App. A). Because in the aged the serum creatinine may not accurately reflect renal function, nomograms and formulas that are routinely employed to guide aminoglycoside therapy and that are based on the value of the serum creatinine alone should be avoided. Patients with pneumonia caused by *Ps. aeruginosa* should receive both an aminoglycoside and either carbenicillin, 450 mg/kg/day IV, ticarcillin, 300 mg/kg/day IV, or a new acylamino penicillin (azocillin or piperacillin) (App. A). When the pneumonia is produced by *Klebsiella,* a cephalosporin (cephalothin, cefazolin, or cefamandole) or a cephamycin (cefoxitin) can be administered in addition to an aminoglycoside; these antibiotics should be given intravenously in doses of 30 mg/kg q4h. Pipercillin and mezlocillin can also be employed with an aminoglycoside in patients with pneumonia due to *Klebsiella*. Elderly patients with nosocomial aspiration pneumonia, in whom sputum analysis proves unrewarding and blood and pleural fluid cultures remain sterile, present a difficult therapeutic problem; in general, such patients should be treated with an aminoglycoside to which the hospital's endogenous aerobic gram-negative flora are susceptible, plus clindamycin (600 mg q6h IV), a cephalosporin, or a new acylamino penicillin.

Supportive Measures

The general supportive measures for patients with nosocomial pneumonia are similar to those outlined for community-acquired infection. Because aged patients with nosocomial pneumonia often require high doses of potentially toxic antimicrobials and are exposed to antibiotic combinations known to produce untoward reactions, these patients must be carefully monitored; see Appendix A for the surveillance procedures that should be followed and for drug-antibiotic interactions that can produce serious consequences.

Pneumonia in the Intensive Care Unit

Elderly patients requiring mechanical ventilatory assistance are likely to develop gram-negative aerobic bacillary pneumonia. This infection results in part from the rapid oropharyngeal and endotracheal tube colonization that invariably occurs in critically ill patients; additionally, the reservoir nebulizers routinely employed in the care of seriously ill patients may generate aerosols contaminated with the more virulent and antibiotic-resistant gram-negative bacilli found in a hospital environment.

A diagnosis of pneumonia is usually established by the demonstration of a new infiltrate on chest roentgenogram in the presence of fever and purulent pulmonary secretions. Other disorders that can mimic bacterial pneumonia in the intubated patient include atelectasis, pulmonary edema, pulmonary emboli, and the adult respiratory distress syndrome. Distinguishing these disorders from bacterial pneumonia can be difficult; the identification of polymorphonuclear leukocytes and gram-negative bacilli on a Gram stain of sputum does not necessarily imply infection. The onset of a pulmonary infection appears to be best detected by a careful daily assessment of the gross and microscopic appearance of the pulmonary secretions and by frequent roentgenographic evaluation.

The general supportive measures and specific antibiotic therapies are identical to those prescribed for patients with hospital-acquired gram-negative pneumonias.

1. Valenti WM, Trudell RG, Bentley DW: Factors predisposing to oropharyngeal colonization with gram-negative bacilli in the aged. *N Engl J Med* 298:1108, 1978.
The prevalence of colonization with aerobic gram-negative bacilli increases with advanced degrees of physical dependence, and those patients who are bedridden or who have respiratory disease are at greatest risk.
2. Phair JP, Kauffman CA, Bjornson A: Investigation of host defense mechanisms in the aged as determinants of nosocomial colonization and pneumonia. *J Reticuloendothel Soc* 23:397, 1977.
Correlations between alterations in host defense mechanisms and the occurrence of colonization with Staphylococcus aureus *and aerobic gram-negative bacilli could not be identified.*
3. Berk SL, et al: Transtracheal aspiration in the severely ill elderly patient with bacterial pneumonia. *J Am Geriatr Soc* 29:228, 1981.
Discusses the safety and value of transtracheal aspiration.
4. Berk SL, Gallemore GM, Smith JK: Nosocomial pneumococcal pneumonia in the elderly. *J Am Geriatr Soc* 29:319, 1981
A total of 20% of aged patients with hospital-acquired pneumonia were infected with Streptococcus pneumonia.
5. Cohen M, et al: Fatal nosocomial Legionnaires' disease: Clinical and epidemiological characteristics. *Ann Intern Med* 90:611, 1979.
Legionellosis should be considered in any aged patient with unexplained nosocomial pneumonia, especially in the setting of an outbreak of enigmatic pulmonary infection.
6. Klimek JJ, et al: Clinical, epidemiologic and bacteriologic observations of an outbreak of methicillin-resistant *Staphylococcus aureus* at a large community hospital. *Am J Med* 61:340, 1976.
Aged patients in the postoperative period or in intensive care units are at risk of developing lower respiratory tract infection due to methicillin-resistant staphylococci.
7. Gleckman RA, Hibert D: Afebrile bacteremia. A phenomenon in geriatric patients. *JAMA* 248:1478, 1982.
Aged patients with afebrile bacteremia are usually debilitated by malignancy and often succumb. Unexplained changes in mental status, the presence of leukocytosis, or other subtle findings represent clues to the presence of bloodborne infection.

32. BACTEREMIA

Anthony L. Esposito and Richard A. Gleckman

Symptoms

The initial clinical manifestations of bacteremia in the elderly are often attributed to some other disease process or are obscured by the presence of concomitant illness. This obscure presentation frequently results in delayed diagnosis and undoubtedly contributes to an excessive mortality. Fever, the hallmark of bacteremia, can be minimal or absent in elderly patients, particularly in the presence of azotemia, uncontrolled diabetes mellitus, hepatic decompensation, corticosteroid therapy, or cachexia. The possibility of infection with bacteremia must be considered whenever an aged patient either develops a slowly progressive, unexplained illness characterized by anorexia, malaise, and weight loss; or experiences an abrupt onset of nausea, vomiting, diaphoresis, agitation, confusion, or stupor. Bacteremia must also be considered when a geriatric patient suddenly develops tachypnea, hypotension, metabolic acidosis, or uncontrolled diabetes; or experiences a rapid deterioration in clinical status in the presence of leukemia, uremia, or immunosuppressive therapy, or following an abdominal or genitourinary surgical procedure.

Diagnosis

Blood cultures represent an invaluable diagnostic procedure that must be performed whenever the possibility of bacteremia arises. Blood for culture should be obtained before the institution of antimicrobial therapy, even when a specific diagnosis appears obvious; for example, although the diagnosis of pneumonia is established by the presence of purulent sputum and a new infiltrate on chest roentgenogram, identification of the causative organisms and, hence, the selection of appropriate antimicrobial therapy can depend exclusively on the isolation of the pathogen from blood. Elderly patients with suspected bacteremia should have 3–4 sets of aerobic and anaerobic blood cultures performed within a 24-hour period. In the case of presumed intravascular infection, in which the bacteremia is continuous (e.g., endocarditis), these cultures can be done at hourly intervals. In the case of presumed abscess or other infection in which bacteremia is intermittent and precedes rigors and fever by 1 hour, multiple blood cultures should be obtained during a shaking chill or prior to the anticipated fever spike. Elderly patients with septic shock should have 2–4 sets of cultures performed within 15–20 minutes. Those patients who are already receiving antimicrobials should have 4–6 pairs of cultures obtained over a 48-hour period; these cultures can be performed in the intervals immediately preceding antibiotic adminstration. The microbiology laboratory should be notified that a patient has recently received antibiotics, so that efforts can be made to neutralize the drug's inhibitory effect on bacterial growth.

The isolation of bacteria from the blood can provide direction for diagnostic investigation when the tissue focus of infection remains obscure. Conversely, knowledge of those pathogens that most frequently cause a specific infection (e.g., cholangitis) permits rational antibiotic selection while culture results are awaited. The organisms most commonly isolated from the blood of aged patients and the tissue sources of sepsis are outlined for both community-acquired bacteremia and nosocomial bacteremia in Appendix A.

Polymicrobic bacteremia occurs in approximately 7% of elderly patients with community-acquired sepsis; in the vast majority of these patients, the tissue focus is cutaneous or abdominal (e.g., cholangitis or perforated viscus). The urinary tract is the most frequently identified tissue source of bacteremia in both community-acquired and nosocomial infection; in hospitalized aged patients, urinary tract sepsis usually occurs in the setting of bladder catheterization or surgical manipulation. The tissue focus of bacteremia cannot be established in a small number of aged patients; these individuals frequently have aplastic anemia, leukemia, or lymphoma.

Septic Shock

Septic shock results from a series of complex pathophysiologic abnormalities that develop within hours of either gram-negative or gram-positive bacteremia. Manifested by fever, hypotension, tachycardia, tachypnea, and mental obtundation, this disorder often appears clinically indistinguishable from the shock syndrome caused by myocardial infarction, gastrointestinal hemorrhage, pulmonary embolism, acute adrenal insufficiency, and pericardial tamponade. Aged patients with septic shock frequently experience pulmonary insufficiency ("shock lung"), gastric hemorrhage, disseminated intravascular coagulation, renal failure, acid-base derangements, and cardiovascular instability. These physiologic abnormalities may result, in part, from the liberation of endotoxin, a lipopolysaccharide component of gram-negative bacilli.

Vigorous supportive measures and antibiotics are essential components in the management of septic shock. Fluid replacement with physiologic saline solutions and volume expansion with albumin must be accomplished rapidly and should be monitored by a central venous catheter or a flow-directed pulmonary artery catheter. Dopamine, a precursor of norepinephrine, is currently considered the vasoactive compound of choice for patients who fail to respond to volume expansion. Dopamine exerts a positive inotropic and chronotropic effect and, in patients with septic shock, usually elevates the cardiac index, stroke volume, and mean aortic root pressure; additionally, dopamine improves renal blood flow and can increase urine output in oliguric patients. Dopamine is administered intravenously at rates of 2–5 μg/kg/min. Serial measurements of arterial blood gases provide an objective assessment of oxygen requirements. An arterial oxygen pressure of greater than 60 mm Hg should be maintained. If, in spite of supplemental oxygen administration, the arterial oxygen pressure decreases to less than 50 mm Hg, intubation and mechanical ventilation are indicated. The use of positive end-expiratory pressure (PEEP) has proved valuable in the management of patients with "shock lung." Because surgical intervention can be the decisive means of eliminating persistent bacteremia and its dire pathophysiologic consequences, an aggressive surgical attitude appears to be essential; abscesses should be drained, obstructions relieved, and necrotic tissue extirpated. Iced saline irrigation is usually successful in arresting gastric hemorrhage; persistent bleeding requires parenteral cimetidine or definitive surgery. Digitalis can reverse the myocardial depression associated with septic shock.

The selection of initial antimicrobial therapy of bacteremic shock is guided primarily by a knowledge of the tissue focus of origin and an awareness of the pathogens usually associated with that focus (App. A). Additional useful information is provided by identifying the bacteremia as community-acquired or nosocomial and by eliciting a history of recent antibiotic exposure.

---

1. Esposito, AL, et al: Community-acquired bacteremia in the elderly: Analysis of one hundred consecutive episodes. *J Am Geriatr Soc* 27:315, 1980.
An analysis of the clinical manifestations, tissue sources of infection, and outcome of bacteremia in aged patients admitted to a suburban hospital.
2. Klastersky J, Carpentier FM, Prevost JM: Significance of antimicrobial synergism for the outcome of gram-negative sepsis. *Am J Med Sci* 273:157, 1977.
Therapy consisting of synergistic combinations of antibiotics appears to improve clinical outcome.
3. Harris JA, Cabbs CG: Persistent gram-negative bacteremia. *Am J Surg* 125:705, 1973.
Intravascular sites of infection and abdominal abscesses may be sources of persistent bacteremia.
4. Anderson, ET, Young LS, Hewitt WL: Simultaneous antibiotic levels in breakthrough gram-negative rod bacteremia. *Am J Med* 61:493, 1976.
Recalcitrant bacteremia may also occur as a result of inappropriate antibiotic therapy or impaired host defense.
5. Kanwar US, et al: Salmonellosis associated with abdominal aortic aneurysms. *Ann Intern Med* 89:931, 1978.
The possibility of an infected aneurysm should be considered in any elderly patient with Salmonella *bacteremia.*
6. Cohen PS, et al: The risk of endothelial infection in adults with *Salmonella* bacteremia. *Ann Intern Med* 89:931, 1978.
Aged patients with Salmonella *bacteremia associated with gastroenteritis, typhoid fever, or other source are at greatest risk for an endothelial surface infection.*

33. SKIN SEPSIS

Anthony L. Esposito and Richard A. Gleckman

The primary management of cutaneous abscesses acquired in the community consists of incision and drainage of the lesion. Routine cultures and antibiotic therapy are not indicated. Patients who have an abscess on an area of the face drained by the cavernous sinus, or who demonstrate systemic toxicity, receive immunosuppressive therapy, or have underlying illness that reduces host defenses should have incision and drainage, aerobic and anaerobic cultures of the abscess, and antibiotic treatment. Initial antimicrobial selection will be determined from interpretation of gram-stained smears and by an awareness of pathogens usually associated with specific sites of infection. For example, *Staphylococcus aureus* and aerobic streptococci cause most hand abscesses; in contrast, perirectal abscesses are usually due to anaerobes, such as bacteroides and streptococci, and gram-negative aerobic bacilli. Blood and wound culture reports form the basis of definitive antibiotic therapy.

Elderly patients with long-standing diabetes mellitus tend to develop neuropathic and arteriosclerotic foot ulcers that serve as portals of entry for soft tissue, bony, and systemic infections. Ulcers complicated by cellulitis have been found to harbor a complex anaerobic-aerobic flora consisting of *Bacteroides, Peptococcus, Clostridia, Staph. aureus,* enterococci, *Escherichia coli,* and *Proteus.* Antibiotic therapy of septic ulcers should be preceded by cultures and Gram's staining.

If the patient with an infected diabetic foot ulcer appears toxic or septic, treatment should consist of cefoxitin (2 gm q4–6h IV) or clindamycin (600 mg q6h IV) plus gentamicin or tobramycin (1.5–1.75 mg/kg q8h IV; see App. A), while the results of blood and tissue cultures are awaited. Antibiotic therapy can be withheld until definitive culture and susceptibility reports are available from those patients who are not seriously ill. Surgical debridement and, on occasion, amputation reduce the morbidity and mortality from these infected ulcers.

Decubitus ulcers have the capability of initiating life-threatening infections. Sepsis associated with decubitus ulcers has been caused by a wide spectrum of organisms, including *Staph. aureus,* aerobic streptococci, *Proteus mirabilis, E. coli, Bacteroides fragilis, Peptococcus* and *Peptostreptococcus.* While definitive ulcer and blood culture reports are awaited, initial therapy of bacteremic patients should consist of clindamycin or cefoxitin and an aminoglycoside (App. A). Aggressive surgical debridement remains an indispensable component of the therapy; indeed, bacteremia may persist in some patients in spite of antibiotic therapy until infected and necrotic tissue is extirpated.

1. Raimer SS, Pursley TV: Office management of viral skin infections in the elderly. *Geriatrics* 36:53, 1981.
Includes a review on the diagnosis and management of herpes zoster and herpes simplex infections.
2. Rose T, Rudolph AH: Identifying and treating bacterial and fungal infections of the skin. *Geriatrics* 29:71, 1978.
Discusses the common cutaneous fungal infections.
3. Ho G Jr, Tice AS, Kaplan SR: Septia bursitis in the prepatellar and olecranon bursae. *Ann Intern Med* 89:21, 1978.
Intravenous antibiotics and bursal fluid drainage constitute optimal therapy.
4. Galpin JE, et al: Sepsis associated with decubitus ulcers. *Am J Med* 61:346, 1976.
Surgical debridement and antibiotics effective against both aerobic and anaerobic bacteria are essential in the management of this complication.
5. Uman SJ, Kunin CM: Needle aspiration in the diagnosis of soft tissue infections. *Arch Intern Med* 135:959, 1975.
This technique is rapid and safe and may facilitate diagnosis.
6. Baxter CR: Surgical management of soft tissue infections. *Surg Clin North Am* 52:1483, 1972.
A comprehensive review of the serious soft tissue infections that require surgical intervention in addition to antimicrobial therapy.

34. FEVER OF UNKNOWN ORIGIN

Anthony L. Esposito and Richard A. Gleckman

Definition

Fever of unknown origin (FUO) refers to a syndrome that is characterized by pyrexia of 38.3°C (101°F) or higher on multiple occasions, that lasts 3 weeks or longer, and that remains undiagnosed after 1 week of in-hospital evaluation. These stringent criteria were developed for adults of all ages; some investigators believe that, for the elderly, the temperature elevation criterion should be lower. The majority of diseases presenting as FUO in the elderly are amenable to specific therapy. Abscesses, bacterial endocarditis, tuberculosis, giant cell arteritis, and pulmonary emboli represent potentially curable entities and account for more than 50% of the serious illnesses producing FUO in these patients. Thus, the diagnostic evaluation of the persistently febrile aged person should be performed in a thorough and expeditious manner, and poorly conceived therapeutic trials must not be allowed to substitute for an appropriate diagnostic evaluation.

A rational approach to the aged patient with FUO is predicated on a knowledge of those disorders whose salient manifestation is fever. Appendix A delineates the most commonly reported causes of FUO in elderly patients. Disorders not specified in Appendix A but acknowledged as etiologies of FUO in the aged include osteomyelitis, disseminated histoplasmosis, rheumatic fever, granulomatous hepatitis, and nonspecific vasculitis. Up to 35% of cases of younger adults with FUO remain undiagnosed in spite of a thorough evaluation; many of these patients eventually experience resolution of fever and during follow-up remain free of disease that might have explained the persistent pyrexia. In contrast, virtually all aged patients with FUO have serious underlying disease.

History and Physical Examination

The initial assessment of a persistently febrile geriatric patient must include a detailed history and a meticulous physical examination. Elements of the past medical history should be carefully noted; for example, a history of nephrolithiasis, diabetes, and recurrent urinary tract infections would suggest a diagnosis of perinephic abscess. Further, an exhaustive review of the remote epidemiologic history must be made; for example, a diagnosis of tuberculosis or brucellosis would be raised in the aged patient with FUO who as a child lived on a farm in Greece and consumed raw milk and dairy products. The significance of poorly characterized or trivial complaints must not be overlooked; vague abdominal discomfort can be the first or only clue to the presence of lymphoma or abscess. Special effort should be made on physical examination to detect epitrochlear lymph nodes, conjunctival petechiae, choroidal tubercles, cardiac murmurs, splenomegaly, abdominal tenderness, and other subtle findings that may provide insight into the nature of the underlying disease and direction for further diagnostic investigation. The importance of repeating the medical history and physical examination cannot be underestimated; virtually all patients with FUO caused by giant cell arteritis eventually develop headache, muscle stiffness, or other highly suggestive symptoms. Since many drugs have the potential to cause fever, the medications that the patient is receiving should be noted, and those that are not essential should be discontinued.

Tests

Initial laboratory tests should include a complete blood count with differential; electrocardiogram; urinalysis; sampling of stool for guaiac; and measurement of erythrocyte sedimentation rate (ESR), serum alkaline phosphatase, serum glutamic oxaloacetic transaminase, and antinuclear antibody, antistreptolysin-O, and rheumatoid factor titers. A monocytosis in the peripheral blood suggests a diagnosis of bacterial endocarditis, tuberculosis, brucellosis, inflammatory bowel disease, solid tumor, or Hodgkin's disease. Persistent lymphocytosis is associated with tuberculosis, infectious mononucleosis, and cytomegalovirus inclusion disease; the latter two infections in the elderly are characterized by persistent fever and by the absence of pharyngitis, lymphadenopathy, or splenomegaly. An elevated ESR is an expected finding in giant cell arteritis, lymphoma, rheumatic fever, and subacute bacterial endocarditis that is unassociated with congestive heart failure. A raised serum alkaline phosphatase level is frequently observed in patients with obstructive or infiltrative disease of the liver, hypernephroma, Hodgkin's disease, giant cell arteritis, and subacute thyroiditis; however, the serum alkaline phosphatase can also be elevated in healthy elderly persons. Rheumatoid factor is present in a significant titer in 50% of patients with bacterial endocarditis of 6 weeks' duration and in 30% of well persons over the age of 64 years; in untreated endocarditis, the titer rises rapidly, but in healthy elderly individuals, it remains stable for years.

Three aerobic and anaerobic blood cultures should be performed on the first and second hospital days; there exists no reason to exceed this number, unless the patient has been receiving antibiotics prior to hospitalization. Cultures of arterial blood and cultures employing hyperosmolar media are not routinely indicated in the initial evaluation of the geriatric patient with FUO. Serum, 5–10 ml, should be secured and frozen for acute phase titer determination. The chest roentgenogram must be carefully reviewed for evidence of previous tuberculous infection (apical fibrosis, pleural or parenchymal calcification) or miliary mottling. Testing with purified protein derivative (PPD-S) should be performed; 90% of patients with extrapulmonary tuberculosis demonstrate a positive reaction, and 60–75% of patients with miliary tuberculosis, including persons with "cryptic" dissemination, manifest a positive reaction on initial testing. A positive response to PPD-S in the elderly patient with FUO is an indication to examine and culture sputum, urine, and gastric washings for *Mycobacterium tuberculosis;* in addition, liver and bone marrow biopsies should be considered early in the evaluation to detect evidence of miliary infection.

Diagnostic procedures should be directed toward investigating specific complaints, physical findings, or laboratory abnormalities; elderly patients tolerate a "shotgun" approach poorly. Among the tests of established value in evaluating elderly patients with FUO are the following: sigmoidoscopy; barium enema; and upper gastrointestinal series with small bowel follow-through to detect evidence of Whipple's disease, tuberculous enteritis, neoplasm, diverticulitis with perforation, Crohn's disease, or idiopathic ulcerative colitis; renal ultrasonography and excretory urography with nephrotomography to detect hypernephroma, tuberculosis, or abscess; ^{99m}Tc sulfur colloid liver-spleen scintiphotography and hepatic ultrasonography to assess hepatic and splenic size and to demonstrate abnormalities suggestive of malignancy or abscess; echocardiography to reveal atrial myxomas or valvular vegetations; computed tomography, ultrasonography, and gallium 67 citrate scintiphotography to detect intraperitoneal and retroperitoneal masses, abscesses, or lymphadenopathy; and perfusion plus ventilatory lung scintiphotography and pulmonary angiography to exclude recurrent pulmonary embolization. A convalescent phase specimen of serum (5–10 ml) should be obtained 3–4 weeks after the initial specimen (acute phase) was secured; if epidemiologic or clinical features suggest the diagnosis of Q fever, cytomegalovirus, Brill-Zinsser disease, toxoplasmosis, brucellosis, or infectious mononucleosis, the paired sera would be submitted for immunologic testing. Liver, bone marrow, lymph node, and temporal artery biopsy represent invasive diagnostic procedures that may be necessary to establish a diagnosis. Temporal artery biopsy should be performed on all elderly patients with FUO: Although the vast majority of patients with this disorder eventually develop headache, myalgias, visual disturbances, or other suggestive symptoms, fever may antedate their appearance by weeks.

Therapeutic Trials and Exploratory Laparotomy

If fever persists and the diagnosis remains obscure, a decision must be made either to discharge the patient, perform an exploratory laparotomy, or initiate a therapeutic trial. The therapeutic trials that have been recommended for elderly patients with FUO include corticosteroids for presumed giant cell arteritis, salicylates for rheumatic fever, heparin for recurrent pulmonary emboli, and antibiotics for tuberculosis or bacterial endocarditis. The mortality and morbidity of aged persons with FUO who are subjected to exploratory laparotomy are significant; nevertheless, because exploration can represent the only means of establishing a definitive diagnosis, elderly patients with objective clinical or laboratory evidence of a pathologic condition in the abdomen should be operated on and should not be relentlessly subjected to invasive diagnostic procedures or multiple therapeutic trials that might delay exploration and accurate diagnosis.

---

1. Esposito AL, Gleckman RA: Fever of unknown origin in the elderly. *J Am Geriatr Soc* 26:498, 1978.
   Abdominal abscesses, bacterial endocarditis, tuberculosis, and giant cell arteritis accounted for more than half of the serious illnesses presenting as FUO.
2. Esposito AL, Gleckman RA: A diagnostic approach to the adult with fever of unknown origin. *Arch Intern Med* 139:575, 1979.
   A comprehensive review.
3. Ghose MK, Shensa S, Lerner PI: Arteritis of the aged and fever of unexplained origin. *Am J Med* 60:429, 1976.
   Anemia, nonspecific liver function abnormalities, and an elevated erythrocyte sedimentation rate are common manifestations of giant cell arteritis.
4. Horwitz CA, et al: Clinical and laboratory evaluation in elderly patients with heterophil-antibody positive infectious mononucleosis. *Am J Med* 61:338, 1976.
   The fever may exceed 3 weeks' duration.
5. Thell R, Martin FH, Edwards JE: Bacterial endocarditis in subjects 60 years of age and older. *Circulation* 51:177, 1979.
   Murmurs are frequently absent in older persons with infective endocarditis.
6. Gleckman RA, Crowley M, Esposito AL: Fever of unknown origin: A view from the community hospital. *Am J Med Sci* 274:21, 1977.
   In aged patients bedridden with obstructive pulmonary disease or heart failure, thrombophlebitis and pulmonary embolism may be manifest by fever alone.

35. POSTOPERATIVE FEVERS

Anthony L. Esposito and Richard A. Gleckman

Diagnosis

Elderly patients frequently experience a low-grade fever immediately following a major surgical procedure; this fever rarely exceeds 37.7°C, resolves spontaneously in 48–72 hours, and appears to be of no clinical significance. When postoperative fever persists, exceeds 38°C, or recurs, or when pyrexia appears for the first time on the third or fourth postoperative day, a thorough investigation must be initiated to determine its etiology. Medications, hematomas, phlebitis, pulmonary disorders, and infections of surgical wounds, intravenous lines, and the urinary tract merit initial consideration. Virtually any drug can evoke a febrile response, and occasionally this response will be accompanied by shaking chills; halothane and methoxyflurane are common anesthetics that can produce a hepatitis manifested primarily by fever. The pulmonary disorders associated with postoperative pyrexia include atelectasis, chemical pneumonitis, bacterial pneumonia, and pulmonary embolus.

In evaluating the postoperatively febrile aged patient, the physician should direct particular attention to the type of anesthesia administered, the temporal relationship of blood transfusions to the fever, the duration of intravenous therapy, the presence of a bladder catheter or endotracheal tube, and, of course, the patient's specific complaints. The physical examination must be meticulous and should be repeated daily; special attention should be paid to the examination of surgical wounds, intravenous sites, and the lungs, heart, abdomen, and extremities. The laboratory tests that should be considered include chest roentgenogram, plain film of the abdomen, urinalysis, complete blood count with total eosinophil count, liver function tests, serum amylase, and serologic tests for cytomegalovirus, Epstein-Barr virus, and hepatitis B virus. Cultures of blood, sputum, urine, and wound drainage should be obtained. Medications that are not essential should be discontinued, and all intravenous lines removed; infected intravenous catheters often fail to demonstrate a purulent discharge or obvious signs of inflammation. The other diagnostic possibilities that should be considered before a patient is subjected to abdominal surgical intervention include bacterial or starch peritonitis, pancreatitis, subphrenic and paracolonic abscesses, and visceral abscesses involving the liver, gallbladder, or pancreas. Diagnostic ultrasound, computed tomography, and gallium citrate scanning are noninvasive procedures that have the potential of detecting these abdominal abscesses.

Therapy

Specific antimicrobial therapy is predicated on the identification of a focus of infection and the isolation of the offending pathogen. Empiric antibiotic therapy should be reserved for those critically ill elderly patients with presumed sepsis or with a suspected abdominal abscess; in such cases antimicrobials should be administered after appropriate cultures have been secured and while further diagnostic procedures are being performed. Empiric therapy should include an aminoglycoside plus a penicillinase-resistant penicillin or a cephalosporin; however, initial treatment for patients with a presumed abdominal infection would consist of ampicillin, an aminoglycoside, and clindamycin or cefoxitin (App. A). If, after further investigation, a tissue focus for infection cannot be identified, and if cultures remain sterile and fever persists, these potentially toxic antibiotics should be discontinued and an alternative diagnosis considered.

1. Roe CF: Surgical aspects of fever. *Curr Probl Surg* 11:1–43, 1968.
   A comprehensive review.
2. Curry CR, Quie PG: Fungal septicemia in patients receiving parenteral hyperalimentation. *N Engl J Med* 285:1221, 1971.
   The isolation of Candida *from the blood of a febrile, postoperative patient receiving hyperalimentation suggests a catheter-related infection and requires removal of the intravenous line.*
3. Stein JM, Pruitt BA: Suppurative thrombophlebitis. *N Engl J Med* 282:1452, 1970.
   Intractable bacteremia with a gram-negative bacillus raises the possibility of either suppurative or nonsuppurative septic thrombophlebitis.

4. Fisher HC, White HM: Biliary tract disease in the aged. *Arch Surg* 63:536, 1951.
Acute calculous or acalculous cholecystitis can complicate extensive surgical procedures.
5. Sutherland RD, et al: Coronary arterial bypass operations without antibiotic coverage. *Chest* 76:174, 1979.
Sternal osteomyelitis, postcardiotomy syndrome, and postperfusion syndrome, which is due to cytomegalovirus or Epstein-Barr virus acquired through blood transfusion, represent causes of postoperative fever unique to patients who have undergone cardiovascular surgery.

VI. CARDIAC DISEASES

36. HYPERTENSION IN THE ELDERLY

Kenneth A. LaBresh and Daniel A. Pietro

The prevalence of hypertension rises with age. Hypertension is an independent risk factor for coronary artery disease, ischemic cerebrovascular disease, intracerebral hemorrhage, aortic aneurysm, congestive heart failure, and peripheral vascular disease both in middle-aged patients and in those over 65.

Recent intervention trials in patients up to age 69 have demonstrated significant reduction in morbidity and mortality when hypertension is effectively treated. Thus, therapy should be initiated for diastolic blood pressures greater than 90 mm Hg and systolic blood pressures greater than 160 mm Hg, as measured on at least three separate occasions, especially if associated with additional risk factors for cardiovascular disease. Reduction of blood pressure below these levels is likely to reduce the incidence of subsequent complications. In addition, blood pressure reduction will lessen symptoms of angina pectoris, congestive heart failure, aortic regurgitation, and mitral regurgitation. Recent evidence suggests that therapy may also reduce morbidity in isolated systolic hypertension. Epidemiologic evidence points to an increased incidence of cerebrovascular complications in these patients and therefore encourages treatment in most cases.

Step-Care Treatment

As with all hypertensive patients, treatment of the elderly should be directed toward obtaining appropriate blood pressure control with the least complexity, expense, and side effects. Elderly patients have a higher incidence of side effects with pharmocologic agents. Therefore, nonpharmacologic intervention, such as weight loss and reduction of dietary sodium, should be pursued initially in mild hypertension (diastolic BP, 90–105 mm Hg). The pharmacologic approach has been organized in a step-care program that is relatively easy to administer. The details are well described in the reviews cited. Some modifications may be required for the geriatric population. The first step is treatment with diuretics alone. Elderly patients are more sensitive to diuretics and develop hypokalemia more easily than younger subjects. Diuretics should, therefore, be started at half the usual initial dose and gradually increased as needed. For patients with normal renal function, thiazides are preferable to furosemide. The use of a thiazide and potassium-sparing diuretic combination improves patient compliance by eliminating the need for potassium supplements, but extreme care must be taken to avoid hyperkalemia, especially in the elderly patient, who may have reduced renal clearance in spite of a normal serum creatinine level.

Step 2 adds an antihypertensive agent to the diuretic. Many of the step 2 agents may result in orthostatic hypotension in older patients because of diminished sympathetic nervous system compensatory mechanisms, so beta-blockers, which are less likely to result in orthostasis, are usually the first choice in step 2. These agents should be avoided in patients with bronchospastic asthma, second- or third-degree heart block, or congestive heart failure and must be used with caution in sick sinus syndrome or sinus bradycardia.

There are a number of new beta-blockers from which to choose. Selective agents such as metoprolol and atenolol produce less bronchoconstriction and may be better tolerated by patients with chronic bronchitis or peripheral vascular disease. In addition, certain beta-blocking agents (e.g., pindolol) have an intrinsic sympathomimetic activity that reduces the likelihood of bradycardia and fatigue, a common side effect in the older patient. For hypertension, all the beta-blockers may be given once or twice daily, to improve compliance. The lipid-soluble agents nadolol and atenolol have longer half-lives, allowing once-daily doses. They also are less likely to produce depression or sleep disturbance.

Step 2 drugs should be started in small initial doses and increased gradually in older patients. Reserpine can cause depression and generally should be avoided in the elderly.

Step 3 drugs (hydralazine or prazosin) combined with a beta-blocker and a diuretic are effective in patients with resistant hypertension. Reflex tachycardia and sodium retention, usually seen with vasodilators, are prevented with this combination. As with step 2 drugs, vasodilators are more likely to produce orthostatic symptoms in the elderly and should be started at reduced doses. In patients with high renin or renovascular hypertension, the converting enzyme inhibitor captopril in combination with a diuretic is particularly useful.

The step 4 drug, guanethidine, blocks the release of norepinephrine. Its antihypertensive effects are augmented by upright posture. In elderly patients this effect may be so marked that it causes severe orthostatic symptoms, making it of little use. When used, its orthostatic effects must be monitored carefully.

For elderly patients without angina, congestive heart failure, or mitral or aortic regurgitation, the usual goal of antihypertensive therapy is to maintain blood pressure in the 150/80–160/90 mm Hg range. With associated ischemia or hemodynamic lesions, further reduction of blood pressure to 100–120 mm Hg systolic may provide additional benefit in reducing symptoms. As always, the management of an asymptomatic but dangerous disease, such as hypertension, must represent a compromise between adverse effects of therapy and ideal blood pressure control. In the vast majority of older patients, blood pressure can be adequately controlled with diuretics and beta-blockers in an uncomplicated, once- or twice-daily regimen.

Follow-up Care. Long-term follow-up care is a major element in successful antihypertensive treatment. In general, patients with the highest initial blood pressures and those with evidence of ischemic or valvular heart disease or renal disease will require the most frequent follow-up. Initial diastolic blood pressures in the 115- to 129-mm Hg range require weekly follow-up while blood pressure is controlled. Patients with initial diastolic pressures of less than 115 mm Hg may be reevaluated at 2- to 6-week intervals. Once blood pressure control is obtained, patients without other complicating diseases may be seen at 2- to 4-month intervals.

Severe Hypertension

Severe hypertension requires a more vigorous approach. Asymptomatic patients with diastolic blood pressure in excess of 130 mm Hg and/or systolic blood pressure greater than 200 mm Hg may be treated using step-care medication but more intensively. In general, they should be hospitalized, and their treatment begun with the use of a step 1 and a step 2 drug simultaneously at twice the usual initial dose. Hydralazine may be added, if necessary, to lower blood pressure below 130 mm Hg diastolic and 200 mm Hg systolic.

Treatment of Hypertensive Emergencies

Hypertensive crisis usually occurs in patients in whom diastolic blood pressures exceed 120 mm Hg. In such patients the pressure should be reduced to normal levels in 1–2 hours. Hypertensive encephalopathy is uncommon but requires prompt recognition and therapy. The major findings in hypertensive encephalopathy are severe headache, confusion, seizures, and coma. Neurologic signs may appear but are usually related to hemorrhagic complication or other CNS lesions. Papilledema is found in most cases.

Aortic dissection presents with intense, sharp, searing pain in the midchest and back. When hypertension is severe, it must be treated rigorously. Aortic dissection may be associated with acute aortic regurgitation, stroke, loss of carotid or brachial pulse, or renal failure.

Cerebral hemorrhage occurs with hypertension. The signs are vomiting, hemiparesis, and bloody spinal fluid. The hypertension should be treated but not lowered precipitously. A component of the acute hypertension follows increased intracranial pressure. Treatment of severe hypertension requires special monitoring and the use of special drugs.

Nitroprusside is now favored in the treatment of hypertensive emergencies. It lowers blood pressure by the combined action of arteriolar and venous smooth muscle dilation. Gastrointestinal and renal blood pressure are maintained; although upright posturing will augment the lowering of blood pressure by venous pooling, the drug is effective in the supine posture. The onset of action is immediate and dissipates within seconds when the drug is stopped. It must be given by intravenous, continuous, controlled infusion with careful monitoring. The usual starting dose is 0.5 μg/kg/min; the maximum that should be reached is 8 μg/kg/min, and most patients will be well controlled by infusions of 2–3 mg/kg/min. Nitroprusside is metabolized to thiocyanate, which is cleared by the kidneys. In patients on long-term infusions, particularly in the setting of renal impairment, toxic effects may develop. These include weakness, fatigue, confusion, slurred speech, nausea, tinnitus, and muscle spasms. Thiocyanate levels should be monitored in patients with renal failure or with more than 48 hours of infusion. Symptoms are generally associated with levels exceeding 10 mg/100 ml. Nitroprusside is unstable when exposed to light. It should be mixed just prior to use and shielded from the light.

Diazoxide is easier to use but less controllable than nitroprusside. The recommended dose of diazoxide is 300 mg, given as a rapid intravenous bolus injection. Diazoxide binds quickly to plasma protein, and this binding may in part be overcome by bolus administration. Rapid lowering of blood pressure to a normal range persists from 2–24 hours. Its major advantage is its ease of administration: Infusion devices are not required. The development of hypotension may be particularly dangerous to older patients. In the case of the elderly, it is recommended that this agent be given as a 50- to 100-mg bolus followed by additional 50- to 100-mg boluses at 5 minute intervals until blood pressure falls.

Other agents are also useful for rapid lowering of blood pressure. Hydralazine is given intramuscularly in an initial dose of 10 mg and has onset of action within 30 minutes. Another choice is trimethaphan (Arfonad), which was used before the introduction of nitroprusside. It is a potent ganglion-blocking agent that requires some head elevation to achieve its effects. It is given by continuous intravenous infusion to titrate the level of blood pressure.

---

1. Kannel WB, Schwarta MJ, McNamara PM: Blood pressure and risk of coronary heart disease. *Dis Chest* 56:43, 1969.
Epidemiologic data from the Framingham study clearly demonstrates increased risk of coronary and cerebrovascular disease in hypertensive patients aged 30–62 years at entry into the study.
2. Kannel WB, et al: Epidemiologic assessment of the role of blood pressure in stroke. *JAMA* 214:301, 1970.
Epidemiologic data from the Framingham study clearly demonstrated increased risk of coronary and cerebrovascular disease in hypertensive patients aged 30–62 years at entry into the study.
3. Veterans Administration Cooperative Study Group on Antihypertensive Agents: Effects of treatment on morbidity in hypertension: Results in patients with diastolic blood pressure averaging 115 through 129 mm Hg. *JAMA* 202:116, 1967.
The first large-scale trial to show that treating hypertension significantly reduces mortality and morbidity.
4. Shekelle RB, Ostfeld AM, Klawans HL: Hypertension and risk of stroke in an elderly population. *Stroke* 5:71, 1974.
An epidemiologic study that shows a significant correlation between systolic hypertension in the elderly and the incidence of stroke.
5. Hypertension detection and follow-up program. Five-year findings of the Hypertension Detection and Follow-up Program. *JAMA* 242:2562, 1979.
Demonstrates that therapy of mild diastolic hypertension (90–104 mm Hg) results in a significant reduction in mortality extending up to age 69.
6. Relman AS: Mild hypertension: No more benign neglect. *N Engl J Med* 302:293, 1980.
Editorial summary of the Hypertension Detection and Follow-up Program.
7. Statement on hypertension in the elderly. Bethesda, Md.: US Department of Health and Human Services, 1980.
States guidelines for treatment goals and the decision to treat that utilize the HDFP data.
8. Report. Joint National Committee on Detection, Evaluation, and Treatment of High Blood Pressure. NIH No. 77-1088. Bethesda, Md.: US Department of Health, Education, and Welfare, 1977.
9. O'Malley K, O'Brien E: Management of hypertension in the elderly. *N Engl J Med* 302:1397, 1980.
A concise summary of the specific problems encountered in elderly patients. Guidelines for therapy where developed prior to publication of the HDFP data.
10. Niarchos AP, Laragh JH: Hypertension in the elderly. *Mod Concepts Cardiovasc Dis* 49:43, 1980.
A review of hypertension emphasizing the use of renin profiling as a guide to therapy.
11. Kirkendall WM, Hammond JJ: Hypertension in the elderly. *Arch Intern Med* 140:1155, 1980.
A careful review of the epidemiologic and intervention data available. Also includes guidelines for treatment and a brief description of pharmacologic agents.

12. Goldberg LJ: Current therapy of hypertension: A pharmacologic approach. *Am J Med* 58:489, 1975.
A general review of the common antihypertensive drugs with particular emphasis on mechanisms of action.
13. Chrysant SG, Frolich ED, Papper S: Why is hypertension so prevalent in the elderly — and how to treat it. *Geriatrics* 31:101, 1976.
One of the earliest reviews of hypertension in this age group.
14. Vestal RE, Wood AJ, Shand DG: Reduced adrenoceptors sensitivity in the elderly. *Clin Pharmacol Ther* 26:181, 1979.
Study demonstrates reduced responsiveness to propranolol and isoproteronol in older subjects. The authors point out, however, that increased plasma levels for similar doses in these subjects partially offsets the reduced clinical response to these agents.
15. Gavras H, Bruner HR, Gavras I: Captopril in the treatment of hypertension. *Ann Intern Med* 95:505, 1981.
A brief summary of the role of converting enzyme inhibitor in the treatment of hypertension.

37. CARDIAC ARRHYTHMIA AND CONDUCTION DISEASE

Daniel A. Pietro

Presentation and Symptoms

Cardiac arrhythmias arise in elderly patients with overt cardiac disease, such as congestive heart failure, coronary artery disease, and hypertension, but often are discovered incidentally in patients without these conditions during a routine physical examination or ECG. The incidence of arrhythmias increases with age, and the stress of a cardiac arrhythmia often is tolerated poorly by the aged patient. The high prevalence of coronary artery disease and other systemic illnesses such as chronic obstructive pulmonary disease (COPD), anemia, and metabolic abnormality no doubt contributes to the high incidence of arrhythmia. In addition, the aging heart is known to have fibrosis and fat deposition in the sinus and intranodal regions, which may add to the risks of arrhythmia. Changes in control of the autonomic nervous system and sensitivity to medication are other factors thought to predispose the elderly patient to cardiac arrhythmias.

The cardiac output decreases at a rate of 1%/yr after middle age. Further reduction in cardiac output from a rhythm disturbance is likely to cause symptoms in the aged patient. For example, flow may be reduced in stenotic vessels that otherwise deliver enough blood to the cerebral, cardiac, renal, or gastrointestinal vessels or vessels of the extremities. When the flow is reduced, the involved organ malfunctions, causing symptoms referable to that organ and thereby masking the role of the cardiac arrhythmia. Arrhythmias may present as palpitations, confusion, sleeplessness, fatigue, congestive heart failure, pulmonary edema, syncope, vague dizziness, angina pectoris, ischemia of an extremity, abdominal angina, myocardial infarction, or sudden death. If the arrhythmia presents with hemodynamic compromise that results in hypotension, shock, confusion, unresponsiveness, angina, or oliguria, rapid determination of the heart rate by apical pulse and ECG will direct therapy.

Diagnosis and Treatment

Limited physiologic reserve in the elderly patient makes it necessary to diagnose and treat the arrhythmia promptly. A full 12 lead ECG should be obtained. If the rhythm is rapid and cannot be determined, the use of the Valsalva maneuver, coughing, gagging, carotid sinus massage, or edrophonium (Tensilon) while running a continuous rhythm strip (on any lead that shows atrial depolarization [P wave]) may not only assist in diagnosis but, in some instances be therapeutic.

The elderly patient is likely to have dysfunction of several organ systems, the manifestations of which may be overlapping. When the patient's condition permits, it is helpful to identify the symptoms associated with the arrhythmia before treatment is undertaken. This may require monitoring in an intensive care unit by telemetry or Holter monitor recording. Correlation of the symptoms and the rhythm disorder is important, because a careful search will often reveal that the symptoms are unrelated to the rhythm disturbance and focus attention on another treatable disorder.

Sinus Tachycardia. Almost always a compensating rhythm in response to stress, sinus tachycardia may occur in the presence of fever, hypotension, sepsis, fecal impaction, dehydration, anxiety, congestive heart failure, or hyperthyroidism. Management is aimed at identifying and treating the underlying cause because use of drugs to decrease the tachycardia without treatment of the underlying cause often further decompensates the patient and may result in hypotension, acidosis, and death.

Atrial Premature Contractions. Atrial premature contractions (APCs) are discovered in more than 10% of elderly patients who have a routine ECG. In most cases, the APCs are asymptomatic and benign. They will often occur more frequently and become multifocal when a patient develops hypoxia, hypotension, congestive heart failure, fever, or electrolyte imbalance. In such cases the treatment should be directed toward the underlying problem. If, after the contributing cause is corrected, the APCs occur more often than 5–10 min and are associated with symptoms, they should be treated in order to control these symptoms and to prevent the development of more significant atrial arrhythmia, e.g., atrial fibrillation or flutter. The drug of choice is quinidine sulfate, 200–400 mg q4–6h PO. Digoxin, procainamide, propranolol, or verapamil are reasonable alternatives if quinidine is ineffective or causes side effects.

Supraventricular Tachycardia. Supraventricular tachycardia (SVT) refers to all tachycardias (ventricular response >105 beats/min) originating at the level of the atrioventricular node or above, i.e., sinus, atrial, or nodal tachycardia. These include atrial flutter, atrial fibrillation, and atrial tachycardia (paroxysmal and nonparoxysmal). The elderly patient with SVT usually has organic heart disease or digitalis toxicity.

If the patient has hypotension, pulmonary edema, or angina, immediate **DC cardioversion** is required. If the patient's condition is stable, however, treatment can begin with sedation—diazepam (Valium), 2–5 mg PO, or phenobarbital, 15–30 mg PO,—and a quiet but not isolated room. Vagal maneuvers or parasympathomimetic drugs are also used to break the SVT, but the patient should have ECG monitoring and emergency drugs readily available before these manipulations are undertaken. Coughing, gagging, and the Valsalva maneuver should be attempted initially. If these produce no effect, then carotid sinus pressure or parasympathomimetic drugs (edrophonium hydrochloride) should be employed. Carotid sinus pressure should be applied with care because of the high incidence of carotid vascular disease in the elderly. When other measures fail, verapamil is the drug of choice, if there is no evidence of congestive heart failure (CHF) is present and left ventricular function is good. Verapamil, 10 mg IV in divided doses (2 mg at a time), will slow ventricular response and often convert SVT to normal sinus rhythm. Diazepam is an alternate treatment and should be given as a total loading dose of 0.75–1.5 mg in divided doses at 2- to 3-hour intervals. The maintenance dose should be adjusted for the patient's age and/or creatinine clearance.

Atrial Fibrillation. Atrial fibrillation (AF) is found on up to 18% of ECGs of hospitalized patients over age 65. The hemodynamic consequences of AF are related to the ventricular response. If the ventricular response is 60–90 beats/min, which allows adequate ventricular filling, then the rhythm is usually well tolerated in the aged. Loss of a synchronized atrial contraction may significantly reduce cardiac output and decompensate patients with cardiomyopathy or valvular heart disease. Elective cardioversion of atrial fibrillation should be considered if the AF has been present less than 6 months and the left atrium is not significantly enlarged. Medical cardioversion with quinidine or procainamide is frequently effective, but DC cardioversion may be necessary in refractory cases. AF is associated with increased thrombus formation, so patients are given anticoagulants for 14–21 days before cardioversion. CHF, pulmonary disease, myocardial infarction, pericarditis, mitral valve disease, hyperthyroidism, and hypoxia may predispose to AF and must be treated to control the ventricular response as well as to maintain a stable rhythm. A slow ventricular response to untreated atrial fibrillation implies atrioventricular node disease, and the use of digoxin or verapamil may cause higher degrees of heart block.

Atrial flutter and **paroxysmal atrial tachycardia** (PAT) occur less frequently in the elderly than atrial fibrillation. These arrhythmias are treated similarly to SVT. Atrial flutter and PAT are less stable rhythms and usually will convert to sinus or atrial fibrillation with or without treatment. Control of the ventricular response (rate, 60–90 beats/min) and correction of underlying conditions are the aims of therapy.

Multifocal Atrial Tachycardia. Multifocal atrial tachycardia is usually seen in severe chronic lung disease or cardiac disease, especially in the elderly. As a rule, the rhythm indicates a poor prognosis when found with pulmonary disease. Improvement of the pulmonary status is the best approach to control of this arrhythmia.

Premature Ventricular Contractions. Premature ventricular contractions (PVCs) are seen on 15–18% of routine ECGs of elderly patients. When there is no cardiac disease and the patient is asymptomatic, PVCs need not be treated unless they are multifocal and occur more often than 8/min. However, if the patient has angina, CHF, or myocardial infarction, and the PVCs are coupled or occur on the T wave (R on T phenomenon), then treatment is recommended. Correction of electrolyte imbalance and treatment of congestive heart failure, coronary artery disease, hypoxia, or digitalis toxicity with quinidine, procainamide, disopyramide, or propranolol improves control of the arrhythmia. Digitalis is useful when CHF is the cause of ventricular arrhythmia; however, be aware that digitalis toxicity often causes PVCs and ventricular arrhythmia in the older patient.

Ventricular Tachycardia. Ventricular tachycardia is a sign of a poor prognosis in the elderly. It is most often seen in acute myocardial infarction but may occur in severe cardiomyopathy, myocarditis, ventricular aneurysm, or drug toxicity, especially from digitalis, quinidine, procainamide, or phenothiazines.

In the elderly patient with ventricular tachycardia, hemodynamic stability usually gives way to rapid deterioration, which requires early and rapid DC cardioversion. The most useful drugs to maintain normal rhythm are lidocaine, procainamide, and bretylium.

Bradycardia-Tachycardia. Bradycardia-tachycardia syndrome (sick sinus syndrome) causes dizziness, vertigo, weakness, palpitations, or syncope. The patient may experience episodic bradyarrhythmia or tachyarrhythmia, which causes symptoms. Although not diagnostic, the most frequent finding on ECG is sinus bradycardia with rates less than 50 beats/min. Atrial fibrillation with a slow ventricular rate also occurs. Documentation of the symptoms and the simultaneous cardiac rhythm, using Holter monitoring (24 hours), telemetry, or ICU observation, should confirm a cause-and-effect relationship. Electrophysiologic evaluation, using sinus node recovery times and His bundle recordings, may help.

Vagal stimulation or drugs that cause or exacerbate bradycardia, such as digoxin, quinidine, reserpine, or beta-blockers, should not be used. Under certain instances, however, digoxin and quinidine may be required to treat the tachyarrhythmia, and the precipitated bradyarrhythmia may require a pacemaker. Indeed, symptomatic bradycardia-tachycardia syndrome is one of the most common indications for permanent cardiac pacing in the elderly.

Heart Block. First-degree atrioventricular heart block in general requires no treatment; however, it may be an early sign of digitalis intoxication and may precede higher degrees of block. Because of the cardiac changes of aging, **second-degree atrioventricular heart block** (Mobitz type I, Wenckebach) may become apparent at rates of 120–130 beats/min and, therefore, manifest itself under conditions of stress in the aged patient, but it is most often caused by digitalis toxicity or inferior myocardial infarction. Mobitz type I second-degree atrioventricular heart block is rarely an indication for a permanent pacemaker. Temporary pacing, however, is often required while an acute myocardial infarction or other condition is treated. Mobitz type II atrioventricular heart block is diagnosed when a sudden unexpected block of a P wave occurs. There is no evidence of progressive P–R prologation. This finding usually indicates a conduction block located below the atrioventricular node in the His bundle system. Mobitz type II atrioventricular heart block is an indication for permanent pacemaker insertion.

Third-degree atrioventricular heart block consists of two types. The first, atrioventricular dissociation, implies a reversible cause such as ischemia, inferior myocardial infarction, or digitalis toxicity. Treatment with atropine or temporary pacemaker insertion will usually be enough until the problem is resolved. Complete heart block, on the other hand, implies an irreversible disconnection between atrial and ventricular activity and is usually associated with progressive conduction system disease. Temporary treatment may be required, but most patients need permanent pacemaker support.

Bundle-branch-block and **fascicular block** are caused by degenerative conduction system disease (Lev's or Lenegre's), ischemic heart disease, hypertensive heart disease, valvular heart disease, and other disorders. The elderly patient with conduction system disease and symptoms must be evaluated. Monitoring via telemetry, Holter monitoring, and electrophysiologic studies may reveal a high degree of block. Permanent pacemaker insertion should be reserved for patients with a documented relationship between bradyarrhythmia and symptoms.

Patients with anterior myocardial infarctions who develop related bifascicular or complete heart block often require temporary and/or permanent pacemaker insertion. Inferior myocardial infarction may be complicated by various degrees of heart block related to ischemia of the atrioventricular node. In most patients with inferior myocardial infarction it is reversible, but treatment with atropine or temporary pacing may be required if the heart rate is less than 50 beats/min or if the patient is symptomatic.

Digitalis Toxicity. Digitalis toxicity can present with varying levels of heart block, PAT with block, severe bradycardia, frequent PVC, multifocal PVC, couplets, or ventricular tachycardia. Diminished renal function, confusion about medication directions, and multiple drug therapy increase the likelihood of digitalis toxicity. Although the presenting arrhythmias can be quite varied, atrial tachycardia with block very likely signifies digitalis toxicity. When this diagnosis is considered, (1) stop all digitalis preparations and (2) correct electrolyte balance and especially maintain a potassium level of 4.5–5.5 mg/100 ml. Potassium may be given (10 mg/hr IV). Serum potassium levels should be monitored frequently. Cardioversion is relatively contraindicated in digitalis toxicity because of an increased incidence of ventricular tachycardia and ventricular fibrillation.

1. Argeuss NS, Rosen EY, Adolph RJ, Fowler WO: Significance of chronic sinus bradycardia in elderly people. *Circulation* 46:924–930, 1972.
   Demonstrates sinus bradycardia in the elderly may be present without cardiac dysfunction. Treatment warrants correlation with symptoms.
2. Ewy GA, et al: Digoxin metabolism in the elderly. *Circulation* 39:449–453, 1969.
   Small study demonstrating the higher concentrations of digoxin seen in elderly patients on maintenance digoxin.
3. Fleg JL, Kennedy HL: Cardiac arrhythmias in a healthy elderly population. *Chest* 81:302–307, 1982.
   Evaluates 98 healthy elderly patients with Holter and demonstrates frequent ventricular and supraventricular ectopy, but rare bradycardia or heart block.
4. Ganu D, Tolentino A, Samet P: Electrophysiologic evaluation of elderly patients with sinus bradycardia. *Ann Intern Med* 90:24–29, 1979.
   Reviews the prognostic importance of electrophysiologic parameters in deciding if pacemaker insertion is indicated. Provides one side of a controversial issue.
5. Ginks W, Leatham A, Siddons H: Prognosis of patients paced for chronic atrioventricular block. *Br Heart J* 41:633–636, 1979.
   Describes 839 patients who were followed after pacemaker insertion for heart block. Evaluates the survival of paced patients and general population.
6. Harris R: Cardiac arrhythmias in the aged, in Caird FI, Dall JLC, Kennely RD (eds): *Cardiology in Old Age.* New York, Plenum Press, 1976, pp 315–346.
   Highlights significant aspects of rhythm changes in the elderly and summarizes treatment.
7. Heger JJ, et al: Cardiac arrhythmia in the elderly. *Cardiovasc Clin* 12:145–159, 1981.
   Reviews some of the features of diagnosis and management of cardiac arrhythmias in the elderly.
8. Mehalich MJ, Fisch C: Electrocardiographic findings in the aged. *Am Heart J* 87:117–128, 1974.
   Reviews the electrocardiographic findings of the aged (73 references).
9. Mehlman DJ, Alnsdorf MF: Antiarrhythmic therapy for the elderly: A two-edged sword. *Geriatrics* 34:29–62, 1979.
   Excellent summary of the topic. Reviews factors that enhance cardiac arrythmias and defines patient risks. Considerable detail on drug therapy.
10. Rubenstein JJ, Schulman CL, Yurchak PM, DeSanctis R: Clinical spectrum of the sick sinus syndrome. *Circulation* 46:5–13, 1972.
    Reviews 56 patients with sick sinus syndrome and reports on the clinical presentation and prognosis.
11. Siddons H: Management of heart block, in Caird FI, Dall JLC, Kennedy RD (eds): *Cardiology of Old Age* New York, Plenum Press, 1976, pp 347–367.
    Discusses the indications for pacing and prognosis of heart block.

38. TREATMENT OF CONGESTIVE HEART FAILURE

Daniel A. Pietro

Congestive heart failure (CHF) is a manifestation of many cardiac problems in the aged. Although ischemic and hypertensive heart disease account for more than 50% of the patients with CHF, valvular heart disease, endocarditis, Paget's disease, thyroid disease, syphilis, senile cardiac amyloidosis, and idiopathic disease are other causes. When there is no identifiable cause of CHF, nonspecific changes of the myocardial collagen associated with aging may be the etiology. The cardiac muscle abnormality is known as *presbycardia* or *senile cardiac disease*. Both young and old patients can have dyspnea on exertion, paroxysmal nocturnal dyspnea, orthopnea, and peripheral edema as the major signs of CHF. Geriatric patients, however, frequently develop wheezing, restlessness, insomnia, confusion, abdominal discomfort, nausea, right upper quadrant discomfort, or sacral edema as the initial presentation. Diminished cardiac output may affect the renal or gastrointestinal system, which cannot tolerate further compromise, so that the symptoms appear to be noncardiac in origin.

The early symptoms of CHF often do not become manifest in the elderly, who are relatively inactive; however, other factors such as fever, infection, arrhythmia, dietary indiscretion, or drug effects may provide enough added stress to precipitate the signs and symptoms of CHF. Correction of these conditions is a necessary step in treatment of the heart failure.

The treatment of congestive heart failure in the aged is similar to that in the younger age groups. The goal of therapy is to decrease cardiac work while improving cardiac output and contractility. In active patients, bed and chair rest alone may result in a significant diuresis. The disappearance of ankle edema, however, may not indicate effective diuresis since fluid is redistributed to the sacral region in the recumbent patient. Measurement of fluid intake and output is a better indicator, but accurate daily weights are more reliable and easier to obtain, especially in the case of an incontinent elderly patient. Prolonged bed rest carries the risk of pulmonary embolism.

Diuretics

Diuretics that reduce volume and blood pressure are often enough to treat CHF in the geriatric patient. Attention to changes in weight, renal function, electrolyte balance, and uric acid levels prevents complications of diuretics in the elderly patient. The physician also must be vigilant for signs of acute urinary retention, orthostatic hypotension, and precipitation of digitalis toxicity, which sometimes are produced by diuretic treatment.

Digitalis

Digitalis preparations play a major role in control of CHF in all age groups, but the risk of digitalis toxicity in the geriatric patient demands special attention. Digoxin, the most widely used of the digitalis preparations, can be given via the intravenous or oral route for the initial loading dose as well as for maintenance therapy. Unlike the treatment of arrhythmias, in which rapid digitalization is important, digitalization in patients with CHF can be done over a 24- to 36-hour period. The usual method calls for a loading dose of 0.75–1.0 mg of digoxin, given in divided doses of 0.25–0.50 mg at 4- to 6-hour intervals. The maintenance dose is 0.125–0.25 mg daily. The loading dose of digoxin is not altered for renal disease, but the maintenance dose is adjusted on the basis of renal clearance, in order to avoid toxicity. Moreover, the serum creatinine in the geriatric patient, because of a reduction in muscle mass with age, may not reflect the degree of renal impairment, so that measurement of creatinine clearance is a better guide in the determination of digoxin maintenance requirements in the aged.

Measurement of serum electrolytes, especially potassium, correction of hypoxia, and adjustment of the dose on the basis of renal function are crucial to reducing the incidence of digoxin toxicity. Digoxin elixir is a valuable method of administering the drug to the elderly patient who has difficulty taking medication or requires an unusual dosage.

Vasodilation

Refractory heart failure that cannot be adequately controlled with the usual treatment approach may improve with venous and arterial dilators, such as nitrates for preload reduction and hydralazine and captopril for afterload reduction. An excessive reduction in preload or afterload, however, may reduce the cardiac output and tissue perfusion, causing clinical deterioration. The vasoactive drugs are titrated to achieve maximal control of symptoms while avoiding hypotension and diminished organ perfusion. Even minor changes in cardiac output can cause decompensation and side effects in elderly patients however. When clinical signs are not clear, it may be necessary to carry out intracardiac hemodynamic assessment in an intensive care unit, in order to determine maximal benefit.

Pulmonary Edema

Acute pulmonary edema is frequently the first **symptomatic** manifestation of cardiac failure in the geriatric patient. One reason for the acute decompensation is that when an elderly patient who is usually at rest is put under stress, the marginally compensated cardiac function decompensates to cause a major symptomatic event. The therapy for pulmonary edema is the same as for younger patients. When the usual treatment is ineffective, it may be necessary to use arteriovasodilators such as nitroprusside. When used with caution, a nitroprusside infusion can rapidly reduce afterload. Monitoring of blood pressure by arterial pressure monitoring and pulmonary artery or pulmonary capillary wedge pressures is needed. The initial dose should be small, 5–10 μg/min, and titrated to maintain a blood pressure of 100–120 systolic. The severe hypotensive effects produced by nitroprusside are especially dangerous in the aged patient because of the risk of myocardial, cerebral, or gastrointestinal infarction. The metabolic products of nitroprusside also can cause thiocyanate toxicity. When a patient has poor hepatic and renal function or is being treated with prolonged high doses of nitroprusside, thiocyanate levels should be measured.

1. Dall JL: Maintenance digoxin in the elderly patients. *Br Med J* 2:705–706, 1970.
   Adverse effects from medication are not uncommon in the elderly. The digitalis glycoside group is a frequent cause of morbidity in these patients. This brief paper demonstrates that many elderly patients on digoxin without evidence of cardiac dysfunction can and should be taken off digitalis preparations.
2. Dock W: Cardiomyopathies of the senescent and senile. *Cardiovasc Clin* 4:362–373, 1972.
   Reviews the evidence for age-related changes in the myocardium. Discusses a possible role in the development of unexplained cardiomyopathy of the aged (presbycardia).
3. Ewy GE, Kapadia GG, Yao L, Lullin M, Marcus FI: Digoxin metabolism in the elderly. *Circulation* 39:449–453, 1969.
   Digoxin toxicity is common in the elderly population. This article demonstrates the need for digoxin dose adjustment even if the serum creatinine is within normal limits. The renal clearance in the elderly is decreased and serum digoxin levels therefore are higher for a given dose.
4. Forrester JS, Waters DD: Hospital treatment of congestive heart failure — management according to hemodynamic profile. *Am J Med* 65:173–180, 1978.
   Demonstrates the role of hemodynamic assessment in designing effective and appropriate therapy for patients with congestive heart failure.
5. Frankl WS: Recognition and management of congestive heart failure. *Geriatrics* 36:92–102, 1981.
   Concise article on acute and chronic congestive heart failure with special emphasis on increased risks in the elderly.
6. Gerstenblith G: Congestive heart failure. *Cardiovasc Clin* 12:131–144, 1981.
   Discusses the physiologic changes associated with aging of the heart. Outlines the possible pitfalls that limit clinicians' ability to recognize congestive failure in the elderly (67 references).
7. Granath A, Jonsson B, Strandell T: Circulation in healthy old men, studied by right heart catheterization at rest and during exercise in supine and sitting position. *Acta Med Scand* 176(Fascile 4):425–446, 1964.
   A very detailed hemodynamic study revealing the changes in stroke volume, cardiac output, cardiac pressures, and vascular resistances that occur in elderly healthy patients.
8. Harris R: Cardiopathy of aging: Are the changes related to congestive heart failure? *Geriatrics* 2:42–46, 1977.

This brief article examines the concept of age-related cardiopathy and concludes that congestive heart failure in the elderly is most often due to typical cardiac lesions (49 references).

9. Harris R: Congestive heart failure, in *Management of Geriatric Cardiovascular Disease. Philadelphia, Lippincott, Harris R: 1970, chap. 13.*
Excellent overview of congestive heart disease in the elderly. Distinguishes etiologic groups according to age. Reviews the common yet often overlooked symptoms of elderly patients.
10. Unverferth OV, Magorien RD, Leier CV: Drug regimens for congestive heart failure. *Geriatrics* 35:26–33, 1980.
Good review of the available therapeutic choices in the treatment of congestive heart failure.

39. CORONARY DISEASE IN THE ELDERLY

Daniel A. Pietro

Angina Pectoris

Coronary artery disease (CAD) is the single most frequent cause of death in the elderly. It is paradoxical that complications from other organ systems affected by CAD often overshadow the cardiac symptoms in the overall management of the elderly patient. The anginal equivalents shortness of breath and gastrointestinal complaints are two familiar examples. CAD may present as angina pectoris, myocardial infarction, or sudden death, but the incidence of silent myocardial infarction is also high.

Hypertension, smoking, diabetes, and a positive family history are risk factors just as in younger patients but are less important as the frequency of CAD increases with age. The male predominance of CAD in the younger age groups also diminishes, and by age 80 the male and female incidence of CAD is equal.

Diagnosis. Angina pectoris is often absent in elderly patients; thus, a high index of suspicion is required to recognize subtle signs of CAD. Dyspnea, epigastric discomfort, breathlessness, arrhythmia, new onset of confusion, unusual giddiness, and syncope may indicate CAD in the elderly patient. Pain caused by CAD may arise in the neck, arm, or shoulder and is often attributed to arthritis; postprandial ischemic discomfort may be confused with hiatal hernia. Since the elderly often have arthritis and hiatal hernia, determination of the true etiology of these symptoms becomes difficult. The usual anginal pattern occurs less frequently in the elderly because of diminished physical activity, an increase in pain threshold, and inadequate reporting because of dementia or confusion.

Laboratory tests do not always solve the diagnostic dilemma. Exercise stress testing is limited in many elderly patients because of peripheral vascular disease, arthritis, neurologic disease, or anxiety. An abnormal baseline ECG with ST–T changes, usual in elderly patients, further limits the use of stress testing. Changes in the ST–T waves associated with symptoms, however, are helpful in the diagnosis. Occasionally, in patients with CAD, abnormal ST–T changes may normalize during symptoms (so-called *pseudonormalization);* this phenomenon points to the diagnosis.

A concomitant disorder, such as anemia, tachyarrhythmia, hyperthyroidism, excessive thyroid replacement, hypoglycemia, hypertension, aortic valve disease, hypoxia, surgical intervention, and sepsis, may precipitate symptomatic coronary artery disease or a myocardial infarction in the elderly. The clinician should **always** consider occult coronary artery disease and its complications when treating the elderly patient, especially if expected response to therapy for other conditions fails.

Treatment

Nitroglycerin. The medical therapy of symptomatic CAD is successful in most patients and reduces the risk of myocardial infarction. Sublingual nitroglycerin (NTG) and the longer-acting oral or transdermal forms are the first choices for treatment of angina, even in the elderly patient. The nitrites reduce myocardial oxygen demand by (1) lowering blood pressure (afterload reduction), (2) reducing ventricular volume (preload reduction) by venous dilatation, and (3) dilatation of collateral branches to diseased coronary arteries. The hypotensive effects of the drug are exacerbated in the elderly by a blunted reflex tachycardia, so when the patient uses NTG he or she should stop activity and sit or lie down. When NTG is first used, it should be given under the supervision of a physician or nurse. The elderly patient should receive a smaller dose initially, and the dose increased until the patient reaches an acceptable balance between the relief of chest discomfort and side effects.

Side effects of NTG include hypotension, headache, flushing of the face and head, and a reflex tachycardia often described as pounding of the heart. If the hypotensive episode is severe, nausea, vomiting, weakness, pallor, diaphoresis, and syncope may occur with it. In spite of these unwanted effects, NTG remains the foundation of treatment.

Beta-adrenergic Blockers. The beta-adrenergic blockers are also useful in treating the symptoms of CAD. Stimulation of the beta-adrenergic receptor sites increases heart rate and cardiac contractility, both of which increase myocardial oxygen requirements. The use of beta-blocking drugs to reduce the myocardial oxygen need has gained wide acceptance in the management of angina pectoris.

The aged patient has a greater risk of side effects to beta-blockers than younger patients. The most bothersome side effects are bradyarrhythmias (especially, marked sinus bradycardia), progressive atrioventricular block, precipitation of congestive heart failure, fatigue, depression, and postural hypotension. The smooth muscles of the respiratory, gastrointestinal, and peripheral vascular systems respond to beta-blockers and cause bronchospasm, nausea, vomiting, and Raynaud's phenomenon. The clinical signs of hypoglycemia, which also may be the result of beta-receptor stimulation, are masked with the use of beta-blockers, so that hypoglycemia may go undiagnosed.

The elderly patient, even with mild congestive heart failure and angina, may benefit from the judicious use of beta-blockers after treatment with digitalis and diuretics. The abrupt withdrawal of beta-blockers, however, may precipitate unstable angina or myocardial infarction.

The use of calcium channel blockers has broadened the therapeutic choices in the treatment of angina. These drugs can be used in place of beta-blockers as initial therapy or can provide an alternate treatment when beta-blockers are not tolerated.

Treatment of Risk Factors. Although risk factor manipulation in the elderly is limited, conditions that may exacerbate angina should be treated aggressively. Treatment of anemia, congestive heart failure, hypertension, tachyarrhythmias, bradyarrhythmias, chronic lung disease, thryoid disease, valvular heart disease (especially aortic stenosis), or fever must be an integral part of the treatment plan. Weight reduction for the obese and avoidance of cigarette smoking may provide significant symptomatic improvement with less medication. Since the elderly are relatively inactive physically, emotional upset, anxiety, and depression are more likely to precipitate anginal symptoms. Therefore, treatment directed at emotional stress may improve the symptoms.

Schedules. The treatment of CAD often demands several drugs in frequent doses, so it is of the utmost importance that the simplest schedules be established. Clear verbal and written instructions indicating medication, dose, and time of dose must be given to the patient or to the person caring for the patient. This written schedule should be conspicuously posted at home and available to the physician at visits to the clinic. This simple practice can reduce markedly the misunderstanding and compliance problems so frequently encountered with the elderly. A chart with the name of the medication dose and a sample pill may be helpful as a visual reminder.

Myocardial Infarction

Symptoms. Like angina, myocardial infarction (MI) in the elderly may present with chest pain and the usual clinical findings. However, 50% of infarctions in elderly patients have other than classic presentations. Myocardial infarction in the elderly causes pain less often than it causes dyspnea, pulmonary edema, and congestive heart failure. "Silent myocardial infarctions," with minimal if any cardiac symptoms, may present as diaphoresis, pallor, hypotension, intensification of heart failure, mental confusion, wheezing, nocturnal cough, or restless agitation with disorientation.

Because of reduced vascular perfusion of other organ systems in elderly patients, a drop in cardiac output from MI may present itself as syncope, seizure, renal failure, or gastrointestinal compromise. The physician must maintain a high index of suspicion for

CAD in the elderly, who so frequently have silent infarction and noncardiac presentations.

The usual ECG findings of MI in the elderly are similar to those in younger patients but are often aberrant. Noninvasive cardiac procedures such as the technetium pyrophosphate scan, thallium scan, and two-dimensional echocardiography have improved our ability to diagnose myocardial infarction in this age group and should be used when the usual ECG and cardiac enzymes are not diagnostic.

Management. Management of an acute myocardial infarction is the same regardless of age. Attention to certain needs, however, will reduce complications in the elderly patient. Frequent verbal contact is very important, as it helps to diminish the confusion and psychosis so often experienced by the elderly in the intensive care unit. The availability of familiar objects or pictures is also of benefit. Careful monitoring for hypotension, respiratory depression, or urinary retention is, of course, necessary.

Elderly patients frequently have a preoccupation with bowel function. Reassurance that daily bowel movements are not necessary may help allay anxiety, and the use of a bedside commode instead of a bedpan is often preferable, provided the patient is moved to and from the commode passively.

Prognosis and Complications. The prognosis following MI depends on the size of the infarction and the general health of the patient. Mortality is increased in elderly patients with blood pressure greater than 200 mm Hg or less than 100 mm Hg, paroxysmal nocturnal dyspnea (PND), prior MI, confusion, cyanosis, arrythmias, blood urea nitrogen (BUN) greater than 100, or other serious disease.

The elderly patient is subject to the same complications related to myocardial infarction as the younger patient but has a higher risk of myocardial rupture and of recurrent subendocardial myocardial infarction. Congestive heart failure, a major complication, occurs in more than 20% of patients 50 years or older with MI. The elderly patient with myocardial infarction is also at risk of developing atrial, nodal, or ventricular arrythmias as well as varying degrees of heart block. In general the elderly tolerate arrythmias poorly, and appropriate treatment often will prevent recurrence of pain and extension of the infarction. Treatment of arrythmia also helps avoid cerebrovascular, renal, and gastrointestinal or extremity compromise, as well as vascular collapse and sudden death.

Reduction of Complications. The physician should also correct hypoxia, electrolyte imbalance (especially K^+, Mg^{+2}, and PO_4), hypotension, and serum pH. Ventricular arrhythmia in the setting of acute myocardial infarction is frequent. Lidocaine, 50–100 mg in a bolus IV (1 mg/kg body weight), followed immediately by a 1–4 mg/min drip, is the first-line drug and often controls the arrythmia. The elderly patient is very sensitive to the central nervous system side effects of lidocaine, which include drowsiness, confusion, somnolence, and seizures, all of which occur more frequently in patients with congestive heart failure. A lower maintenance dose of lidocaine is often required for an elderly MI patient.

It is often difficult to assess the volume status of an elderly patient clinically, but hypotension or shock is a frequent manifestation of myocardial infarction. Shock may follow cardiac failure, hypovolemia, right ventricular infarction, or sepsis with a resultant secondary infarction. The limited physiologic reserve and compromise of other organ systems prevents the elderly patient from adjusting to hypovolemia or other fluid volume stresses. In order to assess the patient's volume status appropriately and to direct fluid therapy, hemodynamic monitoring using the balloon-tipped pulmonary artery catheters should be used **early** in the patient's course. All too often these relatively safe monitoring devices are withheld because of the patient's age. However, it is the elderly patient with blunt compensatory mechanisms and the increased risk to other organs who will benefit most from correct volume assessment and early treatment.

---

1. Berman, ND: The elderly patient in the coronary care unit. *J Am Geriatr Soc* 27:145–151, 1979.
Demonstrates the benefits provided by the appropriate use of intensive care facilities for elderly patients.
2. Biorck G: The biology of myocardial infarction. *Circulation* 37:1071–1085, 1968.
Documents the increasing mortality from myocardial infarction with increasing age. Also demonstrates the decreasing role of gender as a risk factor in CAD in the aged.
3. Burch G: Interesting aspects of geriatric cardiology. *Am Heart J* 89:99–114, 1975.

Overview of geriatric cardiac disease with emphasis on coronary artery disease. Emphasizes the importance of aging process on the manifestations of heart disease in the elderly.

4. Kohn R: Heart and cardiovascular system, in Finch C, Hayflick L (eds): *The Handbook of the Biology of Aging.* New York, Van Nostrand Reinholt, 1977, chap 12, pp 281–317.
Excellent discussion of the physiologic effects of aging on the cardiovascular system.
5. Pathy MS: Clinical features of ischemic heart disease, in Caird FI, Dall JLC, Kennedy RD (eds): *Cardiology in Old Age.* New York, Plenum Press, 1976, pp 193–207.
Details the variety of clinical presentations of myocardial infarction in the elderly.
6. Pathy MS: Clinical presentation of myocardial infarction in the elderly. *Br Heart J* 29:190–199, 1967.
Details the variety of clinical presentations of myocardial infarction in elderly patients.
7. Rodstein M: Heart disease in the aged, in Rossman I (ed): *Clinical Geriatrics.* Philadelphia, Lippincott, 1971, pp 143–163.
Good section on coronary disease that emphasizes the factors that deserve special attention in treating elderly patients with myocardial infarctions.
8. Rothbaum DA: Coronary artery disease. *Cardiovasc Clin* 12:105–118, 1981.
Excellent overview of coronary artery disease in the elderly. Compares features of myocardial infarction and complications between young and old age groups.
9. Semple T, Williams BO: Coronary care for the elderly, in Caird FI, Dall JLC, Kennedy RD (eds): *Cardiology in Old Age.* New York, Plenum Press, 1976, pp 297–312.
Reviews myocardial infarctions in the elderly with particular attention to the requirements of the elderly in the intensive care setting.
10. Wasserburger RA: An electrocardiographic survey of the aged. *Postgrad Med* 58:147, 1975.
Reviews the electrocardiograms of 396 patients aged 75 years or more, demonstrating that 76% have some abnormality.
11. Zeman DF, Rodstein M: Cardiac rupture complicating myocardial infarction. *Arch Intern Med* 105:121–133, 1960.
Documents the high incidence of myocardial rupture as a complication of myocardial infarction in the elderly.

40. VALVULAR DISEASE IN THE ELDERLY

Andrew J. Kemper and Daniel A. Pietro

Significant valvular heart disease usually arises in youth or middle age; however, because of the long natural history of many valvular lesions, the clinician frequently encounters valvular disease in the aged. Cartilaginous degeneration of valvular structures may result in new hemodynamically significant disease. The gradual loss of left ventricular reserve may make previously well-tolerated lesions clinically significant. The aging process itself, which is accompanied by a decrease in vascular elasticity, alters physical findings and makes the clinical diagnosis of the severity of many lesions more difficult. The proper approach to valvular disease in the elderly requires knowledge of the tempo of the disease, the interaction of associated medical conditions, and the potential risk and benefit of medical and surgical intervention. Patients with organic valvular disease usually require prophylaxis for subacute bacterial endocarditis during dental procedures, colonoscopy, sigmoidoscopy, and invasive urologic procedures.

Aortic Stenosis

Aortic stenosis in the elderly is usually caused by degeneration and calcification of a normal tricuspid aortic valve. The patient remains asymptomatic for 10–20 years while the stenosis gradually progresses. The cardinal presenting symptoms of angina pectoris, dyspnea on exertion, exertional syncope, and congestive heart failure do not occur until late in the course of the disease. From the time of presentation, the median survival without definitive surgical intervention is 2–5 years.

The murmur of aortic stenosis is loudest in most cases at the left lower sternal border and radiates to the carotids; however, in the elderly it is often loudest at the apex and can easily be confused with mitral regurgitation. In the elderly, the murmur of severe aortic stenosis can be deceptively soft, while trivial valvular narrowing can be associated with a very loud, musical murmur.

The most reliable physical signs of critical aortic stenosis are a decreased or absent second heart sound and the crescendo-decrescendo quality of the ejection murmur, which peaks in mid- to late systole, when obstruction to outflow is severe. Carotid pulses, which are usually delayed and prolonged in the young with aortic stenosis, are often altered by the loss of vessel elasticity associated with aging and may feel deceptively normal in an older patient.

Aortic valve calcification is almost always present in significant aortic stenosis in the elderly. While the degree of calcification does not have a correlation with the degree of stenosis, the absence of calcification by fluoroscopy virtually rules out this diagnosis in patients over age 65. The ECG shows left ventricular hypertrophy in approximately 75% of patients. Echocardiography can delineate the presence of aortic valve thickening and orifice narrowing as well as associated left ventricular hypertrophy. Although two-dimensional echocardiography can show clearly pliable leaflets with a wide orifice and thus rule out severe aortic stenosis, the intense echoes associated with severe calcification have made more definitive quantification of the degree of stenosis unreliable.

Clinical evaluation of the hemodynamic significance of aortic stenosis in the elderly is difficult because of the presence of concomitant medical conditions. For example, angina pectoris may be due to severe coronary artery disease with trivial aortic stenosis. Likewise, syncope may be due to a seizure disorder, heart block, or sick sinus syndrome, rather than coincident aortic stenosis. Dyspnea on exertion may be due to lung disease or poor left ventricular function. In general, however, it is prudent to proceed to hemodynamic studies in the presence of the cardinal symptoms of aortic stenosis, unless the degree of stenosis can be shown to be clearly trivial by the absence of valvular calcification on fluoroscopy or echocardiographic demonstration of pliable leaflets with a wide orifice.

Unless concurrent severe medical illness prevents operation, no patient should be denied aortic valve replacement for aortic stenosis. With recent surgical advances, aortic valve replacement is a relatively low-risk, remarkably effective, life-prolonging procedure in patients with severe aortic stenosis, regardless of their age. Most surgeons use the porcine aortic valve in elderly patients to avoid the need for long-term anticoagulation.

Obstructive Cardiomyopathy

Obstructive cardiomyopathy (idiopathic hypertrophic subaortic stenosis [IHSS]) is occasionally seen in elderly patients and can usually be distinguished from valvular aortic stenosis on the basis of the accompanying murmur, which increases rather than decreases with the Valsalva maneuver. The echocardiographic finding of increased septal thickness also separates the two disorders. Since the two lesions occasionally coexist, it is sometimes necessary to proceed to cardiac catheterization if calcification of the valve leaflets is seen. For most patients with symptomatic obstructive myopathy, medical therapy with beta-blockade or calcium channel blockers is effective. Since sudden death is a major risk in obstructive myopathy, Holter monitoring is needed to identify dangerous arrhythmia. Antiarrhythmic therapy is indicated, even in the absence of syncopal symptoms, if ventricular couplets or salvos are seen in monitoring.

Aortic Regurgitation

The clinical course of aortic regurgitation differs depending on the chronicity of the lesion. Chronic aortic regurgitation from rheumatic fever, bicuspid aortic valve, or following subacute endocarditis may be asymptomatic for 10–50 years. The course is characterized by a long period of compensated left ventricular dilatation. Eventually left ventricular failure ensues, and dyspnea on exertion and fatigue appear. Acute, severe aortic regurgitation secondary to acute endocarditis, aortic root dilatation, or aortic dissection may present as a catastrophic illness with progressively intractable congestive heart failure without apparent left ventricular dilatation.

The physical signs and laboratory findings in chronic and acute aortic regurgitation are also different. Chronic aortic regurgitation causes a decrescendo murmur located at the left lower sternal border, which persists throughout diastole. In acute regurgitation, the murmur may end well before systole. In chronic cases, the heart is enlarged on the chest x-ray film, and the ECG virtually always shows left ventricular hypertrophy, whereas in acute cases the chest x-ray and ECG are often normal. Echocardiography is helpful in both situations. In chronic regurgitation, an evaluation of the degree of left ventricular dilatation and residual systolic function can be obtained. In acute regurgitation, a small hypercontractile ventricle is seen. Early closure of the mitral valve indicates severe regurgitation in acute regurgitation and usually mandates early surgical intervention. Concomitant aortic valve vegetations, aortic root dilatation, or aortic dissection can often be identified. The radionuclide ventriculogram is helpful in assessing left ventricular function. In acute regurgitation the ejection fraction is often supernormal (>0.70), whereas in chronic regurgitation it is often normal or depressed.

Since patients with a normal (<0.55) ejection fraction and aortic regurgitation have a low operative mortality, valve replacement is almost always indicated in symptomatic, acute aortic regurgitation that does not respond easily to digitalis and diuretics. Elderly patients with chronic aortic regurgitation who have a depressed ejection fraction (<0.50) and show marked ventricular dilatation on the echocardiogram (systolic diameter >5.5 cm) have high surgical mortality and morbidity and often irreversible ventricular dysfunction. Long-term medical therapy with digitalis, diuretics, and afterload reducing agents such as hydralazine is usually the most appropriate treatment for patients with chronic aortic regurgitation and left ventricular dysfunction. In the case of patients who are symptomatic with chronic aortic regurgitation but who have not yet reached the stage of left ventricular dysfunction just described, serious consideration must be given to valve replacement, unless concurrent medical illness is severe. Although operative mortality is relatively high (10%), reversal of left ventricular dysfunction and symptoms is the rule with successful surgery.

Mitral Stenosis

Mitral stenosis, usually a result of rheumatic fever, may be tolerated well into old age. Symptoms and hemodynamic decompensation are usually associated with the development of atrial fibrillation. Thyroid function tests should be done to identify apathetic hyperthyroidism as the cause of atrial fibrillation. In mitral stenosis, M-mode echocardiography shows thickened mitral valve leaflets, and in experienced hands the two-dimensional echocardiogram allows accurate calculation of valve orifice size. Cardiac catheterization is needed to evaluate valve area, left ventricular function, and the presence of concomitant coronary artery disease. A valve area of 1.0 cm^2 or less usually indicates that valve replacement will result in a significant improvement in symptoms of heart failure. Mitral commissurotomy is seldom appropriate for the elderly with mitral stenosis because of the marked valvular calcification usually present.

Medical therapy of mitral stenosis with atrial fibrillation should begin with at least one attempt to restore sinus rhythm, using digoxin and quinidine and, if needed, cardioversion. If normal sinus rhythm cannot be maintained, the rate should be controlled at 70–90 beats/min with digoxin and, if needed, propranolol. Diuresis and other preload reduction with long-acting oral or cutaneous nitrates is also effective in reducing symptoms of pulmonary congestion. For all patients with atrial fibrillation and mitral stenosis, anticoagulation with coumadin should be instituted 3 weeks before cardioversion and continued indefinitely, unless contraindicated, to prevent arterial embolism.

Mitral Regurgitation

The apical holosystolic murmur of mitral regurgitation is a common finding in elderly patients. Mitral regurgitation can be secondary to rheumatic disease or, more commonly in the elderly, to a number of nonrheumatic causes. The intensity of the murmur is not closely correlated with the degree of regurgitation.

In chronic mitral regurgitation echocardiography is helpful in defining the etiology of the lesion and in assessing left ventricular junction. In most cases of rheumatic mitral regurgitation the echocardiogram shows dilatation of the left ventricle and left atrium with thickening of the mitral valve leaflets. The degree of associated mitral stenosis and any other valvular lesions can also be assessed by echocardiography. Because the ventricle is emptying a significant portion of its volume into the low-pressure atrium rather than the high-pressure aorta, the ejection fraction artificially overestimates left ventricular function in chronic mitral regurgitation. Patients with mitral regurgitation who have an ejection fraction of less than 0.55 and marked left ventricular dilatation frequently develop intractable heart failure after valve replacement. Therefore an operation should be performed only if the ventricle is not severely dilated (end-systolic diameter, <5.5 cm by echocardiogram) and if the ejection fraction is well preserved. Chronic mitral regurgitation may be well tolerated for many years, even when poor left ventricular function precludes valve replacement. Standard therapy with digitalis and diuretics, as well as preload reduction therapy with long-acting nitrates and afterload reduction therapy with hydralazine, is effective in ameliorating symptoms of congestion in these patients.

Nonrheumatic mitral regurgitation is common in elderly patients. The major causes are (1) rupture of the chordae tendineae, (2) papillary muscle dysfunction or papillary muscle rupture from myocardial infarction, (3) mitral valve prolapse, (4) calcification of the mitral anulus, and (5) annular dilatation and functional mitral regurgitation secondary to cardiomyopathy.

Rupture of Chordae Tendineae

Rupture of the chordae tendineae is caused by mucoid degeneration of the chordae and usually presents as acute congestive heart failure. When the posterior leaflet is involved, the murmur may radiate to the left or right sternal border and simulate aortic stenosis. In addition, because of the rapid rise in left atrial pressure, it may have a systolic decrescendo rather than the holosystolic quality usual with mitral regurgitation. Most patients remain in sinus rhythm as shown by ECG and have normal heart size on the roentgenogram. Echocardiography shows minimal left ventricular dilatation with hyperdynamic wall motion and may disclose fluttering of the ruptured chordae. The radionuclide ventriculogram shows a supernormal ejection fraction.

Mitral valve replacement is very successful in correcting the hemodynamic lesion and is indicated for patients with preserved left ventricular function in whom symptoms of congestive heart failure are not easily controlled. Nitroprusside infusion or intraaortic balloon counterpulsation is often helpful prior to surgical procedure in stabilizing patients who are severely decompensated.

Papillary Muscle Dysfunction

Papillary muscle dysfunction occurs as a result of myocardial infarction. It is characterized by an apical murmur beginning in early to midsystole, which may radiate to the left sternal border (inferior infarction) or axilla (anterior infarction). This murmur is usually of minimal hemodynamic significance. Symptoms of dyspnea are usually related to poor left ventricular function from a prior infarction rather than to the regurgitant lesion. Some patients may require valve replacement for significant regurgitation and intractable heart failure. Because of depressed left ventricular function, surgical mortality is 25–50% in these patients.

Papillary Muscle Rupture

Myocardial infarction may be complicated by mitral regurgitation from muscle dysfunction, but even more catastrophic is papillary muscle rupture. It usually presents with acute pulmonary edema and shock, with clinical worsening over 24–48 hours. Because cardiac output is low, the systolic murmur may be deceptively soft, often ending before the end of systole. Chaotic fluttering of the mitral leaflet is seen on the echocardiogram. Swan-Ganz catheterization shows giant V waves in the pulmonary capillary wedge tracing, and massive mitral regurgitation is revealed by ventriculography. Nitroprusside infusion, intraaortic counterpulsation, and intravenous pressor agents such as dopamine may allow stabilization. Because the extent of the infarction is often small, left ventricular function is frequently preserved. In this situation, urgent mitral valve replacement and concurrent coronary artery bypass grafting can be performed and should be attempted, as survival with medical therapy alone is unlikely.

Mitral Valve Prolapse

Another mitral regurgitation syndrome that occurs in older age groups is the mitral valve prolapse syndrome. It is characterized by a midsystolic click and late systolic apical murmur and is considered to be a congenital lesion related to laxity of the mitral valve apparatus. Surprisingly, it is initially recognized in many patients in midlife. The echocardiogram shows characteristic buckling of the posterior leaflet of the mitral valve in systole. Although patients occasionally develop significant mitral regurgitation (associated with a holosystolic murmur) the proplapse is seldom of hemodynamic significance, and therapy is directed at control of associated atrial and ventricular arrhythmias. Prophylaxis for bacterial endocarditis is needed except in patients who have a click without an associated murmur. Cerebral emboli occur more frequently in patients with this syndrome than in those with a normal mitral valve. Antiplatelet agents such as aspirin and/or dipyridamole (Persantine) may be of value in preventing repeated embolism.

Mitral Annular Calcification

Mitral annular calcification is a disorder occurring almost exclusively in the elderly. It is usually an incidental finding, seldom necessitating specific therapy. Because the calcification prevents normal annular contraction, however, it is frequently associated with a murmur of mitral regurgitation. Rarely is the regurgitation of hemodynamic significance. Several patients have been identified in whom exuberant calcification has led to functional mitral stenosis. The calcification sometimes may extend into the conducting system, causing a bundle branch or complete heart block. Chest x-ray films may show a C-shaped calcification in the annular area, and echocardiography shows thickening of the anulus behind the mitral valve. Because the leaflets are normal, endocarditis prophylaxis is not needed. Embolism is rare in the absence of atrial fibrillation.

Functional Mitral Regurgitation

Functional mitral regurgitation may also follow left ventricular dilatation from cardiomyopathy, because the dilated, poorly contractile mitral anulus does not allow adequate juxtaposition of the mitral valve leaflets in systole. Patients with cardiomyopathy invariably have cardiomegaly with a markedly depressed radionuclide ejection fraction and an echocardiographically normal mitral valve. Treatment is aimed at control of congestive heart failure. Endocarditis prophylaxis is not indicated.

Atrial Septal Defect

Atrial septal defect of the ostium secundum type usually presents in youth or middle age; however, a number of cases have been described in the elderly. A characteristic fixed splitting of the second heart sound and pulmonary outflow tract murmur are the auscultatory clues. The electrocardiogram shows atrial fibrillation and an incomplete or complete right bundle branch block pattern. Surgical correction is the usual treatment for otherwise healthy patients under 60 years of age who have a large shunt and normal pulmonary vascular resistance. Operative intervention provides a significant symptomatic improvement, and the risk is low. Little information is available for patients over 60 years of age, although most seem to tolerate the lesion and succumb to other diseases. Prophylaxis for endocarditis is not necessary.

---

1. Kotler MN, et al: Bedside diagnosis of organic murmurs in the elderly. *Geriatrics* 36:107–125, 1981.
   Review of pathogenesis of cardiac murmurs with attention to differentiating maneuvers and special pathophysiology of the elderly.
2. Jamieson WRE, et al: Cardiac valve replacement in the elderly: A review of 320 consecutive cases. *Circulation* 64 (suppl 2):177–183, 1981.
   In patients over 65 years of age, low operative mortality was achieved (AVR 4.7%, MVR 11.4%, multiple valves 37.5%) with late deaths at 12.5%/yr and 93.2%/yr of surviving patients remaining in NYHA class I or II.
3. Austen EG, et al: Surgical management of aortic valve disease in the elderly. *JAMA* 211:624–626, 1970.
   In 40 patients with AS over 70 years of age, 32 of whom were NYHA class IV, mortality was 20% and the survivors were all markedly improved.
4. Smith N, et al: Severe aortic stenosis with impaired left ventricular function and clinical heart failure: Results of valve replacement. *Circulation* 58:255–264, 1978.
   Of 19 patients (mean age 65) with severe AS and decreased ejection fraction (mean EF, 0.37), 74% survived 3 years with marked improvement in symptoms and EF (mean,

0.63) after AVR. Heart failure, age, and decreased ejection fraction are not contraindications to surgery in AS.

5. Whiting RB, et al: Idiopathic hypertrophic subaortic stenosis in the elderly. *N Engl J Med* 285:196–200, 1971.
One-third of patients catheterized were older than 60 years of age. Although hemodynamics and symptoms were similar to those in the younger age group, most elderly patients were misdiagnosed as having CAD, MR, or AS.
6. Goldshlager N, et al: The natural history of aortic regurgitation. *Am J Med* 54:577–588, 1973.
Patients with chronic AR become symptomatic im middle or old age with a gradual progression of symptoms over 5 to 10 years. Irreversible left ventricular dysfunction may be present by the time symptoms appear.
7. Morganroth J, et al: Acute severe aortic regurgitation, pathophysiology, clinical recognition and management. *Ann Intern Med* 87:223–232, 1977.
Stresses echocardiography as a method of prompt diagnosis and urges early surgical intervention even in the setting of endocarditis.
8. Ross J Jr: Left ventricular function and the timing of surgical treatment in valvular heart disease. *Ann Intern Med* 94:498–504, 1981.
Review of the determinants of left ventricular function and recommendations for timing surgical intervention.
9. Rahimtolla SH: Valve replacement should not be performed in all asymptomatic patients with severe aortic incompetence. *J Thorac Cardiovasc Surg* 878–890, 1972.
A review of the disorder.
10. Martin RP, et al: Reliability and reproducibility of two-dimensional echocardiographic measurement of the stenotic mitral valve oriface area. *Am J Cardiol* 43:560–568, 1979.
Two-dimensional echo can accurately image mitral valve area; however, proper gain settings and transducer angulation are factors that may limit applicability in inexperienced hands.
11. Stephenson LW, et al: Surgery using cardiopulmonary bypass in the elderly. *Circulation* 58:250–254, 1978.
Discusses the low operative mortality for AVR (10%) compared with the much higher mortality for MVR (57%). Most of the patients in the latter group had chronic mitral regurgitation and heart failure.
12. Mason DT: Afterload reduction and cardiac performance. *Am J Med* 65:106–125, 1978.
Comprehensive review of the concepts of preload and afterload and the relevant drugs that can modify them.
13. Devereaux RB, et al: Mitral valve prolapse. *Circulation* 54:3–14, 1976.
Review of the subject.
14. Korn D, et al: Massive calcification of the mitral annulus: A clinical pathologic study of fourteen cases. *N Engl J Med* 267:900–909, 1962.
Although this disorder is a clinically insignificant finding in up to 10% of the elderly, it can be associated with significant MR, MS, or complete heart block.
15. Rodstern M, et al: Atrial septal defect in the aged. *Circulation* 23:665–674, 1961.
Atrial fibrillation was common in 18 patients aged 65–84 years who had significant ASD. Cyanosis and pulmonary hypertension were rare.
16. Thell R, et al: Bacterial endocarditis in subjects 60 years of age and older. *Circulation* 51:174–182, 1975.
Clinical suspicion of subacute bacterial endocarditis was low (40%) in 42 elderly patients. Although low-grade fever was usually present, murmurs were frequently (37%) absent.

VII. ENDOCRINE DISEASES

41. CARBOHYDRATE METABOLISM AND THE DIAGNOSIS OF DIABETES MELLITUS IN THE ELDERLY

David M. Slovik

Decreased Glucose Tolerance

Glucose tolerance is progressively impaired with advancing age. In nonobese adults, fasting glucose levels increase by approximately 1–2 mg/dl/decade. The small effect of age on fasting glucose concentration has no clinical significance and allows the use of the fasting glucose in diagnosing diabetes in elderly patients. In response to a glucose load, glucose disposal is progressively impaired with advancing age. During an oral glucose tolerance test, a mean increase of 9.5 mg/dl/decade (range, 4–14 mg/dl) occurs for the 1-hour value, and a mean increase of 5.3 mg/dl/decade (range, 1–11 mg/dl) occurs for the 2-hour value. Postprandial glucose concentrations within 1–2 hours of a meal also increase with aging. The glucose values after a glucose challenge are not influenced by gender. The impairment in glucose tolerance with advancing age is also demonstrated by the intravenous glucose tolerance test, the tolbutamide tolerance test, and the oral glucose tolerance test after glucocorticoid administration.

Alterations in insulin secretion, a decrease of the lean body mass, an increase of adipose tissue, poor nutrition, physical inactivity, an increase of proinsulin secretion, and insulin resistance have been proposed to explain the progressive decrease in glucose tolerance with aging. Despite the decline in glucose tolerance with aging, there appears to be no consistent impairment in insulin secretion. The fasting concentration, half-life, and metabolic clearance rates of insulin are generally unaffected by aging. In response to an oral glucose load, there may be a delayed rise in plasma insulin values. In response to intravenous glucose challenges, there appears to be a delay in the acute release of insulin in some aging persons.

With advancing age there is a reduction in the lean body mass (primarily muscle), leading to an increase in the percentage of adipose tissue. Adipose tissue uses less glucose than lean body tissue does, which may account for some of the decrease in glucose disposal with aging. Poor nutrition and physical inactivity also reduce glucose tolerance in the elderly. Proinsulin secretion is increased in elderly subjects and, inasmuch as it has less than one-tenth the biologic activity of insulin, it is possible that a smaller amount of biologically active insulin is available in this age group.

Aging causes a decreased tissue sensitivity to insulin. Since a decrease in hepatic glucose production in response to insulin administration is similar in the young and in the elderly, the muscle and adipose tissue appear to be the sites of insulin resistance with aging. The mechanisms responsible for the reduction in tissue sensitivity with aging are unclear but are probably multifactorial and may be related to an increase in adiposity, a decrease in insulin receptors, impairment in insulin binding, defective glucose transport, and increased values of free fatty acid that may be related to increased obesity in the elderly population. Glucagon release following an arginine infusion is not altered with aging, but the fasting basal glucagon levels are either normal or increased with age. Impairment in fructose and galactose utilization, an increase in the percentage of glycosylated hemoglobin, and an increase in the fasting concentration of human pancreatic polypeptide are also found in elderly patients.

Diagnosis of Diabetes Mellitus

Abnormalities in glucose disposal accompany aging and must be considered when establishing criteria for the diagnosis of diabetes mellitus in elderly patients. In the past, the blood glucose concentrations obtained during an oral glucose tolerance test had to be adjusted for age before the diagnosis of diabetes mellitus could be made in the elderly. In recent years, however, the National Diabetes Data Group of the National Institutes of Health has established new classifications and diagnostic criteria for diabetes mellitus and other categories of glucose intolerance. These criteria take into account age-related alterations in glucose tolerance and therefore can be used for the diagnosis of diabetes mellitus in the elderly.

The diagnostic criteria for diabetes mellitus in a nonpregnant adult include (1) unequivocal elevation of plasma glucose concentration together with the classic symptoms of diabetes, such as polyuria, polydipsia, rapid weight loss, and ketonuria; (2) elevated fasting glucose concentration on more than one occasion: venous plasma glucose of 140 mg/dl or greater, venous whole blood or capillary whole blood glucose of 120 mg/dl or greater; and (3) fasting glucose concentration less than that which is diagnostic of diabetes, but a sustained elevated glucose concentration observed during the oral glucose tolerance test (OGTT). Both the 2-hour sample and some other sample taken between it and the administration of the 75-gm glucose load must meet one of the following criteria: venous plasma glucose of 200 mg/dl or greater, venous whole blood glucose of 180 mg/dl or greater, or capillary whole blood glucose of 200 mg/dl or greater.

The term *impaired glucose tolerance* (IGT) is to be used instead of the previous terms, "asymptomatic diabetes," "chemical diabetes," "subclinical diabetes," "borderline diabetes," and "latent diabetes." To make the diagnosis of IGT in nonpregnant adults, three criteria must be met: (1) the fasting glucose concentration must be below the concentration that is diagnostic for diabetes; (2) the glucose concentration at 2 hours after a 75-gm oral glucose challenge must be between the normal and the diabetic values; and (3) the ½-hour, 1-hour, or 1½-hour glucose value must be unequivocally elevated. Annually, 1–5% of persons with IGT proceed to overt clinical diabetes, although the majority remain in the IGT class for many years or return to normal glucose tolerance. Clinically significant renal and retinal complications of diabetes (microangiopathy) are absent in patients with IGT. Patients seem to have an increased susceptibility to artherosclerotic disease, however, in association with other known risk factors such as hypertension, hyperlipidemia, and adiposity. The physician should attempt to decrease the risk factors for patients with IGT. Glucose tolerance can be improved over the short term by weight loss or caloric restriction, although there is no evidence that treatment of IGT has any long-term impact on the development of clinical diabetes.

Numerous medications (including diuretics and antihypertensive agents, hormonally active agents, psychoactive agents, catecholamine and other neurologically active agents, and analgesic, antipyretic, and antiinflammatory agents) commonly taken by elderly individuals affect glucose homeostasis and may confuse the evaluation of diabetes. In addition, when a glucose tolerance test is necessary, it should be administered only to patients who are otherwise healthy, who are ambulatory, and who are not taking drugs that elevate plasma glucose. The OGTT should be performed in the morning after at least 3 days of unrestricted diet containing 150 gm or more of carbohydrates. The person should have had adequate physical activity and have fasted for at least 10, but not more than 16, hours before the test. Water is permitted during the test, but the patient should remain seated and not smoke. If the above criteria are used and the patient is followed closely, the incorrect diagnosis of diabetes often made in the past will not occur, and those persons who really have an increased risk for diabetes and its related complications will be identified, so that appropriate therapy can be instituted.

1. Agner E, Thorsteinsson B, Eriksen M: Impaired glucose tolerance and diabetes mellitus in elderly subjects. *Diabetes Care* 5:600–604, 1982.
   In a study of 169 subjects tested at age 70 and again at age 80, the 10-year incidence of diabetes mellitus was 20% if impaired glucose tolerance existed at age 70, but only 4% if normal glucose tolerance was present at age 70.
2. Andres R: Aging and diabetes. *Med Clin North Am* 55:835–846, 1971.
   Discussion of glucose tolerance tests and a nomogram for oral GTT to help the diagnosis of diabetes at different ages.
3. Arnetz BB, Kallner A, Theorell T: The influence of aging on hemoglobin A_{1c} (HbA_{1c}). *J Gerontol* 37:648–650, 1982.
   In 48 nondiabetic subjects aged 50–89 years, there was an age-dependent increase in HbA_{1c} values.
4. Berger D, Crowther RC, Floyd JC Jr, Pek S, Fajans SS: Effect of age on fasting plasma levels of pancreatic hormones in man. *J Clin Endocrinol Metab* 47:1183–1189, 1978.
   In 263 healthy subjects, aged 20–69 years, plasma levels of pancreatic polypeptide rose continuously, glucagon levels rose during the third and fourth decade, and insulin levels did not change with advancing age.
5. Davidson MB: The effect of aging on carbohydrate metabolism: A review of the english literature and a practical approach to the diagnosis of diabetes mellitus in the elderly. *Metabolism* 28:688–705, 1979.
   Excellent review.

6. Defronzo RA: Glucose intolerance and aging: Evidence for tissue insensitivity to insulin. *Diabetes* 28:1095–1101, 1979.
With hyperglycemic clamp and euglycemic insulin clamp techniques, the primary factor responsible for the decrease in glucose tolerance with aging is impaired tissue sensitivity to insulin.
7. Duckworth WC, Kitabchi AE: The effect of age on plasma proinsulin-like material after oral glucose. *J Lab Clin Med* 88:359–367, 1976.
After an oral GTT proinsulin-like material was greater in older subjects, suggesting a decreased conversion of proinsulin to insulin or decreased clearance of proinsulin in older subjects.
8. Duckworth WC, Kitabchi AE: Insulin metabolism and degradation. *Endocr Rev* 2:210–233, 1981.
General discussion.
9. Dudl RJ, Ensinck JW: Insulin and glucagon relationships during aging in man. *Metabolism* 26:33–41, 1977.
The glucose disappearance rate was slower, but there were no changes in insulin or glucagon release with aging.
10. Elahi D, Muller DC, Tzankoff SP, Andres R, Tobin JD: Effect of age and obesity on fasting levels of glucose, insulin, glucagon, and growth hormone. *J Gerontol* 37:385–391, 1982.
In 186 male subjects, measurements of the main glucoregulatory hormones in the basal state are not influenced by age, but plasma glucose, insulin, and glucagon levels are influenced by obesity.
11. Golay A, et al: Decreased thermogenic response to an oral glucose load in older subjects. *J Am Geriatr Soc* 31:144–148, 1983.
Decreased glucose-induced thermogenesis in older people may contribute to their decreased energy requirement and an increased propensity to obesity.
12. Horwitz DL: Diabetes and aging. *Am J Clin Nutr* 36:803–808, 1982.
A short, concise review highlighting important points.
13. Jackson RA, et al: Influence of aging on glucose homeostasis. *J Clin Endocrinol Metab* 55:840–848, 1982.
Peripheral glucose uptake in healthy elderly men was one-third that of younger men: and since insulin binding was not reduced in the elderly, the glucose impairment may be due to a postreceptor phenomenon.
14. Kalant N, Leibovici D, Leibovici T, Fukushima N: Effect of age on glucose utilization and responsiveness to insulin in forearm muscle. *J Am Geriatr Soc* 28:304–314, 1980.
The abnormal glucose tolerance seen with advancing age is not due to a decrease in either insulin secretion or insulin stimulation of glucose uptake.
15. Kimmerling G, Javorski WC, Reaven GM: Aging and insulin resistance in a group of nonobese male volunteers. *J Am Geriatr Soc* 25:349–353, 1977.
There was no evidence of any decrease in insulin sensitivity with aging in nonobese subjects.
16. Classification and diagnosis of diabetes mellitus and other categories of glucose intolerance. National Diabetes Data Group. *Diabetes* 28:1039–1057, 1979.
Consensus of an international workshop. A must reading for all physicians involved in the care of patients with diabetes or glucose intolerance.
17. Olefsky JM: Insulin resistance and insulin action: An in vitro and in vivo perspective. *Diabetes* 30:148–162, 1981.
General article including discussion of mechanisms of insulin resistance in obesity.
18. Olefsky JM, Reaven GM: Effects of age and obesity on insulin binding to isolated adipocytes. *Endocrinology* 96:1486–1498, 1975.
In rats, the progressive decrease with age in the ability of adipocytes to bind insulin was due to an increasing adiposity and is associated with a decrease in the number of receptor sites per cell.
19. Pagano G, et al: Insulin resistance in the aged: The role of the peripheral insulin receptors. *Metabolism* 30:46–49, 1981.
A reduction in the number of insulin receptors on target cells may attribute to the insulin resistance seen with aging.
20. Palmer JP, Ensinck JW: Acute-phase insulin secretion and glucose tolerance in young and aged normal men and diabetic patients. *J Clin Endocrinol Metab* 41:498–503, 1975.

Although there was a decrease in the glucose disposal rate in aged normal men, there was no alteration in the acute-phase secretion of insulin in response to glucose.
21. Reaven GM, et al: Does insulin removal rate from plasma decline with age? *Diabetes* 31:670–673, 1982.
This study suggests an age-related decrease in insulin catabolism.
22. Robert JJ, et al: Quantitative aspects of glucose production and metabolism in healthy elderly subjects. *Diabetes* 31:203–211, 1982.
Reduced glucose tolerance in the elderly is associated with changes in glucose uptake by peripheral tissues and possibly impaired insulin efficiency.
23. Swenne I: Effects of aging on the regenerative capacity of the pancreatic beta-cell of the rat. *Diabetes* 32:14–19, 1983.
With aging in the rat, there is a decrease in the number of islet cells able to undergo proliferation.
24. WHO Expert Committee on Diabetes Mellitus: Second report. *WHO Tech Rep Ser* 646:1–80, 1980.
General discussion of diagnosis, classification, epidemiology, complications, and management of diabetes.
25. Williams TF: Diabetes mellitus. *Clin Endocrinol Metab* 10:179–194, 1981.
Review of aging and carbohydrate metabolism as well as diagnosis, clinical picture, and therapy of diabetes mellitus in older patients.

42. COMPLICATIONS OF DIABETES MELLITUS

David M. Slovik

The incidence of diabetes mellitus in the United States has been estimated at between 2% and 5% of the total population. It is also estimated that 8% of the population over age 55 has diabetes and that 80% of all non–insulin-dependent diabetics are older than age 55. Diabetes is associated with long-term morbidity and mortality in the elderly.

Macrovascular Disease

Macrovascular disease in the elderly affects the large blood vessels, causing an increased incidence of myocardial infarction, stroke, and peripheral vascular disease. Arteriosclerotic heart disease appears at an earlier age in diabetics than in nondiabetics. The relative risk of developing a myocardial infarction in the elderly diabetic is several times the usual risk, and there is an increase in "silent" myocardial infarctions. When it is associated with hypertension and advancing age, diabetes significantly increases the chance of stroke.

Peripheral Vascular Disease

Peripheral vascular disease, very common in the elderly diabetic patient, produces significant morbidity. The major risk factors for the development of peripheral vascular disease, in addition to hyperglycemia, are smoking, hyperlipidemia, obesity, and hypertension. Patients with peripheral vascular disease complain of intermittent claudication that progresses to pain at rest. Skin changes, ulcerations, and eventually gangrene occur. The term *diabetic foot* describes a combination of vascular insufficiency, peripheral neuropathy, and infection. When peripheral vascular disease is severe and symptomatic, a bypass operation may be helpful, but involvement of the distal collateral vessels in elderly diabetic patients may prevent it. Meticulous foot care is imperative in the elderly diabetic patient, especially since many of the patients have diabetic peripheral neuropathy, which predisposes to foot ulcers and infections. Diabetic patients should have properly fitting shoes and socks. They should allow nothing to cause blisters or pressure sores on the feet. Lanolin applied daily helps soften the skin. Patients should examine their feet daily for new lesions. The diabetic should never walk barefoot or wear shoes without stockings and should not use chemical agents to remove corns or calluses. The diabetic should avoid injury to the feet from heat or cold and avoid smoking and other risk factors that promote ischemic limb disease. Regular foot and nail care from a trained professional is also a wise preventive measure for the diabetic.

Diabetic Retinopathy

Diabetic retinopathy, a potentially disabling complication of diabetes, is present in over 65% of adult patients who have had diabetes for longer than 10 years. Diabetic retinopathy is divided into **nonproliferative** (background) retinopathy (which includes venous dilatation, microaneurysms, hemorrhages, retinal edema, and exudate formation) and **proliferative** retinopathy (which includes proliferation of fibrovascular tissue from the retina secondary to ischemia, neovascularization, vitreous hemorrhages, and vitreoretinal traction with resultant retinal detachment). Diabetes mellitus is a major cause of blindness and is the most important **systemic** cause of blindness. After 20 years of diabetes, all age groups show a 75–80% frequency of diabetic retinopathy. Proliferative retinopathy accounts for the majority of cases of blindness in young diabetic patients, whereas macular edema from nonproliferative retinopathy accounts for the majority in elderly diabetics. The mean survival of blind diabetic patients is approximately 5–8 years. The major cause of death is nephropathy among blind diabetic patients who die prior to age 60, and arteriosclerotic heart disease among those who die after age 60. Management of retinopathy in the elderly diabetics is directed toward good diabetic control and specific treatment to the eye. Photocoagulation with laser therapy has become a useful tool in improving the symptoms of diabetic retinopathy. Pituitary ablation is rarely used but may benefit a small group of patients with rapidly advancing, florid diabetic retinopathy. Cataracts, which are more common than retinopathy, appear earlier and mature more rapidly in diabetics, and hemorrhagic glaucoma is also a complication of diabetes.

Diabetic Nephropathy

Diabetic nephropathy leads to renal failure, culminating in dialysis, transplantation, or death, in approximately 6–9% of cases of type II diabetes. Diabetic glomerulosclerosis occurs at any age but most often in young patients. The microvascular disease in diabetic patients is associated with a thickening of the capillary basement membrane. In elderly diabetics, the development of renal failure is usually caused by problems other than diabetes. Hypertensive nephrosclerosis, pyelonephritis, papillary necrosis, obstructive uropathy, and administration of intravenous contrast material are frequently causes. Prerenal azotemia is also common in patients with congestive heart failure or diuretic treatment. Good control of blood sugar and hypertension helps in forestalling the development of renal abnormalities. Compared to younger diabetic patients, elderly diabetic patients with severe nephropathy have cardiovascular and other complications that make dialysis or transplantation unfeasible and unrealistic.

Diabetic Neuropathy

There are four syndromes of diabetic neuropathy: distal symmetrical polyneuropathy, autonomic neuropathy, diabetic "amyotrophy," and mononeuropathy.

Distal symmetrical polyneuropathy is the most frequently seen and predominantly involves the lower extremities. A serious complication of peripheral neuropathy in elderly diabetics is loss of sensation in the feet, which can lead to the development of foot ulcers. Pain intensifies at night and is sometimes relieved by pacing the floor, and paresthesias occur. Reduced vibratory sensation and loss of the Achilles reflexes occur with age, so that mild neuropathy is difficult to identify. When the reflexes are known to have been lost in a short time, or knee jerks are absent, neuropathy is easier to diagnose. Tight blood sugar control has not yet been shown to reverse the neuropathy. Phenytoin or carbamazepine may be effective in controlling the severe neuritic pain, if other nonnarcotic analgesics do not succeed.

Autonomic neuropathy can affect the gastrointestinal and genitourinary tracts. Gastrointestinal involvement causes an esophageal neuropathy, gastroparesis diabeticorum, and a diabetic enteropathy that can produce diarrhea alternating with constipation, as well as fecal incontinence. Genitourinary involvement causes a neurogenic bladder. Difficulty in emptying the bladder increases the risk of developing bladder infections and ascending pyelonephritis. Impotence is another complication. Autonomic dysfunction, causing vasomotor instability, anhydrosis, and orthostatic hypotension, occurs in elderly diabetics. Orthostatic hypotension can be relieved by elastic support stockings, a high intake of salt, and fludrocortisone acetate (Florinef) (initially, 50 μg/day). Close medical observation is necessary, in order that elderly patients treated with the drug will avoid fluid overload and cardiac or renal problems.

Diabetic amyotrophy is an asymmetric motor neuropathy that usually develops in older patients. The diabetes is mild and is characterized by an asymmetric progressive weakness and wasting of the muscles of the pelvic girdle and thigh. It is accompanied by pain and variable sensory involvement, but recovery is usually complete in several months.

Mononeuropathy develops suddenly and can involve any nerve, although palsies of the third and sixth cranial nerves are most common. The prognosis is good for full recovery in several months.

Hyperosmolar Nonketotic Coma

Definition. Hyperosmolar nonketotic coma (HNKC) usually develops insidiously over several days or weeks in middle-aged or elderly patients with mild or previously undiagnosed diabetes. HNKC is characterized by a blood sugar concentration greater than 600 mg/dl (often >1,000 mg/dl), a serum osmolality over 350 mOsm/L, and a serum acetone test less than "large" on undiluted serum. Patients with HNKC, in contrast to those with diabetic ketoacidosis (DKA), are usually elderly. The mortality rate, between 40% and 60%, is high because of the age of the patient and the associated medical problems.

Precipitating Factors. The majority of patients with HNKC have recently had some condition that has been the precipitating factor—often in the setting of a chronic illness such as renal or cardiovascular disease. The acute conditions that often provoke HNKC are gram-negative bacterial infection (urinary tract infection and pneumonia), acute myocardial infarction, pancreatitis, gastrointestinal hemorrhage, cerebrovascular accidents, and severe burns. Procedures that increase glucose input into the body, such as total parenteral nutrition and peritoneal dialysis, may also cause HNKC. Diuretics, glucocorticoids, phenytoin, propranolol, cimetidine, and immunosuppressive agents are drugs associated with HNKC.

Clinical and Biochemical Findings. On examination, dehydration, hypotension, and evidence of peripheral vascular collapse are present. Neurologic deficits, even if only minimal, are found in all patients. Half the patients are comatose on admission. Seizures and focal neurologic signs also occur.

In addition to the hyperglycemia and hyperosmolality noted above, serum potassium concentrations may be low (especially if the patient is on diuretics), normal, or high, and the bicarbonate concentration is often decreased to about 18–20 mEq/L. The arterial pH is also a little below normal; values lower than 7.2, however, indicate a severe mixed metabolic acidosis, most likely due to lactic acidosis. Hypernatremia may develop during dehydration and the blood urea nitrogen and creatinine concentrations are typically increased.

Therapy. Treatment of both HNKC and DKA is similar. Early diagnosis is the key to survival. Patients with HNKC are usually more sensitive to insulin than patients with DKA.

Insulin can be administered in small doses by intravenous infusion or parenteral injections. The "low-dose" regimen utilizes an intravenous bolus of 10 to 25 units of regular insulin, which is then followed by an intramuscular, subcutaneous, or intravenous administration of 5–15 units of regular insulin every hour. Patients in shock or who have evidence of decreased perfusion should be given regular insulin intravenously. The dose of insulin is not as critical as careful monitoring and intensive care. If hourly monitoring of blood glucose does not show a significant fall within 2 hours, the dose of insulin should be increased or the way of administering insulin changed to the intravenous route. When the patient's condition stabilizes, usually after 12–24 hours, an intermediate-acting insulin may be given and supplemented with regular insulin as necessary.

Patients with HNKC often have fluid deficits between 8 and 12 liters. About half of the calculated fluid deficit should be replaced during the first 12 hours, with the remainder replaced during the next 24 hours. Hypotonic saline (0.45 normal saline) is the fluid of choice except when cardiovascular collapse demands isotonic saline or other volume expansion.

Bicarbonate is not used unless severe acidosis from associated diseases requires alkali. Because total body stores of potassium are depleted, potassium supplementation is also necessary. With appropriate therapy, many of the presenting neurologic deficits will clear. Diabetic control is usually not difficult in patients who recover from HNKC. Diet alone, oral agents, or low doses of insulin are usually enough. Drugs known to cause carbohydrate intolerance should be given to these patients with caution.

1. Arieff AI, Carroll HJ: Non-ketotic hyperosmolar coma with hyperglycemia: Clinical features, pathophysiology, renal function, acid-base balance, plasma-cerebrospinal fluid equilibria and the effects of therapy. *Medicine* 51:73–94, 1972.
Most patients were middle-aged to elderly, and all had mild diabetes or were not known to be diabetic.
2. Diabetic Retinopathy Study Research Group. Photocoagulation treatment of proliferative diabetic retinopathy: Clinical application of diabetic retinopathy study (DRS) findings, DRS report no. 8. *Ophthalmology* 88:583–600, 1981.
Photocoagulation for the treatment of proliferative diabetic retinopathy reduces the risk of severe visual loss by 50% or more.
3. Ellenberg M: Diabetic neuropathy: Clinical aspects. *Metabolism* 25:1627–1655, 1976.
General review. Diabetic neuropathy is classified into two broad categories: (1) somatic (peripheral) neuropathy, which includes symmetric peripheral neuropathies, asymmetric neuropathies (e.g., mononeuropathies and diabetic amyotrophy), and diabetic neuropathic cachexia; and (2) visceral neuropathy, which includes cranial nerve palsies, gastrointestinal and genitourinary tract dysfunction, and autonomic neuropathy.
4. Feldman M, Schiller LR: Disorders of gastrointestinal motility associated with diabetes mellitus. *Ann Intern Med* 98:378–384, 1983.
In many diabetic patients, GI symptoms are common and are thought to be due to abnormal GI motility, which, in turn, may be a manifestation of diabetic autonomic neuropathy.
5. Gordon EE, Kabadi UM: The hyperglycemic hyperosmolar syndrome. *Am J Med Sci* 271:252–268, 1976.
Review. In the average patient with HNKC, sodium and potassium losses may amount to 300–500 mEq of each. Severe hypokalemia may occur 3–6 hours after the institution of therapy.
6. Jarrett J: Diabetes and the heart: Coronary heart disease. *Clin Endocrinol Metab* 6:389–402, 1977.
Diabetic patients have a greater risk of developing and dying from coronary heart disease than age-matched nondiabetics.
7. Kahn HA, Bradley RF: Prevalence of diabetic retinopathy: Age, sex, and duration of diabetes. *Br J Ophthalmol* 59:345–349, 1975.
The prevalence of retinopathy is positively related to age only for diabetics with a duration of the disease under 10 years.
8. Keller U, Berger W: Prevention of hypophosphatemia by phosphate infusion during treatment of diabetic ketoacidosis and hyperosmolar coma. *Diabetes* 29:87–95, 1980.
Phosphate therapy did not improve the course of patients in diabetic coma and is not a necessary measure in the standard treatment of diabetic coma.
9. Kohner EM, Oakley NW: Diabetic retinopathy. *Metabolism* 24:1085–1102, 1975.
Maculopathy characteristically affects patients with adult-onset nonketotic diabetes and, in those patients over the age of 60, is the most common cause of visual loss.
10. Krosnick A, Podolsky S: Diabetes and sexual dysfunction: Restoring normal ability. *Geriatrics* 36:92–100, 1981.
Impotence in older diabetic men is very common and due chiefly to autonomic neuropathy. The surgical insertion of a penile prosthesis to counteract erectile failure is sometimes helpful.
11. Owens JA Jr: How to treat the diabetic foot. *Geriatrics* 37:57–69, 1982.
The triad of infection, ischemia, and neuropathy involving the foot in diabetic patients can be devastating and lead to amputation if aggressive management is not undertaken.
12. Park R, Arieff AI: Lactic acidosis: Current concepts. *Clin Endocrinol Metab* 12:339–358, 1983.
Review of this disorder, which carries a mortality of over 50%. The use of very high doses of sodium bicarbonate in this disorder has little beneficial effects on overall survival and may worsen blood lactate levels and increase lactate production.
13. Podolsky S: Hyperosmolar nonketotic coma in the elderly diabetic. *Med Clin North Am* 62:815–828, 1978.
Review. This disorder develops insidiously and is characterized by severe dehydration and neurologic findings.

14. Podolsky S: Diagnosis and treatment of sexual dysfunction in the male diabetic *Med Clin North Am* 66:1389–1396, 1982.
Sexual dysfunction is common in long-term diabetic men of all ages. Erectile impotence in the diabetic male may be due to autonomic neuropathy, vascular disease, pharmacologic agents, surgery, and endocrine hypofunction.
15. Schade DS, Eaton RP: Diabetic ketoacidosis—pathogenesis, prevention and therapy. *Clin Endocrinol Metab* 12:321–338, 1983.
Review.
16. Smith IM: Common infections in the elderly diabetic. *Geriatrics* 35:55–58, 1980.
Symptoms of infections are sometimes lacking in elderly diabetic patients, and infections run a more malignant course than in nondiabetic patients.
17. Viskum K: The prognosis of conservatively treated diabetic gangrene. *Acta Med Scand* 185:319–322, 1969.
About one-third of patients who have had an amputation on one leg will require an amputation on the other, initially unaffected leg within 3 years after the first amputation.
18. Zaky DA, Bentley D, Lowy K, Betts RF, Douglas RG Jr: Malignant external otitis: A severe form of otitis in diabetic patients. *Am J Med* 61:298–302, 1976.
This entity seems to occur exclusively in elderly diabetic patients and is characterized by pain and severe tenderness of the tissues around the ear and mastoid, persistent drainage, and the presence of granulation tissue at the junction of the osseous and cartilaginous portions of the external canal.
19. Levin ME, O'Neal LW (eds): *The Diabetic Foot.* St. Louis, Mosby, 1983.
An entire book devoted to this problem.

43. TREATMENT OF DIABETES MELLITUS

David M. Slovik

Diet

The basic principles of therapy for elderly diabetic patients are similar to those for younger diabetic patients. Symptomatic hypoglycemia is much more of a problem in the elderly because of their high incidence of cardiovascular and cerebrovascular disease. Diet remains the hallmark of therapy in type II diabetes. Therapy for the elderly should not disrupt the lifestyle that has developed over many years. The treatment program should take into consideration individual habits, socioeconomic and ethnic constraints, and emotional factors. Elderly diabetics are frequently lonely and depressed, feel isolated, and eat poorly. Medical complications of their age and disease make therapy difficult. Some are unable to walk because of peripheral vascular disease or to remember to take medications as prescribed. To be effective, the therapeutic program must be individualized and uncomplicated, with as little disruption of the patient's lifestyle as possible.

It is estimated that 80% of type II diabetics are overweight, and that the loss of 10–15% of total body weight will cause a significant reduction in glucose intolerance and, in many cases, make pharmacologic therapy unnecessary. Rigid dietary restriction encourages noncompliance in following the diet. Some older persons are unable to understand the diet or may be unable to purchase the correct food because of poverty or inability to get to the store. Some patients have erratic eating habits. Mechanical problems with dentures often necessitate soft food. Changes in intestinal absorption and bowel habits further complicate the situation. Ethnic foods and priorities make selections in the diet harder to estimate. The choice of a diet for the elderly diabetic patient must involve a cooperative effort between the patient and his or her family, dietician, and physician. It must be written out and reviewed on subsequent office visits, giving special consideration to patients with other medical conditions. The total quantity of calories in the diet is more important than the proportion of carbohydrates, proteins, or fats. A diet of 1000–1200 cal/day, if followed, is sufficient for weight loss in most cases. Low-calorie diets are usually followed initially and achieve a short-term reduction in weight, but over a long time they are difficult to follow. For the elderly patient not requiring insulin, the regularity and spacing of the diet are not as crucial as they are for the insulin-dependent diabetic.

Several regularly scheduled meals are still better than one large meal. The diet should contain approximately 40–55% carbohydrate, 15–20% protein, and 25–35% fat. The intake of saturated animal fat, cholesterol, and simple sugars should be reduced, and the amount of fiber should be increased. The use of food-exchange systems is generally not needed.

Exercise

A regular exercise program is also important in the management of diabetes at all ages. Exercise promotes a sense of well-being, helps with weight loss, improves peripheral glucose utilization, and increases insulin receptors. The exercise prescribed for elderly patients should be in accordance with their age and cardiovascular status. Light exercise such as walking is ideal for the older patient.

Assessment of Control of Diabetes Mellitus

Short-term diabetic control is usually assessed by testing of glucose in the urine and periodic determinations of glucose in the blood. Testing of the urine can be inaccurate, however, and varies depending on the renal threshold. Clinitest tablets, which test for reducing substances, may give falsely positive results if a nonglucose reducing substance is present. L-Dopa, alpha-methyldopa, high doses of salicylates, chloral hydrate, probenecid, and several antibiotics in high doses (penicillin, cephalosporin, nalidixic acid, isoniazid, and streptomycin) cause falsely positive results with Clinitest. A falsely negative result can occur with ascorbic acid. Clinistix and Tes-Tape measure glucose but can give falsely negative results with aspirin and L-dopa and in the presence of ketones; however, a correct reading with Clinistix and Tes-Tape can be obtained if only the tip of the paper is used, because the interfering substances migrate more slowly than glucose and allow a chromatographic separation. Home monitoring of blood glucose may be useful in the case of elderly diabetic patients who are difficult to manage. Long-term diabetic control can be assessed by measurement of hemoglobin A_{1c}.

Oral Therapy

The elderly patient without diabetic symptoms, who has persistent postprandial hyperglycemia in the range of 250–300 mg/dl and who is not responsive to dietary therapy, may require either oral hypoglycemic agents or insulin, although there remains controversy as to which of these two to choose. After discontinuing oral hypoglycemic agents, only about 30% of patients need to go back on this medication or start to take insulin. Although oral hypoglycemic agents are less effective than are diet and insulin, they are convenient and well accepted by patients. The prolonged hypoglycemia that occurs following overtreatment with oral agents requires hospitalization and large quantities of glucose. A short-acting oral hypoglycemic agent is preferable. Chlorpropamide is a long-acting oral hypoglycemic agent with a half-life of approximately 36 hours and a biologic effect that can last up to 60 hours. Therefore, if patients become hypoglycemic, they will require prolonged administration of glucose. In addition, chlorpropamide can cause the syndrome of inappropriate antidiuretic hormone (ADH) secretion. Chlorpropamide should be used very cautiously, if at all, for elderly patients and should be avoided when the blood urea nitrogen (BUN) or creatinine is elevated, because it is excreted exclusively by the kidney.

Insulin

Insulin is the treatment of choice for diabetic patients with hyperglycemia and symptoms of polyuria, polydipsia, weight loss, or blurred vision. In addition to human insulin, which is just becoming available, insulin preparations of greater purity have been produced, with a subsequent decline in the incidence of local reactions, insulin allergy and lipoatrophy. It is not yet clear, however, whether the greater purity of the new insulins is clinically significant. Crystalline zinc insulin, also known as "regular" insulin, and semilente insulin are rapidly absorbed after parenteral administration and have a short duration of action, with peak activity 2–4 hours after administration.

Neutral protamine Hagedorn (NPH) insulin and lente insulin are intermediate-acting insulins with a peak activity 6–12 hours after administration. Intermediate-acting insulins are most suitable for controlling the largest number of patients. Long-acting insulin preparations with peak activity 14–24 hours after administration are available. In patients who have received insulin for long periods, the peak effect may be delayed and the duration prolonged.

Of those patients receiving a single morning injection of intermediate-acting insulin, over two-thirds will be adequately controlled. Approximately 16% will have a delayed response, with the nadir of blood sugar concentration between 10:00 P.M. and 5:00 A.M. the night after the injection; these patients are called "late" or "type C" responders. For these patients regular insulin should be added to the morning injection of intermediate-acting insulin. Approximately 16% of patients will have an "early" or "type A" response, with the nadir of blood sugar concentration at or shortly after noon on the day of injection. For these patients there should be a splitting of the dose of intermediate-acting insulin, with approximately two-thirds of the total dose given in the morning and one-third in the late afternoon.

The administration of intermediate-acting insulin in the late afternoon or evening should be followed by a snack before bedtime to prevent nocturnal hypoglycemia. Nocturnal hypoglycemic reactions may lead to early morning reactive hyperglycemia (Somogyi phenomenon) and, if unrecognized, may prompt the incorrect decision to increase insulin. The Somogyi phenomenon is a rebound hyperglycemia after insulin-induced hypoglycemia. It is often difficult to recognize, because the hypoglycemia, being nocturnal, goes unnoticed. Some suggestive symptoms of the Somogyi phenomenon are wide swings in glucose control, night sweats, bad dreams, morning headaches, and insomnia. Once the hypoglycemia is recognized, the insulin dose is reduced 5–10% every 2–3 days.

General Care

In the care of the elderly, care of diabetes often rests with family members or nursing home personnel rather than with the patient. Patients and care-givers should be instructed by health professionals and given information about diet, insulin administration, urine testing, and proper skin and foot care. Instructions as to who should be contacted in case of emergency are necessary, as well as instruction in handling a hypoglycemic reaction. Patients should wear identification tags or carry a cards indicating they have diabetes, especially if they are on insulin.

1. American Diabetes Association. Principles of nutrition and dietary recommendations for individuals with diabetes mellitus: 1979. *Diabetes* 28:1027–1030, 1979.
   The panel suggested some liberalization in carbohydrate intake, preferably as complex carbohydrate (starch associated with fiber).
2. Anderson JW, Midgley WR, Wedman B: Fiber and diabetes. *Diabetes Care* 2:369–379, 1979.
   Persons with diabetes who are eating very low-fiber diets would benefit from an increase in plant fiber intake from whole grains, legumes, and vegetables because these foods lower plasma glucose concentration and decrease glycosuria.
3. Arky R, Wylie-Rosett J, El-Beheri B: Examination of current dietary recommendations for individuals with diabetes mellitus. *Diabetes Care* 5:59–63, 1982.
   The nutrition committees of the American, British, and Canadian Diabetes associations suggest decreasing the fat content and increasing the carbohydrate and fiber content in diabetic meal plans.
4. Bressler R: Should you control blood glucose in the older diabetic? *Geriatrics* 34:41–47, 1979.
   Good blood glucose control does appear to delay or prevent some microvascular complications.
5. Cahill GF Jr, Etzwiler DD, Freinkel N: "Control" and diabetes. *N Engl J Med* 294:1004–1005, 1976.
   Evidence supports the view that the microvascular complications of diabetes are decreased by reduction of blood glucose concentration.
6. Davidson MB: *Diabetes Mellitus: Diagnosis and Treatment.* New York, Wiley, 1981.
   Discussions about general therapeutic principles, treatment, office management, and education.
7. Davidson MB: The case for control in diabetes mellitus. *West J Med* 129:193–200, 1978.
   In diabetic animal models and human studies, microangiopathic complications can be prevented by tight glucose control.

8. Galloway JA: Insulin treatment for the early 80s: Facts and questions about old and new insulins and their usage. *Diabetes Care* 3:615–622, 1980.
Discussion of the use of insulin, including factors that influence insulin's effect, advantages and disadvantages of lente and NPH insulin, and complications of insulin therapy.
9. Home PD, Alberti KGMM: Human insulin. *Clin Endocrinol Metab* 11:453–483, 1982.
The production of human insulin by recombinant DNA technology is a major scientific achievement, but there is little evidence at this time to suggest significant clinical differences between human insulin and highly purified porcine insulin.
10. Kadowaki T, Hagura R, Kajinuma H, Kuzuya N, Yoshida S: Chlorpropamide-induced hyponatremia: Incidence and risk factors. *Diabetes Care* 6:468–471, 1983.
Hyponatremia should be borne in mind in patients receiving chlorpropamide, especially when they are elderly and/or are also receiving thiazide diuretics.
11. Krall LP, Chabot VA: Oral hypoglycemic agent update. *Med Clin North Am* 62:681–694, 1978.
Review.
12. Molnar GD: Clinical evaluation of metabolic control in diabetes. *Diabetes* 27 (suppl 1):216–225, 1978.
Despite the limitations, urine glucose tests are valuable in the management of diabetic patients.
13. Nuttall FQ: Diet and the diabetic patient. *Diabetes Care* 6:197–207, 1983.
It is unknown whether dietary changes significantly delay or prevent long-term complications of diabetes, and it is best to allow diabetic persons to select their own diet and daily meal plan, as long as the nutrient content is adequate.
14. Peacock I, Tattersall R: Methods of self-monitoring of diabetic control. *Clin Endocrinol Metab* 11:485–501, 1982.
The use of home glucose monitoring devices will help establish better control of diabetes.
15. Podolsky S: Management of diabetes in the surgical patient. *Med Clin North Am* 66:1361–1372, 1982.
Hyperosmolar nonketotic coma may develop in surgical patients due to surgical stress, postoperative hyperglycemic drugs, dehydration, and exogenous glucose loads.
16. Raskin P: Diabetic regulation and its relationship to microangiopathy. *Metabolism* 27:235–252, 1978.
Inasmuch as few diabetic patients have ever been rigidly controlled, no convincing clinical evidence supports rigid control of metabolic abnormalities to prevent vascular complications; however, there is also no overwhelming evidence to the contrary. Better studies with rigid control of diabetes will answer this question.
17. Shuman CR: Surgery and diabetes, in Ellenberg M, Rifkin H (eds): *Diabetes Mellitus: Theory and Practice.* New York, Medical Examination Publishing, 1983, pp 679–687.
In diabetic patients who require insulin and need to undergo major surgery, regular insulin may be added to their intravenous infusions, or one-half of the usual dose of insulin (NPH and regular) may be given preoperatively and one-half postoperatively.
18. Soeldner JS: Treatment of diabetes mellitus by devices. *Am J Med* 70:183–194, 1981.
Various insulin delivery systems are being developed in order to provide better control of blood glucose concentration and, hopefully, determine whether tight control of diabetes is important in preventing the late complications of this disease.
19. Sutherland DER, Goetz FC, Najarian JS: Pancreas transplantation. *Clin Endocrinol Metab* 11:549–578, 1982.
During the 15-year period from 1966 to 1981, 183 pancreas transplants were performed, with nearly half being performed in the last 2 years. Although the technical problems are not entirely solved, the major cause of graft failure has been rejection.
20. University Group Diabetes Program. Effects of hypoglycemic agents on vascular complications in patients with adult-onset diabetes: VIII. Evaluation of insulin therapy: Final report. *Diabetes* 31 (suppl 5):1–81, 1982.
The most recent report on the UGDP. Provides a comprehensive evaluation of the effects of insulin treatment on vascular complications. References to the previous reports and a discussion of the UGDP controversy are included.
21. Vranic M, Horvath S, Wahren J (eds): Proceedings of a conference on diabetes and exercise. *Diabetes* 28 (suppl 1):1–113, 1979.
Training programs that result in a diminution of insulin requirements may be most

useful in the control of diabetes, particularly in those patients who do not require insulin therapy.

22. West KM: Diet therapy of diabetes: An analysis of failure. *Ann Intern Med* 79:425–434, 1973.
Diabetic patients rarely understand and follow their diet prescription, yet diet therapy is of considerable potential benefit.
23. Whitehouse FM, Arky RA, Bell DI, Lawrence PA, Freinkel N: Policy statement. The UGDP controversy. *Diabetes* 28:168–170, 1979.
Only data presented in refereed scientific publications concerning the UGDP should be given professional credence; physician judgment on management of maturity-onset diabetic patients should be based on all therapeutic information available; diet therapy is still the prime form of treatment in this group of patients; the choice of a sulfonylurea or insulin is left up to the judgment of physicians after discussion with patients; any formal recommendations on the use of tolbutamide based on initial findings should be held in abeyance until a review of new data is accomplished.
24. University Group Diabetes Program. A study of the effects of hypoglycemic agents on vascular complications in patients with adult-onset diabetes. *Diabetes* 19 (suppl 2):787–830, 1970.
The original report of 823 diabetic patients randomly divided into four treatment groups that showed an increased number of cardiovascular deaths in the tolbutamide group.

44. THYROID FUNCTION AND NONTHYROIDAL ILLNESS IN THE ELDERLY

David M. Slovik

It is unclear whether the diminution of thyroid function with age is the result of the aging process or whether in some way it actually contributes to aging. The thyroid glands from some elderly persons are indistinguishable in size and structure from normal glands in younger subjects; however, other elderly patients have small, atrophic glands with fibrosis, decreased follicle size, and a small round-cell infiltrate.

Thyroid Function Tests

Thyroxine. Thyroxine (T_4) concentrations are usually normal but may be reduced by 15–20% in normal elderly persons. Aging causes a progressive decrease in the metabolic clearance rate (MCR) of T_4 and in the thyroid gland secretion of T_4; however, this decrease does not indicate thyroid gland failure. Neither the free T_4 concentrations nor the **free T_4 index,** an indirect measurement of available free T_4, changes with advancing age. In addition, thyroid-binding proteins do not usually change in healthy elderly individuals.

Triiodothyronine. Approximately 80% of triiodothyronine (T_3) is produced in peripheral tissues from the deiodination of T_4 in the 5′ position; the remaining 20% is produced in the thyroid gland itself. T_3 concentrations decrease with advancing age, although the decline may reflect nonthyroidal illness (NTI) rather than age itself. Inasmuch as the MCR of T_3 appears unchanged, a decrease in the rate of conversion of T_4 to T_3 seems to be responsible for the decreased T_3 concentrations with aging. T_4 can also be deiodinated in the 5 position in peripheral tissues by means of a pathway different from that which produces T_3, with **reverse T_3** (rT_3) thus being formed. About 95–98% of rT_3 is derived from T_4 in peripheral tissues; the remainder is derived from the thyroid gland. Reverse T_3 concentrations do not increase with age in normal elderly patients, although they do increase in elderly patients with NTI.

Thyroid-Stimulating and Thyrotropin-Releasing Hormones. Basal thyroid-stimulating hormone (TSH) values show a slight increase with age, although they usually remain within the normal range. Slight elevations have been reported in up to 8% of elderly patients but may indicate early thyroid gland failure or mild subclinical hypothyroidism. The TSH response to administration of thyrotropin-releasing hormone (TRH) is sometimes blunted in the elderly, particularly in elderly men. Corticosteroids suppress TSH secretion and blunt the response to TRH. The thyroid gland response to exogenous TSH administration is sometimes decreased in the elderly. In elderly women especially, there is a slight increase in low-level antithyroid microsomal and antithyroglobulin antibody titers.

Nonthyroidal Illness

Alterations in thyroid function occur in elderly persons with a variety of nonthyroidal disorders, including systemic illnesses, caloric-deprivation states, surgical procedures, and administration of certain drugs or diagnostic agents, e.g., glucocorticoids, amiodarone, and radiopaque dyes. The abnormalities that result during thyroid function testing may erroneously suggest hypothyroidism or hyperthyroidism to the unwary clinician.

Low T_3 Syndrome. Decreased concentrations of serum T_3 are characteristic of many euthyroid patients with NTI, and the term low T_3 syndrome has been used to describe this selective deficiency of T_3. The low T_3 values result from a decrease in the peripheral conversion of T_4 to T_3. The free T_3 concentration is usually decreased, although it may be in the low normal range. Total and free rT_3 levels are increased in patients with NTI. The production and degradation rates of rT_3 appear normal in NTI. Other characteristics of the low T_3 syndrome include normal T_4 and free T_4 concentration, normal or slightly increased TSH levels, and usually a normal TSH response to TRH.

Low T_3 and Low T_4 Syndrome. Patients with NTI, especially if they are severely ill, may have low T_4 values in addition to low T_3 values. The low T_4 concentration may be caused by changes in (1) thyroidal T_4 secretory rate, (2) protein binding, (3) T_4 transport, and (4) peripheral metabolism of T_4. In NTI the secretion of T_4 from the thyroid appears normal or only slightly decreased, and the peripheral metabolism of T_4 may be increased. It appears, however, that the main reason for the low serum T_4 concentration is an abnormality in the binding of T_4 to serum proteins. This abnormality may be (1) a reduction in one of the binding proteins (thyroxine-binding globulin [TBG], thyroxine-binding prealbumin [TBPA], and albumin); (2) a reduction in the affinity of TBG for T_4; or (3) an inhibitor of thyroid binding that circulates in the blood of some patients with NTI. The **T_3-resin uptake** (T_3R uptake), an indirect measurement of thyroid hormone–binding capacity, is inversely related to the available binding sites. In patients with NTI, the T_3R uptake is usually elevated, indicating a decrease in the thyroid hormone–binding capacity.

The free T_4 index (FT_4I), an estimate of the free T_4 concentration, may give an underestimation of the free T_4 level in euthyroid patients with NTI. On the other hand, the equilibrium dialysis technique may yield an overestimation of free T_4 concentration. There are several other findings characteristic of patients with NTI and low T_4 and low T_3 values: (1) a normal or increased dialyzable fraction of T_3, (2) a decreased or low-normal free T_3 concentration, (3) a normal or increased total and free rT_3 concentration, (4) a normal or slightly increased TSH level, and (5) a normal TSH response to TRH.

Euthyroid Hyperthyroxinemia. *Euthyroid hyperthyroxinemia* refers to an elevation in T_4 concentration in a clinically euthyroid state. It is important to recognize this syndrome in elderly patients, so that the diagnosis of thyrotoxicosis is not mistakenly made and the patient is not treated with potentially harmful medication. Euthyroid hyperthyroxinemia is usually caused by increased thyroid binding due to an acquired increase in thyroid-binding globulin. An inherited abnormality of thyroid hormone–binding proteins is less common. Euthyroid hyperthyroxinemia can be caused by peripheral resistance to thyroid hormones. Transient hyperthyroxinemia can be seen during acute nonthyroidal illnesses, acute psychiatric illness, and after ingestion of certain drugs. The diagnosis of euthyroid hyperthyroxinemia is suggested by a decreased T_3R uptake and a normal calculated free T_4 index. TBG concentration increases in elderly patients with infectious hepatitis, chronic active hepatitis, and primary biliary cirrhosis but not in those with chronic liver disease. Estrogen-producing tumors and exogenous estrogens administered for either menopausal symptoms or prevention of bone loss, as well as 5-fluorouracil and clofibrate, can all increase TBG concentration.

In patients with acute psychiatric symptoms, transient hyperthyroxinemia usually comes from abnormalities in thyroid binding. Restlessness, agitation, nervousness, emotional lability, and tremor may suggest thyrotoxicosis but are also seen in euthyroid patients with psychiatric disorders.

Certain drugs interfere with both thyroid hormone metabolism and regulation of pituitary thyrotropin secretion. Iopanoic acid and ipodate (oral cholecystographic dyes) and amiodarone (an antiarrhythmic drug) contain organic iodine and can increase the serum concentration of T_4, free T_4, rT_3, and TSH as well as the TSH response to TRH; the total

T_3 level is low, however, and the free T_3 either low or normal. The biochemical abnormalities seen with these agents may persist for weeks after their withdrawal.

Patients with elevations in T_4 may have normal or low T_3 concentrations due to NTI. After recovery from the NTI, the T_3 concentration may increase into the thyrotoxic range, although in most cases the T_4 returns to normal and there is no further evidence of thyroid abnormality. The diagnosis of hyperthyroidism in an elderly patient in the setting of acute medical or psychiatric illness and an isolated elevation of serum T_4 can be difficult. A normal TSH response to TRH administration excludes T_4 toxicosis, but an absent or blunted response, usually indicative of thyrotoxicosis, can occur in elderly subjects without thyrotoxicosis and also in some patients with psychiatric or other illnesses. Close clinical and laboratory monitoring of these patients is necessary to either establish or eliminate the diagnosis of hyperthyroidism. A rise in the serum T_3 concentrations into the thyrotoxic range during recovery from the acute illness permits a definitive diagnosis of thyrotoxicosis.

---

1. Azizi F, et al: Pituitary-thyroid responsiveness to intramuscular thyrotropin-releasing hormone based on analysis of serum thyroxine, tri-iodothyronine and thyrotropin concentrations. *N Engl J Med* 292:273–277, 1975.
   Decreased TSH response to TRH administration occurs in older men but not in older women.
2. Bacci V, Schussler GC, Kaplan TB: The relationship between serum triiodothyronine and thyrotropin during systemic illness. *J Clin Endocrinol Metab* 54:1229–1235, 1982.
   During the recovery phase from severe illness, the TSH level may be transiently elevated.
3. Baker SP, Gaffney GW, Shock NW, Landowne M: Physiological responses of five middle-aged and elderly men to repeated administration of thyroid stimulating hormone (thyrotropin; TSH). *J Gerontol* 14:37–47, 1959.
   The thyroid glands of elderly subjects respond normally to TSH administration.
4. Bermudez F, Surks MI, Oppenheimer JH: High incidence of decreased serum triiodothyronine concentration in patients with nonthyroidal disease. *J Clin Endocrinol Metab* 41:27–40, 1975.
   Low serum T_3 levels were found in 70% of euthyroid patients with NTI.
5. Birkhauser M, Burer TH, Bussett R, Burger A: Diagnosis of hyperthyroidism when serum thyroxine alone is raised. *Lancet* 2:53–56, 1977.
   In 31 clinically euthyroid patients with NTI with elevated T_4 and free T_4 and normal T_3 concentrations, classic hyperthyroidism developed in 14 after recovery from intercurrent illness (11 had received iodine-containing preparations), 11 had return of thyroid function test abnormalities to normal in 2–8 weeks, and 6 continued to have elevated T_4 levels but were clinically euthyroid.
6. Borst GC, Eil C, Burman KD: Euthyroid hyperthyroxinemia. *Ann Intern Med* 98:366–378, 1983.
   Review of the various causes of hyperthyroxinemia without thyrotoxicosis.
7. Braverman LE, Dawber NA, Ingbar SH: Observations concerning the binding of thyroid hormones in sera of normal subjects of varying ages. *J Clin Invest* 45:1273–1279, 1966.
   The decreased peripheral turnover of T_4 in the elderly does not result from alterations in the binding of thyroid hormones in the plasma.
8. Britton KE, et al: Is "T_4 toxicosis" a normal biochemical finding in elderly women? *Lancet* 2:141–142, 1975.
   Elevated T_4 levels are a common biochemical finding in euthyroid elderly female hospital patients and do not necessarily indicate hyperthyroidism.
9. Burrows AW, et al: Low serum L-T_3 levels in the elderly sick: Protein binding, thyroid and pituitary responsiveness, and reverse T_3 concentrations. *Clin Endocrinol* 7:289–300, 1977.
   Several factors are important in the pathogenesis of low T_3 levels in NTI, including a shift in monodeiodonation of T_4 from T_3 to rT_3 and hypothalamic-pituitary dysfunction.
10. Burrows AW, et al: Thyroid hormones in the elderly sick: "T_4 euthyroidism." *Br Med J* 4:437–439, 1975.

Elevated levels of T_4 may be seen in elderly sick patients, but the diagnosis of thyroid disease in NTI should not be made on a single test.

11. Caplan RH, Wickus G, Glasser JE, Davis K, Wahner HW: Serum concentrations of the iodothyronines in elderly subjects: Decreased triiodothyronine (T_3) and free T_3 index. *J Am Geriatr Soc* 29:19–24, 1981.
In elderly subjects without complicating illness, a decrease in the total T_3 and free T_3 index is seen, but T_4, free T_4 index, rT_3, and T_2 are unchanged.
12. Chopra IJ: Euthyroid sick syndrome: Abnormalities in circulating thyroid hormones and thyroid hormone physiology in nonthyroidal illness (NTI). *Medical Grand Rounds* 1:201–212, 1982.
General review.
13. Chopra IJ, Solomon DH, Chua Teco GN, Eisenberg JB: An inhibitor of the binding of thyroid hormones to serum proteins is present in extrathyroidal tissues. *Science* 215:407–409, 1982.
The inhibitor is heat-labile and nondialyzable and acts by reducing the binding affinity of thyroid hormones to serum proteins, not by reducing the number of binding sites.
14. Gavin LA, Rosenthal M, Cavalieri RR: The diagnostic dilemma of isolated hyperthyroxinemia in acute illness. *JAMA* 242:251–253, 1979.
In 18 patients with acute illnesses and elevated serum T_4 and free T_4 levels, the serum total T_3 concentration, the T_3/T_4 ratio, and the indirectly measured free T_3 index were the most useful parameters in excluding hyperthyroidism. Of these, the FT_3 index was the most useful, being normal or low in all euthyroid and high in hyperthyroid patients.
15. Gilbert PD: Thyroid function and disease, in Libow LS, Sherman FT (eds): *The Core of Geriatric Medicine.* St. Louis, Mosby, 1981, pp 246–279.
General review of thyroid function changes in the elderly caused by age, thyrotoxicosis, and hypothyroidism.
16. Gregerman RI, Gaffney GW, Shock NW: Thyroxine turnover in euthyroid men with special reference to changes with age. *J Clin Invest* 41:2065–2074, 1962.
The thyroxine degradation rate declines about 50% over the age span of 20–80 years.
17. Havard CWH: The thyroid and aging. *Clin Endocrinol Metab* 10:163–178, 1981.
General review.
18. Hegedus L, et al: The determination of thyroid volume by ultrasound and its relationship to body weight, age, and sex in normal subjects. *J Clin Endocrinol Metab* 56:260–263, 1983.
Significant correlation between thyroid volume and both body weight and age.
19. Ingbar S: The influence of aging on the human thyroid hormone economy, in Greenblatt RB (ed): *Geriatric Endocrinology.* New York, Raven Press, 1978, vol 5 in Aging Series pp 13–31.
General review.
20. Irvine RE, Hodkinson HM: Thyroid disease in old age, in Brocklehurst JC (ed): *Textbook of Geriatric Medicine and Gerontology.* Edinburgh, Churchill Livingstone, 1978, pp 461–494.
General review of thyroid function changes in the elderly caused by age, thyrotoxicosis, and hypothyroidism.
21. Jeffreys PM, Farran HEA, Hoffenberg R, Fraser PM, Hodkinson HM: Thyroid-function tests in the elderly. *Lancet* 1:924–927, 1972.
Abnormal thyroid-function tests in the elderly are due to illness and not the aging process.
22. Kaptein EM, Grieb DA, Spencer CA, Wheeler WS, Nicoloff JT: Thyroxine metabolism in the low thyroxine state of critical nonthyroidal illness. *J Clin Endocrinol Metab* 53:764–771, 1981.
A blunted TSH response to TRH was seen in critically ill patients. This may be secondary to mild pituitary inhibition resulting from elevated glucocorticoid levels.
23. Kaptein EM, Weiner JM, Robinson WJ, Wheeler WS, Nicoloff JT: Relationship of altered thyroid hormone indices to survival in nonthyroidal illnesses. *Clin Endocrinol* 16:565–574, 1982.
Decreased total T_4 levels had the highest correlation with mortality in 195 patients requiring intensive medical therapy.
24. Melmed S, Hershman JM: The thyroid and aging, in Korenman SG (ed): *Endocrine*

Aspects of Aging. New York, Elsevier, 1982, pp 33–53.
General review.

25. Oddie TH, Myhill J, Pirnque FG, Fisher DA: Effect of age and sex on the radioiodine uptake in euthyroid subjects. *J Clin Endocrinol Metab* 28:776–782, 1968.
Average clearance rate for males was lower than for females and decreased with age.
26. Olsen T, Laurberg P, Weeke J: Low serum triiodothyronine and high serum reverse triiodothyronine in old age: An effect of disease, not age. *J Clin Endocrinol Metab* 47:1111–1115, 1978.
Notes identical levels of T_4, T_3, free T_4, free T_3, rT_3, and TSH in serum of young and elderly healthy subjects.
27. Sawin CT, Chopra D, Azizi F, Mannix JE, Bacharach P: The aging thyroid: Increased prevalence of elevated serum thyrotropin levels in the elderly. *JAMA* 242:247–250, 1979.
In 5.9% of 344 relatively healthy persons aged 60 years and older, serum TSH levels were elevated, suggesting mild unrecognized hypothyroidism.
28. Snyder PJ, Utiger RD: Thyrotropin response to thyrotropin releasing hormone in normal females over forty. *J Clin Endocrinol Metab* 34:1096–1098, 1972.
There is no age-related decrease in the TSH response to TRH administration in women.
29. Snyder PJ, Utiger RD: Response to thyrotropin releasing hormone (TRH) in normal man. *J Clin Endocrinol Metab* 34:380–385, 1972.
There is an age-related decrease in TSH response to TRH administration in men.
30. Stoffer RP, Hellwig CAA, Welch JW, McCusker EW: The thyroid gland after age 50. *Geriatrics* 16:435–443, 1961.
Describes anatomic changes in the thyroid with aging.
31. Wartofsky L, Burman KD: Alterations in thyroid function in patients with systemic illness: The "euthyroid sick syndrome." *Endocr Rev* 3:164–217, 1982.
Detailed review with 657 references.
32. Woeber KA, Maddux BA: Thyroid hormone binding in nonthyroidal illness. *Metabolism* 30:412–416, 1981.
Suggests that serum of patients with severe NTI have a nonultrafilterable inhibitor of T_4 binding.

45. HYPERTHYROIDISM

David M. Slovik

Causes

It is estimated that up to 30–35% of all cases of hyperthyroidism occur in patients older than 60. The disease is more common in women than in men. Elderly patients with hyperthyroidism have toxic multinodular goiters more often and Graves' disease less often than the younger patients, and toxic multinodular goiter may be the most common cause of hyperthyroidism in the elderly.

Hyperthyroidism in elderly persons can be caused by toxic multinodular goiter, toxic diffuse goiter (Graves' disease), toxic uninodular goiter, iodine administration (jodbasedow syndrome), exogenous thyroid hormone administration, thyroiditis, and tumors—e.g., follicular carcinoma of the thyroid and thyrotropin-secreting tumors.

General Findings

As many as one-third of elderly hyperthyroid patients do not have goiters, and some may not even have palpable thyroid tissue on clinical examination, unlike younger patients with hyperthyroidism, who invariably have goiters. Although the atypical presentation of hyperthyroidism in the elderly has drawn much attention, the majority of patients are symptomatic, with clinical findings similar to those in the young with hyperthyroidism. Hyperthyroidism often presents in the elderly with symptoms related to a single system, usually the cardiovascular system, although gastrointestinal and neuromuscular symptoms may predominate. The general appearance may suggest chronic illness or apathy, hence the term *apathetic hyperthyroidism*. Many of the hyperkinetic, sympathomimetic manifestations of hyperthyroidism, common in younger patients, are absent or minimal in elderly patients.

Cardiac Abnormalities. More than 40% of hyperthyroid patients over age 60 have heart rates of less than 100 beats/min. Atrial fibrillation is the most common arrhythmia in elderly hyperthyroid patients, although other arrhythmias occur, especially when there is underlying cardiac disease. Atrial fibrillation may be difficult to control with digoxin, even when the thyroid disease is controlled. Congestive heart failure and angina are found in elderly hyperthyroid patients but usually represent an exacerbation of underlying ischemic heart disease.

Ophthalmologic Symptoms. The ophthalmologic manifestations of hyperthyroidism seen in young patients occur much less commonly in elderly hyperthyroid patients. Since the exophthalmos in Graves' disease is believed to be from an autoimmune process, the lower incidence of exophthalmos in the elderly may reflect the higher incidence of toxic multinodular goiter in the elderly.

Gastrointestinal Symptoms. The gastrointestinal manifestations of hyperthyroidism in the elderly, including the triad of anorexia, weight loss, and constipation, suggest an underlying gastrointestinal malignancy. Diarrhea or an increase in the frequency of bowel movements may be the initial complaint.

Neuropsychiatric Symptoms. Neuromuscular or psychiatric symptoms, easily confused with other conditions, may be the presenting manifestation of hyperthyroidism in the elderly. Generalized weakness, marked proximal muscle weakness, and temporal muscle wasting are among the major neuromuscular findings. The fine tremor of hyperthyroidism also occurs in euthyroid elderly persons and therefore may be misleading. Depression and apathy are common psychiatric manifestations. Accelerated bone loss, hypercalcemia, and hypercalciuria may also occur.

Diagnosis

The diagnosis of hyperthyroidism is based on clinical findings and laboratory testing. Elderly hyperthyroid patients usually have elevated total thyroxine (T_4) and free thyroxine concentrations and increased T_3-resin uptake. In hyperthyroidism from Graves' disease, toxic multinodular goiter, or a toxic adenoma, generally the T_4 and triiodothyronine (T_3) concentrations are elevated, but usually the T_3 is elevated out of proportion to the T_4. The additional T_3 is released from the thyroid gland, in addition to the T_3 derived from the conversion of T_4 to T_3 in peripheral tissues. Some persons with hyperthyroidism have normal T_4 concentrations and elevated T_3 concentrations (T_3 toxicosis). Some elderly patients with hyperthyroidism have normal T_3 concentrations despite elevated T_4 concentrations (T_4 toxicosis), which makes the diagnosis of hyperthyroidism difficult (see Chap. 44). The normal T_3 concentrations in this instance may be due to impairment of the peripheral conversion of T_4 to T_3, inasmuch as many of the patients also have nonthyroidal illness. After the concomitant systemic illness improves, the T_3 concentrations may become elevated, and the diagnosis of hyperthyroidism can be made.

Hyperthyroidism (jodbasedow syndrome) may develop in elderly persons after the administration of iodine-containing radiographic contrast materials or medications, and this should always be kept in mind during the evaluation of elderly patients with hyperthyroidism. A normal thyroid-stimulating hormone (TSH) response to the administration of thyrotropin-releasing hormone (TRH) excludes hyperthyroidism; but a blunted response is not diagnostic, because there is a tendency for the response to decrease with age, especially in men.

A radioiodine thyroid scan is helpful in looking at glandular consistency (diffuse enlargement, one nodule or more). The 24-hour radioiodine uptake is usually normal or high in hyperthyroidism due to Graves' disease, toxic multinodular goiter, toxic adenoma, and TSH-producing adenoma; and low or zero in hyperthyroidism due to other causes, e.g., thyroiditis, after iodine administration, or with the factitious ingestion of thyroid medications.

Therapy

Therapy of hyperthyroidism in the elderly generally follows the same principles as for younger patients, except that the elderly are often sicker because of their chronic debilitated state and associated cardiovascular problems. The treatment of choice in elderly hyperthyroid patients is radioactive iodine (RAI) using ^{131}I, which causes progressive thyroid-cell destruction. Avoid giving RAI to acutely ill patients. Before RAI is administered, it is best that the elderly patient be made euthyroid by depletion of thyroid hormone from the thyroid gland with antithyroid drug treatment. In addition, concomitant therapy with a sympatholytic agent (e.g., propranolol) should be given. Iodides are not prescribed before RAI therapy because they may replete the iodide stores in the thyroid gland and increase the likelihood of hyperthyroidism from radiation thyroiditis after RAI administration. They also raise the plasma inorganic-iodide concentration and inhibit the ^{131}I from being taken up by the thyroid gland. Large doses of ^{131}I are needed for toxic multinodular goiters, and repeated doses may be necessary. A radiation-induced thyroiditis may develop within 2 weeks of RAI administration and worsen hyperthyroidism. Three to five days after RAI treatment, thionamides should be restarted and sympatholytics continued. The incidence of post-RAI hypothyroidism increases progressively with time.

The major use of antithyroid drugs is to deplete the thyroid gland of hormone and to render the patient euthyroid so that ^{131}I can be administered. Propylthiouracil and methimazole are the two agents commonly used. Usually a normal metabolic state occurs in 6–8 weeks, but this period varies depending on the size and activity of the thyroid gland and the amount of previously stored hormone. Toxicity with these drugs includes rash, fever, arthralgias, and other minor side effects. Agranulocytosis develops in approximately 0.3–0.6% of cases and usually appears within the first 2 months of therapy. It is more likely to occur in older patients and in patients taking 30 mg or more of methimazole or with any dose of propylthiouracil. Thyroidectomy for hyperthyroidism should be reserved for elderly patients with evidence of respiratory compromise or other local compressive symptoms.

Thyroid Storm

Thyroid storm, a rare medical emergency, can occur following acute illness or stress in an untreated (or undertreated) elderly thyrotoxic patient. Severe hyperpyrexia, tachyarrhythmias, congestive heart failure, and vascular collapse are the major complications of thyroid storm. Treatment consists of the administration of a large loading dose of methimazole or propylthiouracil, followed by an intravenous infusion of potassium iodide. Some patients require large doses of corticosteroids and a sympatholytic agent (e.g., propranolol). Careful cardiac and blood pressure monitoring and supportive measures are also very important. When the acute stress subsides, the iodides and steroids can be discontinued. The antithyroid drugs and propranolol are continued, and when the patient becomes euthyroid, definitive treatment with ^{131}I is given.

1. Bartels EC: Hyperthyroidism in patients over 65. *Geriatrics* 20:459–462, 1965.
   Resting pulse rates below 100 were found in 59% of patients with hyperthyroidism.
2. Bartels EC, Kingsley JW Jr: Hyperthyroidism in patients over sixty. *Geriatrics* 4:333–340, 1949.
   Adenomatous goiter was responsible for hyperthyroidism in about two-thirds of 124 cases, with a female to male ratio of 4 : 1. In elderly hyperthyroid patients a decrease in appetite was more common than an increase in appetite.
3. Braverman LE: Therapeutic considerations. *Clin Endocrinol Metab* 7:221–240, 1978.
   ^{131}I therapy is best for elderly hyperthyroid patients, but careful preparation prior to ^{131}I administration is needed to avoid posttreatment radiation-induced hyperthyroidism.
4. Brun R, Jenny M, Junod JP: L'Hyperthyreuse des Personnes Agees. *Schweiz Med Wochenschr* 108:1504–1510, 1978.
   In 81 thyrotoxic patients over age 60, toxic multinodular goiter was the most common cause (68%) of hyperthyroidism, followed by solitary thyroid nodules (16%) and Graves' disease (16%).
5. Caplan RH, Glasser JE, Davis K, Foster L, Wickus G: Thyroid function tests in elderly hyperthyroid patients. *J Am Geriatr Soc* 26:116–120, 1978.
   The diagnosis of hyperthyroidism in the elderly is difficult, and no single test can be relied upon to exclude the diagnosis; however, TRH tests were not performed in this study.

6. Cooper DS, et al: Agranulocytosis associated with antithyroid drugs: Effects of patient age and drug dose. *Ann Intern Med* 98:26–29, 1983.
Increased risk of agranulocytosis with older age.
7. Cooper DS, Ridgway EC, Maloof F: Unusual types of hyperthyroidism. *Clin Endocrinol Metab* 7:199–220, 1978.
Discussion of hyperthyroidism due to excess TSH secretion, iodine-containing preparations, thyroiditis, thyroid carcinoma, abnormal thyroid stimulators, struma ovarii, and exogenous thyroid hormone.
8. Davis PJ, Davis FB: Hyperthyroidism in patients over the age of 60 years: Clinical features in 85 patients. *Medicine* 53:161–181, 1974.
Excellent review of the clinical findings in thyrotoxicosis in the elderly.
9. Feely J, et al: Propranolol dosage in thyrotoxicosis. *J Clin Endocrinol Metab* 51:658–661, 1980.
The dose of propranolol needed for beta-adrenergic blockade in thyrotoxic patients is quite variable, and many individuals require more than 160 mg/day.
10. Fradkin JE, Wolff J: Iodide-induced thyrotoxicosis. *Medicine* 62:1–20, 1983.
Good review. Elderly subjects with large goiters of long standing are at risk for developing thyrotoxicosis after being administered iodine-containing drugs such as amiodarone and radiographic contrast media.
11. Freund HA, Cooksey WB: Thyrotoxicosis in elderly persons without signs of goiter. *JAMA* 94:1891–1893, 1930.
One of the earliest reports describing 5 patients aged between 50 and 75 years with thyrotoxicosis and lacking classical signs and symptoms. Gastrointestinal symptoms were prominent in this group.
12. Gilbert PD: Thyroid function and disease, in Libow LS, Sherman FT (eds): *The Core of Geriatric Medicine*. St. Louis, Mosby, 1981, pp 246–279.
General review of thyroid function changes in the elderly caused by age, thyrotoxicosis, and hypothyroidism.
13. Gordon M, Gryfe CI: Hyperthyroidism with painless subacute thyroiditis in the elderly. *JAMA* 246:2354–2355, 1981.
Although painless thyroiditis is usually seen in premenopausal women, the authors report 6 elderly patients (61–93 yr) with painless subacute thyroiditis and emphasize the difficulty of diagnosis.
14. Gorman CA: The presentation and management of endocrine ophthalmopathy. *Clin Endocrinol Metab* 7:67–96, 1978.
Depending on the manifestations, treatment of Graves' ophthalmopathy involves protection of the eyes, systemic steroids, radiation therapy, and surgery.
15. Hamburger WW, Lev MW: Masked hyperthyroidism. *JAMA* 94:2050–2056, 1930.
Early report describing 5 patients with hyperthyroidism who lacked typical features of thyroid disease and presented with organic heart disease, diabetes mellitus, or GI distress.
16. Irvine RE, Hodkinson HM: Thyroid disease in old age, in Brocklehurst JC (ed): *Textbook of Geriatric Medicine and Gerontology*. Edinburgh, Churchill Livingstone, 1978, pp 461–494.
General review of thyroid function changes in the elderly caused by age, thyrotoxicosis, and hypothyroidism.
17. Kawabe T, Komiya I, Endo T, Koizumi Y, Yamada T: Hyperthyroidism in the elderly. *J Am Geriatr Soc* 27:152–155, 1979.
The most reliable diagnostic criterion in elderly hyperthyroid patients is a flat TSH response to TRH.
18. Mazzaferri EL, Skillman TG: Thyroid storm: A review of 22 episodes with special emphasis on the use of guanethidine. *Arch Intern Med* 124:684–690, 1969.
Infection was the most common precipitating event, although any stress may be involved. Sometimes no obvious precipitating cause is evident.
19. Menendez C, Rivlin RS: Thyrotoxic crisis and myxedema coma. *Med Clin North Am* 57:1463–1470, 1973.
Discussion about clinical features and therapy.
20. Ryan AJ, Davis PJ: Unusual clinical manifestations of hyperthyroidism in the elderly. *Geriatr Med Today* 2:49–54, 1983.
Unusual CNS manifestations of hyperthyroidism include behavioral changes, convul-

sive disorders, and movements disorders attributable to both corticospinal-tract dysfunction and extrapyramidal-system dysfunction.

21. Schultz AL: Diagnosing and managing hyperthyroidism. *Geriatrics* 33:77–81, 1978. *Long-term treatment of toxic nodular goiter with antithyroid drugs results in a very low permanent remission of hyperthyroidism.*
22. Seed L, Lindsay AM: Hyperthyroidism in the aged: A review of 100 cases over 60 years of age. *Geriatrics* 4:136–145, 1949. *In elderly hyperthyroid patients there is less nervous excitability, exophthalmos is less frequent, and heart failure and atrial fibrillation are more common than in younger patients.*
23. Sterling J, Refetoff S, Selenkow HA: T_3 thyrotoxicosis. *JAMA* 213:571–575, 1970. *The diagnosis of T_3 toxicosis should be suspected in any individual with evidence of hypermetabolism and a normal T_4.*
24. Stiel JN, Hales IB, Reeve TS: Thyrotoxicosis in an elderly population. *Med J Aust* 2:986–988, 1972. *In comparison to young thyrotoxic patients, 136 thyrotoxic patients over 60 years of age had a higher incidence of nodular goiter and atrial fibrillation while nervous system complaints and eye signs were less common.*
25. Sugrue D, McEvoy M, Feely J, Drury MI: Hyperthyroidism in the land of graves: Results of treatment by surgery, radio-iodine and carbimazole in 837 cases. *Q J Med* 49:51–61, 1980. *The relapse rate following a 2-year course of carbimazole was 56% and 62% at 5 and 10 years, respectively, compared with 6% and 10% following surgery, and 3% and 14% after radio-iodine.*
26. Thomas FB, Mazzaferri EL, Skillmann TG: Apathetic thyrotoxicosis: A distinctive clinical and laboratory entity. *Ann Intern Med* 72:679–685, 1970. *Apathetic thyrotoxic patients are older, have a longer duration of symptoms, and a greater weight loss than younger thyrotoxic patients.*

46. HYPOTHYROIDISM

David M. Slovik

Causes

Hypothyroidism often goes undetected in elderly persons, because the symptoms are nonspecific and may be erroneously attributed to the aging process. The incidence of hypothyroidism in the elderly has been estimated to be about 2–4% of hospitalized patients, but this is difficult to judge, because many of the abnormal thyroid function tests may have been due to changes seen with nonthyroidal illnesses (NTI) (see Chap. 44). The major causes of hypothyroidism in the elderly include (1) loss of functional thyroid tissue due to chronic lymphocytic thyroiditis (Hashimoto's thyroiditis), postablative therapy with radioactive iodine for hyperthyroidism, thyroid surgical procedure, and external neck irradiation; (2) defective thyroid hormone biosynthesis and inhibition of thyroid function due to antithyroid drugs, iodide deficiency or iodide excess, or inherited biosynthetic defects; (3) thyrotropin deficiency due either to pituitary disorders (secondary hypothyroidism) or to hypothalamic disorders with thyrotropin-releasing hormone (TRH) deficiency (tertiary hypothyroidism); and (4) peripheral resistance to thyroid hormone action.

Clinical Presentation

General Features. The clinical features of hypothyroidism in the elderly develop insidiously. There are also many characteristics of hypothyroidism that are difficult to discriminate from changes seen in old age. These include constipation, dry skin, lethargy, deafness, cold intolerance, physical and mental slowing, and depression. Important historical features indicating a possible diagnosis of hypothyroidism in the elderly include prior radioiodine therapy or operation for hyperthyroidism; a family history of thyroid disease; a family history of autoimmune disorders, since these may be associated with

Hashimoto's thyroiditis; progression of symptoms characteristic of hypothyroidism; and exquisite sensitivity to drugs, e.g., hypnotics.

Findings in elderly patients with hypothyroidism may differ from those in younger patients, because they combine with those of old age. Weight loss may be more prominent than weight gain in some persons with hypothyroidism. Facial swelling with periorbital edema occurs due to fluid retention. Skin changes include dryness, hyperkeratosis, yellow color due to increased carotene, and vitiligo. The hair also coarsens and thickens, alopecia develops, and there is loss of the lateral third of the eyebrows. The nails become brittle. The voice becomes hoarse, and speech is slow.

Cardiac abnormalities, often hard to distinguish from other cardiac disease in the elderly, include cardiomegaly with pericardial effusions, diminished myocardial contractility, increased preejection period, decreased cardiac output and cardiac index, increased left ventricular end diastolic pressure, bradycardia, hypertension (especially diastolic), decreased blood volume, increased peripheral vascular resistance, and impaired response to catecholamines.

Pulmonary manifestations include alveolar hypoventilation, hypoxia and CO_2 narcosis, sleep apnea, and occult pulmonary infections.

Gastrointestinal manifestations include macroglossia, achlorhydria, hypomotility with ileus, constipation, and obstruction.

Renal abnormalities include decreases in the glomerular filtration rate and free water clearance. Hyponatremia may develop. There is bladder atony, and urinary tract infections develop.

Musculoskeletal abnormalities include a severe myopathy, arthralgias, myalgias and the carpal tunnel syndrome.

Neurologic manifestations include intellectual deterioration, mood alterations including myxedema madness, somnolence, peripheral neuropathy, cerebellar ataxia, sensorineural deafness, and coma. In addition, the deep tendon reflexes may have a delayed relaxation phase, but this may occur in elderly persons who are not hypothyroid.

The metabolism of drugs decreases, especially neuroleptic drugs. Anemia, usually due to a combination of iron, vitamin B_{12}, and folate deficiency, is a common finding in hypothyroidism.

Diagnosis

The diagnosis of hypothyroidism in the elderly should be based on clinical suspicion and laboratory verification. Aging does not significantly influence most thyroid function tests, except perhaps serum triiodothyronine (T_3) concentrations (see Chap. 44). Measurements of T_3 concentrations, however, play no role in the diagnosis of hypothyroidism. **Primary hypothyroidism** is due to an abnormality in the thyroid gland and is characterized by a decrease in total thyroxine (T_4) and free T_4 concentrations, an increase in thyroid-stimulating hormone (TSH), and an exaggerated TSH response to TRH administration. Decreased thyroid reserve, or **prehypothyroidism,** indicates a mild deficiency of thyroid gland reserve; patients have few if any symptoms and normal values of T_4, but elevated TSH values and an exaggerated TSH response to TRH administration.

Secondary hypothyroidism is characterized by a decrease in the T_4 concentration; the TSH levels are not elevated, and there is a flat TSH response to TRH administration.

Tertiary hypothyroidism is characterized by decreased T_4 concentration; the TSH levels are not elevated, and the TSH response to TRH administration is delayed.

Treatment

Hormone Replacement. The treatment of hypothyroidism in the elderly involves slow and cautious hormonal replacement with frequent clinical and laboratory monitoring. Therapy should be initiated with very small doses of exogenous thyroid hormone. Since the half-life of thyroxine is approximately 7 days in normal persons and longer in hypothyroid patients, it will take several weeks for a steady-state concentration of hormone to be reached on any given dose. In the elderly hypothyroid patient, therefore, increases in thyroxine dosage should not be made any more frequently than every three weeks, and only after clinical evaluation of the patient.

There are many thyroid hormone preparations available for chronic replacement, but the preferred preparation is L-thyroxine (L-T_4). L-thyroxine preparations provide physiologic levels of T_3 by allowing the body to convert L-T_4 to T_3 in peripheral tissues. Desiccated animal thyroid preparations contain varying amounts of active iodothyronines and supraphysiologic amounts of T_3 and will make it difficult to monitor therapy. Mixtures of L-T_4 and L-T_3 have no advantage over L-T_4 alone and may supply supraphysiologic doses of L-T_3.

Since hypothyroidism in the elderly develops slowly, and significant other, nonthyroidal illnesses, especially cardiac disease, are often present, the initial dose of L-T_4 in the elderly should be 0.025 mg/day (25 μg). Occasionally, in the case of an elderly patient with significant cardiac disease who also requires thyroid replacement, an initial dose of 0.0125 mg/day may be needed, as well as propranolol, to reduce the myocardial oxygen requirements and prevent angina. The dose of L-T_4 can be increased by 0.0125–0.025 mg/day every 3–4 weeks, depending on the clinical hypothyroid state and cardiac status. The usual replacement dose of L-T_4 varies from 0.10–0.20 mg/day, but lower doses may provide normal replacement, and less than adequate replacement therapy may be necessary for elderly individuals with cardiac disease. To assess the status of replacement, T_4 and TSH levels should be monitored. Elevated TSH levels indicate inadequate replacement, but before any further increase in replacement therapy is made, clinical evaluation is necessary.

Myxedema Coma. Myxedema coma is a medical emergency and is the result of prolonged thyroid hormone deficiency. It occurs primarily in elderly patients, and the mortality is greater than 50%. The syndrome is usually precipitated by acute major medical illnesses, infection, surgical procedure, ingestion of medication (e.g., tranquilizers and sedatives), or other stresses. Patients with myxedema coma present with findings of severe myxedema as well as other systemic complications. The medical complications can be summarized as **"hypo's": hypo**thermia and lack of a febrile response, **hypo**ventilation, **hypo**metabolism of drugs, **hypo**natremia and **hypo**osmolarity, **hypo**tension, **hypo**contractile myocardium, **hypo**adrenalism, **hypo**glycemia, **hypo**volemia, **hypo**tonic bowel, and **hypo**tonic bladder.

Therapy requires the acute management of the medical problem in an intensive care unit. Hypoventilation and respiratory failure require aggressive pulmonary care and assisted pulmonary ventilation. Hypotonic fluids should be avoided, and hypothermia reversed slowly. A diligent search for infection should be done. Hydrocortisone, 200–300 mg/day, should be given during the acute illness. L-Thyroxine is initially administered intravenously in a dose of 200–500 μg, which replaces the total body pool of thyroxine. Thereafter, intravenous doses of 50–100 μg daily will replace the amount of T_4 that is disposed of each day. The risk of giving large doses of L-T_4 to elderly patients is offset by the high mortality associated with this disease. L-T_3 has also been used in the treatment of myxedema coma. Improvement in vital signs usually occurs within 6–12 hours after treatment is initiated, and the patient usually regains consciousness in 24–48 hours. When the patient improves enough to take oral medication, a daily oral maintenance dose of L-T_4 should be prescribed. After clinical improvement, it is necessary to prevent a relapse into myxedema coma that may occur from the premature removal of ventilatory support systems or the inadvertent administration of narcotics or hypnotic drugs.

---

1. Atkinson RL, Dahms WT, Fisher DA, Nichols AL: Occult thyroid disease in an elderly hospitalized population. *J Gerontol* 33:372–376, 1978.
Of 425 hospitalized patients over age 60, unsuspected thyroid disease was found in 10 patients (2.4%), 9 being hypothyroid and 1 hyperthyroid. An additional 11% had abnormal T_4 or TSH levels but were not proved to have thyroid disease.
2. Bahemuka M, Hodkinson HM: Screening for hypothyroidism in elderly inpatients. *Br Med J* 2:601–603, 1975.
In a group of 2,000 geriatric inpatients, hypothyroidism was found in 2.3%, with only one-third having "typical" signs and symptoms.
3. Blum M: Myxedema coma. *Am J Med Sci* 264:432–443, 1972.
Myxedema coma is a medical emergency. It may develop acutely in patients who are mildly hypothyroid and are then exposed to tranquilizers, narcotics, or sedatives.
4. Brennan MD: Thyroid hormones. *Mayo Clin Proc* 55:33–44, 1980.
A comparison of various thyroid hormone preparations was made with the suggestion that L-thyroxine is the preparation of choice for hypothyroidism since crude hormonal preparations made from animals have variable biologic potency and an unphysiologically high T_3 content.

5. Crowley WF Jr, et al: Noninvasive evaluation of cardiac function in hypothyroidism: Response to gradual thyroxine replacement. *N Engl J Med* 296:1–6, 1977.
Slow cautious physiologic thyroid hormone replacement beginning with 25 μg of L-T_4 *will reverse abnormalities in left ventricular function.*
6. Gilbert PD: Thyroid function and disease, in Libow LS, Sherman FT (eds): *The Core of Geriatric Medicine.* St. Louis, Mosby, 1981, pp 246–279.
General review of thyroid function changes in the elderly caused by age, thyrotoxicosis, and hypothyroidism.
7. Ibbertson HK: Hypothyroidism. *Pharmacol Ther* 2:177–196, 1977.
General review. Elderly patients who require thyroid replacement and have coronary artery disease should initially receive 25 μg/day of L-*thyroxine.*
8. Irvine RE, Hodkinson HM: Thyroid disease in old age, in Brocklehurst JC (ed): *Textbook of Geriatric Medicine and Gerontology.* Edinburgh, Churchill Livingstone, 1978, pp 461–494.
Another general review of thyroid function changes in the elderly resulting from thyrotoxicosis, and hypothyroidism.
9. Jellinek EG, Oxon DM: Fits, faints, coma, and dementia in myxedema. *Lancet* 2:1010–1013, 1962.
Among 56 patients with myxedema and neurological complications, 10 presented with epilepsy or syncope, 6 with coma or stupor, and 18 had psychiatric disturbances.
10. Lamberg B-A: Etiology of hypothyroidism. *Clin Endocrinol Metab* 8:3–19, 1979.
Discussion of the various causes of hypothyroidism, including those situations in which hypothyroidism may be transient.
11. Lloyd WH, Goldberg IFL: Incidence of hypothyroidism in the elderly. *Br Med J* 2:1256–1259, 1961.
Out of 3,417 new patients referred to a geriatric unit, 58 cases of hypothyroidism (1.7% incidence) and 17 cases of hyperthyroidism (0.5% incidence) were found.
12. Lloyd WH, Mawdsley C: The face in hypothyroidism. *Med Biol Ill* 17:12–19, 1967.
Facial changes are a constant feature of hypothyroidism, but in two-thirds of patients, especially in the elderly, the changes may be very subtle and easily overlooked.
13. McConahey WM: Diagnosing and treating myxedema and myxedema coma. *Geriatrics* 33:61–66, 1978.
Myxedema coma is rare but often fatal, occurs most often in elderly women, is often mistaken for a chronic debilitating disease, and requires prompt and intensive general medical care and the initial parenteral administration of L-*thyroxine.*
14. Morrow LB: How thyroid disease presents in the elderly. *Geriatrics* 33:42–45, 1978.
In the elderly, ectodermal changes such as loss of eyebrows and thinning or coarsening of the hair become less reliable because similar changes are seen with aging.
15. Porteous WM: Hypothyroidism in elderly hospitalized patients. *NZ Med J* 89:81–83, 1979.
An incidence of hypothyroidism of 3.8% was found in 396 elderly hospitalized patients and the TSH level was the most valuable and reliable screening test.
16. Ray T: What to look for in diagnosing hypothyroidism in elderly patients. *Geriatrics* 32:55–59, 1977.
The clinical presentation of hypothyroidism in the elderly compared to that in younger patients includes the more likely occurrence of drowsiness, lethargy, memory impairment, ataxia, and weight loss.
17. Rosenbaum RL, Barzel US: Levothyroxine replacement dose for primary hypothyroidism decreases with age. *Ann Intern Med* 96:53–55, 1982.
The thyroxine requirement for replacement therapy in primary hypothyroidism decreases with advancing age and in elderly patients. The average replacement dose of levothyroxine was 118 μg/day, compared with 158 μg/day in younger patients.
18. Rosenbaum RL, Barzel US: Clinical hypothyroidism in the elderly — a preventable disorder. *J Am Geriatr Soc* 29:221–223, 1981.
In elderly patients with the "failing thyroid syndrome" (elevated TSH with normal T_4*), the replacement dose of levothyroxine was approximately half that required for patients with clinical hypothyroidism.*
19. Sanders V: Neurological manifestations of myxedema. *N Engl J Med* 266:547–551, 599–603, 1962.
The nervous system is affected in many ways in myxedema, including mental disturbances, paresthesias, cerebellar disorders, headaches, seizures, cranial nerve abnormalities, and myxedema coma.

20. Sawin CT, et al: A comparison of thyroxine and desiccated thyroid in patients with primary hypothyroidism. *Metabolism* 27:1518–1525, 1978.
A daily dose of 100 μg of thyroxine was on the average equal in biologic activity to 100 mg of desiccated thyroid, but there is considerable individual variability.
21. Shopsin B, Shenkman L, Blum M, Hollander CS: Iodine and lithium-induced hypothyroidism: Documentation of synergism. *Am J Med* 55:695–699, 1973.
Lithium and iodine can separately produce hypothyroidism in susceptible individuals but can also act synergistically to produce hypothyroidism.
22. Stock JM, Surks MI, Oppenheimer JH: Replacement dosage of L-thyroxine in hypothyroidism: A re-evaluation. *N Engl J Med* 290:529–533, 1974.
Of 35 patients with primary hypothyroidism, 89% required 100–200 μg/day of levothyroxine with a mean dose of 169 μg/day (2.25 μg/kg).
23. Zwillich CW, Pierson DJ, Hofeldt FD, Lufkin EG, Weil JV: Ventilatory control in myxedema and hypothyroidism. *N Engl J Med* 292:662–665, 1975.
Myxedema and hypothyroidism produce depression of the hypoxic ventilatory drive that is responsive to replacement therapy.

47. ADRENAL FUNCTION IN THE ELDERLY

David M. Slovik

Anatomic Changes

The human adrenal gland does not show significant gross anatomic changes with advancing age, although its weight decreases slightly after age 50. The three zones of the adrenal cortex—fasciculata, reticularis, and glomerulosa—are retained in old age, although the borders between them become somewhat distorted. With advancing age, connective tissue increases, pigment accumulates, and steroid-containing lipids are lost. Nodular hyperplasia of the adrenal cortex occurs with increasing age but does not indicate an overproduction of adrenal hormones. Ultrastructure examination shows mitochondria fragmentation, hyperchromasia, and nuclear vesicle formation.

Adrenal Hormones

Cortisol production is stimulated by adrenocorticotropic hormone (ACTH), which, in turn, is stimulated by corticotropin-releasing factor (CRF), secreted by the hypothalamus. This system is under negative-feedback control and has a circadian rhythm related to the sleep-wake cycle, but both can be overcome by stress. With advancing age, plasma cortisol levels and the diurnal rhythm of cortisol remain unchanged, and the rate of removal of cortisol from the circulation is decreased (prolonged half-life). The reduced cortisol production rate in the elderly may be an adjustment to the slowed metabolic disposal rate for cortisol. The excretion of free cortisol in the urine appears to be unchanged in adults up to age 50. There is an age-related decrease in urinary excretion of the 17-hydroxycorticosteroids (17-OHCS) and the 17-ketogenic steroids (17-KGS); serum levels of cortisol-binding globulin and basal plasma levels of ACTH do not change with age.

Androgen production decreases with advancing age. The urinary excretion of 17-ketosteroids (17-KS) progressively declines to a level that is approximately 50% of the level in young adults. The reduction in urinary 17-KS is greater than the reduction in 17-OHCS. There is a progressive fall of about 50–70% in the plasma levels of dehydroepiandrosterone and androsterone with aging. Androstenedione of adrenal origin decreases in women between the ages of 45 and 50 but remains stable thereafter. Adrenal androgen response to ACTH administration of the elderly is diminished from that of younger subjects.

Production of aldosterone by the zona glomerulosa of the adrenal cortex decreases with advancing age, as does the metabolic clearance rate and plasma concentration. In response to sodium restriction or postural changes, there is a progressive decrease in the adaptive response of aldosterone secretion with aging, and aldosterone levels in elderly subjects may be 30–40% of those seen in young adults. Renin secretion also shows age-related decreases in both baseline levels and stimulated states. By age 80 the level may be 35% lower than it is at age 20. Because of the age-related changes, the diagnosis of hyporeninemic hypoaldosteronism and low-renin hypertension may be difficult to make in elderly patients.

HPA Axis Testing

Dynamic testing of the hypothalamic-pituitary-adrenal (HPA) axis can be performed after administration of insulin, metyrapone, ACTH, or dexamethasone. Insulin-induced hypoglycemia produces similar increases in plasma cortisol levels in young and in elderly persons; however, because of the significant neurologic and cardiovascular risks from insulin-induced hypoglycemia, the test should be used with great caution, if at all, in the elderly. Metyrapone inhibits the adrenal conversion of 11-deoxycortisol to cortisol. The negative-feedback inhibition on the pituitary decreases, resulting in an increase in ACTH secretion that subsequently increases the amount of 11-deoxycortisol produced. The adrenocortical response to metyrapone administration, to dexamethasone suppression, and to ACTH stimulation is similar in both young and elderly subjects. The adrenal response to surgical or medical stress (e.g., acute myocardial infarction) appears to be intact in elderly subjects and not to differ from that in younger subjects. It therefore appears that feedback control over the HPA axis is intact in elderly individuals, and that the inability of elderly persons to handle stress as do younger persons is due to other factors than a diminished adrenal stress response.

Cushing's Syndrome

Cushing's syndrome follows the prolonged overproduction of cortisol from (1) bilateral adrenal hyperplasia secondary to excessive production of ACTH from either the pituitary (Cushing's disease) or ACTH-producing tumors (ectopic ACTH syndrome), (2) adrenal nodular hyperplasia,(3) adrenal tumors, either adenomas or carcinomas, or (4) prolonged exogenous administration of glucocorticoids or ACTH. Probably the most common cause of Cushing's syndrome in the elderly patient is the iatrogenic administration of exogenous glucocorticoids as therapy for other medical disorders. Even small supraphysiologic doses, especially if given in divided doses, will produce Cushing's syndrome. One reason is that synthetic compounds are more weakly bound to plasma proteins, and in the elderly there is a decreased clearance of cortisol from the circulation. Malignant adrenal neoplasms and ectopic ACTH production by other tumors are also more common in the elderly than in younger adults.

There is generally no significant difference between young and elderly patients in the presentation, clinical findings, and diagnostic testing of Cushing's syndrome. Depending on the source of the overproduction of cortisol, surgical excision of the tumor or irradiation of the pituitary gland is usually the treatment of choice. Medical therapy, however, is often necessary in elderly patients (1) for preoperative preparation, (2) as adjuvant therapy, (3) when the patient is unable to be treated by other therapeutic methods, (4) in cases of metastatic disease with ectopic ACTH secretion, or (5) in cases of extensive adrenal carcinoma. Aminoglutethimide, metyrapone, and *o,p′*-DDD all inhibit cortisol production and are therefore helpful in the medical management of excessive cortisol production.

Adrenal Insufficiency

Adrenal insufficiency occurs in both the elderly and the young from the same causes. Causes of primary adrenal insufficiency (Addison's disease) include (1) idiopathic (autoimmune) conditions, (2) tuberculosis, (3) bilateral adrenalectomy, (4) adrenal hemorrhage, (5) metastatic carcinoma, and (6) sepsis and other rare causes. Secondary adrenal insufficiency is due to ACTH deficiency from either hypopituitarism or suppression of the hypothalamic-pituitary-adrenal (HPA) axis by the exogenous administration of glucocorticoids. Hypopituitarism can occur from pituitary or hypothalamic tumors, metastatic tumors to this region, irradiation, surgery, pituitary infarction, infections, or granulomatous diseases.

The signs and symptoms of adrenal insuficiency are often nonspecific and are similar in elderly and young patients. There also is generally no significant difference in the diagnostic testing or treatment of this disorder in different age groups; however, in those patients with primary adrenal insufficiency who in addition to glucocorticoid replacement require mineralocorticoid replacement, close monitoring is necessary because hypertension, edema, fluid retention, congestive heart failure, and hypokalemia may occur with mineralocorticoids.

Isolated aldosterone deficiency is seen in elderly patients with normal cortisol production who have hyporeninism, hyperkalemia, and abnormal renal function. It is probably most frequent in elderly diabetic patients with mild renal failure. The diagnosis is established by demonstrating the failure of plasma renin and aldosterone to rise normally in response to volume depletion and the upright posture; but inasmuch as these responses are blunted in normal elderly persons, the diagnosis of hyporeninemic hypoaldosteronism is more difficult to make in the elderly.

Chronic glucocorticoid therapy is administered in the elderly for a variety of medical disorders. Preparations with the shortest duration of action are less likely to suppress the HPA axis than long-acting ones. Glucocorticoid administration in divided doses will cause a greater therapeutic response, but will also suppress the HPA axis faster than a single daily dose. Oral preparations are generally well absorbed. HPA suppression may occur in patients after as little as 1 week of therapy with the equivalent of 20–30 mg/day of prednisone or after several weeks of small supraphysiologic doses; however, in elderly persons with decreased metabolic clearance of glucocorticoids, lower doses may produce suppression. HPA suppression and side effects from glucocorticoid therapy will be lessened by giving glucocorticoids as a single daily dose in the morning, using short-acting preparations, and, if possible, following an alternate-day schedule. Full recovery from prolonged exposure to large doses of glucocorticoids may take up to 1 year. Until full recovery of the HPA axis has occurred, supplemental glucocorticoids are needed for stress and surgery.

---

1. Axelrod L: Glucocorticoid therapy. *Medicine* 55:39–65, 1976.
Review discussing general principles of long-term glucocorticoid therapy including time course for development of and recovery from hypothalamic-pituitary-adrenal suppression.
2. Baxter JD, Tyrrell JB: The adrenal cortex, in Felig P, Baxter JD, Broadus AE, Frohman LA (eds): *Endocrinology and Metabolism.* New York, McGraw-Hill, 1981, pp 385–510.
A detailed review of adrenal physiology and clinical syndromes.
3. Blichert-Toft M: The adrenal glands in old age, in Greenblatt RB (ed): *Geriatric Endocrinology.* New York, Raven Press, 1978. vol 5 in Aging Series, pp 81–102.
General review of adrenal function in the aging.
4. Blichert-Toft M: Secretion of corticotrophin and somatotrophin by the senescent adenohypophysis in man. *Acta Endocrinol* 78 (suppl 195):1–157, 1975.
Detailed discussion and review suggesting that the function of the glucocorticoid-producing system is decreased in old age as a result of decreased demand for cortisol, with the feedback mechanism remaining intact in old age.
5. Blichert-Toft M, et al: Influence of age on endocrine-metabolic response to surgery. *Ann Surg* 190:761–770, 1979.
Plasma cortisol increased significantly more in elderly than in young subjects during elective inguinal hernia repair, a difference that may be due to a decreased cortisol disposal rate.
6. Cartlidge NEF, Blackman MM, Hall MRP, Hall R: Pituitary function in the elderly. *Gerontol Clin* 12:65–70, 1970.
Normal cortisol response in 8 patients over age 80 to insulin-induced hypoglycemia.
7. Crapo L: Cushing's syndrome: A review of diagnostic tests. *Metabolism* 28:955–977, 1979.
Discussion of the diagnostic tests used for screening and establishing the diagnosis and etiology of Cushing's syndrome.
8. Crilly RG, Marshall DN, Nordin BEC: Effect of age on plasma androstenedione concentration in oophorectomized women. *Clin Endocrinol* 10:199–201, 1979.
Notes an inverse correlation with age but suggests a more discrete change between ages 51 and 55 years.
9. DeFronzo RA: Hyperkalemia and hyporeninemic hypoaldosteronism. *Kidney Int* 17:118–134, 1980.
Review of this syndrome.
10. Dobbie J: Adrenocortical nodular hyperplasia: The aging adrenal. *J Pathol* 99:1–18, 1969.
Adrenocortical nodular hyperplasia is multifocal and may result from focal ischemia due to local arteriopathy.
11. Friedman M, Green MF, Sharland DE: Assessment of hypothalamic-pituitary-adrenal function in the geriatric age group. *J Gerontol* 24:292–297, 1969.
There is no diminution in hypothalamic-pituitary-adrenal function in elderly subjects

as judged by (1) morning cortisol levels and (2) cortisol levels after insulin-induced hypoglycemia, ACTH stimulation, and dexamethasone suppression.

12. Gherondache CN, Romanoff LP, Pincus G: Steroid hormones in aging men, in Gitman L (ed): *Endocrines and Aging*. Springfield, Ill, Thomas, 1967, pp 76–101.
Discusses the metabolism of cortisol, progesterone, androgens, estrogens, and cholesterol in relation to aging in men. The urinary excretion of 17-KS declines gradually with advancing age.
13. Gold EM: The Cushing's syndrome: Changing views of diagnosis and treatment. *Ann Intern Med* 90:829–844, 1979.
General review.
14. Grad B, Rosenberg GM, Liberman H, Trachtenberg J, Kral VA: Diurnal variation of the serum cortisol level of geriatric subjects. *J Gerontol* 26:351–357, 1971.
Elderly subjects maintain a normal diurnal variation of serum cortisol levels.
15. Hamburger C: Normal urinary excretion of neutral 17-ketosteroids with special reference to age and sex variations. *Acta Endocrinol (Copenh)* 1:19–37, 1948.
Notes a progressive decline in 17-ketosteroids with advancing age.
16. Migeon CJ, Keller AR, Lawrence B, Shepard TH II: Dehydroepiandrosterone and androsterone levels in human plasma. Effect of age and sex; day-to-day and diurnal variations. *J Clin Endocrinol Metab* 17:1051–1062, 1957.
In normal males the peak DHA and androsterone levels occurred between 20 and 39 years of age and then showed a rapid, progressive decline.
17. Muggeo M, Fedele D, Tiengo A, Molinari M, Crepaldi G: Human growth hormone and cortisol response to insulin stimulation in aging. *J Gerontol* 30:546–551, 1975.
Adrenal response to intravenous insulin did not change with aging.
18. Nelson DH: *The Adrenal Cortex: Physiological Function and Disease*. In Smith LH Jr (ed): *Major Problems in Internal Medicine*. Philadelphia, Saunders, 1980, vol 18.
Devoted entirely to the adrenal cortex with sections about physiology and clinical syndromes.
19. Phelps KR, Lieberman RL, Oh MS, Carroll HJ: Pathophysiology of the syndrome of hyporeninemic hypoaldosteronism. *Metabolism* 29:186–199, 1980.
Review of this syndrome.
20. Tyrrell JB, Baxter JD: Glucocorticoid therapy, in Felig P, Baxter JD, Broadus AE, Frohman LA (eds): *Endocrinology and Metabolism*. New York, McGraw-Hill, 1981, pp 599–624.
Discussion of the principles related to glucocorticoid therapy.
21. Vermeulen A, Deslypere JP, Schelfhout W, Verdonck L, Rubens R: Adrenocortical function in old age: Response to acute adrenocorticotropin stimulation. *J Clin Endocrinol Metab* 54:187–191, 1982.
Secretion of dehydroepiandrosterone, 17-hydroxypregnenolone, and pregnenolone is impaired in elderly persons.
22. Vihko R: Gas chromatographic-mass spectrometric studies on solvolyzable steroids in human peripheral plasma. *Acta Endocrinol (Copenh)* 52 (suppl 109):1–67, 1966.
With aging there is a decrease in pregnanediol, androsterone, dehydroepiandrosterone, and epiandrosterone.
23. West CD, et al: Adrenocortical function and cortisol metabolism in old age. *J Clin Endocrinol Metab* 21:1197–1207, 1961.
A progressive decrease in the rate of removal of cortisol from the circulation was evident in men over 60 years of age.
24. Wolfsen AR: Aging and the adrenals, in Korenman SG (ed): *Endocrine Aspects of Aging*. New York, Elsevier, 1982, pp 55–79.
General review of adrenal function with aging. Includes a short discussion of clinical syndromes.
25. Xarli VP, et al: Adrenal hemorrhage in the adult. *Medicine* 57:211–221, 1978.
Discussion of clinical significance of bilateral adrenal hemorrhage.
26. Yamaji T, Ibayashi H: Plasma dehydroepiandrosterone sulfate in normal and pathological conditions. *J Clin Endocrinol Metab* 29:273–278, 1969.
Finds a progressive decline in plasma DHA-sulfate with advancing age.

48. GONADAL FUNCTION IN THE ELDERLY MALE

David M. Slovik

Testosterone

With advancing age, beginning usually after age 50, many studies have reported a progressive decline in plasma testosterone concentration. It is unclear, however, whether this decline is caused by unrecognized disease states because some studies of "exceptionally" healthy males did not show any age-related alterations in testosterone concentration. There is considerable individual variation in testosterone concentration among elderly men.

Approximately 45–50% of the testosterone circulating in plasma is bound to a testosterone-binding globulin (TeBG) that is synthesized in the liver. The remaining free, or unbound, fraction is physiologically active. The binding capacity of TeBG increases with advancing age, resulting in an increase in the fraction of TeBG-bound testosterone and a decrease in the concentration of free hormone. Again, there are wide individual variations in free testosterone concentration. Only a small amount of 5-alpha-dihydrotestosterone (DHT) is secreted from the testes, the majority being derived from the conversion, in peripheral tissues, of testosterone to DHT by 5-alpha-reductase. In normal males, circulating concentrations of DHT either are unchanged or show a small decrease with advancing age.

Estrogen and Progesterone

In males, the adrenals and testes are the sources of estrogen and progesterone. Slight elevations in plasma estrone and estradiol levels and even free estradiol levels were previously reported with increasing age, but recent studies in healthy elderly males did not show any age-related changes. Elderly men produce less progesterone and excrete less pregnanetriol than do young men.

Luteinizing and Follicle-Stimulating Hormones

Circulating blood levels of luteinizing hormone (LH) and follicle-stimulating hormone (FSH) increase with age, but the elevations in elderly men are smaller than those of postmenopausal women. Compared with LH, a more consistent and greater increase in FSH is apparent, suggesting that there is more degeneration of seminiferous tubules than decrease in Leydig-cell function. Elderly men respond to gonadotropin-releasing hormone (Gn-RH) administration, but the response is less than that in younger men. The altered gonadotropin dynamics may be related to a decrease in hypothalamic-pituitary feedback sensitivity. Systemic illness and stress (e.g., major operation) may alter gonadotropin dynamics; therefore care must be exercised in interpreting data collected under these conditions. The testicular response to human chorionic gonadotropin (HCG) is diminished in elderly persons.

Prostate

The majority of men over 60 years of age have histologic changes of prostatic hypertrophy and hyperplasia. Elevated male hormonal levels are found in prostatic tissue, whereas benign prostatic hypertrophy (BPH) is absent in elderly males who did not have testicular function because of either castration or the development of hypopituitarism before the age of 40. Circulating levels of androgens do not necessarily reflect end-organ tissue activity, since the tissues themselves have enzymes (e.g., 5-alpha-reductase in prostatic tissue) to convert the hormones into additional products. The most consistent hormonal finding in patients with BPH is the markedly elevated level of DHT in the prostate, which averages three to four times more than those values found in the prostates of normal young men.

Reproductive Capacity

Male reproductive capability is maintained with advancing age. Although degenerative changes in the seminiferous tubules occur with aging, they are scattered, and there remain normal areas of spermatogenesis. The testicular weight and volume decrease with age. Some elderly men have normal sperm counts, whereas others have decreased sperm motility and alterations in sperm number and morphology.

Sexual Function

A decline in sexual function involving libido (sexual drive and desire) and potency occurs frequently in elderly men. This decline is most evident in men over 70 but is found in men in their 60s. Many factors affect libido and potency in elderly men, and even though they may be related to alterations in hormonal balance, they are also influenced by psychological factors, illnesses, medications, and other problems. The sexual activity of elderly men is closely related to the sexual activity of their earlier adult life.

Impotence refers to abnormalities in erectile function and is due to either organic or psychogenic factors. Organic causes include neuropathy and other neurologic disorders, hypogonadism, pharmacologic agents, vascular insufficiency, and genitourinary disorders. Vascular insufficiency from arterial disease is a common cause of impotence in elderly males. Diabetes mellitus, ischemic heart disease, and myocardial infarction are other medical conditions associated with erectile dysfunction in older patients. Drugs associated with erectile dysfunction in elderly men include (1) antihypertensive agents, e.g., alpha-methyldopa, reserpine, spironolactone, guanethidine, and clonidine; (2) psychotropic agents, e.g., phenothiazines, imipramine, and thioridazine; (3) anticholinergic agents; (4) estrogens; and (5) alcohol and narcotics.

Libido declines less than potency in elderly males. In comparison with women who undergo the menopause, the *andropause,* also called "male climacteric," is less dramatic and highly variable. In addition to loss of libido and impotence, symptoms of the andropause include depression, fatigue, irritability, insomnia, decreased attention span, apathy, muscle and joint pain, and headaches. The extent to which each of these factors is related to hormonal deficiency, altered end-organ androgen sensitivity, or other factors is unclear.

Hypogonadism

The diagnosis of hypogonadism in elderly males can be made by the finding of a low testosterone level and a concomitant elevation in plasma LH levels. Although androgen replacement therapy may be helpful in hypogonadal elderly males, the agents promote prostatic growth and therefore should not be administered to males with enlarged or nodular prostates. In addition, oral administration of 17-methylated synthetic androgens may produce liver abnormalities.

1. Albeaux-Fernet M, Bohler CS-S, Karpes AE: Testicular function in the aging male, in Greenblatt RB (ed): *Geriatric Endocrinology.* New York, Raven Press, 1978, vol 5 in Aging Series, pp 201–216.
Review of pathophysiology, hormonal changes, and clinical characteristics of the male climacteric. Androgen therapy may be beneficial in elderly men with hypogonadism and impotence.
2. Baker HWG, et al: Changes in the pituitary-testicular systems with age. *Clin Endocrinol (Oxf)* 5:349–372, 1976.
Detailed study of pituitary-testicular changes in 466 subjects aged 2–101 years. Testicular function declines gradually in men after age 40, but considerable variability exists.
3. Bremner WJ, Vitiello MV, Prinz PN: Loss of circadian rhythmicity in blood testosterone levels with aging in normal men. *J Clin Endocrinol Metab* 56:1278–1281, 1983.
The early morning rise in serum testosterone levels in the young is attenuated or absent in healthy elderly men, and the mean testosterone level for the entire 24-hour day is lower in elderly men.
4. Chieffi M: Effect of testosterone administration on the beard growth of elderly males. *J Gerontol* 4:200–204, 1949.
The administration of testosterone to 11 elderly males without signs of hypogonadism produced a marked increase in beard growth, with the greatest response obtained in 4 weeks.
5. Davidson JM, Kwan M, Greenleaf WJ: Hormonal replacement and sexuality in men. *Clin Endocrinol Metab* 11:599–623, 1982.
Review of hormonal replacement for hyposexuality, including discussions about hormonal changes and sexuality in aging men.
6. Geller J, Albert J: The effect of aging on the prostate, in Korenman SG (ed): *Endocrine Aspects of Aging.* New York, Elsevier, 1982, pp 137–161.
Review of hormonal changes, enzyme activity, and other factors related to changes in the prostate with aging.

7. Gherondache CN, Romanoff LP, Pincus G: Steroid hormones in aging men, in Gitman L (ed): *Endocrines and Aging*. Springfield, Ill, Thomas, 1967, pp 76–101.
Discusses the metabolism of cortisol, progesterone, androgens, estrogens, and cholesterol in relation to the aging process in men.
8. Giusti G, et al: Age-related secretion of androstenedione, testosterone and dihydrotestosterone by the human testis. *Exp Gerontol* 10:241–245, 1975.
With advancing age, the spermatic venous plasma concentration of T and DHT decreased and androstenedione was unchanged.
9. Greenblatt RB, Oettinger M, Bohler CS-S: Estrogen-androgen levels in aging men and women: Therapeutic considerations. *J Am Geriatr Soc* 24:173–178, 1976.
Testosterone levels begin to decrease and LH and FSH levels increase in men in their 40s. In men with climacteric symptoms, androgen replacement may be helpful, but caution must be used.
10. Harman SM, Tsitouras PD: Reproductive hormones in aging men: I. Measurement of sex steroids, basal luteinizing hormone, and Leydig cell response to human chorionic gonadotropin. *J Clin Endocrinol Metab* 51:35–40, 1980.
In normal healthy males from the Baltimore Longitudinal Study, aging was not associated with alterations in serum testosterone, 5-alpha-dihydrotestosterone, estrone, or estradiol, but basal LH levels were increased and there was a diminished testosterone response to hCG stimulation.
11. Harman SM, Tsitouras PD, Costa PT, Blackman MR: Reproductive hormones in aging men: II. Basal pituitary gonadotropins and gonadotropin responses to luteinizing hormone-releasing hormone. *J Clin Endocrinol Metab* 54:547–551, 1982.
In older men there is a decrease in the magnitude of LH and FSH secretory responses to LRH, as well as a delay in the timing of the LH peak.
12. Isurugi K, Fukutani K, Takayasu H, Wakabayashi K, Tamaoki BI: Age-related changes in serum luteinizing hormone (LH) and follicle-stimulating hormone (FSH) levels in normal men. *J Clin Endocrinol Metab* 39:955–957, 1974.
Increases in LH and FSH were noted in normal men beginning in the fifth decade and became more pronounced with advancing age.
13. Kaler LW, Neaves WB: Attrition of the human Leydig cell population with advancing age. *Anat Rec* 192:513–518, 1978.
Total Leydig cell volume and the absolute number of Leydig cells per individual decreased with advancing age.
14. Michal V: Arterial disease as a cause of impotence. *Clin Endocrinol Metab* 11:725–748, 1982.
Discussion of the role of arterial disease as an important cause of impotence in elderly men.
15. Morimoto I, Edmiston A, Horton R: Alteration in the metabolism of dihydrotestosterone in elderly men with prostatic hyperplasia. *J Clin Invest* 66:612–615, 1980.
Elevated DHT concentrations in hyperplastic prostate tissue result from reduced DHT metabolism.
16. Morley JE, Melmed S: Gonadal dysfunction in systemic disorders. *Metabolism* 28:1051–1073, 1979.
A good review of alterations in gonadal function with systemic disorders, since many of these disorders are present in the elderly.
17. Newman G, Nichols CR: Sexual activities and attitudes in older persons. *JAMA* 173:33–35, 1960.
A survey of 250 subjects, aged 60–93 years, showed that 54% of those married were still active sexually; and that although there is a decline in sexual interest and activity with advancing years, cessation of sexual activity in elderly subjects is often due to a decline in physical health of one or both of the marital partners.
18. Rubens R, Dhont M, Vermeulen A: Further studies on Leydig cell function in old age. *J Clin Endocrinol Metab* 39:40–45, 1974.
Gonadotropin levels and pituitary response to LHRH were increased and Leydig cell response to HCG was decreased in healthy elderly males.
19. Shipley RA: The gonads and aging. *J Am Geriatr Soc* 10:26–34, 1962.
Androgen therapy may have effects on muscular performance, but no dramatic rejuvenation is to be expected.

20. Siiteri PK, Wilson JD: Dihydrotestosterone in prostatic hypertrophy: I. The formation and content of dihydrotestosterone in the hypertrophic prostate of man. *J Clin Invest* 49:1737–1745, 1970.
Elevated levels of DHT are present in hypertrophic prostatic tissue, and the local accumulation of DHT may be involved in the pathogenesis of prostatic hypertrophy in man.
21. Snyder PJ, Reitano JF, Utiger RD: Serum LH and FSH responses to synthetic gonadotropin-releasing hormone in normal men. *J Clin Endocrinol Metab* 41:938–945, 1975.
In male senescence there is a decreased LH and FSH response to GnRH administration and evidence of primary Leydig cell failure.
22. Sparrow D, Bosse R, Rowe JW: The influence of age, alcohol consumption, and body build on gonadal function in men. *J Clin Endocrinol Metab* 51:508–512, 1980.
In healthy elderly males from the Normative Aging Study in Boston, there was no effect of age on basal testosterone, free testosterone index, estradiol, or LH, but the testosterone-binding capacity and FSH levels were higher and the DHT levels lower in the elderly.
23. Stearns EL, et al: Declining testicular function with age: Hormonal and clinical correlates. *Am J Med* 57:761–766, 1974.
Testicular length and volume were decreased in 78% and 37%, respectively, of men over age 60 years.
24. Swerdloff RS, Heber D: Effects of aging on male reproductive function, in Korenman SG (ed): *Endocrine Aspects of Aging*. New York: Elsevier, 1982, pp 119–135.
General review on sexual behavior and reproductive hormone function with aging in men.
25. Tsitouras PD, Martin CE, Harman SM: Relationship of serum testosterone to sexual activity in healthy elderly men. *J Gerontol* 37:288–293, 1982.
Although serum testosterone level and ethanol intake may affect sexual activity in older men to some degree, age itself appears to be the most influential variable.
26. Vermeulen A, Rubens R, Verdonck L: Testosterone secretion and metabolism in male senescence. *J Clin Endocrinol Metab* 34:730–735, 1972.
Male senescence is characterized by a decrease in plasma testosterone levels and in the metabolic clearance rate and production of testosterone.
27. Zumoff B, et al: Age variation of the 24-hour mean plasma concentrations of androgens, estrogens, and gonadotropins in normal adult men. *J Clin Endocrinol Metab* 54:534–538, 1982.
The plasma total testosterone concentration showed a slow, continuous decline (35%) with age in 35 healthy adult males, aged 21–85 years, and the free testosterone concentration was closely correlated to the total testosterone level.

49. GONADAL FUNCTION IN THE ELDERLY FEMALE

David M. Slovik

The changes associated with the loss of normal ovarian function are dramatic and are characterized by physiologic and psychological changes associated with the loss of hormonal and reproductive function. The transition period in a woman's life from the cessation of normal reproductive function to senescense is referred to as the *climacteric* or "change of life." It is usually, but not always, associated with symptoms of hormonal deficiency. The *perimenopausal period* is the early stage of ovarian failure, characterized by a shortened menstrual cycle length due to a decrease in the follicular phase, increased frequency of anovulatory cycles, and menstrual irregularity. As ovarian hormonal function decreases, serum gonadotropins increase. The cessation of menstruation is known as the *menopause* and occurs during the climacteric. The median age at which the menopause occurs is about 50 years. The term *postmenopausal,* although vague and difficult to define, can be used to indicate the time from the cessation of menstruation to the onset of senescence.

Decline in Ovarian Function

The senescent ovary is small and fibrotic. The progressive thinning of the ovarian cortex gives it a wrinkled appearance. With increasing age, there is progressive loss of functioning ovarian follicles, and by the time of the menopause, the follicles are unable to respond to even high levels of gonadotropins. The maximum number of oocytes is present by the middle of gestation, but from then on, the number declines continually, most being lost due to atresia, and only a small percentage lost due to ovulation. At the time of the menopause the remaining follicles are in various stages of atresia, although some primordial follicles may be present but disappear thereafter. In many postmenopausal ovaries, the stroma, which is capable of steroid synthesis, becomes increasingly cellular and exhibits nodular or diffuse cortical hyperplasia.

Estrogen-sensitive tissues also show significant changes due to a decline in estrogen stimulation. Atrophy of the vulva, narrowing of the vaginal orifice, and a decrease in the function of the vulvovaginal gland occur. Pruritus is common, and the vulval epithelium is more susceptible to trauma. The vagina becomes shorter and narrower and loses its elasticity. The vaginal epithelium becomes thinner. Vaginal secretions become scant, and an atrophic vaginitis develops, producing symptoms of dyspareunia, ulceration, infection, and vaginal irritation. Vaginal smears show a preponderance of parabasal cells characteristic of the menopause. A decrease in the size of the cervix and in the height of the epithelial cells occurs. The uterus decreases in size and weight. The myometrium becomes thinner, and the endometrium becomes atrophic, although varying degrees of endometrial proliferation and hyperplasia are sometimes present. The fallopian tubes gradually shrink in size. The urethral lining becomes thinner, bladder sphincter tone diminishes, and urinary tract infections increase. The breasts gradually decrease in size and become more flaccid, the alveoli disappear, the duct size diminishes, and the epithelium flattens. After the menopause there is an acceleration in bone loss to levels that will make the bones easily susceptible to fractures later in life.

Estrogens

The loss of ovarian function in the menopause is the best example of endocrine gland senescence. The ovary produces and secretes only a minimal amount of estrogen after the menopause. Estradiol is the major estrogen produced by the ovaries in the reproductive years. In postmenopausal women estradiol levels fall to very low values, and estradiol is then primarily derived from the extraglandular conversion of precursor steroids, inasmuch as estrone and testosterone can be converted in peripheral tissues to estradiol. A small amount is derived from direct adrenal gland secretion. The metabolic clearance rate (MCR) for estradiol is reduced by about 25–30% in postmenopausal women. In the premenopausal woman, estrone is secreted directly from the ovaries, although some is derived from the peripheral conversion of androstenedione, testosterone, and estradiol. In the postmenopausal woman, estrone is the major estrogen and is derived predominantly from the extraglandular conversion of androstenedione. With advancing age, estrone levels decrease, while androstenedione conversion to estrone increases two- to fourfold. The rate of this conversion is altered by such factors as obesity (obese women have higher conversion rates and higher circulating estrogen levels than thin women have). The MCR of estrone is more rapid than that of estradiol, as estrone binds less to proteins. In postmenopausal women, the MCR of estrone decreases, perhaps 20–25%. In addition, the estrone production rate (PR) may decrease.

Progesterone

In premenopausal women, progesterone is secreted almost entirely by the ovary, whereas in postmenopausal women it is of adrenal origin. In postmenopausal women there is a decrease in blood concentrations of progesterone and 17-hydroxyprogesterone, and in urinary pregnanetriol excretion.

Androgens

Androgens are important as a precursor for estrogens in postmenopausal women. In premenopausal women, androgens and their precursors are secreted by the ovary and the adrenal cortex. In postmenopausal women, the ovary loses its ability to aromatize androgens to form estrogens and therefore secretes primarily androgens, while the adrenal gland continues to produce androgens. In pre- and postmenopausal women, androstenedione comes primarily from the adrenal gland, although the ovary contributes some (approximately 20% of the total), and a small amount is derived from the conversion of dehydroepiandrosterone (DHA). Androstenedione is the primary ovarian androgen produced during reproductive life. Plasma androstenedione concentrations decrease after the menopause and with advancing age. The MCR of androstenedione is similar in pre- and postmenopausal women, but its PR declines and its conversion to estrone is more efficient with age.

Testosterone in postmenopausal women comes from a combination of direct secretion, primarily from the ovary, and conversion from androstenedione and DHA. Testosterone levels are only slightly lower in postmenopausal women than they are in premenopausal women; they are, however, lower in postmenopausal women who have had a bilateral oophorectomy than they are in those women who have had a natural menopause. The MCR of testosterone is similar in pre- and postmenopausal women, but the PR is decreased. Because of the loss of ability by the postmenopausal ovary to aromatize sex steroids, the conversion of testosterone to estradiol decreases, and ovarian testosterone secretion is higher in the postmenopausal ovary than in the premenopausal one. The postmenopausal ovary can respond to human chorionic gonadotropin (HCG) stimulation by increasing testosterone and androstenedione output. In both young and old women, DHA is derived almost totally from the adrenal cortex, but the plasma concentration in the elderly is approximately 40% of that found in younger women.

Gonadotropins

Long before the final menstrual period, ovarian function begins to decline. The changes in the hypothalamic-pituitary axis that occur during the perimenopausal period and the menopause appear to be secondary to gonadal failure. Several years before the cessation of menses, the ovary becomes less responsive to gonadotropin stimulation. Decreasing ovarian function releases the negative-feedback inhibition on the pituitary gonadotropes, and the first detectable manifestation of decreasing reproductive function is a gradual increase in plasma follicle-stimulating hormone (FSH), occurring despite normal ovulatory cycles. Some time after the FSH levels rise, luteinizing hormone (LH) levels begin to increase. In the postmenopausal period the elevations in serum FSH and LH levels are dramatic. FSH levels are higher and more consistently elevated than LH levels. Within 2–3 years of the natural menopause, gonadotropin levels reach a maximum in the circulation; they then decline over the next 30 years to values of approximately 40–50% of the maximum level achieved. In premenopausal women who have had removal of both ovaries, the gonadotropin levels rise within days of operation. Severe illness, however, with or without weight loss, may suppress gonadotropin levels in postmenopausal women. In both young and old women, gonadotropins are secreted in a pulsatile pattern, but the amplitude is much greater in older women as a result of increased release of gonadotropin-releasing hormone (Gn-RH) from the hypothalamus and enhanced pituitary responsiveness to Gn-RH. In postmenopausal women, the plasma Gn-RH levels are elevated.

Symptoms

A majority of women experience some symptoms related to the loss of gonadal function, but there is great individual variation. Some women do not experience any symptoms that can be definitely attributed to loss of hormonal function. Short-term problems include atrophic changes in the genitourinary, vasomotor, emotional, and sexual symptoms, whereas long-term problems are related to severe bone loss and the development of osteoporosis. The most common symptom of the climacteric is the sudden, episodic hot flush described as a sensation of warmth and heat. It is often accompanied by diaphoresis. In over 80% of women, hot flushes are present for more than 1 year, and in over 25% they persist for more than 5 years; however, these hot flushes are variable in frequency, duration, and intensity. The flushing sensation is most prominent in the head, neck, upper chest, and back and sometimes is preceded by a very short-lasting pressure sensation in the head. The mechanisms responsible for the vasomotor symptoms are still not clear and cannot be totally explained by either low estradiol levels or high gonadotropin levels. It appears that the hot flush is a central rather than peripherally mediated disturbance.

Other symptoms include night sweats, insomnia, headaches, and palpitations. Irritability, anxiety, mood fluctuations, memory changes, decreased concentration, decreased energy and motivational drive, and depression have all been associated with the climacteric. Some of these problems are relieved with estrogen therapy. Declining sexual interest occurs in the menopause. There is no clear correlation between sexual symptoms and plasma hormone levels, and perhaps depression may be partly responsible for the decreased libido. Women who enjoyed sex in their younger years are more likely to maintain sexual response through the menopause.

Symptoms caused by atrophic changes in the genitourinary tract include dyspareunia, vaginitis, urinary urgency and frequency, and incontinence. Due to a decrease in the muscle tone of the pelvic floor, cystocele, rectocele, and uterine prolapse occur. Symptoms related to vasomotor instability and emotional factors usually improve within several years of the menopause. Problems related to atrophic and degenerative organ changes will continue and often increase with senescence. Estrogens can be given to those women with severe menopausal symptoms that adversely affect their lifestyle. The lowest dose necessary to relieve the menopausal symptoms should be administered on a cyclic program for the shortest possible time. The long-term use of estrogens to prevent bone loss is discussed in Chap. 79.

---

1. Abraham GE, Lobotsky J, Lloyd CW: Metabolism of testosterone and androstenedione in normal and ovariectomized women. *J Clin Invest* 48:696–703, 1969.
The metabolic clearance rate and production rate of testosterone were lower, but the MCR was similar and the PR lower for androstenedione in ovariectomized as compared with normal women.
2. Asch RH, Greenblatt RB: The aging ovary: Morphologic and endocrine correlations, in Greenblatt RB (ed): *Geriatric Endocrinology. New York, Raven Press, 1978, vol 5 in Aging Series, pp 141–164.*
General review of hormonal changes in the aging ovary, including a discussion of estrogen, progesterone, and androgen metabolism. Also includes discussion of hormone-producing tumors of the aging ovary.
3. Campbell S, Whitehead M: Estrogen therapy and the postmenopausal syndrome. *Clin Obstet Gynecol* 4:31–47, 1977.
In patients with moderate or severe postmenopausal symptoms, a significant improvement in well-being, both psychological and symptomatic, can be achieved with estrogen therapy.
4. Chakravarti S, et al: Hormonal profiles after the menopause. *Br Med J* 2:784–786, 1976.
Peak gonadotropin levels are found 2 to 3 years after the menopause but then gradually decline in the next 3 decades to values that were 40–50% of the maximal levels.
5. Chang RJ, Judd HL: The ovary after menopause. *Clin Obstet Gynecol* 24:181–191, 1981.
Circulating estradiol levels characteristic of menopause may not be established until 6 months or more after the cessation of menses.
6. Coble YD Jr, Kohler PO, Cargille CM, Ross GT: Production rates and metabolic clearance rates of human follicle-stimulating hormone in premenopausal and postmenopausal women. *J Clin Invest* 48:359–363, 1969.
There was a 15-fold increase in FSH production in postmenopausal women, and only 3–5% of the total FSH production appeared in the urine in a biologically active form.
7. Crilly RG, Marshall DH, Nordin BEC: Effect of age on plasma androstenedione concentration in oophorectomized women. *Clin Endocrinol (Oxf)* 10:199–201, 1979.
Finds a significant inverse correlation with age, but a discrete change in the first half of the sixth decade rather than a continuous fall with advancing age.
8. Dennerstein L, Burrows GD: Hormonal replacement therapy and sexuality in women. *Clin Endocrinol Metab* 11:661–679, 1982.
Estrogen therapy has a stimulatory effect on sexual interest, vaginal lubrication, enjoyment, and orgasmic frequency in oophorectomized women.
9. Hallstrom T: Sexuality in the climacteric. *Clin Obstet Gynecol* 4:227–239, 1977.
The impairment of sexual function in postmenopausal women, in addition to being due to biologic factors, also is due to significant psychosocial factors.

10. Hemsell DL, Grodin JM, Brenner PF, Siiteri PK, MacDonald PC: Plasma precursors of estrogen: II. Correlation of the extent of conversion of plasma androstenedione to estrone with age. *J Clin Endocrinol Metab* 38:476–479, 1974.
In women of advancing age, there is a progressive increase in the efficiency with which circulating androstenedione is converted to estrone.
11. Kohler PO, Ross GT, Odell WD: Metabolic clearance and production rates of human luteinizing hormone in pre- and postmenopausal Women. *J Clin Invest* 47:38–47, 1968.
The metabolic clearance rate for LH was similar in premenopausal and postmenopausal women.
12. Monroe SE, Menon KMJ: Changes in reproductive hormone secretion during the climacteric and postmenopausal periods. *Clin Obstet Gynecol* 20:113–122, 1977.
In the postmenopausal ovary, the stroma is the only remaining functional compartment, and androgens are produced that may serve as precursors for estrogen biosynthesis in peripheral tissues.
13. Rakoff AE, Nowroozi K: The female climacteric, in Greenblatt RB (ed): *Geriatric Endocrinology.* New York, Raven Press, 1978, vol 5 in Aging Series, pp 165–190.
Review, including a discussion of morphologic changes in the ovary and other reproductive organs, hormonal changes of menopause, and therapy for menopausal symptoms.
14. Sherman BM, West JH, Korenman SG: The menopausal transition: Analysis of LH, FSH, estradiol and progesterone concentrations during menstrual cycles of older women. *J Clin Endocrinol Metab* 42:629–636, 1976.
During the menopausal transition period, there is variability of menstrual cycle length and elevated FSH levels with normal LH levels.
15. Studd JWW, Thom MH: Ovarian failure and aging. *Clin Endocrinol Metab* 10:89–113, 1981.
General review of hormonal changes, symptoms (vasomotor, emotional, sexual), and treatment of the menopause.
16. Vaughn TC, Hammond CB: Estrogen replacement therapy. *Clin Obstet Gynecol* 24:253–283, 1981.
General discussion of endocrinologic changes of the climacteric and the benefits and risks of estrogen replacement therapy. Although estrogen therapy is not without risk, its use should not be withheld from appropriately selected, symptomatic patients.
17. Vermeulen A: The hormonal activity of the postmenopausal ovary. *J Clin Endocrinol Metab* 42:247–253, 1976.
The postmenopausal ovary is responsible for about 50% of plasma testosterone and 30% of androstenedione levels.
18. Vermeulen A, Verdonck L: Sex hormone concentrations in post-menopausal women: Relation to obesity, fat mass, age and years post-menopause. *Clin Endocrinol (Oxf)* 9:59–66, 1978.
A significant correlation was found between plasma estrone levels and the degree of obesity and fat mass.
19. Warren MP, Siris ES, Petrovich C: The influence of severe illness on gonadotropin secretion in the postmenopausal female. *J Clin Endocrinol Metab* 45:99–104, 1977.
Gonadotropin secretion may be suppressed in severely ill postmenopausal women with or without weight loss.
20. Wide L, Hobson BM: Qualitative difference in follicle-stimulating hormone activity in the pituitaries of young women compared to that of men and elderly women. *J Clin Endocrinol Metab* 56:371–375, 1983.
FSH in the pituitaries from young women has biologic activity that is qualitatively different from that of FSH in men and in elderly women.
21. Yen SSC, Tsai CC, Naftolin F, Vandenberg G, Ajabor L: Pulsatile patterns of gonadotropin release in subjects with and without ovarian function. *J Clin Endocrinol Metab* 34:671–675, 1972.
Qualitative and quantitative differences in the pulsatile pattern of gonadotropins, observed between different phases of the cycle and between subjects with or without ovarian function, provide evidence that ovarian steroids modulate the frequency and magnitude of gonadotropins by the pituitary gland.

50. DISORDERS OF THE ANTERIOR PITUITARY GLAND

David M. Slovik

Our knowledge of neuroendocrinology has vastly increased in recent years, but our understanding of many aspects of the human nervous and endocrine system is still scant. Feedback control of the hypothalamic-pituitary axis is complex under normal circumstances but is even more difficult to understand in the elderly because of concomitant illnesses, drug ingestion, and age-related changes.

Growth Hormone Secretion

Growth hormone (GH) secretion is under the control of two hypothalamic hormones: growth hormone–releasing factor and an inhibiting factor (somatostatin). These peptides are produced in the medial basal hypothalamus, released into the hypophyseoportal circulation, and transported to the anterior pituitary gland. The hypothalamic peptides are in turn regulated by adjacent neurons. Factors that stimulate GH secretion include exercise, stress, insulin-induced hypoglycemia, dopaminergic agonists (e.g., L-dopa), alpha-adrenergic agonists (e.g., clonidine), beta-adrenergic antagonists (e.g., propranolol), serotoninergic precursors (e.g., L-tryptophan), arginine, glucagon, and vasopressin. GH secretion is inhibited by dopaminergic antagonists (e.g., phenothiazines), alpha-adrenergic antagonists (e.g., phentolamine), beta-adrenergic stimulation (e.g., isoproterenol), serotoninergic inhibitors (e.g., methysergide and cyproheptadine), glucocorticoids, medroxyprogesterone, obesity, and hyperglycemia. GH secretion is pulsatile, with maximal bursts occurring during the first 2 hours of sleep. In the elderly, there is a loss of the normal sleep-related GH peaks, a decrease in the 24-hour secretion of GH, and fasting basal GH concentrations that are either lower than or similar to values found in younger individuals. Basal GH concentrations are lower in males than in females.

GH secretion can be stimulated by (1) insulin-induced hypoglycemia (which should be avoided in elderly patients and in patients with coronary artery disease, cerebrovascular disease, and seizure disorders), (2) arginine, (3) L-dopa, and (4) glucagon. L-Arginine is infused over 30 minutes in a dose of 0.5 gm/kg body weight, up to 30 gm. GH values are obtained at 0, 30, 60, 90, and 120 minutes; and normal subjects show a rise in plasma GH levels of 5–7 ng/ml. L-Dopa is given in a dose of 500 mg PO. GH values are obtained at 0, 30, 60, and 120 minutes, and, in normal subjects, show a rise of greater than 5 ng/ml. Side effects such as nausea, vertigo, and slight orthostatic hypotension frequently occur with L-dopa. Glucagon is given in a dose of 1 mg IM. GH values are obtained at 0, 60, 90, 120, 150, and 180 minutes; an increase of 7 ng/ml in males and of 10 ng/ml in females is normal. GH secretion in response to stimulation appears to be intact in most elderly individuals.

Acromegaly

Acromegaly has similar features in all age groups, except that in the elderly, the initial presentation is less frequent than in younger patients. Major clinical features include headaches, acral growth, prognathism, hyperhidrosis, osteoarthritis, generalized visceromegaly, impaired glucose tolerance, cardiac abnormalities, carpal tunnel syndrome, and hypermetabolism. The diagnosis is confirmed by demonstration of elevated GH levels that are not suppressible and may even show a paradoxic increase with exogenous glucose administration. Enlargement of the sella turcica is usually evident on skull x-rays, and computerized tomography (CT) scanning of the sella turcica will show enlargement of the pituitary as well as suprasellar and parasellar extension, if it is present. Therapeutic alternatives include surgical removal, conventional external irradiation of the pituitary gland, proton-beam irradiation, radiation implants, and cryohypophysectomy. Bromocriptine, a long-acting dopamine agonist, paradoxically lowers GH secretion in acromegaly, and, although GH levels do not usually return to normal with bromocriptine, many acromegalic patients report improvement in clinical symptoms with this therapy.

Hyperprolactinemia

Prolactin (PRL) is unique among pituitary hormones, because it is under tonic inhibitory control. It appears that dopamine is the major prolactin-inhibitory factor. Substances that increase prolactin release include thyrotropin-releasing hormone (TRH), serotoninergic compounds (e.g., L-tryptophan), estrogens, dopaminergic blockers (e.g., metoclopramide), opiate agonists, psychotropic drugs (e.g., phenothiazines), reserpine, alpha-methyldopa, and derivatives of gamma-aminobutyric acid (GABA). Prolactin values rise during the late hours of sleep and are secreted in 4–9 pulses/day. Prolactin concentrations also rise during stress.

Pathologic states associated with hyperprolactinemia include prolactin-secreting pituitary tumors, acromegaly, hypothalamic disorders, hypothyroidism, renal failure, liver disease, and chest wall trauma. The clinical manifestations of hyperprolactinemia include galactorrhea, anovulation, or amenorrhea in younger females and hypogonadism, impotence, decreased libido, and gynecomastia in males. Little is known about changes in prolactin secretion with advancing age. Prolactin levels are higher in females than in males and have been reported as either decreasing or remaining the same with advancing age in women and tending to increase with advancing age in men. TRH administration produces a greater prolactin response in older women than in men, and although the magnitude of the peak response is similar in young and elderly persons, in the elderly the time to reach the peak and the rate of decrease are delayed. Skull x-rays of the sella turcica and CT scanning of the sella turcica will demonstrate either microadenomas or macroadenomas. Therapy of patients with prolactin-secreting pituitary tumors includes bromocriptine administration, surgical intervention, and proton-beam or conventional radiotherapy.

Hypopituitarism

Hypopituitarism may result from hypothalamic or pituitary tumors, pituitary infarction or hemorrhage, infiltrative diseases, granulomatous diseases, infection, surgical procedure, or irradiation. Patients with hypopituitarism, in addition to treatment of the underlying disorder, are treated with appropriate adrenal and thyroid replacement, but gonadal hormone therapy is usually not required in the elderly.

Discussion of the hypothalamic-pituitary axis and the thyroid, adrenal glands, and gonads are found in Chaps. 44–49.

1. Carlson HE, Gillin JC, Gorden P, Snyder F: Absence of sleep-related growth hormone peaks in aged normal subjects and in acromegaly. *J Clin Endocrinol Metab* 34:1102–1105, 1972.
A sleep-associated peak in GH concentration was absent in 4 of 6 normal subjects over age 50.
2. Cartlidge NEF, Black MM, Hall MRP, Hall R: Pituitary function in the elderly. *Gerontol Clin* 12:65–70, 1970.
In response to insulin-induced hypoglycemia, elderly patients over the age of 80 had a normal growth hormone and ACTH response.
3. Christy NP, Warren MP: Disease syndromes of the hypothalamus and anterior pituitary, in DeGroot LJ, et al (eds): *Endocrinology.* New York, Grune & Stratton, 1979, pp 215–252.
General review that discusses the various clinical syndromes associated with hypopituitarism and hyperpituitarism.
4. Cohen KL: Metabolic, endocrine, and drug-induced interference with pituitary function tests: A review. *Metabolism* 26:1165–1177, 1977.
Review of multiple factors that interfere with the assessment of pituitary function.
5. del Pozo E, Brownell J: Prolactin: I. Mechanism of control, peripheral actions and modifications by drugs. *Horm Res* 10:143–172, 1979.
A number of drugs can modify prolactin secretion, mainly by acting on the dopaminergic control mechanism.
6. Dilman VM, Anisimov VN: Hypothalamic mechanisms of aging and of specific age pathology: I. Sensitivity threshold of hypothalamo-pituitary complex to homeostatic stimuli in the reproductive system. *Exp Gerontol* 14:161–174, 1979.
Notes an age-associated increase in the sensitivity threshold of the hypothalamopituitary complex to inhibition by estrogens.
7. Dilman VM, Ostroumova MN, Tsyrlina EV: Hypothalamic mechanisms of aging and of specific age pathology: II. On the sensitivity threshold of hypothalamo-pituitary complex to homeostatic stimuli in adaptive homeostasis. *Exp Gerontol* 14:175–181, 1979.

Notes on age-associated increase in the sensitivity threshold of the hypothalamopituitary complex to inhibition by glucocorticoids.

8. Dudl RJ, Ensinck JW, Palmer HE, Williams RH: Effect of age on growth hormone secretion in man. *J Clin Endocrinol Metab* 37:11–16, 1973.
Plasma GH levels after an overnight fast, after a glucose "pulse," and following arginine infusion were not significantly altered with age in 44 men, aged 22–81 years.
9. Everitt AV, Burgess JA: Growth hormone and aging, in Everitt AV, Burgess JA (eds): *Hypothalamus, Pituitary and Aging.* Springfield, Ill, Thomas, 1976, pp 464–475.
In elderly subjects of both sexes, sleep-related serum GH peaks are usually absent, and as a result the 24-hour secretion of GH is diminished. However, there is no good evidence that senescence is due to a lack of GH.
10. Finkelstein JW, Roffwarg HP, Boyar RM, Kream J, Hellman L: Age-related change in the twenty-four–hour spontaneous secretion of growth hormone. *J Clin Endocrinol Metab* 35:665–670, 1972.
Notes an age-related decrease in the 24-hour secretion of GH.
11. Greenblatt RB, Natrajan PK, Tzingounis V: Role of the hypothalamus in the aging woman. *J Am Geriatr Soc* 27:97–103, 1979.
The hypothalamic-pituitary axis appears to remain fractionally intact well into old age.
12. Jadresic A, et al: The acromegaly syndrome: Relation between clinical features, growth hormone values, and radiologic characteristics of the pituitary tumors. *Q J Med* 51:189–204, 1982.
Patients with acromegaly present most frequently around the fourth decade of life. In this study, approximately 8% of patients were over age 60 and none over age 68.
13. Kalk WJ, Vinik AI, Pimstone BL, Jackson WPU: Growth hormone response to hypoglycemia in the elderly. *J Gerontol* 28:431–433, 1973.
The mean GH response to insulin-induced hypoglycemia was similar in both young and elderly subjects, although elderly females had a significantly lower GH response than their male counterparts.
14. Klijn JGM, Lamberts SWJ, de Jong FH, van Dongen KJ, Birkenhager JC: Interrelationships between tumor size, age, plasma growth hormone and incidence of extrasellar extension in acromegalic patients. *Acta Endocrinol (Copenh)* 95:289–297, 1980.
In acromegalic patients there was a negative correlation between tumor size and age that contrasted with that in patients who had prolactinomas.
15. Lazarus L, Eastman CJ: Assessment of hypothalamic pituitary function in old age, in Everitt AV, Burgess JA (eds): *Hypothalamus, Pituitary and Aging.* Springfield, Ill, Thomas, 1976, pp 97–122.
Dynamic testing of the pituitary has not revealed any significant impairment of pituitary hormone reserve with age.
16. Meites J: Changes in neuroendocrine control of anterior pituitary function during aging. *Neuroendocrinology* 34:151–156, 1982.
In aged rats, evidence supports a reduced ability of the hypothalamopituitary system to secrete LH, FSH, GH, biologically active TSH, and possibly ACTH.
17. Mills TM, Mahesh VB: Pituitary function in the aged, in Greenblatt RB (ed): *Geriatric Endocrinology.* New York, Raven Press, 1978, vol 5 in Aging Series, pp 1–11.
Review that primarily focuses on the hypothalamic-pituitary-ovary axis in menopause.
18. Sandberg H, Yoshimine N, Maeda S, Symons D, Zavodnick J: Effects of an oral glucose load on serum immunoreactive insulin, free fatty acid, growth hormone and blood sugar levels in young and elderly subjects. *J Am Geriatr Soc* 21:433–439, 1973.
GH levels in the fasting state and 1–2 hours after a glucose load were significantly higher in elderly males than in younger males.
19. Thorner MO: Prolactin. *Clin Endocrinol Metab* 6:201–222, 1977.
General review of prolactin physiology and discussion of clinical disorders of hyperprolactinemia.
20. Vekemans M, Robyn C: Influence of age on serum prolactin levels in women and men. *Br Med J* 4:738–739, 1975.
Prolactin levels in subjects aged from 18–65 years showed a steady decline in women and a rising trend in men with advancing age.
21. Vidalon C, et al: Age-related changes in growth hormones in non-diabetic women. *J Am Geriatr Soc* 21:253–255, 1973.

Older nonobese women have GH levels that are lower than younger nonobese women, although such age-related differences were not evident in obese women.

22. Vigneri R, Goldfine ID: Pharmacologic therapy of patient with pituitary tumors secreting prolactin, growth hormone and adrenocorticotropin. *Adv Intern Med* 25:69–89, 1980.
Over 75% of acromegalic patients treated with bromocriptine will have a 50% reduction in growth hormone values.
23. von Werder K, Eversmann T, Rjosk H-K, Fahlbusch R: Treatment of hyperprolactinemia, in Ganong WF, Martini L (eds): *Frontiers in Neuroendocrinology.* New York, Raven Press, 1982, vol 7, pp 123–159.
Neurosurgical procedures almost inevitably fail to normalize extremely elevated prolactin levels in patients with large macroprolactinomas.
24. Yamaji T, Shimamot K, Ishibashi M, Kosaka K, Orimo H: Effect of age and sex on circulating and pituitary prolactin levels in human. *Acta Endocrinol (Copenh)* 83:711–719, 1976.
Finds no effect of age on serum prolactin concentrations, although the peak prolactin response to TRH was delayed in the older groups.

51. DISORDERS OF THE POSTERIOR PITUITARY GLAND

David M. Slovik

Antidiuretic Hormone

Antidiuretic hormone (ADH, arginine vasopressin) is synthesized in the supraoptic nuclei of the hypothalamus, transported through the axons of the neurohypophyseal tract along with a carrier protein, neurophysin, and stored in the posterior pituitary gland. The major role of ADH is the conservation of water through promotion of water reabsorption by the distal convoluted tubules and collecting tubules in the kidney. The release of ADH into the circulation is influenced by changes in the osmolality of the blood, changes in blood volume, and psychogenic and other factors. Osmoreceptors, located in the hypothalamus, respond to a 1–2% increase in plasma osmolality to produce an increase in the synthesis and release of ADH. Volume receptors in the left atrium and baroreceptors in the aorta and carotid arteries respond to a decrease in plasma volume by sending impulses to the hypothalamus to increase ADH release.

ADH release is also stimulated by emotional stress, severe pain, and pharmacologic agents including nicotine, morphine, chlorpropamide, barbiturates, cyclophosphamide, vincristine, clofibrate, beta-adrenergic agents, and tricyclic antidepressants. ADH release is inhibited by ethanol, atropine, and alpha-adrenergic agents. Basal plasma concentrations of ADH are usually similar in young and old persons, but after hypertonic saline infusions, elderly persons release more ADH than younger persons do. In response to intravenous ethanol administration, plasma ADH concentrations fall progressively in young persons but only transiently in older persons. In response to orthostasis, a failure to release ADH is more common in the elderly than in the young.

Diabetes Insipidus

Causes. Diabetes insipidus (DI) results from either inadequate secretion of ADH (central DI) or inability of the renal tubules to respond to ADH (nephrogenic DI). The major clinical features are polyuria and polydipsia. In elderly patients, however, the commonest cause of polyuria and polydipsia is **diabetes mellitus.** Central DI may be caused by (1) idiopathic factors; (2) hereditary disorders; (3) tumors, including pituitary tumors, craniopharyngiomas, and metastatic tumors; (4) granulomatous diseases; (5) infections; and (6) trauma, including head injury and operation. Nephrogenic DI may be caused by (1) hereditary renal disorders; (2) chronic renal disease, including complications from obstructive uropathy, renal transplant, and acute tubular necrosis; (3) hypercalcemia; (4) hypokalemia; and (5) drugs, e.g., lithium, demethylchlortetracycline, and methoxyflurane (an anesthetic agent).

Patients with DI fail to increase urine osmolality adequately in response to increases in serum osmolality. Elderly patients may suffer dehydration and hypernatremia when they have inadequate water, e.g., during periods of unconsciousness, during a surgical procedure, or after head trauma. Hypertonic solutions increase the osmolality in these patients and should be avoided, unless adequate free water or hypotonic fluids are given simultaneously.

Diagnosis. DI is diagnosed by demonstration of an inability to concentrate the urine appropriately after several hours of water deprivation. At the end of this period, a significant increase in urine osmolality in response to vasopressin administration will identify central DI, inasmuch as nephrogenic DI will not respond. Although hypertonic saline infusions can also be used to demonstrate DI, the test is dangerous for elderly patients, especially those who are unable to tolerate a large saline load.

Senescent rats are known to have a form of DI in which ADH secretion is impaired. The secretion failure can be correlated with the reduced neurosecretor content in the posterior pituitary gland, and the impaired ability to concentrate urine is reversed with ADH administration. Elderly humans, unlike elderly rats, do not show evidence of central DI. They do have a decreased ability to concentrate urine in response to water deprivation, but this defect appears to be renal in origin and related to a decrease in the glomerular filtration rate.

Treatment. Treatment of diabetes insipidus requires the administration of vasopressin or other drugs to augment the renal responsiveness to endogenous vasopressin. A synthetic analog of arginine vasopressin, 1-desamino-8-arginine vasopressin (DDAVP), is a very effective form of therapy for central DI. It is instilled intranasally in a single dose of 10–20 μg (0.1 or 0.2 ml of the 100 μg/ml solution) and is effective for 12–24 hours. An injectable form of DDAVP is now available. DDAVP may also be used diagnostically at the end of the water-deprivation testing, to distinguish between central DI and nephrogenic DI. Lysine vasopressin is a nasal spray that is effective for 4–6 hours. Aqueous vasopressin in a dose of 5 or 10 units IM or SC is used for diagnostic purposes and for the acute control of DI after pituitary surgery. Vasopressin tannate in oil, in a dose of 2.5 or 5.0 units IM, can provide relief of polyuria for 24–72 hours. Oral drugs such as chlorpropamide, clofibrate, and carbamazepine decrease urinary volume in patients with DI and some endogenous ADH, but, because of side effects, should be used with caution, if at all, in the elderly.

Syndrome of Inappropriate ADH Secretion

Definition and Causes. The syndrome of inappropriate ADH secretion (SIADH) causes hyponatremia in the elderly and is due to the inappropriate secretion of ADH despite a decrease in serum osmolality. The diagnostic criteria are (1) hyponatremia and hypoosmolality of plasma; (2) inappropriately high urine osmolality in the setting of plasma hypotonicity; (3) absence of hypovolemia, congestive heart failure, and cirrhosis; and (4) normal renal, adrenal, and thyroid function. Plasma or urinary vasopressin levels may be clearly elevated or within the normal range but inappropriately high for the degree of serum hypoosmolality. Urinary sodium excretion reflects the dietary sodium intake and is generally greater than 20 mEq/liter, although it can fall below this in the setting of severe dietary sodium restriction. The causes of SIADH include malignant conditions, nonmalignant pulmonary disease, central nervous system disorders, drugs, and positive-pressure breathing. Oat cell carcinoma of the lung is the tumor most frequently associated with the ectopic production of ADH. Carcinoma of the pancreas, duodenum, ureter, lung (in addition to oat cell carcinoma), and prostate; and thymomas, bronchial carcinoids, and lymphomas have all been associated with SIADH. Other causes are nonneoplastic pulmonary diseases, including tuberculosis, pneumonia, and lung abscesses; central nervous system disorders, including subdural hematomas, subarachnoid hemorrhages, cerebral atrophy, meningitis, abscesses, head trauma, and tumors; drugs, including chlorpropamide, vincristine, cyclophosphamide, narcotics, barbiturates, general anesthesia, carbamazepine, nicotine, clofibrate, and tricyclic antidepressants. Disorders associated with impaired renal water handling, such as cirrhosis, congestive heart failure, renal failure, adrenal insufficiency, and myxedema, can also produce hyponatremia.

Clinical Course. The clinical manifestations of SIADH are those due to hyponatremia. Hyponatremia usually develops slowly, and few symptoms are evident until the serum sodium concentration falls below 120 mEq/liter. Early clinical manifestations include anorexia, nausea, vomiting, irritability, drowsiness, and personality changes. Muscle weakness, confusion, lethargy, seizures, stupor, coma, and death follow untreated cases. Patients with SIADH generally have no peripheral edema.

Treatment. Treatment of the SIADH consists of water restriction and, with this alone, the serum sodium concentration can usually be maintained in or near the normal range. Demeclocycline and lithium may also be used in the treatment of the SIADH, inasmuch as both are capable of inducing a state of partial nephrogenic DI by interfering with the action of ADH on the distal nephron. Demeclocycline is preferred, because lithium has greater toxicity and less consistent efficacy. Demeclocycline is given 600–1200 mg/day, in divided doses. In the critically ill patient with hyponatremia-induced seizures or coma, hypertonic saline (3%) can be administered to raise the serum sodium concentration temporarily. Especially in elderly persons, however, the administration of hypertonic saline carries the risk of fluid overload and congestive heart failure. In order to prevent fluid overload, furosemide can be administered IV (initial dose, approximately 1 mg/kg), while urinary sodium and potassium losses are replaced by hypertonic saline with potassium supplements. This treatment can be of considerable help, especially to elderly patients with life-threatening hyponatremia. After the serum sodium concentration has been partly or totally corrected, hypotonic fluids, if used, should be administered cautiously, to prevent the recurrence of severe hyponatremia.

1. DeTroyer A, Demanet JC: Clinical, biological and pathogenic features of the syndrome of inappropriate secretion of antidiuretic hormone: A review of 26 cases with marked hyponatremia. *Q J Med* 45:521–531, 1976.
   Neurologic manifestations including changes in consciousness, extrapyramidal signs, asterixis, and seizures were the presenting findings in 18 of 26 patients.
2. Dunihue FW: Reduced juxtaglomerular cell granularity, pituitary neurosecretory material, and width of zone glomerulosa in aging rats. *Endocrinology* 77:948–951, 1965.
   A reduction in the content of neurosecretory material in the posterior lobe of the pituitary gland was found in old rats compared with young rats.
3. Edwards CRW: Vasopressin and oxytocin in health and disease. *Clin Endocrinol Metab* 6:223–259, 1977.
   General review of vasopressin, including discussions of diabetes insipidus and the syndrome of inappropriate ADH secretion.
4. Forrest JN Jr, et al: Superiority of demeclocycline over lithium in the treatment of chronic syndrome of inappropriate secretion of antidiuretic hormone. *N Engl J Med* 298:173–177, 1978.
   Demeclocycline (600–1200 mg/day) restored serum sodium concentration to 139 mEq/liter from 122 mEq/liter within 5–14 days in 10 patients with chronic SIADH.
5. Frolkis VV, Bezrukov VV, Duplenko YK, Genis ED: The hypothalamus in aging. *Exp Gerontol* 7:169–184, 1972.
   A reduction in neurosecretory activity in the hypothalamo-hypophyseal system occurs with aging in animals.
6. Helderman JH, et al: The response of arginine vasopressin to intravenous ethanol and hypertonic saline in man: The impact of aging. *J Gerontol* 33:39–47, 1978.
   Osmoreceptor sensitivity, expressed as the slope of the changes in AVP on the changes in serum osmolality, was significantly greater in the old than in the young subjects.
7. Kleeman CR, Berl T: The neurohypophysial hormones: Vasopressin, in DeGroot LJ, et al (eds): *Endocrinology.* New York, Grune & Stratton, 1979, pp 253–275.
   Review of water metabolism, vasopressin physiology, and the clinical syndromes associated with hypernatremia and hyponatremia.
8. Lewis WH, Alving AS: Changes with age in the renal function in adult men: I. Clearance of urea. II. Amount of urea nitrogen in the blood. III. Concentrating ability of the kidneys. *Am J Physiol* 123:500–515, 1938.
   Finds that urinary concentrating ability declines with advancing age.
9. Lindeman RD, Lee TD Jr, Yiengst MJ, Shock NW: Influence of age, renal disease, hypertension, diuretics and calcium on the antidiuretic responses to suboptimal infusions of vasopressin. *J Lab Clin Med* 68:206–223, 1966.
   The renal responsiveness to ADH is not appreciably altered by age. However, the urinary concentrating ability decreases with advancing age.
10. Miller JH, Shock NW: Age differences in the renal tubular response to antidiuretic hormone. *J Gerontol* 8:446–450, 1953.
    Older individuals have an impaired ability of the distal tubule to respond to ADH.
11. Moses AM, Notman DD: Diabetes insipidus and syndrome of inappropriate antidi-

uretic hormone secretion (SIADH). *Adv Intern Med* 27:73–100, 1982.
Review. DDAVP is the most convenient and effective form of therapy for most patients with central diabetes insipidus. Patients with chronic SIADH may show satisfactory improvement in hyponatremia when declomycin is administered as 900–1,200 mg/day in divided doses.

12. Mukherjee AP, Coni NK, Davison W: Osmoreceptor function among the elderly. *Gerontol Clin* 15:227–233, 1973.
Only 1 of 6 elderly subjects showed a normal response to the challenge of fluid deprivation.
13. Robertson GL: Diseases of the posterior pituitary, in Felig P, Baxter JD, Broadus AE, Frohman LA (eds): *Endocrinology and Metabolism.* New York, McGraw-Hill, 1981, pp 251–277.
General review.
14. Rowe JW, Minaker KL, Sparrow D, Robertson GL: Age-related failure of volume-pressure-mediated vasopressin release. *J Clin Endocrinol Metab* 54:661–664, 1982.
Failure to release arginine vasopressin in response to orthostasis is more common in the elderly than in the young.
15. Turkington MR, Everitt AV: The neurohypophysis and aging with special reference to the antidiuretic hormone, in Everitt AV, Burgess JA (eds): *Hypothalamus, Pituitary and Aging.* Springfield, Ill, Thomas, 1976, pp 123–136.
The neurohypophysis of the old Wistar rat has an impaired ability to secrete ADH.

VIII. GASTROINTESTINAL DISEASES

52. ESOPHAGEAL DISORDERS

Sanjiv Chopra and Richard L. Curtis

Gastric Reflux

Reflux esophagitis is a disorder frequently found in the elderly. The most important determinant of gastric reflux into the esophagus appears to be an inadequate lower esophageal sphincter. Hiatus hernia, the frequency of which increases linearly with age (incidence at age 70 yr, 50%), does not have a close correlation with reflux symptoms such as heartburn, esophageal bleeding, and aspiration. Rarely, odynophagia and esophageal spasm, also reflux symptoms, are confused with angina pectoris. Dysphagia from peptic stricture formation may occur in the absence of a prior history of symptoms of reflux.

Presbyesophagus

Presbyesophagus is the clinical syndrome of abnormal esophageal motility, consequent to the aging process. Manometric studies have demonstrated, however, that subjects older than 70 years have a diminished amplitude of propulsive contractions but that the remainder of the peristaltic complex is intact. In addition, the incidence of abnormal nonperistaltic, spontaneous contractions is similar to that in younger control subjects. The previous notion of a specific motility defect related to aging has thus been challenged, and diverse illnesses such as diabetes mellitus, Parkinson's disease, peripheral neuropathy, and senile dementia have been implicated in the pathogenesis of disordered motility.

Motility Disorders

Dysphagia is the subjective awareness of solid or liquid food being lodged in the esophagus. Dysphagia is **never** psychogenic or physiologic. Therefore, its presence should provoke a systematic search for its etiology. Dysphagia may be the result of disordered motility or of mechanical obstruction.

There are several characteristic clues to the motility disorders, one of which is dysphagia for liquids as well as solids, with intermittent rather than progressive symptoms. Dysphagia may occur when drinking cold liquids in particular. Often, repeated swallowing, throwing the head or shoulders back, and the Valsalva maneuver provide relief. The primary defect in motility disorders may involve striated muscle, as in myasthenia gravis and polymyositis. Abnormality of the central or peripheral nervous system also may produce motility disorders. Examples are Parkinson's disease, pseudobulbar palsy, and diabetes mellitus. Smooth muscle may also be involved, as in achalasia, scleroderma, or hollow visceral myopathy.

Achalasia

Fewer than 15% of cases of classic achalasia begin after age 60. The composite picture of achalasia in elderly patients with a brief duration of symptoms and marked weight loss suggests secondary achalasia, most often from gastric carcinoma. Cricopharyngeal achalasia, on the other hand, is almost exclusively a disorder affecting elderly patients. A prominent indentation of the barium column is seen at the level of the cricopharyngeal muscle. The condition often results in inanition and pulmonary aspiration. Cricopharyngeal myotomy is the treatment of choice.

Carcinoma

Carcinoma of the esophagus, which obstructs the passage, is the commonest cause of progressive dysphagia in the elderly. Other mechanical causes of dysphagia include webs, rings, Zenker's diverticulum, and benign esophageal strictures. Extrinsic compression by mediastinal tumors or aberrant vessels (dysphagia lusoria) is a rare cause of dysphagia.

Dysphagia in an elderly patient should be assumed to indicate carcinoma unless proved otherwise. Risk factors associated with esophageal carcinoma include alcohol, smoking, lye strictures, ionizing radiation, achalasia, Barrett's esophagus, tylosis, and the Plummer-Vinson syndrome. Dysphagia (initially for liquids), odynophagia, back pain, and weight loss are the usual symptoms of carcinoma. Elderly patients sometimes present only with weight loss, minimizing or denying their esophageal symptoms, and ascribing the problem to ill-fitting dentures. Such patients subconsciously alter their eating habits and subsist on baby food, a historical clue to obstruction often obtained only in retrospect.

Barium swallow followed by endoscopy with biopsy and brush cytology will establish the diagnosis in most instances. Exfoliative "wash" cytology appears to be the single most effective method of obtaining positive results. If wash cytology is the only positive test obtained from a patient with dysphagia and an esophageal stricture, however, evaluation of the tracheobronchial tree should be carried out, since malignant cells may originate from a lung or pharyngeal lesion.

Treatment of esophageal cancer in general is palliative. Only 20% of patients are candidates for surgical cure. The modality of therapy (surgical procedure, radiotherapy, or chemotherapy) is dictated by the site of the carcinoma, its extent, and the availability of good surgical intervention or megavoltage radiotherapy.

---

1. Cohen S: Motor disorders of the esophagus. *N Engl J Med* 301:184, 1979.
   Excellent review of esophageal motility disorders.
2. Cohen S, Lipshutz W: Lower esophageal sphincter dysfunction in achalasia. *Gastroenterology* 61:814, 1971.
   Comparison of 20 normals and 16 patients before and after pneumatic dilation.
3. Dodds WA, Hogan WJ, Miller WN: Reflux esophagitis. *Am J Dig Dis* 21:49, 1976.
   Review of the determinants of esophagitis, methods of diagnosis, and modes of therapy.
4. Hallis JF, Castell DO: Esophageal function in elderly men: A new look at presbyesophagus. *Ann Intern Med* 80:371, 1974.
   Study of 21 elderly male patients demonstrating that disordered motility is more likely a result of disease than of age.
5. Heimlich AJ, O'Connor TW: Vascular dysphagia; Cancer is not always the culprit. *Geriatrics* 34:93, 1979.
   Presentation of 4 cases and review of the literature.
6. Palmer ED: Disorders of the cricopharyngeus muscle: A review. *Gastroenterology* 71:510, 1976.
   A review of the anatomy and physiology of the cricopharyngeus muscle and a discussion of the more important disorders affecting the upper esophagus.
7. Pope CE: Pathophysiology and diagnosis of reflux esophagitis. *Gastroenterology* 70:445, 1976.
   Defines reflux esophagitis, reviews the determinants of reflux, and discusses the diagnosis of reflux esophagitis.
8. Soergel KH, Zboralske FF, Amberg JR: Presbyesophagus: Esophageal motility in nonagenerians. *J Clin Invest* 43:1472, 1964.
   A group of 15 nonagenerians with complicating illnesses such as senile dementia and diabetes were noted to have defects of primary peristalsis. Tertiary contractions, delayed esophageal emptying, and esophageal dilatation were prominent abnormalities on barium swallow.
9. Tucker HJ Snape WJ Jr, Cohen S: Achalasia secondary to carcinoma: Manometric and clinical features. *Ann Intern Med* 89:315, 1978.
   Authors report carcinoma-induced achalasia in association with pancreatic, bronchogenic, and gastric carcinoma. Manometric features are identical to those of primary achalasia.
10. Vantrappen G, Janssens J, Hellemans J, Coremans G: Achalasia, diffuse esophageal spasm, and related motility disorders. *Gastroenterology* 76:450, 1979.
    Includes evidence suggesting the existence of intermediate types of motility disorders and showing that achalasia and diffuse esophageal spasm are part of a spectrum of related disorders.

53. UPPER GASTROINTESTINAL BLEEDING

Sanjiv Chopra and Richard L. Curtis

Common causes of upper gastrointestinal bleeding in the elderly include peptic ulcer, gastritis (aspirin, alcohol), Mallory-Weiss tears, gastric or esophageal carcinoma, and esophageal varices. Regardless of the site or the cause of hemorrhage, the risk of mortality from GI hemorrhage is highest in elderly patients.

Emergency Measures

Immediate supportive measures may often save the patient's life. Among the emergency procedures are the establishment of intravenous lines (control venous pressure [CVP] monitoring desirable); aspiration of stomach contents with a large-bore tube; and lavage with ice-cold water, if active bleeding is present. Blood products should be given as necessary to correct volume depletion and coagulation defects—as ascertained by determination of prothrombin time (PT), partial prothrombin time (PPT), platelet count, and bleeding time. The magnitude of blood loss may be established by assessing blood pressure, pulse, degree of cyanosis, pallor, excessive thirst, Hb and Hct, central venous pressure (CVP) reading, and nature of nasogastric aspirate.

Diagnosis

In any case of upper GI bleeding an adequate history and physical examination are essential. Information should be obtained as to a previous history or symptoms suggestive of ulcer disease; a drug history (aspirin, alcohol, chemotherapy, coumadin); as well as a history of weight loss, dysphagia, or previous upper gastrointestinal hemorrhage. Examination of the skin and mucous membranes may reveal spider nevi, petechiae, palmar erythema, acanthosis nigricans, and telangiectasias. The presence of hepatomegaly, splenomegaly, or ascites may provide further clues to the diagnosis.

Treatment

Therapy requires a team approach at the onset. Passage of an Ewald tube may not only demonstrate the bleeding but allow for ice-water lavage, which may stop the hemorrhage. Usually upper GI panendoscopy provides the diagnosis. Occasionally hemorrhage may be so brisk as to prevent visual diagnosis and require selective angiography. An upper GI series during the period of active GI hemorrhage is to be discouraged, as demonstration of varices or an ulcer need not imply that the lesion seen is responsible for the bleeding. Furthermore, an upper GI examination will often fail to demonstrate the presence of gastritis, a Mallory-Weiss tear, or active ulceration in a deformed bulb, and the presence of barium in the gut may prevent diagnosis by upper endoscopy or angiography.

Once the diagnosis has been established, specific therapy can be instituted. Intravenous vasopressin (Pitressin), beginning at 0.2 μ/min, has been shown to be effective in controlling hemorrhage from varices and perhaps gastritis. Occasionally tamponade with a Sengstaken-Blakemore tube may be required for control of variceal hemorrhage. Hemorrhage from a Mallory-Weiss tear will usually cease with conservative therapy, although an occasional patient may continue to bleed unless the tear is oversewn. Selective intraarterial infusion of Pitressin is an alternative form of treatment. Recently, embolotherapy, electrocoagulation, and laser phototherapy have been employed for control of bleeding. Availability of these techniques is limited, and their efficacy over more conventional therapy remains to be proved. In the event that GI bleeding continues, emergency surgical intervention should not be delayed. Indications for emergency intervention include bleeding at a rate of greater than 3 units q8h after initial resuscitative efforts; recurrent hemorrhage, particularly from peptic ulcer disease or varices; and the requirement of more than 6 units of blood in an elderly patient with continued bleeding.

1. Chang FC, Drake JE, Farha GJ: Massive upper gastrointestinal hemorrhage in the elderly. *Am J Surg* 134:721, 1977.
A retrospective study demonstrating that vigorous resuscitative efforts and early surgical intervention reduced operative mortality to 5%.
2. Kaplans MS, et al: Surgical management of upper gastrointestinal bleeding in the aged patient. *Am J Gastroenterol* 58:109, 1972.
Greatly increased mortality occurred with greater than 2,500 cc bleeding and age over 75 years. Mortality for partial gastrectomy (14%) was similar to that for vagotomy and pyloroplasty (18%).
3. Schuller KFR, Truelove SC, Williams DG: Haematemesis and malaena, with special reference to factors influencing the outcome. *Br Med J* 2:7, 1970.
The mortality was 16% in patients over the age of 60, as compared with 3% in the younger age groups.

54. INTESTINAL OBSTRUCTION

Sanjiv Chopra and Richard L. Curtis

Intestinal obstruction is a major cause of abdominal pain in elderly patients. Incarcerated hernias are the single most frequent cause of bowel obstruction and account for about one-third of the cases in patients 65 or older. Every elderly patient with abdominal pain should be examined for the presence of hernias. The overall mortality for hernia-related obstructions approaches 20%. Small bowel obstruction is often caused by adhesions from previous abdominal surgical procedures, no matter how trivial or remote.

In the case of a woman over 70 years of age with bowel obstruction, who does not have an external hernia or scars related to a previous laparotomy, gallstone ileus should be strongly considered as the cause of obstruction. Gallstone ileus occurs from impaction of a gallstone, 2.5 cm in diameter or larger, in the intestinal lumen, after it has entered the bowel through a cholecystenteric fistula. The advanced age of the patient and the intermittency of symptoms—caused by temporary occlusion of the lumen at one spot, followed by dislodgment of the stone and passage further along—can lead to a delay in diagnosis and a mortality of 20–30%. On roentgenograms of the abdomen, air is seen in the biliary tree. The risk of recurrent gallstone ileus is less than 5%, and treatment should be directed primarily at removal of the obstructing gallstone through an enterotomy, which is then closed. Cholecystectomy and surgical repair of the fistula is not done acutely; most fistulas close spontaneously.

In an elderly patient, obstruction of the large bowel is most often related to the presence of a malignant neoplasm. Constipation or abdominal distention may be the only clues. In general, colonic obstruction produces less fluid and electrolyte disturbance than mechanical small bowel obstruction. Volvulus of the sigmoid and diverticulitis are next in frequency as causes of large bowel obstruction in the elderly. Pain, abdominal distention, and obstipation are the usual clinical clues. A plain film of the abdomen will often demonstrate a massively dilated sigmoid in the shape of an inverted U in patients with sigmoid volvulus. Barium enema examination reveals a characteristic "bird's beak" appearance caused by the funneled narrowing of the barium column at the site of the volvulus. Sigmoidoscopy may be therapeutic, if one observes an explosive discharge of feces and gas during the procedure. Close observation is required to detect symptoms or signs of compromise to the vascular integrity of the bowel.

1. Andersson A, Zederfeldt B: Gallstone ileus. *Acta Chir Scand* 135:713, 1969.
Reports 44 cases and discusses symptomatology, treatment, and prognosis.
2. Greene WW: Bowel obstruction in the aged patient. *Am J Surg* 118:541, 1972.
Reviews 300 cases of bowel obstruction in patients over the age of 65 years. The incidence is evenly distributed into small bowel, large bowel, and hernia-related disorders.
3. Raf L, Spangen L: Gallstone ileus. *Acta Chir Scand* 137:665, 1971.
Describes the clinical course of 66 patients with gallstone ileus and emphasizes the tendency for spontaneous closure of the fistula between the gallbladder and intestine.

55. GASTRITIS AND PEPTIC ULCER

Sanjiv Chopra and Richard L. Curtis

Changes in gastric emptying as a function of aging have not been studied, but gastric emptying has been shown to be prolonged in atrophic gastritis and carcinoma, disorders that are frequent in the elderly population. Acid secretion also appears to decline with increasing age.

Atrophic Gastritis

The prevalence of chronic atrophic gastritis increases with advancing age. Pathologically there is thinning of the gastric mucosa and muscular wall. The mucosa is infiltrated with lymphocytes, plasma cells, and eosinophils; gastric glands are scant or absent. As the process becomes worse, the gastric mucosa is replaced by an intestinal type of mucosa with crypts and villi. Two types of atrophic gastritis have been described. **Type A** is characterized by achlorhydria and pernicious anemia, a positive test for parietal cell and intrinsic factor antibodies, and normal antral histologic findings. High serum gastrin levels have been reported in type A but not in type B. Gastric cancer, gastrointestinal symptoms, or overt hemorrhage may complicate this form of atrophic gastritis, but they are relatively uncommon.

In the **type B** form of atrophic gastritis, achlorhydria is also present, but tests for parietal cell and intrinsic factor antibodies are absent. Biopsy of the antrum demonstrates gastritis. Most importantly, the incidence of gastric carcinoma appears to be far more common in this form of atrophic gastritis than in type A. Clearly, however, both varieties may be complicated by gastric carcinoma, and annual surveillance by an upper GI series or endoscopy is a reasonable plan. It is not certain at present, though, that enhanced surveillance and early surgical intervention will produce an increase in survival rates.

Peptic Ulcer

The incidence of peptic ulcer disease in the United States is approximately three million annually, and about 20% of peptic ulcers appear for the first time in individuals older than 60 years. Duodenal ulcer is four times more frequent than gastric ulcer in the younger age group, but the proportion of gastric to duodenal ulcer increases with increasing age so that by age 70 the two types have a similar incidence.

Age-related Factors. Absence of a prior history and a lack of flagrant symptoms contribute to misdiagnosis and mismanagement in the elderly patient. Peptic ulcer in the elderly is often associated with complications. As many as 25% of patients older than 60 admitted to the hospital for peptic ulcer disease require surgical intervention for bleeding, perforation, or obstruction. Mortality is more closely related to age than to any other single factor, with 80% of all ulcer deaths occurring in the elderly. An increased incidence of gastric ulcer is associated with aspirin use, which is common in the elderly. Moreover, the patient may not report the use of aspirin unless asked specifically.

Treatment. There are several therapeutic choices in the management of gastric ulcers. Antacids appear to relieve pain and accelerate ulcer healing. Side effects can be devastating in the elderly population, however, especially osmotic diarrhea and hypermagnesemia associated with magnesium hydroxide. Magnesium-containing antacids are contraindicated in the face of chronic renal failure. Other side effects include hypophosphatemia from the binding of phosphate in the intestinal lumen by aluminum hydroxide, acid rebound and hypercalcemia from calcium-containing antacids in large doses, and salt overload from sodium-containing antacids.

H_2-receptor antagonists such as cimetidine and ranitidine are potent agents that suppress gastric acid secretion. They are used for a 6- to 8-week course of treatment of duodenal ulcer disease, and cimetidine has recently been approved for the treatment of gastric ulcer. Their use in hypersecretory states such as gastrinomas (Zollinger-Ellison syndrome) and systemic mastocytosis is more clearly established. Mental confusion and agranulocytosis can be complications of this drug therapy in the elderly. Anticholinergics are best avoided in treatment of elderly patients because, they may cause complications of tachycardia, urinary retention, flushing, constipation, and mental confusion.

Treatment includes antacids for gastric ulcer disease and antacids or cimetidine for duodenal ulcer. The choice of drug will depend on cost, patient compliance, complicating illnesses, and adverse reactions.

Other agents such as bismuth, carbenoxolone, and prostaglandins are not yet available. The prostaglandins may expedite ulcer healing through acid reduction and unique cytoprotective properties. Recently, sucralfate, a sulfated polysaccharide, has been shown to be an effective agent in the treatment of duodenal ulcer.

Surgical intervention is usually reserved for ulcer patients with perforation, obstruction, or significant hemorrhage. Hemorrhage is significant when hemoglobin is less than 9 gm/100 ml and (1) more than 1,500 ml is required to restore blood volume, or (2) the patient is unable to tolerate gastrointestinal bleeding, or (3) there is a second bleed in the hospital. Nonhealing gastric ulcers are often operated on to rule out malignancy, which occurs in approximately 5% of gastric ulcers. The type of surgical procedure depends on the individual.

1. Burkett DH: When do you recommend surgery for peptic ulcer? *Geriatrics* 36:83, 1981.
Reviews the indications for surgery in elderly patients with peptic ulcer disease.
2. Byrd BF, Richie RE, Thomison JB: Surgical operations for peptic ulcer in the geriatric patient. *Ann Surg* 159:787, 1964.
Notes a mortality of 4% for elective procedures, but one of 26% for emergency procedures.
3. Donaldson GA, Jarrett F: Perforated gastroduodenal ulcer disease at the Massachusetts General Hospital from 1952 to 1970. *Am J Surg* 120:306, 1970.
Patients over the age of 60 years suffered increased mortality as compared with younger patients.
4. Finkelstein W, Isselbacher KJ: Cimetidine. *N Engl J Med* 299:992, 1978.
A concise but thorough review article dealing with the current uses of the drug in the treatment of peptic ulcer disease and related acid-peptic disorders.
5. Grossman MI, et al: Peptic ulcer: New therapies, new diseases. *Ann Intern Med* 95:609–627, 1981.
Excellent review article highlighting results of recent epidemiologic studies, the search for new genetic markers, and our understanding of physiologic abnormalities. Newer medical and surgical treatments are discussed.
6. McGuigan JE: A consideration of the adverse effects of cimetidine. *Gastroenterology* 80:181, 1981.
A critical appraisal and commentary on the adverse effects that have been described in association with administration of cimetidine.
7. Narayanan M, Steinheber FU: The changing face of peptic ulcer in the elderly. *Med Clin North Am* 60:1159, 1976.
Excellent article highlighting the higher complication rate of peptic ulcer disease in elderly patients.
8. Strickland RG, Mackay IR: A reappraisal of the nature and significance of chronic atrophic gastritis. *Dig Dis Sci* 18:426, 1973.
Progress report reviewing nature and clinical significance of chronic atrophic gastritis.

56. DIVERTICULOSIS AND INFLAMMATORY BOWEL DISEASE

Sanjiv Chopra and Richard L. Curtis

Idiopathic inflammatory bowel disease refers to ulcerative colitis and to Crohn's disease. Both are disorders of unknown etiology that affect the bowel, although they sometimes also involve the hepatobiliary system, kidneys, joints, skin, mucous membranes, and eyes. The extraintestinal manifestations may predate the intestinal symptoms and can flare up at a time of inactive intestinal disease.

Ulcerative Colitis

Approximately 10% of individuals with ulcerative colitis have the onset after age 60 years. The disease may be more severe in older patients, but in most instances the symptoms, clinical course, and response to treatment are similar to those of younger patients.

About 25% of patients over age 50 years have pancolitis; in the remainder involvement is limited to the left colon or rectosigmoid. Symptoms include abdominal pain, diarrhea, rectal bleeding, and weight loss. Arthritis, uveitis, and erythema nodosum affect some; fever is usually mild or absent. Many patients are initially misdiagnosed as having neoplastic or diverticular disease of the colon. Proctosigmoidoscopy and biopsy demonstrate friability, erythema, or ulcerations, which help make the diagnosis. Barium enema studies performed when the patient is not acutely ill will usually rule out diverticular disease and carcinoma of the colon. Ischemic colitis rarely involves the distal sigmoid and rectum, owing to the rich vascular supply to these areas. Stool cultures are necessary to exclude *Salmonella, Campylobacter,* and *Clostridium difficile.* The last may occasionally complicate known inflammatory bowel disease and produce clinical exacerbations. Most patients will respond to Azulfidine (sulfasalazine) or steroid enemas (hydrocortisone hemisuccinate, 50–100 mg, given as a daily enema). Patients with severe ulcerative colitis may require oral steroids or parenteral therapy with hydrocortisone, 50–100 mg IV q6h. Such patients usually require systemic corticosteroid therapy for 6–8 weeks. About 5–

10% of elderly patients with colitis develop a fulminant disease. Treatment should include fluid replacement, blood transfusions, broad-spectrum antibiotics, intravenous steroids, and good surgical backup. Opiates, anticholinergics, and barium enema or colonoscopic examination are contraindicated. Worsening of the clinical situation or failure to improve within 3–4 days is an indication for emergency surgery.

Crohn's Disease

Crohn's disease, traditionally thought to affect young individuals, seems, from recent epidemiologic studies, to have a bimodal age incidence, with a first peak around the third decade and a second around age 70. Many elderly patients are women with Crohn's colitis. Involvement of the ileum (regional enteritis) affects the younger patients predominantly.

Abdominal pain, diarrhea, and gastrointestinal bleeding are the usual symptoms. The disease is most frequently misdiagnosed as carcinoma of the colon or diverticular disease. It can be distinguished from ulcerative colitis in about 80% of cases through clinical information, sigmoidoscopy, rectal biopsy, barium enema examination, and colonoscopy with biopsies.

Treatment is similar to that for ulcerative colitis and consists of Azulfidine and prednisone. In more fulminant disease, ACTH or intravenous hydrocortisone is used. Surgical intervention may be necessary for intractable perianal disease, intestinal obstruction, toxic megacolon, or severe disease unresponsive to medical therapy. Metronidazole (Flagyl) appears to offer some promise of healing fistulas caused by regional enteritis.

Diverticulosis

Diverticulosis refers to the mere presence of uninflamed diverticula of the colon, which are acquired herniations of the colonic mucosa and submucosa through the muscular layers of the colonic wall, in close proximity to penetrating nutrient arteries (vasa recta). The incidence of diverticular disease increases with advancing age, such that diverticulosis, rarely found in individuals younger than 30 years of age, is found in approximately 50% of patients over the age of 60 years. Epidemiologic studies suggest an increased prevalence in developed nations, whose populations by and large ingest less dietary fiber.

Patients with diverticulosis often complain of constipation or a long-standing history of alternating constipation and diarrhea. Bleeding from diverticular disease is sudden, massive, painless, and bright red. Blood clots from the rectum also are found in elderly patients, who often have underlying hypertension and atherosclerosis. The bleeding subsides spontaneously in 80% of cases. Continued bleeding calls for angiography to localize the site of bleeding, most often located in the right colon, and for infusion of Pitressin (vasopressin). When stable, such patients should be thoroughly evaluated by endoscopic and barium contrast studies to rule out other lesions. Recurrent bleeding occurs days or months later in about 20% of patients.

Diverticulitis

Diverticulitis refers to a perforation of a diverticulum with the formation of a pericolic abscess. Left lower quadrant pain ("left-sided appendicitis"), fever, nausea, vomiting, and constipation are the usual symptoms. A mass may be palpated. Inflammation contiguous to the bladder may produce symptoms simulating a urinary tract infection. Laboratory studies reveal leukocytosis, and occasionally red cells and white cells in the urine. An intravenous pyelogram may help rule out a primary renal disorder or involvement of the ureter by the inflammatory mass (pericolic abscess). Treatment with intravenous fluids, antimicrobials, and nasogastric suction (for obstruction) should be instituted after the diagnosis has been made clinically. It is appropriate to seek surgical consultation from the start. Complications include fistula formation, colonic obstruction, intraabdominal abscesses, and peritonitis.

Lower gastrointestinal bleeding is most often secondary to diverticulosis, polyps, carcinoma, inflammatory bowel disease, ischemic bowel disease, or hemorrhoids. In recent years, however, recurrent gastrointestinal bleeding of unclear etiology has been identified. It is found in patients who have had many negative barium studies and unrewarding laparotomies, during which some have even undergone gastric resections. After exclusion of upper GI bleeding and of the diseases most likely to cause lower GI bleeding, colonoscopy and/or angiography should be performed to look for angiodysplasias (hemangiomas and vascular ectasias), most often located in the cecum and ascending colon. Most patients are elderly (average age in one report, 70 years), and many have aortic stenosis (both calcific and rheumatic). If the patient's condition permits an operation, a right hemicolectomy should be performed. Alternatively, treatment via colonoscopic electrocoagulation may be attempted. Occasionally bleeding recurs, suggesting that the angiodysplasia was an incidental finding and the true source of recurrent bleeding remains to be identified.

---

1. Adams RT: The barium enema as treatment for massive diverticular bleeding. *Dis Colon Rectum* 17:439, 1974.
   Of 38 patients suspected of having diverticular disease as the source of their massive bleeding, 37 had cessation following barium enema. The incidence of rebleeding was 5%.
2. Almy TP, Howell DA: Diverticular disease of the colon. *N Engl J Med* 302:324, 1980.
   Excellent review of prevalence, natural history, complications, and therapy.
3. Bartlett JG, et al: Antibiotic-associated pseudomembranous colitis due to toxin-producing clostridia. *N Engl J Med* 298:531, 1978.
   This study demonstrated the relationship between toxin-producing clostridia and pseudomembranous colitis.
4. Bartlett JG, et al: Symptomatic relapse after oral vancomycin therapy of antibiotic-associated pseudomembranous colitis. *Gastroenterology* 78:431, 1980.
   Among 20 patients studied, 14% had symptomatic relapse. Most patients responded to a second course of therapy.
5. Crohn's disease in the elderly: A diagnostic problem, editorial. *Br Med J* 3:188–189, 1973.
   The difficulty of diagnosis and differentiation from diverticulitis are stressed: absence of diverticula, presence of bleeding, anal lesions, or extraintestinal complications should suggest Crohn's disease.
6. Eisenberg RL, Montgomery CK, Margulis AR: Colitis in the elderly: Ischemic colitis mimicking ulcerative and granulomatous colitis. *Am J Roentgenol* 133:1113, 1979.
   Ischemic colitis may demonstrate radiologic features similar to those of inflammatory bowel disease.
7. Fras I, Litin EM, Bartholomew LG: Mental symptoms as an aid in the elderly diagnosis of carcinoma of the pancreas. *Gastroenterology* 55:191, 1968.
   A high incidence of depression, anxiety, and premonitions of serious illness was found in 46 patients with carcinoma of the pancreas.
8. George WL: Antimicrobial agent-associated colitis and diarrhea. *Compr Ther* 7:33, 1981.
   Good current review.
9. Greenstein AJ, et al: Cancer in universal and left-sided ulcerative colitis: Factors determining risk. *Gastroenterology* 77:290, 1979.
   Patients with left-sided disease developed cancer at a median duration from the onset of colitis of 37 years, while those with universal colitis had a median duration of 20 years.
10. Hermann RE, Cooperman AM: Cancer of the pancreas. *N Engl J Med* 301:482, 1979.
    Analyzes methods of diagnostic evaluation and current modes of therapy. Resectability rate is less than 10%.
11. Larson DM, Masters SS, Spiro HM: Medical and surgical therapy in diverticular disease: A comparative study. *Gastroenterology* 71:734, 1976.
    A retrospective analysis of 132 patients with documented acute diverticulitis. For 75% of the patients, acute diverticulitis occurred as a single episode that responded to either medical or surgical treatment.
12. Law DH, Steinberg H, Sleisinger MH: Ulcerative colitis with onset after the age of fifty. *Gastroenterology* 4:457, 1961.
    Study of 30 patients aged over 50 years with a strikingly high incidence of misdiagnosis on presentation. The disease was likely to be limited to the rectum and/or rectosigmoid colon.
13. Meyers MA, Alonso DA, Baer JW: Pathogenesis of massively bleeding colonic diverticulosis: New observations. *Am J Roentgenol* 127:901, 1976.
    Authors present evidence that suggests that traumatic factors arising within the diverticular or colonic lumen induce changes in the arterial wall that predispose to rupture and bleeding. There is no evidence of accompanying diverticulitis.

14. Rusch V, Simonowitz DA: Crohn's disease in the older patient. *Surg Gynecol Obstet* 150:184, 1980.
Comparison of the clinical course of patients who were under and over the age of 50 referred for operations.
15. Shapiro PA, et al: Crohn's disease in the elderly. *Am J Gastroenterol* 76:132, 1981.
Only hospitalized patients were evaluated; however, symptoms, signs, laboratory data, and x-rays were similar to those of younger patients.
16. Stanley RJ, Melson GL, Tedesco FJ, Saylor JL: Plain film findings in severe pseudomembranous colitis. *Radiology* 118:7, 1976.
Moderate gaseous distention of the colon with wide transverse bands of thickened bowel wall and thumbprinting are common.
17. Surowicz, CM, et al: Rectal biopsy in the diagnosis of Crohn's disease: Value of multiple biopsies and serial sectioning. *Gastroenterology* 80:66, 1981.
Rectal biopsy revealed granulomas in 28% of patients with Crohn's colitis. No granulomas were seen in normals or patients with ulcerative colitis.
18. Trnka Y, LaMont JT: Association of clostridium difficile toxin with symptomatic relapse of chronic inflammatory bowel disease. *Gastroenterology* 80:693, 1981.
In a prospective study of 59 patients with inflammatory bowel disease, 11 (19%) had C. difficile toxin in their stools. The presence of the toxin correlated strongly with underlying disease activity. Vancomycin therapy appeared to be beneficial.
19. Watson DW: Pancreatic carcinoma. *Am J Dig Dis* 15:767, 1970.
Discussion of usual and unusual manifestations of pancreatic carcinoma as well as of surgical therapy.
20. Watts J McK, deDombal FT, Watkinson G, Goligher JC: Long term prognosis of ulcerative colitis. *Br Med J* 1:1447, 1966.
The mortality in the group of patients aged over 60 years was 4.9%/yr (higher than in the younger age groups).

57. VASCULAR DISEASE OF THE BOWEL

Sanjiv Chopra and Richard L. Curtis

A diminution of blood flow to the intestine, whether secondary to primary atherosclerotic disease, emboli, or vasculitis, causes disorders ranging from episodes of ischemic colitis to fatal infarction of the bowel. Anatomic, physiologic, and temporal factors dictate the pattern of intestinal involvement. Blood flow and oxygen content are critical to adequate tissue oxygenation. Thus, local oxygen requirements may increase significantly following a meal and explain the characteristic postprandial discomfort of persons with abdominal angina. The rate of occlusion of major blood vessels will influence the development of collateral circulation. Vasculitis primarily affects smaller vessels and is more apt to cause a segmental infarction. Arterial emboli most frequently lodge in the superior mesenteric artery because of its oblique take-off from the abdominal aorta.

Abdominal Angina

Abdominal angina is characterized by intermittent dull or cramping abdominal pain, occurring 15–10 minutes after a meal and lasting for several hours. The patients are usually elderly and have evidence of advanced arteriosclerotic disease elsewhere in the body, with hypertension or diabetes mellitus. A fear of eating develops, and pronounced weight loss ensues. The presence or absence of an abdominal bruit is of no diagnostic aid. Barium contrast studies are of little help. Mesenteric angiography reveals greater than 50% stenosis of at least two of the three major splanchnic vessels (celiac, superior mesenteric, and inferior mesenteric arteries) and, often, evidence of collateral flow. Angiography, however, only supports a clinical diagnosis, as it evaluates vessel patency or diameter and not blood flow, which is the critical determinant of adequacy of tissue oxygenation. Bypass, endarterectomy, and reimplantation procedures sometimes have been effective in relieving pain and correcting malabsorption. The decision to operate is a difficult one and often is made after other abdominal pathologic conditions have been excluded.

Whether surgical correction prevents subsequent acute intestinal infarction has not been proved conclusively.

Mesenteric Embolization

Mesenteric embolization occurs most commonly in patients with rheumatic or arteriosclerotic heart disease with mural thrombi. Occasionally emboli arise from vegetations of bacterial endocarditis, valvular prostheses, atrial myxomas, or arteriosclerotic plaques. The onset is usually abrupt, with severe abdominal pain, nausea, vomiting, and diarrhea. Gastrointestinal bleeding and evidence of intestinal obstruction may be absent initially, and objective findings are minimal, with a paucity of abdominal signs.

Laparotomy and embolectomy should be carried out early. Preoperative angiography may be desirable. Occasionally it is not possible to determine whether the occlusion is embolic or thrombotic. In that case a surgical procedure will be required to make the definite diagnosis. Embolectomy is performed prior to assessment of intestinal viability. A "second look" operation may be necessary for persistant abdominal symptoms or a recheck of intestinal viability.

Mesenteric Thrombosis

Mesenteric thrombosis often has a less sudden onset than mesenteric arterial embolism, because preexisting collateral blood flow is often present. Approximately 50% of patients with acute thrombotic infarction of the intestine will have an antecedent history of abdominal angina. Leukocytosis, hemoconcentration, elevation of serum amylase, and evidence of gastrointestinal bleeding support the clinical diagnosis. Dilatation of the bowel, air-fluid levels, "thumbprinting" (intramural hemorrhage and edema of the bowel wall), and air in the portal vein are useful but late radiologic clues. Angiography may be useful early in the course of such an illness. Frequently, complete occlusion is revealed in a patient with abdominal pain; however, such "occlusion" may be seen in patients who are entirely asymptomatic and therefore be coincidental to the current findings. When the patient has signs of peritonitis, angiography may cause an unnecessary delay in surgical management.

After supportive measures (nasogastric suction, correction of fluid and electrolyte imbalance, appropriate blood and fresh frozen plasma replacement, and antibiotic therapy) have been instituted, a surgical procedure should be performed. Necrotic bowel should be removed and revascularization of remaining viable bowel attempted. A "second look" operation 12–36 hours after the initial exploration is usually necessary to remove additional nonviable bowel. The advanced age of most patients, the presence of concomitant life-threatening cardiac, pulmonary, renal, or cerebrovascular disorders, and the nonspecific early presentation of these syndromes produce a mortality rate of 60–70%.

Nonocclusive Intestinal Infarction

Nonocclusive intestinal infarction has been recognized with increasing frequency as a cause of visceral ischemia, accounting for 30% of cases of intestinal infarction. The term *nonocclusive* is used because there is no occlusion of the **major** arteries. Usually, however, there is occlusion of the arterioles, capillaries, and venules. Many patients are elderly and have severe congestive heart failure, hypotension, or hypoxemia. Digitalis glycoside preparations, known to cause mesenteric vasoconstriction, may precipitate the problem. The pathogenesis is splanchnic vasoconstriction precipitated by decreases in cardiac output, hypotension, dehydration, and vasopressors. The clinical syndrome is similar to that of occlusive mesenteric vascular disease. Early angiography may be beneficial in (1) excluding thrombotic or embolic occlusions; and (2) revealing an angiographic pattern relatively specific for this syndrome, namely, narrowed, irregular branches of the superior mesenteric artery, spasm of the arcades, and impaired filling of the intramural vessels; and (3) providing the option of preoperative or nonoperative management via intraarterial vasodilator therapy (papaverine, phenoxybenzamine, prostaglandin E^1). Mortality is in the range of 80–90%, owing to the high incidence of complicating illnesses, advanced age, and inadequate available therapy.

Ischemic Colitis

Ischemic colitis occurs in patients in their sixth decade or older who have evidence of atherosclerosis. The abrupt onset of lower abdominal crampy pain and diarrhea in an elderly patient is more likely to represent an episode of ischemic colitis than inflammatory bowel disease. The syndrome is variable in its extent, severity, and prognosis, ranging from segmental ischemia of the "watershed" areas (splenic flexure and rectosigmoid) to catastrophic "toxic dilatation" of the colon and even colonic infarction. Sigmoidoscopy may show proctitis, discrete ulcers, or polypoid blue-black nodular masses. Rectal biopsy may show ischemic necrosis but is often nonspecific, with variable ulceration, crypt-abscess formation, and submucosal inflammation. "Thumbprinting" is seen on plain films or barium enema examination. The acute onset and rapid resolution help separate this diagnosis from inflammatory bowel disease. Full recovery is common, but occasionally a stricture will ensue and require resection.

Abdominal Aortic Aneurysms

The true frequency of significant abdominal aortic aneurysms in the elderly patient is not known. Abdominal aneurysms represent an important public health challenge in the elderly, however, since they are easily recognizable, ready reparable, and potentially lethal if left untreated. Most patients are asymptomatic, and thus routine palpation of the abdominal aortic pulse should be mandatory in examination of patients older than 50 years. A pulsatile, expansile mass in the epigastrium, with or without a bruit, should suggest the diagnosis. About two-thirds of abdominal aneurysms can be seen because of calcifications on cross-table lateral films of the abdomen. Gray scale ultrasonography is also useful in establishing the diameter of the aneurysm.

Complications include *leakage* and *rupture*—the latter accounting for 1 of every 250 deaths in people over age 50 years in one retrospective study. Patients with symptomatic aneurysms larger than 7 cm in diameter should have elective surgical intervention (mortality is several times higher when the procedure is done as an emergency, 35–85% compared to the usual 3–7% for elective operations), provided they are not very poor operative risks.

Mycotic aneurysms of the aorta account for less than 3% of abdominal aneurysms. Salmonellosis makes up a large proportion of such aneurysms. Forty-five percent of patients with abdominal aortic salmonellosis have had previous graft procedures, and sixty-five percent are 60 years of age or older. About half the patients have a characteristic triad of unexplained fever, back pain, and a pulsatile abdominal mass. Blood cultures usually grow *Salmonella*. Despite appropriate antibiotic therapy, graft infection occurs in 20% of cases and overall mortality is high.

Intestinal Vasculitis

Intestinal vasculitis may be subdivided into primary and secondary forms. Primary vasculitis, typified by polyarteritis nodosa, causes a lesion dependent on the distribution of the involved vessels, their size, and the collateral blood supply. Vasculitis may cause partial villous atrophy, stricture formation, or a diffuse enterocolitis. Frequently the patient presents with symptoms of intermittent small bowel obstruction. Bacterial overgrowth may occur concomitantly in the dilated proximal segment. X-ray features depend on the degree of intestinal involvement and may mimic Crohn's disease. Laparotomy with intestinal resection is needed when there are peritoneal findings. Nasogastric suction and steroids are used when there are no peritoneal signs. Chronic small bowel obstruction may require a limited resection.

---

1. Boley SJ, et al: On the nature and etiology of vascular ectasias of the colon: Degenerative lesions of aging. *Gastroenterology* 72:650, 1977.
   Discusses evidence suggesting that vascular ectasias develop as a degenerative process of aging, are multiple, and may be the most common cause of major lower GI bleeding in the elderly.
2. Boley S, Brandt L, Veith F: Ischemic disorders of the intestines. *Curr Probl Surg* 15:6, 1979.
   Excellent review of the physiology, pathophysiology, clinical manifestations, and therapy.
3. Britt L, Cheek R, Nonocclusive mesenteric vascular disease: Clinical and experimental observation. *Ann Surg* 169:705, 1969.
   Notes a changing character of bowel sounds that varies from those characteristic of ileus to normal. The typical patient was elderly with a history of ASCVD, arrhyth-

mias, and CHF on digitalis. The presence or absence of necrotic bowel could not be determined clinically.

4. Bynum TE, Jacobson ED: Non-occlusive intestinal ischemia. *Arch Intern Med* 139:281, 1979.
Concise editorial reviewing the pathophysiology of this entity.
5. Eklof B, Hoerels J, Ihse I: The surgical treatment of chronic intestinal ischemia. *Ann Surg* 187:318, 1978.
Classic symptoms include postprandial pain in the upper abdomen after 20–30 minutes, with weight loss due to malabsorption or fear of eating. Restoration of flow to one of the three arteries is sufficient because of the extensive collateral circulation.
6. Friedman SA: Common manifestations of degenerative arterial disease. *Med Clin North Am* 60:1079, 1976.
Excellent article focusing on some common clinical problems in elderly patients with an emphasis on approach to therapy. Concise and well-written section on abdominal aortic aneurysms.
7. Marston A: Diagnosis and management of intestinal ischemia. *Ann R Coll Surg Engl* 50:29, 1972.
Good overview of the problems of management and diagnosis, although most current modes of therapy are not discussed.
8. Mendelowitz DS, Ramstedt R, Yao JST, Bergan JJ: Abdominal aortic salmonellosis. *Surgery* 85:514, 1979.
Presents a case report of salmonella mycotic abdominal aorta aneurysm and reviews 24 previously published cases. Emphasis is placed on modes of presentation, diagnosis, and surgical management.
9. Smith GW: Lower GI bleeding in the elderly: Diverticulosis and angiodysplasia as dominant causes. *Postgrad Med* 69:36, 1981.
Discusses characteristics of bleeding in each disorder with an emphasis on diverticular bleeding as arterial, acute, and severe, as compared with angiodysplastic bleeding, which is venous, less severe, and recurrent.
10. Vellar I, Doyle J: Acute mesenteric ischemia. *Aust NZ J Surg* 47:54, 1977.
Of the patients studied, 71% had SMA thrombosis while only 18% had bloody diarrhea. Any cardiac patient developing unexplained GI hemorrhage, abdominal distention, or abdominal pain should be considered to be possibly suffering from the low output syndrome.
11. Weaver GA, et al: Gastrointestinal angiodysplasia associated with aortic valve disease: Part of a spectrum of angiodysplasia of the gut. *Gastroenterology* 77:1, 1979.
Of the 12 patients reported, 6 shared in common gastric or duodenal angiodysplasias, aortic valvular disease, and advanced age. On rare occasions angiodysplasias of the UGI tract may be a source of bleeding.
12. Williams LF: Vascular insufficiency of the intestines. *Gastroenterology* 61:757, 1971.
"Progress" article reviewing the pathophysiology, clinical diagnosis, and therapy of the wide spectrum of intestinal vascular disorders.

58. COLONIC AND RECTAL CARCINOMA

Sanjiv Chopra and Richard L. Curtis

Colonic and rectal carcinoma, representing 15% of all malignant neoplasms, is the second most frequent malignant disease in the United States. Over 80,000 new cases are diagnosed each year in patients who are usually in their sixth and seventh decades of life.

The cardinal symptoms are abdominal pain, change in bowel habits, rectal bleeding, and weight loss. Blood in the stool of an elderly patient must be assumed to be due to cancer of the large bowel until proved otherwise. Sigmoidoscopy and barium enema should be performed to localize the tumor. Rectal bleeding should never be ascribed simply to the presence of hemorrhoids. Neoplasms of the right side of the colon tend to be large, polypoid, fungating, and friable; patients are often anemic. Left-sided neoplasms are more scirrhous and apt to lead to obstructive symptoms. Diarrhea and tenesmus occur frequently in patients with distal colonic lesions. Gross bleeding, common in left colon tumor, is infrequent in right-sided lesions, particularly cecal tumors.

Digital examination of the rectum combined with sigmoidoscopy will identify approximately 50% of large bowel cancers. Barium enema examination after a thorough cleansing of the bowel will identify most lesions. Diagnostic colonoscopy can help to evaluate an equivocal lesion; obtain a specimen for histologic examination; evaluate synchronous lesions; or screen high-risk individuals with longstanding ulcerative colitis, family histories of colonic carcinoma, or previous histories of polyps or carcinoma of the colon. An elevated CEA level has no special relevance to colonic carcinoma per se and has to be evaluated in light of the overall clinical situation. It may aid, however, in the early detection of recurrent disease following removal of a colonic carcinoma.

Many adenocarcinomas of the colon and rectum arise from adenomatous polyps. Polyps within reach of the sigmoidoscope should be excised. More distant polyps either greater than 1–2 cm in diameter or villous, should be removed by colonoscopy or laparotomy. Colonoscopic removal of a polyp on a stalk may be considered a cure if there is no invasion of the base of the stalk by carcinoma. If there is invasion of the base, removal by a standard operation is recommended.

The primary treatment of adenocarcinoma of the colon is surgical. Preoperative radiotherapy does not necessarily improve chances of resection by decreasing tumor bulk, nor does it favorably influence survival. Palliative bowel resections are indicated to alleviate obstruction and to control hemorrhage or pain. For elderly patients with rectal carcinoma and concomitant disease, fulguration (often several staged treatments) may provide sufficient palliation.

1. Copeland EM, Miller LD, Jones RS: Prognostic factors in carcinoma of the colon and rectum. *Am J Surg* 116:875, 1968.
   Study of 1,084 patients.
2. Fras I, Litin EM, Bartholomew LG: Mental symptoms as an aid in the early diagnosis of carcinoma of the pancreas. *Gastroenterology* 55:191, 1968.
   A high incidence of depression, anxiety, and premonitions of serious illness was found in 46 patients with carcinoma of the pancreas.
3. Glenn F, McSherry CK: Obstruction and perforation in colorectal cancer. *Ann Surg* 173:983, 1971.
   Both obstruction and perforation in colorectal cancer are associated with high operative mortality and low 5-year survival rates.
4. Hermann RE, Cooperman AM: Cancer of the pancreas. *N Engl J Med* 301:482, 1979.
   Methods of diagnostic evaluation and current modes of therapy are analyzed. Resectability rate is less than 10%.
5. Linos DA, et al: Cholecystectomy and carcinoma of the colon. *Lancet* 3:381, 1981.
   Data are presented that support the hypothesis that cholecystectomy is a predisposing factor in the development of colonic carcinoma.
6. Watson DW: Pancreatic carcinoma. *Am J Dig Dis* 15:767, 1970.
   Discussion of usual and unusual manifestations of pancreatic carcinoma, as well as of surgical therapy.
7. Winawer SJ, Sherlock P, Miller DC: Screening for colon cancer. *Gastroenterology* 70:783, 1976.
   Reviews risk factors and techniques for diagnosis, along with an approach to the diagnosis of colorectal carcinoma.
8. Wolf WI, et al: Comparison of colonoscopy and the contrast enema in five hundred patients with colorectal disease. *Am J Surg* 129:181, 1975.
   Colonoscopy proved effective in diagnosing polyps and ruling out false positive radiologic diagnoses.

59. GASTRIC CARCINOMA

Sanjiv Chopra and Richard L. Curtis

Gastric carcinoma is a dismal disease, with an overall 5-year survival rate of less than 10%. Fortunately, for unexplained reasons the incidence of gastric adenocarcinoma has

declined dramatically over the last 3–4 decades. Atrophic gastritis (type B) and intestinal metaplasia represent precancerous conditions. Gastric cancer occurs more often in patients with blood group A, individuals over 50, and in certain families. Countries such as Japan and Chile have very high incidence rates, whereas the incidence is low in the United States, Canada, New Zealand, and tropical countries. Migrants from high- to low-risk nations maintain their increased susceptibility, while the risk to their offspring parallels that of inhabitants of the new homeland.

Symptoms include anorexia, abdominal discomfort with pain, early satiety, weight loss, dysphagia, and symptoms referable to anemia. Metastatic spread may involve the liver, lungs, bone, brain, supraclavicular glands, ovary (Krukenberg's tumor), pelvis, and rectum (Blumer's shelf). Diagnosis may be suggested by barium contrast studies and is most often established by gastroscopy with biopsy or by gastric cytology. Acid studies are of no practical value except in the instance of gastric ulcer, in which case achlorhydria almost always signifies the ulcer to be malignant.

Gastric carcinoma occurs with increased frequency in elderly patients who have had gastric surgical procedures (most often Billroth II gastric resection) for benign ulcer disease. The operation may antedate the detection of carcinoma in the gastric stump by 10–20 years. No consistent pattern of histologic changes in the gastric mucosa as an early indication of malignant transformation has yet been identified. Fiberoptic gastroscopy with multiple biopsies (12–20) should be performed, even in the absence of endoscopic features to suggest malignancy, and the patients may benefit from repeated routine surveillance endoscopic procedures. Subtotal gastrectomy with resection of associated lymph nodes or total gastrectomy is the only procedure with a potential for cure of gastric cancer.

See Selected Readings, Chap. 58.

60. HEPATIC DISEASE

Sanjiv Chopra and Richard L. Curtis

The single most important cause of persistent jaundice is malignant obstruction of the biliary tree, most often related to pancreatic carcinoma. Other causes of jaundice include drug-induced hepatitis (Tables 60-1 and 60-2), congestive heart failure, severe bacterial infections, shock, and primary and metastatic tumors of the liver. Viral hepatitis is an uncommon cause of jaundice in the elderly but is important to recognize, as misdiagnosis may have disastrous consequences.

Viral Hepatitis

Many cases of viral hepatitis are related to transfusions and are from the non-A, non-B group of viruses. The incidence of posttransfusion type B hepatitis has decreased markedly with the institution of third-generation screening tests and increased usage of volunteer blood. Symptoms of viral hepatitis may be insidious, and the profound anorexia and lassitude characteristically seen in younger patients may be lacking. Cholestatic features, such as persistent jaundice and pruritis, may be prominent and suggest extrahepatic obstruction. Abdominal pain may be marked, and exploratory laparotomy (done on the mistaken assumption that the patient has biliary tract disease rather than acute viral hepatitis) carries a prohibitive morbidity and mortality. Edema, ascites, and encephalopathy may be more common in patients over the age of 40 years, and reflect the presence of submassive hepatic necrosis, a histologic lesion supposed to be more frequent in the older age group. The single most important prognostic factor in fulminant hepatic failure (important causes include viral hepatitis and drug hepatitis) is advanced age. Mortality is markedly increased in patients over 40 years of age. Concomitant underlying debilitating disease or malignancy will further increase the fatality rate.

Drug-Related Jaundice

Drug-related jaundice occurs almost as frequently as viral hepatitis in the elderly. Hepatotoxins may be classified as intrinsic (predictable) or idiosyncratic (unpredictable).

Table 60-1. Acute drug-induced hepatic injury

Histological Classification	Clinical Aspect	Examples
Cytotoxic		
Necrotic	Severe hepatitis-like illness; may be fatal	INH Halothane
Steatotic	Resembles acute fatty liver of pregnancy and Reye's syndrome	Tetracycline
Cholestatic	Simulates extrahepatic obstructive jaundice	Chlorpromazine Erythromycin estolate Testosterone
Mixed (cytotoxic and cholestatic)	Variable	Sulfonamides Para-aminosalicylic acid Phenylbutazone

Table 60-2. Chronic drug-induced hepatic injury

Types of Chronic Liver Disease	Drugs
Chronic active hepatitis	Oxyphenisatin, INH, methyldopa, nitrofurantoin, sulfonamides
Cirrhosis	Methotrexate, INH, methyldopa, chlorpromazine, arsenicals, tolbutamide
Peliosis hepatis (blood-filled cystic lesions)	Anabolic steroids
Neoplasms	
Adenoma	Anabolic steroids
Carcinoma	Anabolic steroids
Angiosarcoma	Arsenic, thorotrast, vinyl chloride
Budd-Chiari syndrome	Chemotherapeutic agents

INH = isoniazid.

Intrinsic hepatotoxins are highly toxic to exposed individuals, are characterized by a relatively brief period between exposure and advent of illness, cause an apparent dose-dependent injury, and reproduce toxicity in experimental animals. Examples of intrinsic toxins are carbon tetrachloride, yellow phosphorus, *Amanita phalloides,* and arsenicals. Idiosyncratic hepatotoxins, on the other hand, are toxic in only a small number of exposed individuals, involve a relatively long latent period prior to the development of symptoms, show no relationship between dose and liver injury, and are not toxic in laboratory animals. Fever, rash, and eosinophilia are frequently present. Examples include sulfonamides, *para*-aminosalicylic acid (PAS), phenothiazines, methyldopa, halothane, isoniazid (INH), and oxyphenisatin.

The liver biopsy may show a cholestatic, cytotoxic, or a mixed pattern for either type of injury. The cholestatic form of hepatic injury may mimic extrahepatic obstructive jaundice and is associated with chlorpromazine or erythromycin estolate. The hepatic injury may be acute and occasionally fulminant, as with halothane or tetracycline; chronic injury (chronic active hepatitis) is seen with methyldopa, oxyphenisatin, and INH. Cirrhosis has been described following the use of methotrexate, INH, methyldopa, arsenicals, and tolbutamide.

Two aspects of drug-related hepatitis should be emphasized. First, the incidence of hepatotoxicity from a drug may increase with advancing age. Thus, significant liver damage with INH seldom has been seen in patients under 20 years of age and rises linearly with increasing age, varying from 0.3% between the ages of 20 and 34 years to 2–3% at 50 years and older. Second, drug-induced hepatic disease causes less than 5% of all acute liver disease but is still responsible for 20–30% of fulminant hepatic failure.

1. Chalmers TC, Koff RS, Grady GF: A note on fatality in serum hepatitis. *Gastroenterology* 49:22, 1965.
Review of published data suggesting that elderly patients with serum hepatitis have a markedly increased mortality.
2. Harville DD, Summerskill WHJ: Surgery in acute hepatitis. Causes and effects. *JAMA* 184:257, 1963.
Cholestatic viral hepatitis in elderly patients can simulate extrahepatic obstruction. Surgery in such patients carries a high morbidity and mortality.
3. Maddrey WC, Boitnott JK: Drug-induced chronic liver disease. *Gastroenterology* 72:1348, 1977.
Review article that examines the evidence associating commonly used therapeutic agents with the development of chronic liver disease.
4. Zimmerman HJ (ed): Drug-induced liver disease. *Semin Liv Dis* 1:91, 1981.
Entire issue devoted to drug-induced liver disease. Articles cover drug-induced chronic liver disease, isoniazid- and halothane-induced liver disease, and hepatic lesions caused by steroids.
5. Mitchell JR, et al: Isoniazid liver injury: Clinical spectrum, pathology, and probable pathogenesis. *Ann Intern Med* 84:181, 1976.
Excellent review of the literature by those involved in unravelling the "isoniazid story."
6. Trey C, Lipworth L, Davidson CS: Parameters influencing survival in the first 318 patients reported to the fulminant hepatic failure surveillance study. *Gastroenterology* 58:306, 1970.
Survival from fulminant hepatic failure decreased dramatically in patients over the age of 45 years.
7. Zimmerman HJ: *Hepatotoxicity: The Adverse Effects of Drugs and Other Chemicals on the Liver.* New York, Appleton-Century-Crofts, 1978, pp 3–121, 310–390.
Excellent, authoritative book on the subject of drug hepatotoxicity.

61. HEPATIC FAILURE

Sanjiv Chopra and Richard L. Curtis

Massive or submassive necrosis of the liver results in a clinical syndrome characterized by encephalopathy, ascites, and jaundice. Causes include viral and drug-induced liver injury, severe congestive heart failure, and hypotension. Hepatic infarction (as in periarteritis nodosa) and tumors affecting the liver are rare causes of severe hepatic disease.

Hepatic Coma

Etiology. The exact mechanism responsible for hepatic coma is not known. Ammonia is the traditional villain and has fascinated investigators since it was shown that susceptible cirrhotics developed hepatic coma after ingestion of ammonium chloride. The correlation between levels of blood ammonia and severity of encephalopathy is poor, however. Other putative factors include methylmercaptan (responsible for characteristic fetor hepaticus), biogenic amines (octopamine), short-chain fatty acids, and alpha-ketoglutarate.

Recent investigations have focused on the altered ratio of aromatic to branched-chain amino acids. This ratio may influence entry of tryptophan and phenylalanine into the brain, leading to increased serotonin synthesis, decreased catecholamine production, and subsequent coma.

Symptoms. Staging of hepatic encephalopathy is clinically helpful. In stage I, symptoms include euphoria, restlessness, confusion, and an altered sleep rhythm. Asterixis may be present; the EEG is usually normal. Mortality averages 25%. Patients with stage

II encephalopathy are generally drowsy much of the time and show asterixis. The EEG shows generalized slowing. Predominating features of stage III encephalopathy are stupor and incoherence. The patient is arousable with stimulation, however, and when the patient can cooperate, asterixis is evident. Encephalopathy has reached stage IV when the patient is no longer arousable. Deep noxious stimuli may produce a response, however. Decerebrate or decorticate rigidity occurs regularly in hepatic coma. The mortality in the second and third stages is around 60% and is as high as 90% in stage IV.

Metabolic abnormalities are noted frequently in hepatic failure and include alkalosis as well as acidosis. Hyponatremia is a common feature. Impaired hemostasis may follow the decreased synthesis of factors I, II, V, VII, IX, and X. Thrombocytopenia and low-grade disseminated intravascular coagulation (DIC) may also complicate severe liver failure.

Gastrointestinal bleeding occurs in 50% of the patients and is the cause of death in 30%. Sites of bleeding include the esophagus, stomach, and duodenum. Esophageal varices are the source of hemorrhage in less than 50% of cases. Renal failure may be a result of acute tubular necrosis or hepatorenal syndrome. Septicemia may be associated with aspiration pneumonia, urinary tract infection, or spontaneous bacterial peritonitis. Malaise, altered mental status including frank hepatic coma, and diffuse abdominal pain may be presenting features of spontaneous bacterial peritonitis. Ascites is a sine qua non for this condition. Fever of hypothermia is common. Hypoglycemia from decreased glycogen stores and impaired glyconeogenesis occurs in 5–10% of patients. Hypotension, cardiac arrhythmias, and cerebral edema are frequent preterminal events.

Treatment. Maintenance of vital functions and treatment of complications are currently the only form of therapy effective in hepatic failure. Dietary management consists of low protein and sufficient caloric intake, with avoidance of routine hyperalimentation formulas. Attempts at dietary manipulation with provision of branched-chain amino acids have produced equivocal results. Neomycin, 4–8 gm PO, PR, or via nasogastric tube, is helpful. Recently, lactulose, 30–45 cc tid, has been shown to be as efficacious as neomycin in the treatment of hepatic encephalopathy. Heroic measures such as plasmaphoresis, administration of hepatitis B immunoglobulin, and hepatic transplantation are of unproved efficacy and impractical in elderly patients.

Prognosis. The single most important prognostic factor in hepatic failure is **advanced age,** as patients older than 40 have the highest mortality. The prognosis also appears to depend on the severity of the encephalopathy. Laboratory features such as prothrombin time, serum albumin, and fetoprotein levels do **not** predict survival in **individual** cases.

Portosystemic Encephalopathy

Patients with portosystemic encephalopathy generally have advanced (and often progressive) liver disease; yet the prognosis is considerably better than in hepatic coma secondary to massive hepatic necrosis. Portosystemic encephalopathy may arise in 20–30% of patients with surgically created shunts.

Etiology. Onset is often insidious, and the correct diagnosis may not be made. Hepatic coma is often induced by some precipitating event or physiologic derangement, which may appear trivial. If recognized and treated, the syndrome is reversible.

A condition called acquired, non-Wilsonian hepatocerebral degeneration characterized by dementia, dysarthria, choreoathetosis, grimacing, and head tremor may be present in addition to other features of portosystemic encephalopathy. Occasionally a spastic paraparesis develops.

Gastrointestinal hemorrhage provides a substrate for increased ammonia production. Protein levels rise to 15–20 gm/100 ml blood, and resultant hypovolemia produces decreased cerebral, hepatic, and renal perfusion. Diuretics produce encephalopathy by inducing hypokalemic alkalosis, increasing renal vein ammonia output, and enhancing transfer of ammonia across the blood-brain barrier. Over-vigorous diuresis (and paracentesis) may lead to hypovolemia and prerenal azotemia. Usage of tranquilizers, sedatives, and hypnotics may result in encephalopathy by producing a direct depressive effect on the brain. Infection results in increased tissue catabolism, increased endogenous nitrogen load and increased ammonia production. Uremia as well as a high-protein diet increases the amount of urea available for bacterial breakdown in the gastrointestinal tract and therefore results in increased ammonia production. With progressive hepatocellular disease and surgical shunts, there is a failure to detoxify nitrogenous and other products from the gastrointestinal tract.

Treatment. The management of hepatic encephalopathy includes identifying and treating precipitating causes. CNS-depressing drugs should be avoided. Dietary protein should be reduced initially to zero, and adequate calories should be provided. Protein may be increased by 10–20 gm every other day. Following improvement, vegetable protein may be better tolerated by and beneficial to some patients with portosystemic encephalopathy. Vitamins may be necessary. Ketoanalogs of essential amino acids may be beneficial.

Drugs play an important role in the therapy of hepatic encephalopathy. Neomycin, 4–8 mg/day, may be given orally or via nasogastric tube and will decrease urease-producing intestinal flora. Although neomycin is a time-honored modality, its **optimal** dose, route of administration (PO, by retention enema, or the two in combination) and effect on gut flora as ascertained by modern cultural techniques has not been determined. Approximately 2–3% of administered dose is absorbed. Side effects include diarrhea, ototoxicity, and nephrotoxicity.

Lactulose is as effective as neomycin plus sorbitol in the treatment of portosystemic encephalopathy. It is a synthetic, nonabsorbable sugar that is hydrolyzed by colonic bacteria to form lactic and acetic acids. It causes an osmotic diarrhea and lowers the pH of the stool. Lactulose may work by trapping ammonia (pH), decreasing bacterial production of ammonia, or increasing bacterial utilization of ammonia. The dose is 30–45 ml tid or qid (end point, 2–3 soft bowel movements daily, with stool pH < 6.0). Lactulose is less expensive than neomycin and is not toxic. Occasionally patients will benefit from one drug and not the other.

Other drugs, such as L-dopa and bromocriptine, have not shown unequivocal benefit; although the bromocriptine has been useful in treating patients with the syndrome of acquired non-Wilsonian hepatocerebral degeneration.

Colon bypass has been advocated as effective long-term therapy, but in one control study this maneuver was not of any substantial benefit. The procedure carries a high operative and postoperative mortality rate, and may give rise to cephalad bacterial colonization of the small bowel may occur.

---

1. Conn HO, Lieberthal MM: *The Hepatic Coma Syndromes and Lactulose.* Baltimore, Williams & Wilkins, 1978.
Clinical findings and course, pathogenesis, and current management of hepatic encephalopathy are reviewed in Chaps. 1 and 2.
2. Fischer JE: Portasystemic encephalopathy, in Wright R, Alberti KGMM, Karran S, Millward-Sadler GH (eds): *Liver and Biliary Disease.* Philadelphia, Saunders, 1979, pp 973–1001.
Evidence presented that suggests crucial role for appropriate nutritional support in hepatic encephalopathy.
3. Hoyumpa AM Jr, et al: Hepatic encephalopathy. *Gastroenterology* 76:184, 1979.
4. Misra P: Hepatic encephalopathy. *Med Clin North Am* 65:209, 1981.
In the elderly, chronic hepatic encephalopathy may occur in the absence of overt signs of liver disease.

62. HEPATOCELLULAR CARCINOMA

Sanjiv Chopra and Richard L. Curtis

Primary Hepatocellular Carcinoma

Primary hepatocellular carcinoma is rare in the United States and western Europe, accounting for 1–2% of all malignancies. Etiologic associations include hepatitis B virus infection, hemochromatosis, macronodular cirrhosis, alcoholic cirrhosis, alpha$_1$-antitrypsin deficiency, and chemical compounds such as thorotrast, *Senecio* alkaloids, and oral estrogenic compounds. Between 30% and 80% of patients with primary hepatocellular carcinoma have cirrhosis. Hepatoma complicating Wilson's disease and primary biliary cirrhosis is extremely rare, however. Most patients in the United States are middle-aged or elderly; incidence peaks in the sixth and seventh decades.

Diagnosis. Signs and symptoms of neoplasia such as weight loss, anorexia, and weakness are present in 30% of patients; another 30% have had cirrhosis and present with unexplained clinical deterioration. Persistent pyrexia, an abdominal catastrophe (hemoperitoneum), or one or more of the many systemic manifestations of hepatoma—hypercalcemia, hypoglycemia, erythrocytosis, carcinoid, and porphyria cutanea tarda—may be predominant in the clinical presentation. Between 10% and 20% of hepatomas are discovered as incidental findings at laparotomy or autopsy. Physical examination will often reveal the stigmata of chronic liver disease: A firm, tender mass with a bruit is highly suggestive. The diagnosis is often suspected on clinical grounds.

Radionuclide scanning is generally unhelpful, although the yield with gallium scans is allegedly very high. An alpha-fetoprotein level higher than 500 ng/ml in an adult patient is virtually diagnostic. Liver biopsy, if feasible, remains the definitive means of establishing the diagnosis. Angiography may be characteristic but is not pathognomonic; its usefulness lies in determining feasibility of resection. Inanition, gastrointestinal bleeding, infection, and hepatic coma are the usual complicating features. Metastasis occurs most frequently to the lungs.

Treatment. Therapy consists of curative resection (usually contraindicated for patients with cirrhosis, severe jaundice, or ascites), radiotherapy, or chemotherapy (systemic or regional hepatic arterial infusion) but is rarely effective in prolonging survival. Median survival for patients who do not undergo resection is less than 6 months.

Hepatic Metastasis

Diagnosis. Metastatic involvement of the liver by tumor is a late feature of many malignancies and is far more common than primary carcinoma of the liver. Hepatic involvement has been reported in up to 50% of patients dying from malignant diseases. Neoplasms metastasizing to the liver most often originate in the gastrointestinal tract, pancreas, lungs, breasts, kidneys, ovaries, and skin.

Metastases tend to be multiple. Histologically, the majority of metastatic tumors are adenoplastic or anaplastic carcinoma. Symptoms include fever (common in renal metastases), weight loss, anorexia, malaise, and fatigue. Unusual manifestations of metastatic involvement are (1) vague right upper quadrant pain, occasionally rather distressing, secondary to neural involvement, and (2) bleeding from esophageal varices consequent to portal hypertension. Hepatomegaly, often tender, nodular, and very firm, is present in most patients. A friction rub may be audible. Jaundice is a late sign and portends a poor prognosis in the absence of metastases to the porta hepatis. Laboratory manifestations include an increase in the alkaline phosphatase and lactic dehydrogenase levels. Severe lactic acidosis resistant to the usual modes of therapy has also been described, most commonly in association with leukemia, lymphoma, or oat cell carcinoma metastatic to the liver.

Diagnosis depends on direct-imaging techniques. Liver scintiphotography is generally positive in 80% of patients with metastatic liver disease; with false-negative results are caused by lesions smaller than 2 cm. False-positive findings have been reported as a result of enlarged lymph nodes in the porta hepatis, cysts, diffuse nonmalignant disease, and abscesses. Ultrasonography will detect metastases in excess of 2 cm in diameter. The majority of hepatic metastases exhibit echo amplitudes below those of normal hepatic parenchyma (breast and lung), while intestinal metastases appear to be hyperechoic. Metastases usually appear as areas of diminished density on CT scanning of the liver. Confirmation of the diagnosis usually depends on laparotomy or percutaneous liver biopsy. The latter is usually positive in 50–80% of cases, especially when two passes are made through the liver.

Included in the differential diagnosis are abscesses, cysts, benign tumors, primary hepatoma, and infiltrative or storage diseases.

Prognosis and Treatment. The prognosis depends most heavily on the extent of liver involvement. Those patients with involvement of both lobes of the liver by colorectal primary tumors have 5–7% 1-year survival rate, as compared to 60% survival for patients with only solitary masses.

There is little effective treatment. Patients with solitary or localized metastases may be candidates for partial hepatic resection. Systemic chemotherapy may be palliative.

1. Alpert E, et al: Primary hepatic tumor. *Gastroenterology* 74:759, 1978.
2. Blumberg BS, London WT: Hepatitis B virus and the prevention of primary hepatocellular carcinoma. *N Engl J Med* 304:782, 1981.

Editorial succinctly summarizing the evidence that persistent infection with HBV is required for the development of most cases of primary hepatocellular carcinoma.

3. Chan CH: Primary carcinoma of the liver. *Med Clin North Am* 59:989, 1975.
4. Fenster LF, Klatskin G: Manifestations of metastatic tumors of the liver. A study of 81 patients subjected to needle biopsy. *Am J Med* 31:238, 1961.
Delineates the clinical and laboratory features of metastatic tumors of the liver.
5. Ihdle DC, Sherlock P, Winawer SJ, Fortner JG: Clinical manifestations of hepatoma. A review of 6 years experience at a cancer-hospital. *Am J Med* 56:83, 1974.
Articles 1 to 3 discuss the common clinical manifestations of primary hepatocellular carcinoma.
6. Margolis S, Homcy C: Systemic manifestations of hepatoma. *Medicine* 51:381, 1972.
Reviews the broad spectrum of systemic manifestations and stresses the practical value of recognition of such syndromes.
7. Wepsic MT, Kirkpatrick A: Alpha fetoprotein and its relevance to human disease. *Gastroenterology* 77:787, 1979.
Excellent review article.

63. GALLBLADDER DISEASE

Sanjiv Chopra and Richard L. Curtis

Gallstones

It is estimated that 10% of men and 20% of women between the ages of 55 and 65 years have gallstones, and that the incidence increases steadily with age. Symptoms may be minimal and nonspecific. Clinical features usually consist of abdominal pain, localized tenderness in the right upper quadrant, nausea, and vomiting. Murphy's sign (pain and inspiratory arrest when the patient takes a deep breath) may be present. A tender mass in the right upper quadrant is an unusual finding and should suggest emphysematous cholecystitis, localized perforation of the gallbladder, or carcinoma of the gallbladder with superimposed acute or chronic cholecystitis. The clinical picture may resemble acute pancreatitis when there is impaction of a stone at the ampulla of Vater. Liver function studies give variable results in cholelithiasis.

A normal oral cholecystogram during an acute illness excludes acute cholecystitis. Plain films of the abdomen may reveal opaque gallstones or air in the wall and lumen of the gallbladder (emphysematous cholecystitis). A HIDA scan demonstrating a functioning gallbladder effectively rules out acute cholecystitis. Ultrasound and CT scans support the diagnosis if they clearly demonstrate gallstones (positive in 80–90% of cases). Endoscopic retrograde cannulation of the pancreas and biliary tree (ERCP) and/or "skinny" needle transhepatic cholangiography may be necessary preoperatively to establish the nonpatency of the biliary tree and precisely localize the obstruction.

Management is usually surgical, consisting of cholecystectomy with or without exploration of the common duct. Cholecystostomy may be the procedure of choice in elderly debilitated patients with common duct stones, although stones will recur in 50% of such patients. The prognosis of acute cholecystitis is highly dependent on complicating medical illness with morbidity predominantly determined by the cardiac status of patients. Emergency cholecystectomy is associated with a higher mortality than elective cholecystectomy. Finally, medical management of gallstones with chenodeoxycholic acid and ursodeoxycholic acid may be attempted in an effort to dissolve nonopaque gallstones in patients with functioning gallbladders.

Gallbladder Carcinoma

Carcinoma of the gallbladder is a rare but uniformly fatal disorder that has its peak incidence in the sixth and seventh decades. Gallstones are associated in 60–90% of cases, but a cause-and-effect relationship has not been established. Symptoms are nonspecific and may resemble those of chronic cholelithiasis. Diagnosis is often made at surgery. Cholecystectomy and wedge resection of adjacent liver tissue are recommended for small lesions with minimal liver invasion. Median survival in most cases is less than 12 months, with death occurring secondary to inanition and local spread.

Bile Duct Carcinoma

Carcinoma of the extrahepatic bile ducts is unique in that, of all gallbladder and biliary tract disorders, it is the only one with a male predominance. The mean age of patients is 65 years.

Risk factors include gallstones, bile acids, chemicals (benzidine), parasitic infestations (*Clonorchis sinensis*), and inflammatory bowel disease. Patients with ulcerative colitis have a ten times greater risk of bile duct carcinoma than unselected populations, their mean age is two decades younger, and proctocolectomy does not obviate the risk.

Although bile duct carcinoma is biologically a slow-growing tumor, it carries a poor prognosis, because jaundice, often the presenting manifestation (95%), signals advanced disease; also its proximity to vital adjacent structures may make it unresectable. Differential diagnosis includes other causes of extrahepatic biliary obstruction (stones, strictures, and carcinoma of the pancreas or ampulla) as well as sclerosing cholangitis and primary biliary cirrhosis, which is more common in females. Pruritus often antedates development of jaundice, and the antimitochondrial antibody is present in 95% of patients with primary biliary cirrhosis.

Total resection for cure is possible, if the lesion is limited to the right or left hepatic duct or to the distal portion of the bile duct. Palliation for relief of pruritus and jaundice may be achieved by establishing free flow of bile into the intestine. Percutaneous transhepatic drainage of the biliary tract has recently been described. This procedure is useful in obtaining a biliary cytologic or biopsy specimen, thus obviating the need for surgical exploration to establish a definitive diagnosis of malignancy. Continuous drainage of bile in inoperable cases can be achieved. In elderly, debilitated patients with obstructive jaundice and significant hepatic dysfunction, it may also serve as a preliminary step for decompression prior to surgery. Unfortunately, palliative procedures, despite decompression of the biliary tree, are associated with a 25–50% incidence of subsequent sepsis.

---

1. Adson MA: Carcinoma of the gallbladder. *Surg Clin North Am* 53:1203, 1973.
   Reviews 112 patients with gallbladder carcinoma. Most cases are not correctly diagnosed preoperatively; about 25% of patients are potentially curable.
2. Gaines RD: Surgery for gallbladder disease in the elderly. *Geriatrics* 32:71, 1977.
   Reviews the incidence and clinical features of cholelithiasis in elderly patients and discusses the indications for surgery.
3. Haff RC, Butcher HR Jr, Ballinger WF: Factors influencing morbidity in biliary tract operations. *Surg Gynecol Obstet* 132:195, 1971.
   Morbidity in patients over the age of 60 years is determined by the degree of underlying cardiac disease.
4. Hermann RE, Martin JC: Biliary disease and advancing age. *Geriatrics* 24:138, 1969.
   There is a two-fold increased incidence of gallbladder carcinoma in patients over the age of 60 years with gallstones when compared to younger patients.
5. Ibach JR Jr, Hume HA, Erb WH: Cholecystectomy in the aged. *Surg Gynecol Obstet* 126:523, 1968.
   Emergency cholecystectomy is associated with a higher mortality than is an elective procedure.
6. Ritchie JK, et al: Biliary tract carcinoma associated with ulcerative colitis. *Q J Med* 43:263, 1974.
   There is an increased incidence of biliary tract carcinoma in patients with ulcerative colitis. Most patients had a long history of colitis.
7. Steiger E, Seltzer MH, Rosato FE: Cholecystectomy in the aged. *Ann Surg* 174:142, 1971.
   Reviews authors' experience with cholecystectomy in 51 patients aged 75 years and older. The operative mortality was 8%.

64. PANCREATITIS

Sanjiv Chopra and Richard L. Curtis

Acute Pancreatitis

Acute pancreatitis in the elderly is notable for its association with different etiologic factors and a higher morbidity and mortality than in younger age groups. The most common associated clinical entity is cholelithiasis. Gallstone-induced pancreatitis does not, however, lead to chronic pancreatitis. Acute pancreatitis is seen in as many as 10% of all patients with carcinoma of the pancreas.

Symptoms. The cardinal symptom of pancreatitis is pain, which is present in 95% of patients. Classically the pain is located in the midepigastrium and left upper quadrant; it radiates to the back in 50% of patients. Diffuse abdominal pain may occur as well, even in the absence of generalized peritonitis. Right upper quadrant pain may predominate. Nausea, vomiting, and fever occur in 75% of cases. Other manifestations include hypovolemic shock from exudation of plasma into the retroperitoneum, "third spacing" in the gastrointestinal tract from ileus, hemorrhage, and the activation of the kallikrein system with peripheral vasodilatation. Neurologic symptoms of confusion, disorientation, and coma may predominate in the elderly, especially if the patient develops diabetic coma. Physical findings include abdominal tenderness in the midepigastrium and left upper quadrant, with involuntary guarding.

Persistent and spiking fevers suggest pancreatic abscess or ascending cholangitis. The patient may have atelectatic rales or dullness at the base of the lung (usually left) as a result of sympathetic pleural effusion. Rarely, the adult respiratory distress syndrome occurs, with symptoms and signs of hypoxemia. Hypocalcemia may cause a positive Chvostek's or Trousseau's sign.

Diagnosis. An elevated serum amylase level is helpful in diagnosis but is neither specific nor sensitive. Amylase is elevated 2–12 hours after onset, generally returning to normal after 3–4 days. An amylase creatinine clearance ratio of greater than 5% further supports the diagnosis. Such values are also seen in diabetic ketoacidosis and thermal burns, however. A persistently high amylase may indicate the presence of a pseudocyst. An elevated bilirubin occurs in 20% of patients. High bilirubin levels suggest extrahepatic obstruction from common bile duct stones or obstructing carcinoma of the pancreas. The incidence of hypocalcemia has a correlation with the severity of the disease process and may be from an inadequate parathyroid response, hypoalbuminemia, or loss of calcium as soap into the peripancreatic region. A normal calcium level during the course of acute pancreatitis in fact is suggestive of preceding hypercalcemia. Hyperlipoproteinemia may be present as a result of pancreatitis or may indicate a basic metabolic defect (types I, IV, and V are associated with pancreatitis).

The diagnosis depends on an index of suspicion based on the clinical findings, supportive laboratory data, and x-ray findings. The latter tend to be nonspecific and include a sentinel loop of bowel overlying the pancreas, the soap-bubble appearance of an abscess in the region of the pancreas, and pancreatic calcification. Visualization of the gallbladder may be impossible in 50% of patients with pancreatitis, even in the absence of cholecystitis. Ultrasonography or CT scan reveals an edematous pancreas in 90% of patients. ERCP (endoscopic cannulation of the pancreas and biliary tree) is contraindicated in the presence of acute pancreatitis, as it is capable of inducing fatal pancreatitis in this situation or converting a bland phlegmon to an abscess.

Treatment. Medical management consists of intravenous replacement of appropriate fluids, nasogastric suction, and analgesic therapy. Unproved therapies include Trasylol (a trypsin inhibitor), prophylactic antibiotics, anticholinergics, and glucagon. Surgical therapy should be instituted if there is evidence of associated biliary tract obstruction or if the pancreatitis is severe and unresponsive to medical management. Pseudocysts can be followed by ultrasonography, and most resolve spontaneously within 2 months. Surgical therapy is indicated for progressive enlargement, rupture, or hemorrhage into the cyst.

Overall mortality in acute pancreatitis is approximately 15%, and in elderly patients it may approach 30–50%.

Pancreatic Carcinoma

Pancreatic carcinoma is the second most common cause of death due to gastrointestinal carcinoma (cancer of the colon is the first). It is the fifth leading cause of cancer death in the United States, and it is estimated that 20,000–25,000 new cases are diagnosed each year. For inexplicable reasons its incidence appears to be increasing. The mean age at time of diagnosis is in the sixth decade. Suspected risk factors include smoking; increased coffee consumption; heavy ethanol intake; diabetes mellitus; chemicals such as benzidine, urea, and methylnitrosourethane; and chronic calcific pancreatitis. Males are affected twice as often as females.

Diagnosis. Initial symptoms are often vague and nonspecific. Depression may be a predominant feature. The classic triad of pain, weight loss, and progressive jaundice is a late feature. Glucose intolerance, gastrointestinal bleeding (from direct tumor invasion of the stomach, splenic vein thrombosis, and subsequent development of gastric and esophageal varices), migratory thrombophlebitis, subcutaneous fat necrosis, and acute pancreatitis are uncommon features of this malignancy. Physical examination will often reveal signs of weight loss, jaundice, hepatomegaly, and a palpable gallbladder (Courvoisier's sign).

Laboratory diagnosis may reveal anemia, elevated blood glucose, and an elevated sedimentation rate. Hyperbilirubinemia is common in the late stages. An elevated carcinoembryonic antigen is seen in more than 90% of patients with pancreatic carcinoma. Recent diagnostic techniques of abdominal ultrasound, CT scanning, endoscopic retrograde pancreatography, and selective angiography have permitted an accurate preoperative diagnosis. The role of percutaneous needle biopsy or aspiration cytology (guided by ultrasound or CT scan) in diagnosing pancreatic carcinoma and affecting the clinical outcome needs to be objectively evaluated.

Prognosis. The prognosis of pancreatic carcinoma is dismal. There is no satisfactory treatment in most cases. It is unusual to diagnose early resectable lesions, and the operative mortality for pancreaticoduodenectomy (Whipple operation) is 10–20%. Survival at 5 years is 10–15%. Palliative operations to relieve jaundice and itching may bring substantial comfort to the patient. Dietary manipulation, pancreatic enzyme replacement, and insulin therapy are useful adjuncts.

Pancreatic Cholera

In 1958, Verner and Morrison described the association of a non–beta-cell adenoma, profuse watery diarrhea, and hypokalemia in the absence of gastric hypersecretion. This entity has been subsequently designated as *pancreatic cholera, WDHA* (watery diarrhea, hypokalemia, histamine-fast achlorhydria), and *apudoma,* subtype *vipoma.*

There are several case reports of individuals in their fifth to seventh decades with this syndrome. The diagnosis should be suspected when patients have a *secretory* diarrhea. Clues to a secretory diarrhea include profuse watery diarrhea with stool volumes exceeding 1 liter/day and persistence of diarrhea despite fasting.

In pancreatic cholera, laboratory values often reveal severe hypokalemic acidosis, fecal $K+$ 100–400 mEq/day, and dehydration. Stool osmolality is similar to plasma osmolality and is accounted for almost totally by multiplying by 2 the sum of the sodium and potassium concentration of the stool. Basal and histamine-fast achlorhydria and hypercalcemia are not uncommon. Steatorrhea is minimal or absent.

Vasoactive intestinal peptide (VIP) concentrations may be high, but similar concentrations have been seen in patients with surreptitious laxative abuse and on diuretic therapy.

Response to corticosteroids or indomethacin reinforces the clinical suspicion.

Other causes of secretory diarrhea, such as villous adenoma, Zollinger-Ellison syndrome (gastrinoma), medullary carcinoma of the thyroid, carcinoid, oat cell lung carcinoma, and ganglioneuroblastoma, should be looked for. VIP may be responsible for the diarrhea in the last two conditions. Surreptitious laxative abuse must be sought for assiduously. Intestinal perfusion studies may be in order.

Localization of the tumor by roentgenography, ultrasonography, and angiography should be attempted but is successful in only about one-third of cases. Surgical exploration is often necessary to establish the diagnosis. Treatment is aimed at restoring the acid-base and electrolyte imbalance, resection of solitary tumor (cure), or attempting palliation by subtotal or total pancreatectomy despite evidence of metastases. Corticosteroids and indomethacin may be effective in controlling diarrhea. Regression of tumor mass and abatement of diarrhea has followed treatment with streptozocin in a few cases.

1. Banks PA: Acute pancreatitis. *Gastroenterology* 61:382, 1971.
2. Graham DY, Johnson CD, Bentlif PS, Kelsey JR: Islet cell carcinoma, pancreatic cholera, and vasoactive intestinal peptide. *Ann Intern Med* 83:782, 1975.
   Discussion of 3 patients with pancreatic cholera and evidence implicating elevated levels of vasoactive intestinal peptide as the cause.
3. Jacobs ML, et al: Acute pancreatitis: Analysis of factors influencing survival. *Ann Surg* 185:43, 1977.

Analyzes abnormalities on physical examination and laboratory results that portend poor prognoses.

4. Krejs GT, Walsh JH, Morawski SG, Fordtran JS: Intestinal perfusion studies and plasma VIP concentrations in patients with pancreatic cholera syndrome and surreptitious ingestion of laxatives and diuretics. *Am J Dig Dis* 22:280, 1977.
   Good review of secretory pattern seen in pancreatic cholera.
5. Mallory A, Kern F Jr: Drug-induced pancreatitis: A critical review. *Gastroenterology* 78:813, 1980.
   Review of available literature linking a variety of drugs with acute pancreatitis.
6. Nakayama T, Ikeda A, Okuda K: Percutaneous transhepatic drainage of the biliary tract. Technique and results in 104 cases. *Gastroenterology* 74:554, 1978.
   Reports authors' experience with 104 patients, 84 of whom had malignant lesions producing extrahepatic biliary tract obstruction.
7. Rambaud JC, et al: Pancreatic cholera: Studies on tumoral secretions and pathophysiology of diarrhea. *Gastroenterology* 69:110, 1975.
   The small intestine is the site of water and electrolyte losses with the colon reabsorbing high amounts of water and sodium.
8. Sato T, et al: Preoperative determination of operability in carcinoma of the pancreas and the periampullary region. *Ann Surg* 168:876, 1968.
   Reviews 201 cases. Pancreaticoduodenectomy could be performed in only 11–13% of patients with symptoms for longer than 3 months, as opposed to in 56% of those with a duration of less than 3 months.
9. Warshaw AL: Acute pancreatitis. *View. Dig. Dis.* 9:5, 1977.
   Readings 1 and 2 are authoritative reviews of the etiology, pathophysiology, clinical features, and treatment of acute pancreatitis.
10. Warshaw AL, Fuller AF Jr: Specificity of increased renal clearance of amylase in diagnosis of acute pancreatitis. *N Engl J Med* 292:325, 1975.
   The renal clearance of amylase increased sharply in acute pancreatitis but not in most other situations associated with hyperamylasemia.
11. Warshaw AL, et al: The pathogenesis of pulmonary edema in acute pancreatitis. *Ann Surg* 182:505, 1975.
   Acute pulmonary edema developed in 8 percent of patients with acute pancreatitis. This distinctive form of pulmonary injury is caused by a loss of integrity of the alveolar capillary membrane.

IX. PULMONARY DISEASES

65. ASPIRATION PNEUMONIA

Robert Brown and Steven M. Scharf

Causes

Pneumonitis is a common sequel of the aspiration of endogenous secretions or exogenous substances into the lungs. Predisposing to aspiration are conditions that affect the level of consciousness such as neurologic disorders (including seizures), sedative drugs, alcohol abuse, and general anesthesia. Gastrointestinal disorders such as abnormalities of deglutition (perhaps secondary to a stroke), esophageal diverticula, and hiatus hernia may cause recurrent aspiration. The presence of a nasogastric, endotracheal, or tracheostomy tube may disrupt sphincter mechanisms that normally protect against aspiration. Finally, although uncommon among younger patients, chronic aspiration of oily materials occurs in many elderly patients who use mineral oil, oil-based laxatives, or oily nose drops. This is because the oily substances may pass through the pharynx and larynx and into the lungs without stimulating a reflex cough response. Once in the lungs, they insidiously cause a chemical pneumonitis that on chest x-ray may simulate a lung mass, a chronic interstitial process, or a wide variety of other conditions.

Symptoms and Treatment

The consequences of aspiration depend on the nature of the inoculum. Aspiration of large solid particles may cause asphyxia and sudden death (so-called *café coronary*). Aphonia is often a clue to the diagnosis. Aspiration of somewhat smaller particles causes bronchial obstruction, leading to dyspnea, wheezing, and postobstructive atelectasis. In the latter cases, removal of foreign bodies via a rigid bronchoscope is the treatment of choice. When aspirated, gastric contents of pH $\leq$ 2.5 cause, within 2–12 hours, a chemical pneumonitis characterized by cough, dyspnea, tachycardia, rales and wheezes, and abnormal gas exchange (Mendelson's syndrome). Treatment is largely supportive and includes oxygen, bronchodilators, chest physiotherapy, and, when necessary, endotracheal intubation and mechanically assisted ventilation. Positive end-expiratory pressure is often needed to maintain adequate oxygenation.

The role of corticosteroids and antibiotics in the management of chemical pneumonitis due to aspiration of gastric contents is controversial. The best studies fail to demonstrate any benefit from the use of corticosteroids, and these agents may even hasten the appearance of gram-negative superinfection in the lung. In all cases, sputum cultures should be monitored for evidence of bacterial pneumonitis superimposed on chemical pneumonitis.

We recommend use of antimicrobial agents when the patient who has aspirated has carious teeth or chronic gingivitis. Antibiotic coverage should be given for the anaerobic organisms associated with these disorders. Penicillin is the drug of choice, although some organisms may be resistant (*Bacillus fragilis, Bacteroides melaninogenicus*). Oddly, it is not clear that the presence of resistant organisms diminishes the effectiveness of penicillin, although this is probably because many different organisms are aspirated and only a few are penicillin-resistant. Should clinical improvement not occur within 3 days to a week, clindamycin is an alternative antimicrobial agent to use. Due to colonization of the oropharynx, hospital- or nursinghome–acquired aspiration pneumonia may often involve gram-negative organisms and, in the presence of rapidly progressive disease, a regimen including an aminoglycoside in combination with a semisynthetic penicillin or a cephalosporin is indicated. The choice of antimicrobial agents depends on the prevalence of specific organisms found in different institutions and on results of sputum cultures (see also Chaps. 30, 31).

Prevention

Assiduous attempts should be made to prevent aspiration pneumonia. Unconscious patients in whom protection of the upper airway is compromised should undergo elective endotracheal intubation. Nasogastric tubes should be used only when necessary and removed as soon as possible. In some centers, antacids or cimetidine is administered to patients considered at high risk for aspiration. This is done in order to elevate the pH of gastric contents, so that damage to the lungs will be minimized if aspiration does occur. Patients with esophageal and gastric disorders that predispose to recurrent aspiration should sleep in a semiseated position, or should have their beds elevated such that the head is 8 inches or more above the feet. If recurrent aspiration remains a problem, and there is respiratory decompensation, a surgical procedure to correct the primary disorder is indicated. Lipoid pneumonia can be prevented by avoiding the use of oily nose drops and laxatives.

1. Garb JL, Brown RB, Garb JR, Tuthill RW: Differences in etiology of pneumonias in nursing home and community patients. *J Am Med Assoc* 240:2169–2172, 1978.
2. Johanson WG, Pierce AK, Sanford JP, Thomas GD: Nosocomial respirtory infections with gram negative bacilli. *Ann Intern Med* 77:701–706, 1972.
These are important papers for understanding the basis of the choice to use antibiotics in different patient groups with pneumonia.
3. Bynum LJ, Pierce AK: Pulmonary aspiration of gastric contents. *Am Rev Respir Dis* 114:1129–1136, 1976.
4. Wolfe JE, Bone RC, Ruth WE: Effects of corticosteroids in the treatment of patients with gastric aspiration. *Am J Med* 63:719–722, 1977.
These two papers provide important information on the etiologic factors, consequences, and management of aspiration pneumonitis.

66. PULMONARY EMBOLISM

Robert Brown and Steven M. Scharf

Pulmonary embolus, sometimes called the "silent killer," is common in elderly patients. The frequency of nonfatal emboli is close to 20 in 1,000 older patients and that of fatal emboli is close to 5 in 1,000. This is because of conditions associated with aging that predispose to thrombus formation, i.e., immobility, congestive heart failure, venous stasis, and hypercoagulable states. The presenting symptoms may be classic—pleuritic chest pain, dyspnea, tachypnea, and hemoptysis of sudden onset—or unusual, such as syncope and hypotension. Rales and fever (101–102°F) also occur. A loud pulmonic closure and right-sided gallop are helpful signs.

Diagnosis

The source of the emboli may be obvious as in the case of deep venous thrombosis of the legs (the source in more than 90% of cases); or not obvious, such as the ovarian veins, right atrium (in association with atrial fibrillation), and thigh veins. In elderly patients, furthermore, recurrent emboli may precede a large embolus and be characterized clinically only by dyspnea and tachypnea. Most of the classic diagnostic criteria—right heart strain on the ECG, wedge-shaped shadow on chest x-ray, and increased LDH and bilirubin with a normal transaminase—are rarely present in the elderly. Arterial hypoxemia is common in elderly patients, especially in the presence of congestive heart failure and pneumonia. An acute decrease in arterial PO_2 unassociated with the usual conditions helps to suggest the diagnosis of pulmonary emboli. Even large emboli, however, can occur with relatively good preservation of arterial PO_2. Perfusion lung scanning is often not very helpful, but a normal perfusion scan makes pulmonary embolus unlikely. The presence of perfusion defects is often difficult to interpret, especially in the presence of chronic obstructive pulmonary disease (COPD), congestive heart failure, pneumonia, asthma, and carcinoma. Even the addition of a ventilation scan, to look for segmental areas of high ventilation-perfusion ratios, may not be helpful in the case of the elderly, especially those with coexistent respiratory disorders. Pulmonary angiography is the best method of diagnosing emboli; but it has a definite but low morbidity and mortality, so it should be reserved for cases in which a therapeutic decision hinges on the diagnosis.

Since the major source of emboli is deep venous thrombosis of the leg veins, several methods have been developed to detect this condition. Radioactive fibrinogen labeling, Doppler ultrasound, impedance plethysmography, and venography are most commonly used. Venography is the most specific but has the highest morbidity.

The rate of resolution of pulmonary emboli is variable. Large clots can break up within a few hours and not be visible with angiography or perfusion scanning. The final resolution, however, may take several weeks.

Treatment

The treatment is anticoagulation to prevent further clotting in the affected veins. Heparin is the treatment of choice in the acute phase. Continuous infusion of heparin to maintain a partial thromboplastin time (PTT), or clotting time, of 2–2½ times the normal value is the favored method of therapy. A loading dose of 3000–5000 units is given intravenously and followed by 100 units/hr by continuous infusion. The infusion rate can be varied to bring about the desired PTT or clotting time. Intermittent doses of 5000–7500 units IV q4h are also sometimes given, but complications from bleeding are more common with this method. Contraindications to heparin therapy include a bleeding diathesis, active bleeding site (GI or otherwise), and severe hypertension. Aspirin or other antiplatelet agents should be discontinued. After a few days of heparin therapy, anticoagulation with Coumadin can be started. With Coumadin, prothrombin time (PT) should stay within 2–2½ times the normal value. Heparin can be discontinued when the PT is adequately elevated. Orally administered anticoagulants should be continued for 2–4 months, long enough to allow the primary thrombotic process to clear. Patients may require lifetime anticoagulation, if the source does not resolve.

The use of subcutaneous heparin in "mini-doses," i.e., 5000 units bid or tid, has been advocated as an effective prophylactic measure for patients subjected to prolonged periods of bed rest postoperatively or following acute illness. Chronically bedridden patients rarely develop deep venous thrombosis after the initial period.

Patients with acute massive embolism in whom pressors and fluids do not maintain blood pressure may require a pulmonary embolectomy.

Patients with recurrent emboli from the legs while on adequate anticoagulation, patients for whom anticoagulation is contraindicated, and patients having a near-fatal pulmonary embolus should be considered for inferior vena cava ligation or passage of an umbrella into the inferior vena cava. Such patients usually develop venous stasis in the lower extremities postoperatively and may require anticoagulation and/or diuretics as adjuvant therapy.

---

1. McNeil BJ: A diagnostic strategy using ventilation-perfusion studies in patients suspect for pulmonary embolism. *J Nucl Med* 17:613–616, 1976.
2. Salzman EW, Deykin D, Shaprio RM, Rosenberg R: Management of heparin therapy. *N Engl J Med* 292:1046–1050, 1975.
3. Sasahara AA: Current problems in pulmonary embolism: Introduction, in Sasahara AA, et al: *Pulmonary Emboli*. New York, Grune & Stratton, 1975.
4. Szucs MM, et al: Diagnostic sensitivity of laboratory findings in acute pulmonary embolism. *Ann Intern Med* 74:161–166, 1971.
5. Urokinase-streptokinase embolism trial. Phase II results. Cooperative Study. *J Am Med Assoc* 229:1606–1613, 1974.
   These papers provide an excellent review of major issues related to the diagnosis and management of pulmonary thromboembolic disease.

67. CHRONIC OBSTRUCTIVE PULMONARY DISEASE

Robert Brown and Steven M. Scharf

The term *chronic obstructive pulmonary disease* (COPD) refers to a spectrum of diseases in which chronic, relatively irreversible obstruction to air flow is the single common denominator. This group of diseases are distinguished from asthma, which is a disease characterized by reversible episodic airway obstruction. Patients with COPD may also have a significant "asthmatic" (i.e., episodic, partially reversible) component.

Etiology and Clinical Picture

COPD is responsible for approximately 20,000–30,000 deaths annually in the United States. The condition is clearly related to cigarette smoking and, in general, the greater the smoking history, the greater the impairment clinically and physiologically. Quantification of the smoking history by number of "pack-years" (i.e., packs smoked daily times the number of years smoking) is useful historical information. Patients usually present in their fifth decade, unless the disease is associated with a genetic disorder such as cystic fibrosis or $alpha_1$-antitrypsin deficiency.

There are two main types of presentation of COPD. These are chronic bronchitis (CB) and emphysema (E). Patients with CB have mucous gland hyperplasia, chronic inflammation, and mucous plugging of the bronchial tree. They have low PaO_2 because of uneven ventilation-perfusion relationships in the lung and because of hypoventilation. The latter leads to increases in arterial $PaCO_2$. Patients with emphysema have abnormal enlargement of air spaces (parenchyma), associated with destruction of alveolar walls. Since collagen and elastic fibers are destroyed, the elasticity of the lung is reduced, and this leads to hyperinflation. The fact that both alveolar walls and capillary beds are destroyed together tends to keep the distribution of ventilation-perfusion relationships more normal. As compared to the patient with severe CB, the patient with E has, therefore, relatively well-preserved arterial PaO_2. Hypoventilation is not a prominent feature, and $PaCO_2$ is normal. The main complaint of the patient with CB (also called the "blue bloater" because of cyanosis) is cough and sputum production, while the major complaint of the patient with E (also called the "pink puffer," because arterial saturation is relatively normal at rest) is severe dyspnea on mild exertion. Most patients with COPD have elements of both CB and E clinically, physiologically, and pathologically.

Physical examination of patients with COPD may reveal tachypnea, cyanosis, plethora, low diaphragms that move little with inspiration, wheezing, and/or diminished breath sounds.

Pulmonary function studies show flow rates (FEV_1, MMFR) lower than the age-adjusted normal range. The ratio of the FEV_1 to vital capacity (VC) is very helpful for characterizing airway obstruction. Normal patients less than 50 years old can expire at least 80% of their VC in the first second of a forced expiration. Patients over 60 years old can expire at least 75% of their VC in the first second (FEV_1/FVC = 75%). A ratio of FEV_1/FVC of 65–75% indicates mild obstruction, 50–65% is moderate obstruction, and less than 50% is severe obstruction.

In general, in COPD the pathologic processes are irreversible. Optimal medical management, however, can reverse some of the physiologic deficiencies and can often improve the quality of life for affected patients.

Management

Principles of management of COPD are similar for the elderly and for the young. The elderly, however, often have concurrent illnesses that complicate therapy.

It seems self-evident that patients should stop injuring their lungs with tobacco smoke. This, in general, is very difficult to do. Nicotine is an addictive stimulant that the patient may refuse to discontinue. If this is the case, he or she should be encouraged to reduce tobacco consumption as much as possible.

Antibiotics. Patients with CB have chronically inflamed airways in which the normal defense mechanisms malfunction. Acute exacerbations of infection are common and are usually heralded by an increase in cough and sputum production and a change in sputum color from white to yellow or green. These symptoms should be treated early. Viral bronchitis commonly evolves into bacterial bronchitis, and most patients with changed cough and sputum should be treated with antibiotics. Oral medication is most commonly used, but intravenous drugs allow larger doses to be administered to very ill patients. The most common pathogens are *Streptococcus pneumoniae* and *Hemophilus influenzae*. Ampicillin, tetracycline, and erythromycin, 1–2 gm/day PO in 4 divided doses, are the usual antibiotics. A mixture of trimethoprim and sulfisoxazole is also used by some. The course of therapy should be at least 7 days. At times the use of chronic antibiotic therapy has been advocated, especially for patients with continuous pyogenic infection. Although no effect on mortality has been demonstrated, there is a reduction in morbidity as measured by time missed from work due to exacerbations of respiratory infection. At present it is most accurate to say that the role of chronic antibiotic therapy is not known but may be of benefit to selected patients.

Immunization. In addition to antibiotics, immunization of moderately to severely ill patients with polyvalent influenza vaccine and antipneumococcal vaccine (Pneumovax) seems prudent. Viral and bacterial pneumonias can have devastating effects on patients with COPD.

Bronchodilators. The use of bronchodilator agents should be a cornerstone of therapy in COPD. Patients with moderate to severe airway obstruction usually benefit symptomatically from regular doses of bronchodilator drugs. Small doses given at infrequent intervals are not particularly useful. With adequate doses, improvement in dyspnea, lessening of cough, and increased clearance of bothersome secretions is possible.

Many commercial preparations of oral bronchodilators contain a methylxanthine (aminophylline or theophylline) in addition to a number of other ingredients of uncertain efficacy. The methylxanthine is the primary ingredient and, if mixed preparations are used, dosage should be based on the aminophylline content of the medication. Appendix B contains information concerning many common bronchodilator agents.

In general, a rational bronchodilator program is based on the use of a methylxanthine agent and/or a beta-adrenergic sympathomimetic. Severely affected patients should have both. The effectiveness as well as the toxicity of the methylxanthine preparations is related to the blood level. The optimal therapeutic range is 10–20 μg/ml. This is the range in which therapeutic efficacy is maximized and toxicity is minimized for most patients. It should be remembered, however, that individual variability is great; blood levels of less than 10μg/ml may be toxic for some patients, and levels greater than 20μg/ml may not be toxic for others.

For younger patients the adequate levels can be achieved with a loading dose of aminophylline equal to 5.6 mg/kg BW followed by a maintenance of 0.9 mg/kg/hr [30]. For elderly patients (> 60 yr) the maintenance dose should be lowered to 0.6–0.7 mg/kg/hr, and for patients with liver disease or congestive heart failure, the dose should be reduced to 0.4–0.5 mg/kg/hr. When oral therapy is initiated, the loading dose is not needed. Blood levels are useful in determining whether or not therapeutic levels are achieved with a given dose.

Beta-adrenergic agents are available in oral and inhaled form. If the patient is capable of using an inhaled agent, that is the preferred form. Careful instruction in the use of the inhaler is needed. The patient should exhale fully, then, while inhaling deeply (**not before** initiating inhalation), press the release mechanism of the inhaler and hold his or her breath near total lung capacity (TLC) for 5–10 seconds. Since there are potent $beta_2$ (i.e., bronchial tree–specific) agents now available, there is little reason to risk cardiac ($beta_1$) side effects by using epinephrine or isoproterenol. Patients who cannot use the inhalers may benefit from nebulization of 0.5 cc of an agent (isoetharine or salbutamol) in 2.5 ml saline, breathing in the vapors via a face mask or hand-held nebulizer. Corticosteroids have not been shown to be efficacious in most cases of COPD. This is in contrast to asthma, in which corticosteroids may be very helpful. Some patients with a diagnosis of COPD who have episodic bronchospasm or eosinophilia are demonstrable may be misdiagnosed asthmatics and may benefit from steroids. Furthermore, when standard methods of treatment of COPD fail, corticosteroids are sometimes used, occasionally with success. Apparent improvement may be due to steroid-induced euphoria, and one should follow pulmonary function to document real benefit.

Hydration. The role of hydration in the treatment of COPD has been emphasized greatly, but little evidence exists that hydration above the physiologic norm enhances sputum expectoration or decreases sputum vicosity. Indeed, hydration should be used with caution, since it may precipitate congestive heart failure in elderly patients. Dehydration seems to decrease mucous transport velocity, and it is probably prudent to suggest that the patient should not become dehydrated. In this regard, excessive use of diuretics may be detrimental. Furthermore, use of diuretic agents often leads to potassium depletion and hypochloremic alkalosis, which may precipitate arrhythmias, decreased cerebral blood flow, and decreased central respiratory drive. Careful supplementation with potassium chloride should be undertaken if levels of serum $K+$ fall.

Management of Secretions. For patients with copious daily sputum production, clearance of secretions and opening of plugged airways is helpful in reducing potential foci of infection and in improving ventilation-perfusion balance. Bronchodilators are important in this regard, as is a well-developed cough from a deep inspiration. Postural drainage may be helpful if secretions come from a particular area of the lung, as in the case of localized bronchiectasis. Percussion with encouragement to cough is helpful to many patients. The chronic use of intermittent positive-pressure breathing (IPPB) has not been shown to be of benefit, and we do not recommend it. Indeed, nebulized saline or water may even precipitate bronchospasm in some patients.

Low-Flow Oxygen. Cases of chronic hypoxemia (PO_2 <55) the use of low-flow (1–2 L/min) oxygen for at least 12 hours daily has been shown to reduce pulmonary arterial pressures and thus alleviate cor pulmonale. Use of O_2 at night may also reduce sleep-induced hypoxemia and decrease insomnia. A patient whose arterial PO_2 is reduced significantly during exercise benefits from a portable O_2 apparatus. Home O_2 is expensive, but it often reduces the frequency of hospitalization and thus is often cost-effective.

Breathing Exercises. Much attention has been devoted to the use of various breathing exercises. In patients with COPD and hyperinflation, both the diaphragm and the inspiratory muscles of the rib cage operate at a mechanical disadvantage, such that there is a decrease in the mechanincal efficiency of these muscles. Pursed-lips breathing, in which the patient inhales deeply, concentrating on pressing his abdomen outward and then exhales through pursed lips, has been shown to increase arterial PO_2 and to decrease the subjective sensation of dyspnea in many patients. The mechanism responsible for these effects is not fully understood, but it may be related to the deep inspiration taken beforehand or to prevention of bronchial collapse.

Management of Acute Respiratory Failure. Acute respiratory failure complicating chronic respiratory failure is an ominous sign in patients with COPD. It may be precipitated by an acute infection, cardiac failure, increased bronchial obstruction, or the use of respiratory depressants. The inital symptoms may be cough and sputum production, breathlessness, and reduced exercise tolerance. Warning signs are labored breathing, tachypnea, wheezes, use of accessory muscles of respiration, and manifestations of cor pulmonale. Arterial PO_2 is decreased, and PCO_2 may be decreased or increased relative to the patient's norm. If the PCO_2 is sufficiently increased, somnolence and confusion may dominate the clinical picture. Management includes bronchodilators (methylxanthine plus a beta-adrenergic agent), physiotherapy, low-flow O_2 (1–2 one/min) in order to increase PO_2 with only a minimal effect on PCO_2, antibiotics to treat infection, and diuretics if indicated. Sedatives and tranquilizers should be scrupulously avoided. Intubation should be avoided unless absolutely necessary. The indications for intubation of patients with acute or chronic respiratory failure are (1) inability of the patient to cooperate, e.g., from severe obtundation; and (2) respiratory acidosis leading to a pH of less than 7.2. The level of the PCO_2 per se is not critical to the decision to intubate.

Management of Arrhythmias. Patients with acute or chronic respiratory failure are likely to develop cardiac arrhythmias. Most important of these are multifocal atrial tachycardia, ventricular premature contractions, ventricular tachyarrhythmias, and atrial fibrillation. The usual antiarrhythmic medications are used, but measures directed at alleviating hypoxemia, acid-base disturbances, electrolyte imbalance, pleural effusion, and pneumothorax also are needed. Furthermore, drugs used in the treatment of airway obstruction may contribute to the genesis of arrhythmias, for instance, beta-adrenergic agents (especially non–$beta_2$-selective agents) and methylxanthines. Fluorocarbons, the "inert" component of many aerosolized medications, are also arrhythmogenic.

---

1. Francis RS, Spicer CC: Chemotherapy in chronic bronchitis. *Br Med J* 1:297–303, 1960.
2. Value of chemoprophylaxis and chemotherapy in early chronic bronchitis. British Medical Research Council Study: *Br Med J* 1:1317–1322, 1966.
   These papers provide the basis for empirically using broad-spectrum antibiotic therapy in chronic bronchitis and emphysema.
3. The health consequence of smoking. Department of Health, Education and Welfare, *Chronic Obstructive Bronchopulmonary Disease. Report of the Surgeon General,1971.* Washington, DC, US Government Printing Office, 1972, chap. 3.
   A tell-tale documentation of the enormous epidemiologic effect of tobacco abuse.
4. Haas H, Morris JF, Samson S, Kitbourn JP, Kim PJ: Bacterial flora of the respiratory tract in chronic bronchitis: Comparison of transtracheal, fiber bronchoscopic, and oropharyngeal sampling methods. *Am Rev Respir Dis* 116:41–47, 1977.
   An important paper for understanding the problems related to obtaining the best possible data on which to base the antibiotic therapy of lung infection.
5. Jusko WJ, Koup JR, Vance JW, Schentag JJ, Kuritzky P: Intravenous theophylline therapy: Nomogram guidelines. *Ann Intern Med* 86:400–404, 1977.
6. Tenko PA, Olgivie RI: Rational intravenous doses of theophylline. *N Engl J Med* 289:600–603, 1973.
   Guidelines and principles are outlined in these references for proper administration of theophylline preparations.
7. Abraham AS, Cole RB, Bishop JM: Reversal of pulmonary hypertension by prolonged

oxygen administration to patients with chronic bronchitis. *Circ Res* 23:147–157, 1968.

8. Stewart BN, Hood CI, Block AJ: Long-term results of continuous oxygen therapy at sea level. *Chest* 68:486–492, 1975.
   These are early studies providing the impetus for more recent controlled trials of home oxygen therapy, each demonstrating an improved survival with oxygen use.
9. Gutierrez AC, Vincent RG, Bakshi S, Takita H: Radio-isotope scans in the evaluation of metastatic bronchogenic carcinoma. *J Thorac Cardiovasc Surg* 69:934–941, 1975.
10. McNeil BJ, Weichselbaum R, Paulser SG: Fallacy of the five-year survival in lung cancer. *N Engl J Med* 299:1397–1401, 1978.
11. Phillips TL, Miller RJ: Should asymptomatic patients with inoperable bronchogenic carcinoma receive immediate radiotherapy?—Yes, editorial. *Am Rev Respir Dis* 117:405–410, 1978.
12. Weiss RB: Small-cell carcinoma of the lung: Therapeutic management. *Ann Intern Med* 88:522–531, 1978.
    These papers are selected to address common controversies in the diagnosis and management of lung cancer.
13. Mueller RE, Petty TL, Fittey GF: Ventilation and arterial blood gas changes induced by pursed lips breathing. *J Appl Physiol* 28:784–789, 1970.
    Useful in understanding the mechanical effects of pursed lip breathing.
14. Sahn SA: Corticosteroids in chronic bronchitis and pulmonary emphysema. *Chest* 73:389–395, 1978.
    Some of the controversies related to corticosteroid therapy in chronic obstructive pulmonary disease are discussed.
15. Cherniack R, Svanhill E: Long-term use of intermittent positive pressure breathing (IPPB) in chronic obstructive pulmonary disease. *Am Rev Respir Dis* 113:721–728, 1976.
    One of the papers used as the basis of the rejection of IPPB as a useful therapy in COPD.
16. Chopra SK, et al: Effects of hydration and physical therapy on tracheal transport velocity. *Am Rev Respir Dis* 115:1009–1014, 1977.
    One of the few papers evaluating the question whether hydration really affects the pulmonary secretions.
17. Flowers NC, Horan LG: Nonanoxic aerosol arrhythmias. *J Am Med Assoc* 219:33–40, 1972.
    Arrhythmias may occur as a result of different forms of therapy in COPD, e.g., drugs. This paper outlines yet another potential cause.

X. DISEASES OF BONE AND JOINT

68. OSTEOARTHRITIS

Edward W. Campion

Osteoarthritis (OA) or degenerative joint disease is a condition of degeneration of the smooth hyaline cartilage surfaces that normally allow nearly friction-free joint movement. More than half of persons over age 60 have evidence of OA. It ranges from mild to devastatingly severe. The rate of progression varies remarkably. Severe osteoarthritis is not merely part of the normal aging process. The "nothing can be done about it" approach leads to unnecessary suffering and disability.

Symptoms

The cardinal symptom of significant OA is joint pain on weight bearing. The spine is commonly involved, and disorders of gait are often the result. Disabling OA frequently involves a hip or knee, producing a "quickstep" limp on the affected, painful side. Advanced OA of the hip gives an *adductor lurch* to the gait, tilting the upper body over the weakened hip. Going down stairs, the patient leads with the bad leg, but drags it behind when climbing stairs. Abnormal mobility and deformities add to the problems of osteoarthritis. Significant OA in the hip causes thigh muscle atrophy, with a reduced circumference compared to the contralateral side. Range of motion, especially internal rotation, is limited, and produces pain and crepitance (grating). OA of the knee produces irregular bony enlargement, usually with an effusion. Asymmetric cartilage loss causes either a *genu varus* ("bowleg") or *genu valgus* ("knock-knee") deformity. Gross knee instability, usually in the medio-lateral plane, indicates accompanying ligament or meniscal damage with marked functional limitation. Ankles are rarely involved by OA. Hallux valgus, the common deformity of the great toe, creates little functional limitation, but it may demand a specially fitted shoe and measures to prevent pressure ulcers.

Contractures at heel cords, hamstrings, and hip flexors may worsen the disability from OA. Neurologic sensory deficits predispose to severe OA and produce Charcot joints. OA may also develop after previous trauma to a joint, including fracture, infection, or inflammatory arthritis. Obesity and mechanical malalignment of weight bearing both predispose to OA. In atypical and unusually severe cases of OA, appropriate tests are needed to identify known causes of secondary OA. The differential diagnosis includes hemochromatosis, acromegaly, Gaucher's disease, Cushing's syndrome, chondrocalcinosis, and ochronosis.

There is no detectable abnormality in blood or urine in OA. The sedimentation rate is normal. Rheumatoid factor is of no help in the diagnosis. Joint fluid analysis can help confirm the diagnosis of OA and rule out any suspicion of rheumatoid arthritis, gout, pseudogout, or infection. On average, OA joint fluid has 600 WBC/mm^3 (range, 100–3,000) with few polymorphonuclear leukocytes. The joint fluid in OA has no crystals, and cultures are sterile. The mucin test gives a good clot in dilute acetic acid. A joint fluid with more than 3,000 WBC/mm^3 points to a diagnosis other than OA. X-ray films in advancing OA show loss of joint space, subchondral sclerosis, and reactive bony overgrowth (osteophytes) at joint margins.

The presence of OA clinically or on a roentgenogram in no way rules out other diagnoses. In fact, elderly patients with gout, rheumatoid arthritis, or joint infection frequently have coincidental OA on their x-ray films, but this should not mislead the clinician. Pseudogout also commonly complicates OA. Acute inflammation about a joint and pain unrelated to weight bearing are not part of OA. Joint fluid analysis is usually necessary to establish the correct diagnosis. Systemic symptoms such as fever, weight loss, and anemia should never be attributed to OA.

Management

Relief of Symptoms. The primary goal of management is to lessen discomfort in involved joints while taking measures to retard progression of OA. Symptomatic improvement can usually be achieved with aspirin (600–1,200 mg qid), but nonsteroidal antiinflammatory agents may be better tolerated by some patients. Simple analgesics such as acetaminophen (650–1,300 mg bid or tid) also may be of use in controlling symptoms. Narcotics are inadvisable, and systemic steroids are never indicated for OA.

Weight reduction brings surprising improvement in moderate OA. In general, joints should be protected from excessive trauma that may hasten OA. Improved body mechanics may both improve function and retard progression of OA. Physical therapy can reduce contractures and strengthen supporting musculature with active, non–weight-bearing exercises against resistance. Many other rehabilitation measures are useful, including ramps, grab bars, and reaching devices. A cane, for example, held in the opposite hand helps unload stress from an involved hip or knee. Crutches or a walker also help in more severe cases. Properly fitted braces may stabilize a weakened knee or ankle.

Steroid Injections. Intraarticular steroids do not stop the progress of OA and may actually accelerate it. In addition, the procedure carries a small risk of infection, even with careful sterile technique. Symptomatic relief may result, but it lasts only several weeks. In special circumstances, however, such as to facilitate physical therapy and reambulation for the elderly patient with severe OA, the temporary improvement may justify use of intraarticular steroids. Three injections annually in a single joint is the maximum. A joint about to be operated on or one with prosthetic components already in it should not receive an injection. **Never** give an injection into a hip joint.

Surgical Intervention. Surgical management of osteoarthritis has progressed dramatically with the development of joint reconstruction. The major indications for surgical intervention are severe pain, functional disability, and large analgesic requirements. Joint reconstruction is appropriate only for a severely impaired joint that shows major changes roentgenographically. Patients functioning well with mild arthritis should not be referred for operation. Surgical intervention must come, however, before the patient becomes nonambulatory and has atrophied musculature. The most common surgical procedure in OA is total hip replacement with a polyethylene acetabulum and metal femoral head and stem. Hip replacement is usually successful even for patients in the ninth decade. It has replaced most former types of arthroplasty and arthrodesis (see Chap. 71.) Total knee replacements are being done now on elderly patients, with very good results. The complications are principally infection ($< 1\%$), loosening, and patellofemoral pain. Joint resurfacing procedures are being developed but remain experimental.

Before going to the operating room the patient needs to be in optimal medical and nutritional condition. Preoperative physical therapy strengthens musculature, improves balance, and greatly facilitates postoperative success. Careful explanation preoperatively improves postoperative compliance and motivation. Elderly patients with multiple problems may require several weeks of intensive physical therapy after hip or knee replacement. Some may temporarily regress in their functional level under the stress of hospitalization. Close, caring, and expert supervision by the orthopedist and the primary medical physician is mandatory.

Erosive Osteoarthritis

Erosive osteoarthritis (EOA) is a form of osteoarthritis that strikes older women and resembles rheumatoid arthritis in some of its features. EOA begins in middle-aged and elderly patients with pain, swelling, and tenderness in the small joints of the hands, especially in the distal and proximal interphalangeal joints. White females, particularly of northern European descent, are at greatest risk, and often there is a family history of EOA. By physical examination the hands affected by EOA may be indistinguishable from those typical of rheumatoid arthritis. EOA, however, usually spares the metacarpal phalangeal joints. Rheumatoid factor and the sedimentation rate are normal in EOA, and roentgenograms show a pattern of sclerosis and bone proliferation entirely different from that of rheumatoid arthritis.

Erosive osteoarthritis may be acutely severe in some patients but generally "burns out" to become less painful with time. The deformity may be striking, but usually there is not major permanent functional loss in the hands. EOA leaves the hard swollen knuckles known as Heberden's and Bouchard's nodes at the distal interphalangeal and proximal interphalangeal joints respectively. Medical treatment is aimed at symptoms. Local heat, aspirin, and nonsteroidal antiinflammatory agents are useful. Gold, penicillamine, and systemic steroids are not indicated. Patients may need painstaking reassurance that they do not have rheumatoid arthritis.

1. Peter JB, et al: Erosive osteoarthritis of the hands. *Arthritis Rheum* 9:365, 1966.
Acute inflammation may mimic rheumatoid arthritis.

2. Hernborg JS, Linden B, Nilsson BE: Chondrocalcinosis of the knee: A secondary finding in osteoarthritis of the knee. *Geriatrics* 32:123, 1977.
Evidence of chondrocalcinosis developed in the course of 23% of the patients.
3. Kellgren JH, Moore R: Generalized osteoarthritis and Heberden's nodes. *Br Med J* 1:181, 1952.
Classic description of a primary form of osteoarthritis that may be in part genetically determined.
4. Heimmann WG, Freiberger RH: Avascular necrosis of femoral and humeral heads after high-dosage corticosteroid therapy. *N Engl J Med* 263:672, 1960.
Discusses steroids as the cause of cartilage damage and osteoarthritis.
5. Stross JK, Mikkelsen WM: Educating patients with osteoarthritis. *J Rheumatol* 4:313, 1977.
Describes cost effectiveness of patient education for older arthritics.
6. Moskowitz RW: Management of osteoarthritis. *Bull Rheum Dis* 31:31, 1981.
Salicylates and nonsteroidals have major roles and may retard cartilage damage.
7. Casscells SW: Gross pathologic changes in knee joint of aged individuals: Study of 300 cases. *Clin Orthop* 132:225, 1978.
Examination at postmortem shows most aged knees to be normal or nearly normal.
8. Solomon L: Patterns of osteoarthritis of the hip. *J Bone Joint Surg (Br)* 58B:176, 1976.
Osteoarthritis may be secondary to trauma or to associated diseases.
9. Gresham GE, Rathey VK: Osteoarthritis in the knees of aged persons. *JAMA* 233:168, 1975.
Some patients have x-ray abnormalities without associated symptoms or limitation.
10. Mankin HJ: The reaction of articular cartilage to injury and osteoarthritis. *N Engl J Med* 291:1285, 1335, 1974.
A review of the biology of normal cartilage and the metabolic abnormalities in osteoarthritis.
11. Howell DS, Talbott JH (eds): Osteoarthritis symposium. *Semin Arthritis Rheum* (suppl) 11:1, 1981.
An authoritative update on research into the pathogenesis of osteoarthritis.
12. Peyron JG: Epidemiologic and etiologic approach to osteoarthritis. *Semin Arthritis Rheum* 8:288, 1979.
Obesity predisposes patients to osteoarthritis of the knee but not of the hip.
13. Mikkelson WM, Dodge HJ, Duff IF, Kato H: Estimates of the prevalence of rheumatic diseases in the population of Tecumseh, Michigan, 1959–60. *J Chronic Dis* 20:351, 1967.
Over a third of women over 60 years had evidence of osteoarthritis.

69. RHEUMATOID ARTHRITIS

Edward W. Campion

Rheumatoid arthritis (RA) is a chronic systemic disease with peak age of onset in the 40s. Most elderly persons with RA have complications from long-standing disease. It has been estimated that as many as 5% of elderly patients have had RA, although the degree of severity varies tremendously. RA may begin at any age, but in the elderly, it affects males as frequently as females, whereas in younger patients its incidence is greater in women. Newly developing RA in the elderly may emerge slowly, but usually it progresses explosively from the very start.

Symptoms

Patients may experience months of fatigue, morning stiffness, and vague arthralgias before developing multiple inflamed painful joints. Small joints of the hands and feet are commonly involved first. Joints become inflamed symmetrically in an additive pattern. Careful examination can usually distinguish RA from the coexisting osteoarthritis (OA) that is so common in elderly patients. Distinguishing signs are palmar erythema, tenderness of joints to direct palpation, warmth of overlying skin, and thickened synovium (joint lining). The distribution of the arthritis is also a clue. In the hands, RA affects wrists, proximal interphalangeal and metacarpal phalangeal joints but rarely the distal interphalangeal joints. Shoulder tenderness and MTP tenderness are typical of RA but not of OA. Rheumatoid nodules accompany more severe disease developing on extensor surfaces in about 20% of RA cases. Moderate to marked lymphadenopathy is also common in RA.

Laboratory and Roentgenographic Findings

Laboratory findings in RA are not specific but reinforce the clinical impression. The sedimentation rate is usually elevated and parallels the course of inflammation. A moderate normochromic, normocytic anemia that does not respond to iron is common in active RA. Severe, active RA also depresses serum albumin and elevates serum globulins. Rheumatoid factor (RF), an IgM immunoglobulin directed against IgG, is present in most patients with classic RA. The latex method of assessing RF has a false-positive rate as high as 40% in normal patients over age 60, so its usefulness is limited in older patients. High titers of RF as found by the more specific *bentonite method* have a more consistent correlation with pathologic conditions. The RF alone never establishes a diagnosis of RA, however, as it may be negative in unequivocal RA. A positive RF is not specific for RA. Pulmonary fibrosis, cryoglobulinemia, tuberculosis, sarcoidosis, subacute bacterial endocarditis, chronic active hepatitis, and systemic lupus erythematosus (SLE) all may yield positive RF.

Roentgenograms are helpful in diagnosing and monitoring RA. Hand films with juxtaarticular demineralization and multiple bony erosions typify advancing RA and clearly distinguish it from erosive osteoarthritis (see Chap. 68). Erosion of distal clavicles and of ulnar styloids is classic for RA. Careful analysis of joint fluid readily distinguishes RA from OA. In RA the joint fluid has 3000–50,000 WBC/mm^3, with polymorphonuclear leukocytes predominating. In dilute acetic acid a poor mucin clot forms. On the other hand, joint fluid in OA has less than 3000 WBC/mm^3 and forms a good mucin clot. In addition, joint fluid complement is decreased in RA but not in OA. In the older patient with both RA and OA, the joint fluid has the characteristics of RA. Older patients with advanced RA frequently have positive antinuclear antibody (ANA) without clinical lupus.

A positive finding of rheumatoid factor and nonspecific joint findings are never sufficient to diagnose RA. Symmetric, inflammatory polyarthritis in the older patient may also be caused by inflammatory bowel disease, SLE, polymyositis, psoriasis, hepatitis, sarcoidosis, or drugs such as hydralazine and procainamide. Arthritis consistently confined to a single joint is rarely caused by RA in the elderly. As a diagnostic rule, fever in an older patient should never be attributed to RA. The presence of OA in no way rules out RA, since many older people have both.

Complications

Complications of RA are at times as serious as the underlying arthritis. Perhaps the most harmful complication is the development of an attitude by the physician or patient that RA will inevitably progress to render the patient crippled and helpless. In fact, RA with its onset in old age has a **better** prognosis than does RA developing in the earlier years. Remissions are most common in RA of recent and acute onset. Pressure sores, contractures, and muscle wasting are other avoidable complications that develop rapidly if the RA patient is confined to bed without a proper rehabilitation program.

A feared complication of RA in the cervical spine is subluxation of cervical vertebrae with cord compression and quadriparesis. Amyloid deposition complicates some RA of long duration. Bacterial sepsis within a rheumatoid joint is a threat recognized only when the physician with a high index of suspicion taps the inflamed rheumatoid joint and obtains a culture.

Sicca complex symptoms of dry mouth and dry, gritty eyes (*Sjögren's syndrome*) are associated with an increased risk of lymphoproliferative malignancies. Prompt treatment with artificial tears (q2–4h) avoids infection and ulceration of the cornea. Felty's syndrome adds to RA granulocytopenia, splenomegaly, and an increased risk of infection and leg ulcers. RA of the lung may produce pleurisy, pleural effusions, pulmonary fibrosis, or rheumatoid pulmonary nodules that mimic carcinoma. Rheumatoid vasculitis, whose most common features are multiple superficial ulcerations and mononeuritis multiplex, arises in fewer than 10% of cases of RA. Penicillamine or immunosuppressives may be effective in RA vasculitis.

Treatment

Therapy in RA requires a long-term commitment by a group of experienced professionals. The RA patient benefits most when cared for by a team of physician, nurse, physical therapist, occupational therapist, recreational therapist, and social worker. Goals are to maintain maximal mobility, muscle mass, joint integrity, functional independence, and quality of life. Well-timed rest periods are an essential part of RA therapeutic programs. Rest increases endurance and function while decreasing inflammation and protecting the joints.

Determination and cautious optimism are essential. Virtually every RA patient can be helped in some way to become more comfortable and self-sufficient. The most precious asset is the patient's determination in the face of adversity. Physical and social measures often provide major relief for the patient. A rehabilitation team can evaluate the elderly RA patient's home situation and detect unrecognized barriers and dangers. The home visit is particularly useful for the debilitated patient about to make a difficult transition from hospital to home. Adaptations can make the home safer and more functional. Raised toilet seats, tub chairs, nonslip tub mats, and handrails make a bathroom accessible for the RA patient. Push-button phones, intercoms, and doorway buzzers ensure safety and communication. Scatter rugs, steps, raised thresholds, conventional doorknobs, low chairs, and high beds are particular hazards to be altered. The kitchen can be restructured for the RA patient with adapted faucet handles, jar openers, and reaching devices.

Physical Therapy. Physical therapy must be used appropriately. Severely inflamed joints are rested, splinted, and put through full range of motion three times daily. Hot packs (20 min bid) help lessen the synovitis of large joints, but when the weight of hot packs is too uncomfortable, inflamed joints can be painted with hot paraffin. When there is less acute inflammation, regular assisted exercises prevent contractures at heel cords, knees, and hips. Gently resistive exercises develop quadriceps, hip flexors, and hip abductors. The patient's balance and mobility improve through supervised ambulation with parallel bars, walker, quad cane, and, finally, stick cane. Assistive devices frequently require adaptation to accommodate RA deformities in the upper extremities. An unstable joint may be stabilized by bracing, with special caution used to protect the skin. Molded Philadelphia cervical collars help neck pain or instability but do not lessen the need for utmost precaution to avoid trauma.

Occupational Therapy. Every elderly person with RA can benefit from occupational therapy (OT), evaluation, and instruction. The goals of OT are to maximize functional ability and protect joint function. RA in the hands and wrists improves with hot paraffin applications (20 min bid) and splinting in the position of function. Regular range-of-motion exercises greatly preserve shoulder function. OT programs teach patients new techniques in those activities of daily living that are crucial for maintaining independence. For the patient with severe RA, dressing, bathing, toileting, food preparation, eating, writing, and reading may once again be possible through appropriate OT. Adaptive devices must be offered tactfully, recognizing that patients may initially see them as unpleasant stigmata of debility and as threats to self-esteem. Frequently useful aids are a long-handled comb, long-handled sponge, button hook, dressing hook, and reaching device, as well as thick-handled eating utensils and jar openers. A full OT evaluation in the home should recommend how to adapt the environment to fit the elderly RA patient.

Medical Therapy.

Salicylates. In the medical therapy of RA, salicylates remain the principle antiinflammatory and analgesic agent. To be effective they must be taken consistently in adequate doses. Buffered aspirin, 600–1,200 mg qid with food, is adequate for most elderly patients. Salicylate toxicity is all too common in the elderly. It must be recognized in patients who develop ataxia, tinnitus, deafness, confusion, or respiratory alkalosis. Severe cases of toxicity may progress to a life-threatening metabolic acidosis. The best prevention is monitoring to keep serum salicylate levels in the therapeutic range (15–25 mg/100 ml, 2 hr after dose). Elderly patients may have a toxic reaction from unknowingly adding aspirin containing over-the-counter arthritis preparations to their other medications. The most common serious side effects from aspirin are gastric irritation and hemorrhagic gastritis. Stool guaiac testing should be performed at least twice a year to detect occult bleeding.

Enteric-coated aspirin causes less gastric irritation but its absorption may be erratic. Peptic ulcer disease and recent GI bleeding are contraindications to the use of any salicylate or nonsteroidal preparations. Aspirin is dangerous to patients anticoagulated with Coumadin. *Magnesium choline salicylate* (such as Trilisate, 500–1,000 mg bid) may be given with greater safety to patients receiving anticoagulants.

Nonsteroidal Antiinflammatory Agents. The nonsteroidal antiinflammatory drugs have become increasingly popular in the treatment of arthritis. Nevertheless, they are **all** more expensive, and have no proved greater therapeutic efficacy, than aspirin. They do offer more convenient dosage regimens, and some patients find particular benefit from a particular nonsteroidal agent. These drugs may cause gastric irritation and bleeding and are potentially dangerous to anticoagulated patients. They may give rise to fluid retention, worsen congestive heart failure, and cause toxicity similar to salicylism. In addition, they may be nephrotoxic, particularly in patients with prior renal impairment.

Unlike the case of aspirin, serum levels are not available for the nonsteroidal inflammatory drugs. Indomethacin, a potent antiinflammatory drug, is poorly tolerated by elderly patients. It causes dizziness, disorientation, and severe headaches. It is not advised for chronic administration. Ibuprofen may have less gastric irritation than aspirin. Naproxen has the convenience of a long half-life so it can be prescribed in a bid dose. Sulindac may cause less gastric irritation and have less adverse effect on renal perfusion. Tolmetin may have less antiplatelet effect than aspirin.

Gold. Gold salts have been proved to induce remission in some patients with RA. Gold is reserved for patients with progressive, inflammatory RA that has not been adequately controlled by 6–12 months of conventional therapy. Age is **not** a contraindication to gold therapy. Although gold has serious potential toxicity, it is generally well tolerated by older patients. The benefits from gold are not expected until 3–6 months after start of treatment. If pain, joint inflammation, morning stiffness, sedimentation rate, hematocrit, and albumin have not improved at that time, the therapy is discontinued. Prior to each gold injection the physician must examine the patient carefully and stop the drug (1) if an eczematous, itchy **rash** has appeared on the trunk or elsewhere; (2) if there is proteinuria; or (3) if there is thrombocytopenia or leukopenia. Directly after a gold injection elderly patients occasionally experience untoward reactions, which consist of transient flushing, shortness of breath, and hypotension. Switching gold preparations may avert further reactions.

The two preparations available are gold sodium thiomalat (Myochrysine) and gold thioglucose (Solganal). After a 5-mg test dose for idosyncrasy, therapy is started with 25 mg IM. If no signs of toxicity have appeared one week later, weekly injections of 50 mg IM are given for 20 weeks. Very elderly patients or those weighing less than 45 kg are given 25-mg weekly doses. After 20 weekly doses, if the patient has responded favorably, injections are given every other week for 10 doses, every 3 weeks for 5 doses, and monthly from then on. As long as the patient receives gold, he or she must be monitored for potentially serious toxicity to skin, bone marrow, or kidney. Patients with severe active RA who have not improved on gold or who cannot tolerate it can be treated with penicillamine. Penicillamine can induce marked improvement after 3–6 months of therapy, but its potential toxicities are severe: rash, leukopenia, thrombocytopenia, nephrotoxicity, and a myasthenia-like syndrome. Renal impairment and penicillin allergy are contraindications. Elderly patients require reduced doses of penicillamine and frequently experience dyspepsia or loss of taste from it. Penicillamine should be reserved for patients with refractory, progressive RA.

Cytotoxic Drugs. Cytotoxic drugs offer some patients with severe RA a chance of improvement. Cyclophosphamide and azathioprine are effective in RA, but their potential toxicity requires that they be reserved for the most severe, actively progressive cases, after all else has failed. Elderly patients seem particularly sensitive to the nausea, alopecia, and bone marrow suppression associated with the cytotoxic agents, but azathioprine can be well tolerated if begun in low doses of 25–50 mg per day. Immunosuppressives are especially helpful in controlling vascular complications such as skin ulcers.

Steroids. Systemic steroids can bring rapid and impressive symptomatic improvement of inflammatory RA, but they do not retard progression of the joint damage, and the side effects of chronic steroid use may be severe. Osteoporosis, infection, cataracts, skin breakdown, psychosis, aseptic necrosis, protein-wasting, and worsening of hypertension, diabetes, or congestive heart failure are all potential complications. Despite their serious disadvantages, steroids used at the proper time may prevent the elderly RA patient from becoming immobilized and bedridden. Steroids are sometimes the only drugs well tolerated by an elderly RA patient.

Complications can be reduced by using the smallest dose possible. Alternate-day steroids cause less suppression of the hypothalamic-adrenal mechanism, but many RA patients find the days between doses intolerably painful. Giving the lowest single daily dose possible, in the early morning, helps reduce morbidity. On a daily basis even 5 mg of prednisone can alleviate much inflammation and pain. Doses larger than 10 mg should be avoided entirely. Concurrent aspirin or nonsteroidal antiinflammatory therapy lowers the steroid requirement in RA. The physician must always attempt to reduce steroids to the lowest effective dose. It is best to taper steroids slowly, by less than 20% of the total dose weekly. Supplemental steroids are mandatory for acute stress until full adrenal function returns.

Calcium and vitamin D supplements may slow steroid-induced osteoporosis. Occasional use of intraarticular steroid injections gives prompt symptomatic relief in particularly inflamed RA joints. Scrupulous sterile technique is necessary to minimize chances of introducing infection, which occurs in about 1 in 5000 injections. Three yearly injections in a single joint is the maximum under most circumstances.

Surgical Reconstruction. Tremendous advances in reconstructive orthopedic surgical procedures have allowed restoration of function and alleviation of pain in badly damaged joints, even in very elderly patients. Surgical intervention must be properly timed before the patient is bedridden and begins to atrophy. Resection of painful, protruding metatarsal heads is a simple procedure that can restore comfort and preserved mobility. Total hip replacement (or arthroplasty) and total knee replacement have excellent results in elderly patients when done by orthopedic teams experienced in RA joint reconstruction. Skilled preoperative and postoperative care increases success. Fusion (or arthrodesis) of an unstable wrist can restore effective hand function. Hand function can be improved surgically with tendon transfers, thumb fusion, joint prostheses, and debridement of synovium. An operation should not be performed merely to improve the appearance of a deformed but functional hand, however. Replacement prostheses for wrist, elbow, shoulder, and ankle are now available. Surgical synovectomy to prevent future joint damage remains controversial and is rarely indicated for the elderly RA patient.

Supportive Care. Despite all medical and surgical maneuvers, some elderly patients with long-standing RA must live with extreme crippling disability. Consistent, caring management by the physician can greatly enhance the quality of life of those patients. Very modest goals can be set, so that some progress is possible. Reaching even minor goals is important for the patient. Depression is common and may require psychiatric and pharmacologic treatment. Nutrition is frequently inadequate because of steroid-wasting, difficulty in food preparation, depression, and actual discomfort from eating.

The physician should recognize that health professionals have a tendency to avoid severely crippled patients and should encourage them to remain committed and understanding. Periodic reassessment of the patient by the entire rehabilitation team helps to keep solvable problems in focus and shows the patient that a plan is being followed. In fact "rheumatoid cachexia" may improve significantly with physical rehabilitation, intensive nutritional supplementation, and favorable responses to gold and other medical therapies.

---

1. Short CL, Bauer W, Reynolds WE: *Rheumatoid Arthritis*. Cambridge, Mass, Harvard University Press, 1957.
Classic study of the manifestations and progression of the natural history of the disease.
2. Brown JW, Sones DA: The onset of rheumatoid arthritis in the aged. *J Am Geriatr Soc* 10:873, 1967.
Myalgias and systemic symptoms are prominent early in presentation.
3. Carrigan AB: Benign rheumatoid arthritis of the aged. *Br Med J* 2:55, 1974.
Prognosis is favorable for new onset disease in old age.
4. Zvaifler NJ: Rheumatoid synovitis: An extravascular immune complex disease. *Arthritis Rheum* 17:297, 1974.
Reviews the immunopathology underlying rheumatoid disease.

5. Gordon DA, Stein JL, Broder I. The extraarticular features of rheumatoid arthritis. *Am J Med* 54:445, 1973.
Emphasizes the systemic nature of the disease and involvement beyond the joints.
6. Hunder GG, Bunch TW: Treatment of rheumatoid arthritis. *Bull Rheum Dis* 32:1, 1982.
Review of the basics of management, including alternative drug regimens.
7. Pearson CM, et al: Diagnosis and treatment of erosive rheumatoid arthritis and other forms of joint destruction. *Ann Intern Med* 82:241, 1975.
Discussion of management strategies and differential diagnosis.
8. Hall AP: The decision to operate in rheumatoid arthritis. *Ortho Clin North Am* 6:675, 1975.
Age is not a contraindication to major joint replacement.
9. Jette AM: Improving patient cooperation with arthritis treatment regimens. *Arthritis Rheum* 25:447, 1982.
Develops strategies for "poor compliance," which is often the result of ambiguous or ineffective communication.
10. Meenan RF, et al: The costs of rheumatoid arthritis. *Arthritis Rheum* 21:827, 1978.
Analyzes the breakdown of health care costs, which averaged $2,319 per year per patient.
11. Meenan RF, et al: The impact of chronic disease: A sociomedical profile of rheumatoid arthritis. *Arthritis Rheum* 24:544.
Presents evidence of the need for an effective multidisciplinary approach.
12. Rogers MP, Liang MH, Partridge AJ: Psychological care of the adult with rheumatoid arthritis. *Ann Intern Med* 96:344, 1982.
Dynamics and strategies for the crucially important emotional aspects of chronically disabled patients.
13. Karsh J, et al: Lymphopheresis in rheumatoid arthritis. *Arthritis Rheum* 24:867, 1981.
A randomized trial of a recently discovered and apparently effective therapy for rheumatoid disease.
14. Gottlieb NL: Chrysotherapy. *Bull Rheum Dis* 27:912, 1977.
Presents details of gold therapy, along with its risks and benefits.
15. Wilkens RF, Watson MA, Paxson CS: Low dose pulse therapy in rheumatoid arthritis. *J Rheumatol* 7:501, 1980.
This immunosuppressive appeared effective in the majority of severely arthritic patients in a uncontrolled trial.
16. Kimberly RP, et al: Reduction of renal function by newer nonsteroidal anti-inflammatory drugs. *Ann J Med* 64:804, 1978.
The consequences of prostaglandin inhibition may be less benign than is generally recognized.
17. Kassan SS, Thomas TL, Moutsopoulos HM: Increased risk of lymphoma in sicca syndrome. *Ann Intern Med* 89:888, 1978.
Incidence appears increased 44 times for those with long-standing Sjögren's syndrome.

70. GOUT AND PSEUDOGOUT

Edward W. Campion

The most common forms of acute arthritis in the elderly are the crystal-induced attacks of gout and pseudogout. Proper management can promptly alleviate the excruciating, immobilizing pain of these disorders and avoid needless morbidity.

Acute Gout

Diagnosis. A warm, red, painful, swollen joint is the rule in acute gout. Multiple joints may be involved, usually assymetrically in the lower extremities. The differential diagnosis based on the clinical picture includes gout; pseudogout; septic arthritis; and an acute flare of RA, SLE, or psoriatic arthritis. An acutely inflamed joint with overlying erythema should not simply be presumed to be due to gout. Sepsis must be considered, and the joint fluid cultured.

Elevated serum uric acid alone never constitutes a diagnosis of gout, but patients with uric acid levels above 9 mg/100 ml are clearly at increased risk for gout. Uric acid is elevated by thiazide diuretics but does not rise with advancing age. A definite diagnosis of gout can only be made by demonstrating, under a polarized light microscope, needle-shaped sodium urate crystals in the joint fluid. With a red compensator, sodium urate crystals have negative birefringence. The joint fluid is inflammatory, with up to 100,000 WBC/mm^3.

Medical Management. Medical management of acute gout aims at reducing inflammation and pain. This can be accomplished promptly by a short course of a nonsteroidal antiinflammatory drug, beginning with a large dose and tapering it over 3–5 days. Aspirin should **not** be used in acute gout. Indomethacin is effective, as are ibuprofen and naproxen. Any of these medications may cause confusion in a susceptible elderly patient. None should be given to anticoagulated patients or patients with a history of GI bleeding. It is being recognized increasingly that nonsteroidal drugs can adversely affect kidney function, particularly in patients with preexisting renal insufficiency.

Oral colchicine is effective in acute gout but often creates an unacceptable amount of diarrhea, which is distressing and even dangerous for the older patient. Intravenous colchicine, however, may be used effectively in acute attacks. A dose of 1–2 mg in 10 ml of normal saline is given IV, with care taken to avoid extravasation into the subcutaneous tissue. If relief is not obtained within 8 hours, 0.5–1.0 mg may be administered then repeated in 8 hours if necessary. The total dose of IV colchicine given to the elderly should not exceed 3 mg during a single treatment course. Colchicine should not be given orally and intravenously at the same time. It also must not be given to patients with renal failure. Excessive doses of IV colchicine cause bone marrow suppression.

Intraarticular steroids may also be useful in arresting a persistent gouty attack and may help the older patient who tolerates oral antiinflammatory agents poorly. Before intraarticular steroids are given, the diagnosis must be established unequivocally and sepsis ruled out. Systemic steroids have no role in the management of gout. Most patients require no treatment except during the acute attack.

Tophaceous Gout

Ironically, gout is hardest to recognize when it appears in its severest form. Advanced tophaceous gout may even be mistaken for rheumatoid arthritis. The correct diagnosis is made by demonstrating urate crystals in material aspirated from joints or from tophi. The tophi are small lumpy white-crested nodules on the ears, over the distal interphalangeal joints, or over the olecranon process, where they may be mistaken for rheumatoid nodules. Patients with tophaceous gout should be kept on allopurinol, 200–400 mg qd, to protect against joint destruction and gouty nephropathy. The allopurinol dose should be adjusted to keep the serum uric acid below 5 mg/100 ml. Urinary uric acid levels identify patients in danger of the uric acid nephropathy and kidney stones that develop in 15–20% of gout patients. A 24-hour excretion of more than 800 mg of uric acid should be treated preventively with allopurinol to inhibit purine breakdown.

Patients with multiple recurrent attacks of gout may be helped by allopurinol. The other major indications for chronic allopurinol are a history of uric acid kidney stones, a uric acid excretion greater than 800 mg daily, tophaceous gout, and the need to protect against the acute urate nephropathy that may accompany purine breakdown with chemotherapy for certain malignancies. Hyperuricemia may result from obesity, thiazide diuretics, aspirin in low doses, or decline of renal function. Totally asymptomatic hyperuricemia is common and is usually best left untreated. Unless there is a history of kidney stones or excessive urinary uric acid excretion, allopurinol is not used. Intervention should be reserved for the acute attack.

A stigma attached to gout bothers some old patients, who feel gout is the consequence of immoral overindulgence. No dietary restrictions are necessary except for the rare patient who feasts regularly on purine-laden foods such as anchovies, liver, kidney, and sweetbreads. General weight reduction may, however, reduce the serum uric acid level.

Pseudogout

Pseudogout is another crystal-induced arthritis but is caused by calcium pyrophosphate crystals rather than by urate. Clinically it may be indistinguishable from gout, acutely causing red, swollen, painful joints. Pseudogout generally strikes older patients, particularly in wrists and knees affected with osteoarthritis. Roentgenograms often demonstrate a fine line of calcification within the cartilage (*chondrocalcinosis*), which predisposes patients to pseudogout attacks. The diagnosis is established by demonstration of calcium pyrophosphate crystals in fluid from an affected joint. The crystals differ from urate in that they are squarish or rhomboid in shape rather than needlelike. By polarized microscopy with a red compensator they have positive birefringence. Pseudogout may be found in association with diabetes mellitus, hyperparathyroidism, hypothyroidism, or hemochromatosis.

The medical management of pseudogout uses short courses of nonsteroidal antiinflammatory agents for acute flares. Colchicine is not recommended, because the response to it is variable. Allopurinol has no use in pseudogout. With the diagnosis clearly established and sepsis ruled out, intraarticular steroids help greatly in severe or persistent cases.

---

1. Fox IH, Kelley WN: Management of gout. *JAMA* 242:351, 1979.
Acute attacks may be managed with nonsteroidals or colchicine, either by mouth or intravenously.
2. Wyngaarden JB, Kelley WN: *Hyperuricemia and Gout.* New York, Grune & Stratton, 1976.
Authoritative and encyclopedic review of gout.
3. Wallace SL, et al: Selected data on primary gout. *Bull Rheum Dis* 29:992, 1979.
Triggering events may be medical illness, trauma, or recent surgery.
4. Yu TF, Gutman AB: Efficacy of colchicine prophylaxis in gout. *Ann Intern Med* 55:179, 1961.
Recurrent gouty attacks can be curbed by colchicine in low maintenance doses.
5. Hadler NM, et al: Acute polyarticular gout. *Am J Med* 56:715, 1974.
Gout may produce a polyarthritis with fever and leukocytosis.
6. Berger L, Yu T: Renal function in gout. *Am J Med* 59:605, 1975.
Long-term follow-up shows little renal damage ascribable to gout alone.
7. Liang MH, Fries JF: Asymptomatic hyperuricemia: The case for conservative management. *Ann Intern Med* 88:666, 1978.
Summary of arguments against treating elevated uric acid in the absence of renal disease.
8. Yost RL, et al: Selected physiologic and drug effects on serum uric acid levels in an elderly population. *J Am Geriatr Soc* 29:273, 1981.
Measures of obesity best predict hyperuricemia in the elderly.
9. Messerli FH, et al: Serum uric acid in essential hypertension: An indicator of renal vascular involvement. *Ann Intern Med* 93:817, 1980.
Even mildly decrease renal blood flow appears to elevate uric acid.
10. Fessel WJ, Barr GD: Uric acid, lean body weight and creatinine interactions. *Semin Arthritis Rheum* 7:115, 1977.
Analysis of 78 variables shows little relation of age to uric acid levels.
11. McCarty DM: Calcium pyrophosphate dihydrate crystal deposition disease. *Clin Rheum Dis* 3:61, 1977.
The clinical spectrum of the pseudogout syndrome.
12. Schumacher HR, et al: Arthritis associated with apatite crystals. *Ann Intern Med* 87:411, 1977.
This newly described acute arthritis looks like gout clinically but is caused by much smaller hydroxyapatite crystals.
13. McCarty DJ, Kohn N, Faires JS: The significance of calcium pyrophosphate crystals in the synovial fluid of arthritic patients: "Pseudogout syndrome." *Ann Intern Med* 56:711, 1962.
Classic description of the acute syndrome that is a common arthritis in the elderly.
14. Ellman MH, Levin B: Chondrocalcinosis in elderly persons. *Arthritis Rheum* 18:43, 1975.
Calcified cartilage predisposes patients to attacks of acute pseudogout.
15. O'Duffy JD: Clinical studies of acute pseudogout attacks: Comments on prevalence, predispositions and treatment. *Arthritis Rheum* 19:349, 1976.
Sudden drops in serum calcium may precipitate acute attacks.

16. Ellman MH, Brown NL, Levin B: Prevalence of knee chondrocalcinosis in hospital and clinic patients aged 50 or older. *J Am Geriatr Soc* 29:189, 1981.
In patients over age 65, 15% have chondrocalcinosis by x-ray, but it is usually asymptomatic.

71. HIP FRACTURES

Edward W. Campion

Incidence

Hip fracture is the most common major complication of osteoporosis. With current orthopedic techniques nearly all hip fracture patients can regain full mobility with a stable, pain-free hip. No patient with an acute hip fracture should be presumed too old or too frail for orthopedic repair of the hip. Approximately 150,000 patients annually in the United States fracture their hips. The incidence doubles every 5 years past age 65. By age 90, nearly one-third of all females have had a hip fracture. Postmenopausal osteoporosis increases the hip fracture rate for women, making it more than double that of men. The risk of osteoporotic fractures increases in persons with rheumatoid arthritis, diabetes, alcoholism, Cushing's syndrome, epilepsy, and chronic obstructive lung disease. Osteoporosis also is worsened by immobilization, malnutrition, and calcium deficiency.

Emergency Care

Severely osteoporotic bone fractures with only minor trauma or with no apparent trauma at all. Therefore, hip pain in the elderly patient means a fracture until proved otherwise. A fall is the explanation reported for most fractured hips, although a convincing reason for the fall is often not apparent. Cardiac and neurologic work-up may be indicated.

After the fracture the patient lies in obvious pain that may be referred to the groin, thigh, or medial knee. The involved leg is shortened and externally rotated. There may be ecchymoses over the hip, but large amounts of bleeding are uncommon in hip fractures, unlike the case in fractures of the femoral shaft. Primary management of the fracture aims at keeping the pain and deformity to a minimum. The patient should be transported by stretcher with the leg immobilized. Roentgenograms establish the diagnosis, and range of motion should **not** be assayed. Analgesia sufficient to make the patient comfortable is given parenterally. Referral for orthopedic evaluation must be prompt, since complication rates increase steadily with delay. The more debilitated the patient, the more urgent is surgical intervention. Careful examination for other injuries should be made. Head injury and fractures of wrist, humerus, or ribs often accompany a fractured hip. Medical complications may include dehydration, hypothermia, pneumonia, and congestive heart failure or diabetes out of control.

Orthopedic Repair

The best treatment for patients who have been ambulatory is prompt orthopedic repair, generally with a single operation within 24 hours. The operation relieves pain in over 95% of cases, and most patients are restored to their previous level of function. After uncomplicated procedures, patients are out of bed and moving within 72 hours. The alternative to a surgical procedure, 6–8 weeks of traction and bed rest, has frequent and major complications. It is now generally discouraged. Operation entails open reduction and internal fixation to stabilize the fracture. Intertrochanteric and subtrochanteric fractures generally receive open reduction and internal fixation with a permanent plate, pins, or compression screw. If the viability of the femoral head is threatened, either a Moore's prosthesis or a total hip replacement may be used.

Total Hip Replacement. Whether for hip fracture or for arthritis, the long-term results of total hip replacement (THR) in the elderly have been excellent. The complications that may develop early in the course include deep vein thrombophlebitis, hemorrhage, and infection of the prosthesis. The most common late complication is loosening of the prosthesis, which may show up on x-ray films in 25% of THRs by the end of 5 years. Loosening, however, is symptomatic in only about 3% of patients. Loosening may be a clue to deep infection. The risk of THR infection appears to be increased in patients with rheumatoid arthritis and in patients undergoing a second or third hip operation. Infection may not be apparent until weeks or months after surgical intervention, when fever, hip pain, tenderness, and erythema develop. Massive lysis of the bone supporting the THR and protrusion inward of the acetabular component are additional, less common, complications. Heterotopic formation may become excessive and restrict motion of the THR, especially in spondylitis and in Paget's disease. Dislocation of the THR is uncommon and can be prevented by safety precautions taught by physical therapy. The problem of excessive wear of THR after years of use is less a problem in the elderly than in very active younger patients.

Complications. The revolution in orthopedic techniques for hip fractures has greatly reduced complications. Overall inpatient mortality is less than 10%. Close cooperation between medical and orthopedic teams ensures the best outcome for the patient. Blood loss during the surgical procedure is always considerable. Patients receive at least 2–4 units of blood replacement intraoperatively. Signs of fluid overload or a need for further transfusion may develop in the elderly patient. About 50% of hip fracture patients develop clots in the deep veins of the leg. These are usually silent clinically but may progress to frank thrombophlebitis or pulmonary emboli. It remains controversial whether to administer prophylactic anticoagulation before operation at the price of increased intraoperative bleeding. Aspirin prophylaxis (600 mg bid) is used frequently. The complications of pressure sores can be avoided by early mobilization, good nursing care, and proper nutrition. Acute confusional syndromes postoperatively generally resolve with orientation, mobilization, and correction of underlying metabolic, infectious, or pharmacologic precipitants.

A persistently painful hip months after the fracture may be the result of movement of a metal fixation device, infection, refracture, or aseptic necrosis with accelerated osteoarthritis. Inflammatory capsulitis or bursitis may cause pain overlying the hip. Heterotopic bone formation (myositis ossificans) sometimes develops in the soft tissues over the hip. It may be uncomfortable and limit motion.

Rehabilitation. It takes approximately 12 weeks for a hip fracture to heal, but most patients can begin to stand 2–3 days after operation. Rehabilitation teaches proper gait and protection of the vulnerable hip. The timing of progression from no weight bearing to partial to full weight bearing varies with type of fracture and repair. Hospital length of stay averages 3 weeks. Some patients, however, progress slowly and require prolonged therapy from a skilled rehabilitation team.

Attitude is an important determinant of eventual success. Some patients regress temporarily. Previously unrecognized medical or psychiatric problems may emerge, requiring evaluation and treatment. Family members may underestimate the rehabilitation potential of their elder relative. Elderly patients are especially sensitive to periods of immobility. A desire for bed rest "to get my strength back" is counterproductive and may delay ambulation to the point where the patient becomes bedfast. Previous problems with feet, knees, upper extremities, vision, or hearing take on new importance under the demands of rehabilitation. The patient often feels fearful he or she will fall again.

A skillful rehabilitation team can coax back confidence in the reluctant patient. Considerable conditioning may be required to establish sufficient endurance to permit a partial weight-bearing gait using assistive devices. There may be flares of osteoarthritis in the knees or bursitis in the shoulders. Long-handled shoehorns, elastic shoe laces, and grab bars in the bathroom help preserve function safely. The leg on the side of the fracture is often shorter when measured carefully. A lift added to the shoe can improve stability and avoid discomfort. Toward the end of the rehabilitation phase, a home visit by the rehabilitation team accompanied by the elderly patient helps to correct hazards and ensure a safe, successful return home.

1. Miller CW: Survival and ambulation following hip fracture. *J Bone Joint Surg (Am)* 60:930, 1978.

   Improved surgical techniques have greatly improved patient survival.

2. Evans JG, Prudham D, Wandless I: A prospective study of fractured proximal femur: Factors predisposing to survival. *Age Ageing* 8:246, 1979.

Emphasizes the relation of patients' prior level of function to outcome.

3. Keene JS, Anderson CA: Hip fractures in the elderly. *JAMA* 248:564, 1982.
   Develops a rating scale to define those at greatest risk for institutionalization after a fractured hip.
4. Garraway WM, et al: Limb fractures in a defined population. *Mayo Clin Proc* 54:701, 1979.
   Femoral fractures accounted for 62.5% of total hospital days for fractures.
5. Niemann KM, Mankin HJ: Fractures about the hip in the elderly indigent patient. *Geriatrics* 23:150, 1968.
   Even in high-risk patients pathologic fractures appear rarely.
6. Alfram PA: An epidemiological study of cervical and trochanteric fractures of the femur in an urban population. *Acta Orthop Scand* 65: (Suppl) 1, 1964.
   Documents increasing fracture rates with increasing age over a 13-year study.
7. Sherk HH: The treatment of hip fractures in institutionalized patients. *Orthop Clin North Am* 5:543, 1974.
   Prior disability adversely affects patient outcomes.
8. Braatz J, Pine A: Therapy and rehabilitation for psychiatric-geriatric patients with hip fracture. *Geriatrics* 27:101, 1972.
   Practical approaches to rehabilitation in multi-problem elderly hip fracture patients.
9. Hielema FJ: Epidemiology of hip fracture. *Phys Ther* 59:1221, 1979.
   Review of data from the perspective of physical therapy.
10. Weiss NS, et al: Decreased risk of fractures of the hip and lower forearm with postmenopausal use of estrogen. *N Engl J Med* 303:1195, 1980.
    A case-control study showing decreased risk of fractures in women taking estrogen.
11. Aloia JF: Exercise and skeletal health. *J Am Geriatr Soc* 29:104, 1981.
    Exercise can prevent involutional bone loss.
12. Overstall PW: Prevention of falls in the elderly. *J Am Geriatr Soc* 28:481, 1980.
    Emphasizes disorders of balance as the cause of most falls and fractures.
13. Riggs BL, et al: Effect of the fluoride/calcium regimen on vertebral fracture occurrence in post-menopausal osteoporosis. *N Engl J Med* 306:446, 1982.
    Although not a randomized study, supplemental treatment appears to decrease fracture rates.
14. Harris WH: Total hip replacement. *N Engl J Med* 297:650, 1977.
    Good to excellent results occur in 90% of patients.

72. ANKYLOSING SPONDYLITIS

Edward W. Campion

Clinical Picture

Ankylosing spondylitis (AS) is a common inflammatory arthritis affecting primarily the axial skeleton. It usually appears by the fourth decade with chronic back pain and stiffness, conjunctivitis, and peripheral inflammatory arthritis. By age 70 the prevalence of spondylitis is 529/100,000, with a 3 : 1 male predominance. Most elderly patients with AS have advanced, unmistakable disease with a frozen spine that is disabling but no longer painful. Spondylitis may develop in the setting of psoriasis, ulcerative colitis, Crohn's disease, or Reiter's syndrome. X-ray films in advanced ankylosing spondylitis show a "bamboo spine" and obliteration of the sacroiliac joints. The genetic marker HLA-B27 antigen is present in 90% of AS patients but in only 6% of the general population.

Treatment

The complications of an immobile spine and destruction of large joints cause the major problems in elderly AS patients. There is little need for antiinflammatory drugs in the advanced, "burnt-out" stage of the disease. Steroids should be avoided. Physical therapy can improve range of motion in hips and shoulders and maximize respiratory function. Safe mobility is a major concern. Occupational therapy provides assistive devices to improve the patient's ability and safety in daily functions. Surgical intervention is indicated only for selected patients with severe spinal deformities. Radiotherapy is no longer given for ankylosing spondylitis. Those older patients who received radiotherapy in the past have an increased risk of malignancy.

Complications

Major complications of long-standing AS include defects in the cardiac conducting system and aortic insufficiency, for which appropriate endocarditis prophylaxis is indicated. Pulmonary insufficiency may develop as a result of fibrosis and loss of chest expansion. Destructive arthritis of the hips and shoulders is most disabling. Surgical intervention may be needed for destructive hip disease in AS but is frequently complicated by heterotopic bone formation. Falls are another threat that can lead to devastating fractures of the brittle, fused spine. A cauda equina syndrome develops in some AS patients, and amyloid has been found in others.

1. McEwen C, DiTata D, Lingg C: Ankylosing spondylitis and spondylitis accompanying ulcerative colitis, regional enteritis, psoriasis, and Reiter's disease. *Arthritis Rheum* 14:291, 1971.
   Classic study of the diseases associated with spondylitis.
2. Resnick D, et al: Diffuse idiopathic skeletal hyperostosis. *Semin Arthritis Rheum* 7:153, 1978.
   This condition of older males may mimic spondylitis.
3. Radford EP, Doll R, Smith PG: Mortality among patients with ankylosing spondylitis not given x-ray therapy. *N Engl J Med* 297:572, 1977.
   A controversial study describing increased mortality from many causes.
4. Calin A, et al: Clinical history as a screening test for ankylosing spondylitis. *JAMA* 237:2613, 1977.
   Development of sensitive and specific indicators of spondylitis.
5. Cohen JM, et al: Increased risk for spondylitis stigmata in apparently healthy HL-AW 27 men. *Ann Intern Med* 84:1, 1976.
   The genetic predisposition is strong although clinical expression varies.
6. Kaprove RE, et al: Ankylosing spondylitis: Survival in men with and without radiotherapy. *Arthritis Rheum* 23:57, 1980.
   Spondylitis with past irradiation was shown to reduce survival in this 25-year follow-up.
7. Calin A, Marks S: Management of ankylosing spondylitis. *Bull Rheum Dis* 31:25, 1981.
   Education, counseling, and exercises can alleviate much of the morbidity.
8. Hunter T, Dubo H: Spinal fractures complicating ankylosing spondylitis. *Ann Intern Med* 88:546, 1978.
   Fracture identification may be difficult in advanced spondylitis.

73. SEPTIC ARTHRITIS, BURSITIS, AND JOINT TUMORS

Edward W. Campion

Septic Arthritis

Septic arthritis can destroy a joint rapidly if not identified and treated promptly. Particularly in the elderly, signs may be subtle. Infection can linger for weeks undetected in a joint unless specifically sought. Untreated, it can lead to life-threatening sepsis.

Diagnostic Features. Septic arthritis must be sought particularly in a compromised host (such as an immunosuppressed patient) and a compromised joint (such as one badly damaged by rheumatoid arthritis). Patients usually but not always have fever and an elevated white blood count. The cardinal features are localized pain, swelling, tenderness, effusion, and erythema. Several joints may be involved in sepsis. A septic joint may be the result of infection acquired from penetrating trauma, unsterile joint taps, or orthopedic surgical procedure. Septic joints may develop as a result of bacteremia from a source elsewhere in a body, such as an infected heart valve. Most elderly patients have septic arthritis concurrently with other joint disorders, such as RA, OA, and previous surgical procedure on the joints.

The diagnosis can be made only by tapping the suspected joints and culturing the fluid for both aerobes and anerobes. Joint fluid WBC counts in sepsis generally exceed 25,000/ mm^3, with polymorphonuclear leukocytes predominating. Glucose in the joint fluid is depressed. Blood cultures are positive only in a minority of cases.

The most common organism in the elderly is *Staphylococcus aureus,* although streptococci and gram-negative organisms are also found. Tuberculosis should be suspected and cultured in patients with prior TB, who are on steroids or who have chronic "sterile" inflammatory effusions. Synovial biopsy may be required to establish the diagnosis.

Treatment. Treatment of septic arthritis hinges on adequate use of specific antibiotics. Most cases require 4–6 weeks of IV antibiotics selected for the sensitivities of the particular pathogen. Repeated joint aspirations are helpful therapeutically. Serial cultures and WBC counts of joint fluid help ensure that treatment is sufficient. Open drainage is occasionally necessary. Prosthetic implants generally must be removed from an infected joint. Septic arthritis in severely deformed joints may extend into adjacent bone and therefore require prolonged treatment for osteomyelitis.

Bursitis

Differential Diagnosis. Acute bursitis is common in older patients and may be misdiagnosed as osteoarthritis, muscle strain, or a "pinched nerve." In the shoulder subdeltoid bursitis produces tenderness and extreme pain with abduction. Tenderness anteriorly in the shoulder aggravated by pronation of the forearm is characteristic of bicipital tendinitis. In the elderly, however, shoulder pain also arises commonly from disorders of the cervical spine. Exquisite point tenderness over the lateral aspect of the elbow is found in epicondylitis ("tennis elbow"). Severe hip pain with point tenderness over the greater trochanter appears with trochanteric bursitis. Marked tenderness and inflammation over the inner inferior aspect of the knee is the clue to anserine bursitis. Costochondritis (Tietze's syndrome) is inflammation of the costochondral junction, which produces chest pain that may be mistaken for cardiac pain. A careful examination localizes the tenderness to the costochondral junction. A variant of bursitis, *periarthritis calcarea,* produces acute pain and inflammation usually around one of the small joints of the hand or wrist. Correct diagnosis depends on recognizing the fine calcifications visible adjacent to the joint on the x-ray film. Roentgenograms of other types of bursitis may show calcific deposits or no abnormality at all.

Treatment. Bursitis or periarthritis responds well to short courses of indomethacin or other nonsteroidal, antiinflammatory drugs. With severe symptoms the quickest and most appreciated relief comes with careful local injection of a long-acting steroid preparation (such as triamcinolone hexacetonide) into the point of maximum tenderness. Injection is of particular benefit to the elderly patient who experiences intolerable side effects from antiinflammatory drugs. Sepsis must always be ruled out prior to injection of steroids.

Joint Tumors

Primary tumors arising from within a joint are rare. When they do occur, they mimic a monarticular arthritis. Lesions in the bone or soft tissue adjacent to a joint may also produce joint pain that is misinterpreted as arthritis. Therefore the elderly patient with persistent monarticular pain or a destructive bone lesion requires evaluation to establish a definite diagnosis.

The major tumors in and around joints are (1) pigmented villonodular synovitis, a locally destructive lesion that does not metastasize; a clue to diagnosis is brown-black joint fluid; (2) lipoma arborescens, also locally destructive, which arises in the setting of osteoarthritis; (3) synovial sarcomas, rare but highly malignant, which arise from surrounding soft tissue and invade a joint; (4) primary bone tumors, such as giant cell tumors and sarcomas that may give pain referred to a joint; (5) metastatic carcinomas to bone adjacent to a joint, which may be misinterpreted as arthritis; and (6) pulmonary tumors, which may produce at the end of the long bones a reactive periostitis (hypertrophic pulmonary osteoarthropathy), which mimics a polyarthritis.

The diagnosis of joint tumor can often be made without opening the joint surgically. Xeroradiograms and CT scans aid the roentgenographic interpretation of bone and soft tissue masses. A needle biopsy can be performed in some cases to obtain a tissue diagnosis. Biopsy of intraarticular lesions may also be done through the arthroscope with very little morbidity. Treatment is determined by the biopsy results. Malignant lesions require radical excision or amputation, if there is a chance of a cure. Locally destructive nonmalignant lesions can often be removed through the arthroscope.

1. Wallace R, Cohen AS: Tuberculous arthritis. *Am J Med* 61:277, 1976.
   Synovial biopsy and fluid cultures are most sensitive diagnostic maneuvers.
2. Goldenberg DL, Cohen AS: Acute infectious arthritis. *Am J Med* 60:369, 1976.
   Prior arthritis and infected extraarticular source are predispositions.
3. Ho G, Su EY: Antibiotic therapy of septic bursitis. *Arthritis Rheum* 24:905, 1981.
   Prompt diagnosis and frequent aspiration improve success rates.
4. Swezey RL, Spiegel TM: Evaluation and treatment of local musculoskeletal disorders in elderly patients. *Geriatrics* 34:56, 1979.
   The soft tissue syndromes may create secondary disabilities unless treated promptly.
5. Brown BB: Diagnosis and therapy of common myofacial syndromes. *JAMA* 239:646, 1978.
   Fibrositis and bursitis may create excruciating discomfort that is highly treatable.
6. Smythe HA: Non-articular rheumatism and the fibrositis syndrome, in Hollander KL, McCarty DJ (eds): *Arthritis and Allied Conditions*. Philadelphia, Lea & Febiger, 1972.
   Thorough review of the many soft tissue syndromes that are common in the elderly.
7. McCarty DJ: A basic guide to arthrocentesis. *Hosp Med* 4:77, 1968.
   An expert's guide to tapping virtually any joint.
8. Gottlieb NH, Riskin WG: Complications of local corticosteroid injections. *JAMA* 243:1547.
   Tendon rupture and infection are definite hazards.
9. Schiller AL: Tumors and tumor-like lesions involving joints, in Kelley WN (ed): *Textbook of Rheumatology*. Philadelphia, Saunders, 1981.
   Authoritative summary of the complex array of joint tumors.
10. Colabro JJ: Cancer and arthritis. *Arthritis Rheum* 10:553, 1967.
    Musculoskeletal symptoms may be the clue to an occult neoplasm.
11. Chunstensen JH, Paulsen JO: Synovial chondromatosis. *Acta Orthop Scand* 46:919, 1975.
    These intraarticular tumors are benign but may impair joint function.

74. CERVICAL SPONDYLOSIS

Thomas M. Walshe

Cervical spondylosis is an abnormality of the cervical spine caused by bone degeneration of the vertebral bodies and intervertebral discs. The bony degenerative changes create deformities of the spinal canal and of the neuroforamina, leading to compression of the spinal cord and roots. Degenerated intervertebral disc material that herniates through the anulus also may entrap the cervical nerves, or ridge formations in the spinal canal may narrow the space so that the spinal cord is compressed. Moreover, deformity of the spinal canal may alter the vascular supply to the spinal cord and its roots, but a clear vascular abnormality has not been identified pathologically in cervical spondylosis. Other bone disorders, such as osteoporosis, are not associated with root or cord compression, although they may cause chronic back pain.

Signs

Cervical degenerative arthritis, the underlying cause of cervical spondylosis, is very common in patients over 50, and the incidence increases with age. One of the most common causes of neurologic signs unaccompanied by symptoms in elderly patients is occult cervical spondylosis. Many elderly people who are asymptomatic may have slightly increased reflexes, upgoing toes, or minor sensory disturbances that are relatable to root or cord compression from degenerative spinal changes. Asymptomatic elderly patients who have neurologic manifestations, such as a Babinski sign, abnormal deep tendon reflex, or sensory disturbance, can be shown to have the roentgenographic changes of cervical spondylosis either on plain films or on myelograms. Such patients have no complaints and may erroneously be diagnosed as having cerebrovascular disease or other neurologic syndromes. Skeletal abnormalities other than degenerative arthritis tend to cause spondylosis in younger patients. Paget's disease of bone is an exception. Other disorders cause degenerative joint disease, usually in the low back, where weight bearing is greatest. Tabes dorsalis and diabetic neuropathy are examples of conditions that cause vertebral defects (Charcot joints), which in turn may cause root and spinal cord entrapments. Tumors metastatic to the vertebral canal or to the meninges should also be considered in evaluating patients with signs of root and cord compression. CT scan shows tumor and bony invasion. A radionuclide bone scan is also helpful in identifying bony metastases. Ankylosing spondylitis, when associated with fractures of the vertebrae, may cause neurologic signs, but uncomplicated cases do not show clear neurologic abnormalities. Rheumatoid arthritis also causes cervical myelopathy in patients with severe disease. Subluxation of the first cervical vertebra is a risk in rheumatoid arthritis and can be identified on plain films of the neck.

Clinical Course

The clinical syndrome of cervical spondylosis usually begins with pain in the neck and shoulders. Radiation of the pain into the shoulder, arm, or occipital region of the head is a frequent complaint. Two distinct neurologic syndromes are associated with cervical spondylosis: a root entrapment syndrome and a cord compression syndrome.

Root Entrapment Syndrome. When root entrapment occurs, the patient usually complains of pain and numbness in the upper extremities. Sensory and motor signs easily identified on examination include muscle-wasting and deficient reaction to pinprick, vibration, or other sensory modalities. The pain begins proximally and spreads toward the hand. The roots affected most often are the lower cervical (C_6–C_7). The syndrome is usually unilateral or worse on one side, and there may be reflex asymmetry with an absent biceps or triceps jerk.

Cord Compression Syndrome. When the spinal cord is compressed, the syndrome is different. Pain may be more diffuse or even absent. There is usually bilateral hyperreflexia in the upper and lower extremities. Babinski signs and a segmental sensory level indicate the spinal cord localization. Sense of vibration and joint position may be affected more than pain from a pinprick, and bladder dysfunction occurs in advanced cases. In the most subtle cases there are only brisk reflexes and a painful sensory abnormality that may show no objective signs.

Root and Cord Involvement. If both root and cord are involved, the two syndromes may be combined. When there is prominent muscle-wasting from the radiculopathy and some spasticity from the cord compression, cervical spondylosis may be confused with amyotrophic lateral sclerosis (ALS). In most cases of cervical spondylosis, however, there is a clear sensory disturbance and pain, findings not associated with ALS. Unlike ALS, cervical spondylosis does not affect the muscles of the pharynx, jaw, or tongue.

Roentgenographic Diagnosis

When patients with cervical spondylosis present with pain only, or with a sensory disturbance alone, the diagnosis remains uncertain clinically until myelography demonstrates cord compression. The clinical history in elderly patients is almost always one of gradual weakness and spasticity, with failure of gait. Cervical spondylosis is rarely an acute problem, except when trauma causes it to become suddenly worse. Patients who have a narrowed canal but no symptoms may develop an acute spinal cord syndrome or root syndrome following trauma or hyperextension of the neck. In the average case, however, the signs and symptoms of cervical spondylosis appear slowly over months or years. Patients with cervical spondylosis, unlike those with lesions from stroke or other cerebral events, have no signs relatable to the brainstem or above. When patients have abnormalities in higher cortical function or in the cranial nerves, the diagnosis of cervical spondylosis must be reconsidered. Cervical spondylosis and other neurologic illnesses occur together in elderly patients, making the interpretation of the clinical findings difficult at times. A careful history and examination can sometimes help, but myelography or computed tomography is usually needed, if there is a suspicion of symptomatic spondylosis.

Plain films of the cervical spine often show degenerative bone changes in asymptomatic elderly patients. Roentgenographic changes are helpful only when they match the clinical findings, since there is not a complete correlation between roentgenographic abnormality and clinical symptomatology. The diagnosis of cervical spondylosis affecting the nervous system must rest on the clinical findings more than on the roentgenographic changes.

The AP diameter of the cervical spinal canal as measured on plain lateral roentgenograms of the neck is normally greater than 17 mm. In significant cervical spondylosis the canal diameter is less than 14 mm. Cord compression almost always shows as narrowing of the canal on lateral neck films. In general, the cervical canal is considered "wide enough" when its diameter is equal to the width of the vertebral centrum. When it is less than 80% of the width, one should suspect significant spondylosis. About two-thirds of patients with symptoms of cervical spondylosis show a narrowing of the spinal canal or of the neuroforamina. Patients with root compression alone, however, may have normal canal diameter. The diagnosis can be made with certainty by contrast myelography, which demonstrates an anatomic lesion that can be correlated with the clinical findings and symptoms. Myelographic studies are done when a patient is a surgical candidate and has neurologic signs or severe pain. When the diagnosis is suspected, a period of bed rest may relieve the complaints without recourse to surgery.

Treatment

The prognosis for patients who have symptomatic cervical spondylosis depends on the degree of canal stenosis and the severity of the cord compression. Most elderly patients with minimal signs and symptoms can be managed with bed rest, a flat sleeping surface, and nonnarcotic analgesics. A soft cervical collar may help to immobilize the neck and reduce muscle spasm. The collar also prevents sudden extension and flexion movements. Head traction using 2–3 pounds of weight is sometimes useful in patients who have pain as a prominent symptom.

Narcotic analgesics have no place in the chronic treatment of neck and back pain, although they may help in the short term while the patient is being treated with bed rest. Aspirin and sedatives are sometimes of help in reducing the muscle spasm and arthritic pains associated with spondylosis. Elderly patients, however, sometimes become confused when treated with sedatives and bed rest.

When a narrowing of the spinal canal is associated with neurologic findings at the same level, laminectomy is the definitive treatment, even for the elderly, since the neurologic deficit is usually reversible after successful operation. Younger patients have better results from laminectomy, but other factors such as duration of symptoms and severity of neurologic signs are also important in determining success. Even moderately severe deficits that have been present for only a few months may be reversed in some cases.

The appropriate surgical approach depends on the patient and the surgeon. Cervical laminectomy with various modifications has been used traditionally, but anterior approaches are also employed. The overall results are variable, and the operation is reserved for patients who have clear neurologic findings and an obvious lesion on the myelogram.

---

1. Adams CBT, Logue V: Studies in cervical spondylotic myelopathy. *Brain* 94:557–594, 1971.
   Clinical and pathologic review.
2. Brain WR, Wilkenson M (eds): *Cervical Spondylosis and Other Diseases of the Cervical Spine.* Philadelphia, Saunders, 1967.
   A complete review.
3. Brownwell B, Hughes JT: Necropsy observations on the damage to the nervous system in degenerative disease of the cervical spine. *Proc Fifth Int Congress Neuropathol* 1:551–554, 1975.
   The autopsy study that documents the prevalence of spondylitic myelopathy.
4. Burrows EH: The sagittal diameter of the spinal canal in cervical spondylosis. *Clin Radiol* 14:77–86, 1963.
   In 300 normals the diameter was about 17 mm; in patients with cervical spondylosis it was 15 mm.
5. Ehni G: Neurological disorders associated with skeletal changes, in Fields WS (ed):

Neurological and Sensory Disorders in the Elderly. Chicago, Year Book, 1975, pp 33–50.
A very good review based on personal experience.

6. Lawrence JS, Brenner JM, Bier F: Osteoarthrosis: Prevalence in the population and relationship between symptoms and x-ray changes. *Ann Rheum Dis* 25:1, 1966.
X-ray changes do not always fit the clinical signs.
7. Mayfield FH: Cervical spondylosis: A source of pain, parathesias, paralysis and plaintiffs, is it traumatic? (Scudder Oration). *Bull Am Coll Surg* 51:6–10, 1966.
An editorial that discusses the social and legal aspects of spine disease.
8. Mayfield FH: Cervical spondylotic radiculopathy and myelopathy, in Thompson RA, Green JR (eds): *Advances in Neurology.* New York, Raven Press, 1979, vol 22, pp 307–321.
Good discussion of the surgical techniques.
9. McRae DL: The significance of abnormalities of the cervical spine. *Am J Roentgen* 84:3, 1960.
Again, x-ray changes alone do not mean trouble.
10. Nakano KK, Schoene WC, Baker RA, Dawson DM: The cervical myelopathy associated with rheumatoid arthritis: Analysis of 32 patients with two postmortem cases. *Ann Neurol* 3:144–151, 1978.
Describes the anterior subluxation that occurs late in the course of rheumatoid arthritis.
11. Nurick S: The natural history and the results of surgical treatment of the spinal cord disorder associated with cervical spondylosis. *Brain* 95:101–108, 1972.
Notes success in using laminectomy.
12. Nurick S: The pathogenesis of spinal cord disorder associated with cervical spondylosis. *Brain* 95:87–100, 1972.
A discussion of the mechanism of cord compression and the role of canal diameter.
13. Pallis C, Jones AM, Spillane JD: Cervical spondylosis: Incidence and implications. *Brain* 77:274–289, 1954.
Early description of the syndromes.
14. Sheehan S, Bauer RB, Meyer JS: Vertebral artery compression in cervical spondylosis. *Neurology* 10:968–986, 1960.
Vascular compromise remains controversial and perhaps less common than this paper suggests.
15. Stoltmann HF, Blackwood W: The role of the ligamenta flava in the pathogenesis of myelopathy in cervical spondylosis. *Brain* 87:45, 1964.
Helps to explain why the cord is compressed in some cases.

75. LUMBAR SPONDYLOSIS

Thomas M. Walshe

Causes

Degenerative arthritis causes bony deformity and canal narrowing in the lumbar region, just as in the cervical area. Most lumbar stenosis and spondylosis is caused by degenerative joint disease, but neuropathic conditions such as tabes dorsalis and diabetic neuropathy also cause degenerative bone changes in the weight-bearing lumbar region. A narrow lumbar canal is known to complicate spondylolisthesis, particularly after an operation on the back. Laminectomy, fusions, chemonucleolysis, trauma, Paget's disease, and certain congenital malformations have also been identified as the foundation of lumbar stenosis.

Incidence

Lumbar stenosis and spondylosis occur about one-tenth as frequently as lumbar discopathy, but in the population over 60 they are more common than discopathy. About two-thirds of patients with symptomatic lumbar stenosis are older than 60 years, and about 15% are over 70. On the other hand, a ruptured disc without stenosis of the canal is most common in the 35- to 45-year age group. Symptomatic lumbar stenosis is about as common as symptomatic cervical spondylosis. Lumbar spondylosis strikes men more than women and follows trauma in only about one-fourth of patients. The complaints are usually present for years before the diagnosis becomes clear.

Symptoms

Symptomatic lumbar stenosis is caused usually by a combination of disc herniation, spondylosis, and canal stenosis. Developmental stenosis of the lumbar canal alone is an unusual cause of symptoms.

The diameter of the lumbar canal varies among individuals, so that persons with large lumbar canals even with extensive degenerative changes in the bone may not have neurologic deficits. On the other hand, patients who begin with narrow canals and develop degenerative joint disease may experience symptoms.

The lumbar canal space contains the cauda equina, which is surrounded by the dura, the intervertebral disc material, and the ligamenta flava. Thickening and abnormalities of the surrounding structures can further encroach upon the bony canal space. When the canal is narrowed, the cauda equina, which begins at the high lumbar area, may be crushed, causing pain and leg weakness. The syndrome of lumbar spondylosis or lumbar stenosis, therefore, is primarily one of lower spinal root symptomatology. The pathophysiologic picture is not completely understood, but in some cases a failure of the posterior spinal ligaments, usually in the L_4–L_5 region may allow the L_4 vertebra to move over the L_5 vertebra, thus scissoring off the lumbar canal and causing intermittent signs and symptoms.

Pain is the most prominent complaint associated with lumbar spinal stenosis and is usually in the back, but at times the patient complains of painful muscle cramps in the legs. The pain in the legs may be unilateral or bilateral and sometimes radiates from the back to the foot. Muscle-wasting in the legs without back pain occasionally happens but is distinctly uncommon. A few patients with spinal stenosis experience numbness and tingling without other complaints. Impotence and urinary incontinence sometimes develop. The onset may be acute, gradual, or progressive over years. A few patients suffer a remitting, relapsing course that is very difficult to diagnose clinically.

A complete cauda equina syndrome with paraparesis, sensory loss, and urinary incontinence sometimes arises late in the disease. Weakness of one or both legs without complete paralysis is the usual finding. The physical signs associated with lumbar stenosis vary with the severity of the lesion. Depressed ankle jerks and knee jerks are found, with weakness of the anterior tibial, extensor hallucis, and triceps surae muscles. Patients gradually become unable to walk and have hypoesthesia in the lower extremities. Pain with straight leg flexion is uncommon, but extension of the legs from the prone position may cause pain. Indeed, exacerbation of back and leg pain by posture and exercise is a distinctive sign in lumbar stenosis. An exaggerated lordotic posture may precipitate or worsen the pain and neurologic complaints.

Differential Diagnosis

Leg pain in lumbar spondylosis and in peripheral vascular disease are both associated with exercise and therefore may be hard to distinguish from each other. Neurogenic claudication can be separated from vascular claudication by observation of several features: Femoral and distal pulses are usually present in neurogenic cases, and there are no distal vascular trophic changes. Abdominal and large vessel bruits are more commonly found in vascular claudication than in neurogenic cases. The pain in neurogenic claudication starts when the patient assumes the erect posture and is made worse with extension of the back. The pain in vascular claudication is usually found in the contracting muscles of the calf and thigh, rather than in the limbs. Body position improves the cauda equina lesions, especially when the back is flexed. Vascular disease causing claudication does not improve with position but depends entirely upon extent of exercise. Patients with normal pulses in the legs before and after exercise almost never have vascular claudication. In a rare patient, however, neurogenic and vascular claudication coexist.

The diagnosis is made when contrast myelography or computed tomography shows abnormalities at the level of clinical dysfunction. Just as in cervical spondylosis, roentgenographic abnormalities alone do not constitute the diagnosis. In lumbar stenosis, plain films almost always show bone changes. Myelograms show complete canal block or partial block from the ventral or lateral deformities inside the canal. The extent of the neurologic deficit depends on the rapidity and degree of encroachment.

Treatment

The treatment of lumbar stenosis depends on the severity of the syndrome. When the pain is disabling or neurologic signs are progressing, a wide laminectomy and facetectomy above and below the stenotic areas as seen on the myelogram is the procedure of choice. When complaints are less severe and there are no neurologic findings, bed rest, analgesics, and reduction of activity may reduce the symptoms. Surgical intervention is most helpful when the deficit is not complete and has less chance of success when there are severe neurologic findings.

1. Blau JN, Logue V: Intermittent claudication of the cauda equina. *Lancet* 1:1081–1086, 1961.
   Intermittent pain and paresthesia in the legs, which describes the syndrome well, were reported in 6 patients.
2. Blau JN, Logue V: The natural history of intermittent claudication of the cauda equina. A long-term follow-up study. *Brain* 101:211–22, 1978.
3. Brish A, Lerner MA, Braham J: Intermittent claudication from compression of cauda equina by a narrowed spinal canal. *J Neurosurg* 21:207–211, 1964.
   Reports 2 cases.
4. Dyck P, Pheasant HC, Doyle JB, Rieder JJ: Intermittent cauda equina compression syndrome. *Spine* 2:75–81, 1977.
   A report of 30 cases.
5. Epstein JA, Epstein BS, Lavine L: Nerve root compression associated with narrowing of the lumbar spinal canal. *J Neurol Neurosurg Psychiatry* 25:165–176, 1962.
   Patients with narrow canals have more problem with discopathy. This is a good review of the anatomic changes.
6. Lancourt JE, Glenn WV, Wiltse LL: Multiplanar computerized tomography in the normal spine and in the diagnosis of spinal stenosis. *Spine* 4:379–390, 1979.
   Computer tomography can precisely localize lesions in the lumbar spine.
7. Porter RW, Wilks M, Ottewell D: Measurement of the spinal canal by diagnostic ultrasound. *J Bone Joint Surg* 60B:481–484, 1978.
   A neat trick.
8. Verbiest H: *Neurogenic Intermittent Claudication with Special Reference to Stenosis of the Lumbar Vertebral Canal.* New York, Elsevier, 1976.
   An experienced review of the subject.
9. Verbiest H: A radicular syndrome from developmental narrowing of the lumbar vertebral canal. *J Bone Joint Surg* 36B:230–237, 1954.
   The earliest description of 7 cases.
10. Weinstein PR, Ehini G, Wilson CB: *Lumbar Spondylosis: Diagnosis, Management and Surgical Treatment.* Chicago, Yearbook, 1977.
11. Wilson CB, Echni G, Groumus J: Neurogenic intermittent claudication. *Clin Neurosurg* 18:62–85, 1970.
    Separates the vascular from the neurogenic types of leg pain.
12. *Clin Orthop* 115:1, 1976.
    Entire subject is covered in 23 articles.

76. SYSTEMIC LUPUS ERYTHEMATOSUS

Edward W. Campion

Symptoms

Systemic lupus erythematosus (SLE), principally a disease of younger people, has its onset in late life in about 15% of cases. In addition, many patients with SLE of earlier onset survive to carry the disease into old age. SLE must be suspected in patients with polyarthritis, pleurisy, pericarditis, discoid or erythematous skin rashes, leukopenia, hemolytic anemia, thrombocytopenia, persistent unexplained fever, seizures, or deteriorating renal function. In some elderly subjects the only initial clinical clue to SLE is depression and malaise. The alopecia of SLE, unlike normal age-related hair loss, is patchy, with scarring. SLE tends to be more insidious and indolent in the elderly than in the young, but it can be very aggressive, particularly in elderly blacks.

Diagnosis

The most sensitive serologic test for SLE is antinuclear antibody (ANA). It gives positive results in 99% of definite cases of SLE. It is not specific, however. Many older patients have positive ANA test results with no detectable disease. The lupus erythematosus preparation is more specific but is expensive and inappropriate as an initial screening test for SLE. Anti-double-stranded DNA antibodies are the most specific serologic test for SLE but are of low sensitivity. Skin biopsy showing immune complexes at the dermal-epidermal junction is also highly specific for SLE. Other laboratory clues to SLE are leukopenia, thrombocytopenia, hemolytic anemia, a biologic false-positive test for syphilis, elevated SGOT, elevated CPK, proteinuria, and hematuria.

False-positive ANA's test results are common in the elderly and do not constitute a diagnosis of SLE. Specific laboratory and clinical manifestations must be present for a diagnosis of SLE. Some drugs, particularly procainamide and hydralazine, produce positive ANA results and a syndrome nearly identical with SLE, which usually regresses when the drug is stopped. A speckled pattern on the ANA test points to the diagnosis of mixed connective tissue disease, a milder SLE variant that rarely endangers kidneys or CNS. The polyarthritis of SLE occasionally may be so severe as to be mistaken for rheumatoid arthritis. SLE in the elderly has a generally good prognosis, with a 5-year survival rate of 92%. Physicians must be ready to correct the mistaken impression of some SLE patients that their disease is rapidly and invariably fatal. Many flares of SLE will subside with simply rest and aspirin. No known therapy is curative. Excessive corticosteroids may sometimes be more hazardous than the disease itself, especially in the elderly.

Treatment

Hydrochloroquine may improve the polyarthritis and skin rashes of SLE. Because of the drug's possible retinal toxicity, however, regular ophthalmologic surveillance is required for those taking it. Corticosteroids improve the thrombocytopenia, hemolytic anemia, pleuropericarditis, severe arthritis, and malaise. Since steroid side effects are dose-related, the dose and duration should be the absolute minimum required. Tapering of steroids should always be gradual (< 20% dose reduction weekly) to prevent flare-ups. Management of lupus nephritis remains controversial and demands specialty consultation. High-dose corticosteroids and cytotoxic drugs may be of benefit in selected cases.

Complications

Serious infections often complicate SLE. Influenza and pneumococcal vaccination are recommended. Fever is frequently a manifestation of SLE itself, but thorough investigation is required to identify possible underlying infection in the compromised host. Other complications include myopathy, asceptic necrosis of bone, pleurisy, malaise, and depression. Atherosclerotic heart disease is a major cause of death in SLE. Conscientious treatment of hypertension and discontinuation of smoking may lessen that risk. SLE patients should avoid excessive sun exposure and use sunscreens containing PABA to avoid exacerbation of the rash. Complications due to chronic steroid–induced osteoporosis may be reduced by calcium and vitamin D supplementation.

---

1. Decker JL, et al: Systemic lupus erythematosus. *Ann Intern Med* 82:391, 1975.
   Detailed review of the varied clinical manifestations.
2. Ropes MW: *Systemic Lupus Erythematosus.* Cambridge, Mass, Harvard University Press, 1976.
   Classic study of lupus over several decades.
3. Baker SB, Rovira JR, Campion EW, Mills JA: Late onset systemic lupus erythematosus. *Am J Med* 66:727, 1979.
   The disease becomes less aggressive in older patients.
4. Ballou SP, Khan MA, Kushner I: Clinical features of systemic lupus erythematosus: Differences related to race and age of onset. *Arthritis Rheum* 25:55, 1982.
   Older patients had less hypocomplementemia and improved survival.

5. Wallace DJ, Bluestone R, Klinenberg JR: The biology of aging and the immune system. *Bull Rheum Dis* 32:13, 1982.
Reviews complexities of immunology and aging, and their impact on disease in the elderly.
6. McDuffie FC, Bunch TW: Immunologic tests in the diagnosis of rheumatic disease. *Bull Rheum Dis* 27:900, 906.
False-positive test rates increase in the elderly.
7. Sharp GC: Mixed connective tissue disease. *Bull Rheum Dis* 25:828, 1974.
Classic description of an overlap syndrome that may look like SLE, scleroderma, or polymyositis.
8. Axelrod L: Glucocorticoid therapy. *Medicine* 55:39, 1976.
Elderly patients are particularly at risk for adverse effects from steroids.

77. GIANT CELL ARTERITIS AND POLYMYALGIA RHEUMATICA

Edward W. Campion

Giant cell arteritis (GCA temporal arteritis) is rarely seen in patients under 50 years old. It is a potentially devastating disorder when the primary lesion leads to inflammatory destruction and thrombosis of retinal, cerebral, or other critical arteries. Sudden blindness is a feared and not uncommon complication. When giant cell arteritis is identified early, the thrombotic complications can usually be prevented. The average annual incidence of giant cell arteritis is 11.7 in 100,000 persons over 50 years. It is clearly a disease of the elderly, with a median age of 75 years at diagnosis. GCA strikes whites more often than blacks and women twice as frequently as men.

Symptoms

Headaches affect 90% of patients with GCA. Elderly patients with new onset of headaches should be screened for arteritis. The headaches are generally severe and localize to the scalp itself, particularly the temples. Visual symptoms such as blurring, diplopia, and transient or permanent visual loss result when arteritis compromises blood supply to the retina or optic nerve. Visual disturbance affects 40% of patients, with sudden total blindness in some cases. Symptoms of polymyalgia rheumatica are frequently associated with GCA.

Giant cell arteritis usually causes constitutional symptoms such as weight loss, malaise, confusion, and depression. Fever is common; in fact, fever of unknown origin may be the sole presenting sign of GCA. Claudication of jaw, arm, or tongue may be a clue to the diagnosis. Large artery involvement, including aortic dissection occurs in about 15% of cases. The temporal arteries may feel swollen and nodular and have absent pulsations. Occasionally frank necrosis of the scalp develops. Joints are not affected by GCA. The Westergren sedimentation rate is almost always over 50 mm/hr and frequently over 100 mm/hr. Over half of patients with active GCA have anemia, which in some cases is profound, as well as mild leukocytosis and elevated liver function test results. Urinalysis may show red blood cells, but clinically significant renal involvement is rare. Rheumatoid factor and ANA tests are of no help in the diagnosis.

Diagnosis

Diagnosis is made by temporal artery biopsy, which is simple and safe. Whenever possible, biopsy is done prior to steroid therapy and is taken from the side of maximal symptoms. Multiple sections should be examined pathologically because of "skip lesions." A negative biopsy does not absolutely rule out GCA. Some cases in which there are strong clinical findings may warrant multiple biopsies.

Treatment

Prompt treatment is important to avert complications. Visual symptoms in patients with evidence of GCA constitute a medical emergency. Prednisone, 60–80 mg qd is begun at once. Temporal artery biopsy should be done within 3 days. Patients with a positive biopsy but without visual symptoms are begun on prednisone 40 mg qd. When the sedimentation rate returns to normal and symptoms subside, the daily prednisone dose is gradually reduced by not more than 5 mg weekly. Daily steroids (≥7.5 mg prednisone) should be continued for at least one full year and will arrest most GCA completely. Steroid administration every other day is not effective in GCA. A few patients require low prednisone doses for several years to control the disease and to preserve vision. If the original symptoms recur, the sedimentation rate rises, or the polymyalgia syndrome develops, increasing the prednisone dose usually helps. Patients on prednisone should be treated with vitamin D and calcium to minimize steroid-induced osteoporosis.

Polymyalgia Rheumatica

Polymalgia rheumatica (PMR) is a distinct syndrome of proximal muscular aching pain with an elevated sedimentation rate, which occurs in the elderly. There is an associated occult giant cell arteritis in about 40% of patients with PMR. The typical patient complains of pain with marked stiffness about the neck, shoulder girdle, and proximal thighs. There may be low-grade fever, weight loss, anemia, and perhaps symptoms of accompanying giant cell arteritis. Patients with PMR are often frustrated and depressed. Some become labeled as merely excessive complainers. There are no characteristic physical findings of PMR. The joints are not inflamed, and muscular strength is normal, although there may be tenderness and guarding. The essential laboratory finding is a Westergren sedimentation rate of greater than 50 mm/hr. CPK and thyroid function tests are normal. Rheumatoid factor is usually negative. Disorders that resemble polymyalgia rheumatica are hypothyroidism, depression, polymyositis, occult malignancy, cervical spondylitis, and the prodrome of rheumatoid arthritis. A brief therapeutic trial of prednisone, 10 mg qhs for 4 days, usually gives dramatic relief of PMR symptoms but will not change the other disorders. Temporal artery biopsy is recommended in all patients with definite PMR. Those with a positive biopsy are treated as described above. Uncomplicated PMR responds to 7.5–15 mg qd of prednisone. As the sedimentation rate returns to normal, the dose is slowly reduced. After a year it is usually possible gradually to discontinue steroids altogether. Some patients may require prolonged therapy for recurring symptoms.

1. Hamilton CR, Shelly WM, Tumulty PA: Giant cell arteritis: Including temporal arteritis and polymyalgia rheumatica. *Medicine* 50:1, 1971.
   Classic summary of this puzzling disease of the elderly.
2. Wilske KR, Healy LA: Polymyalgia rheumatica: A manifestation of giant cell arteritis. *Ann Intern Med* 66:77, 1967.
   Myalgias in the elderly may be the major diagnostic clue.
3. Healy LA, Wilske KR: The systemic manifestations of temporal arteritis. New York, Grune & Stratton, 1979.
   Emphasizes the systemic disease manifestation.
4. Klein RG, Hunder GG, Stanson AW: Large artery involvement in giant cell arteritis. *Ann Intern Med* 83:806, 1975.
   About 10% of cases are complicated by aortitis.
5. Hunder GG, Allen GL: Giant cell arteritis: A review. *Bull Rheum Dis* 29:980, 1979.
   Excellent review of varied presentations from headache to hemiplegia.
6. Enzmann D, Scot WR: Intracranial involvement of giant cell arteritis. *Neurology* 27:794, 1977.
   Focal deficits or confusional syndromes may result.
7. Goodman BW: Temporal arteritis. *Am J Med* 67:839, 1979.
   Manifestations vary from face pain to fever to sudden blindness.
8. Bengtsson B, Malmval B: The epidemiology of giant cell arteritis including temporal arteritis and polymyalgia rheumatica. *Arthritis Rheum* 24:899, 1981.
   The disease is being recognized in the elderly as more common than once thought.
9. Huston KA, et al: Temporal arteritis. *Ann Intern Med* 88:162, 1978.
   The epidemiology of the disease over 25 years in a Minnesota county.
10. Fauci AS: The spectrum of vasculitis: Clinical, pathologic, immunologic and therapeutic considerations. *Ann Intern Med* 89:660, 1978.
    Update on the vasculitic syndromes that are becoming increasingly treatable.
11. Calamia KT, Hunder GG: Giant cell arteritis presenting as fever of unknown origin. *Arthritis Rheum* 23:660, 1980.

Nearly half of the patients had fever; some were undiagnosed for weeks.

12. Liang GC, Simkin PA, Mannik M: Immunoglobulins in temporal arteritis. *Ann Intern Med* 81:19, 1974.
Details patterns of antibody deposition in the pathogenesis.
13. Miller LD, Stevens MB: Skeletal manifestations of polymyalgia rheumatica. *JAMA* 240:27, 1978.
Sternoclavicular inflammation was a prominent diagnostic clue.
14. Spiera H, Davison S: Long-term follow-up of polymyalgia rheumatica. *Mt Sinai J Med* 45:225, 1978.
Low-dose steroids usually avert complications safely.

78. POLYMYOSITIS

Edward W. Campion

Presentation

Polymyositis is an inflammatory myopathy that sometimes strikes elderly patients and that may be a clue to an occult malignancy. When the skin is involved, it is termed *dermatomyositis*. Polymyositis may appear as an acute fulminant myopathy of rapid onset with myoglobinuria or as a subacute to chronic disorder. At times it appears as muscular weakness in association with manifestations of scleroderma, lupus erythematosus, or mixed connective tissue disease. When polymyositis appears in association with an underlying malignancy, it may either precede or follow the emergence of the neoplasm. About 20% of polymyositis patients over age 50 are found to have malignancies.

Symptoms

The symptoms of polymyositis are usually related principally to muscle weakness, but constitutional symptoms of fever, weight loss, periorbital edema, polyarthritis, and Raynaud's phenomena may also be present. Dysphagia with aspiration may be a particularly difficult manifestation to treat. The principal muscles affected are those of the proximal limbs, neck, and shoulder girdle, with lesser involvement of distal musculature. There is usually no pain in the muscles, although some patients have muscle aching with tenderness. Atrophy usually occurs late in the disorder, if ever. The skin lesions may range from mild subcutaneous edema in the periorbital regions to a generalized angry erythematous eruption that is both dramatic and disabling. Skin involvement is confined to the knuckles, face, and upper trunk.

Differential Diagnosis

In the elderly patient, myopathy is sometimes overlooked or attributed to coexisting pathologic conditions or to aging itself. Only with careful questioning and testing can one be sure there is a specific decline in motor power. The neck is usually involved in polymyositis but is rarely affected in neuropathies. Hip flexors are also more often weak in myopathies than in neuropathies. Elevation of creatine phosphokinase (CPK) is a sensitive laboratory indicator of muscle breakdown. The sedimentation rate is often elevated in myositis. Electrophysiologic studies usually illustrate only the nonspecific changes of myopathy. Muscle biopsy is most helpful when obtained from an affected muscle. A negative muscle biopsy does not eliminate the possibility of the disease. Disorders such as thyroid myopathy, polymyalgia rheumatica, amyotrophic lateral sclerosis, myasthenia gravis, lupus erythematosus, Cushing's disease, and the muscular dystrophies must be considered in the differential diagnosis.

Treatment

Acute polymyositis is a fulminant disease that may be fatal. Complications may include myocarditis, respiratory failure, severe dysphagia, or renal failure from myoglobinuria. In the elderly, the course is frequently more insidious and slowly progressive. If the myopathy is mild, little or no treatment is necessary.

In cases of rapidly progressive myopathy or severe myopathy, corticosteroids are usually helpful in bringing on remission. Prednisone is given in daily doses of 40–60 mg until the clinical symptoms and muscle enzymes begin to come under control. Then the drug is tapered as the patient is followed for clinical or chemical relapse. A steroid-induced myopathy may become superimposed upon a case of chronically treated polymyositis. Steroid-induced myopathy generally does not raise the enzymes and should improve with a trial of reduced steroids. Immunosuppressive drugs such as methotrexate can be used in refractory and severe progressive myopathy. Side effects of immunosuppressives are not uncommon in the elderly, demanding great caution and reduced doses. Early intensive physical therapy can improve functional outcome and prevent contractures.

Risk of Malignancy

The incidence of malignancy in polymyositis is at least five times greater than in the general population and is greatest in older patients, particularly males. Patients without stigmata of connective tissue disease are at higher risk for malignancy. A thorough search of occult malignancy is recommended in all cases of elderly patients with polymyositis. When a resectable malignancy is found, the myositis may resolve following surgical intervention. Some studies find the association is stronger in dermatomyositis than in polymyositis. The most commonly found tumors are those of lung, colon, ovary, and breast.

1. Bohan A, et al: Computer-assisted analysis of 153 patients with polymyositis and dermatomyositis. *Medicine* 56:255, 1977.
   Separates fact from fancy in analyzing a classic study.
2. Bohan A, Peter JB: Polymyositis and dermatomyositis. *N Engl J Med* 292:344, 403, 1975.
   The differential diagnosis in the elderly becomes complex.
3. Metzger AL, et al: Polymyositis and dermatomyositis: Combined methotrexate and corticosteroid therapy. *Ann Intern Med* 81:182, 1974.
   In refractory cases immunosuppressives can lessen the steroid requirements and steroid complications.
4. Gottdiener J, et al: Cardiac manifestations in polymyositis. *Am J Cardiol* 41:1141, 1978.
   Conduction abnormalities, arrhythmias, and ventricular dysfunction may be severe complications.
5. Barnes BE: Dermatomyositis and malignancy. *Ann Intern Med* 84:68, 1976.
   Analysis describing greater than fivefold increased risk of cancer, especially of breast, lung, ovary, and stomach.
6. DeVere R, Bradley WB: Polymyositis: Its presentation, morbidity and mortality. *Brain* 98:637, 1975.
   Outcomes range from total recovery to persisting severe myopathy.
7. Hunt TE: Practical considerations in the rehabilitation of the aged. *J Am Geriatr Soc* 28:59, 1980.
   Rehabilitation is crucial for those who develop a chronic myopathy.

79. OSTEOPOROSIS

David M. Slovik

Osteoporosis refers to a group of disorders of varying etiology that are characterized by a decrease in bone mass per unit volume below the point needed to maintain the structural integrity and mechanical support of the bone. The bone that is present has a normal ratio of mineral to matrix.

Causes of Bone Loss

Skeletal maturity and the maximal bone mass are normally achieved by 25–30 years of age. Bone loss occurs in all parts of the skeleton, although unequally. Cross-sectional studies have shown that, for normal women, overall bone loss throughout life can approximate 42% in the lumbar spine (predominantly trabecular bone), 39% in the mid-radius (90% cortical bone), and 39% in the distal radius (approximately 75% cortical and 25% trabecular bone). Women with osteoporosis and vertebral compression fractures have the lowest vertebral bone mass. For normal men, the rate of decrease is much lower.

The causes of osteoporosis and age-related bone loss are not well understood, but genetic traits, the maximal bone mass attained at skeletal maturity, exercise, and nutrition and hormonal factors are important. The maximal bone mass attained at skeletal maturity is very important, inasmuch as persons who have attained a greater bone mass at that time have a lower incidence of osteoporosis. The same rate of bone loss in two individuals will have less effect in the one with a larger skeleton. Exercise and physical activity are important in bone development and in preventing subsequent bone loss. Immobilization accelerates bone loss, as does weightlessness during space flights. Exercise programs may prevent bone loss and possibly increase bone mass in the elderly.

The role of calcium intake on the attainment of maximal bone mass, bone loss, and the development of osteoporosis is still not clear. Many large-scale epidemiologic studies have not demonstrated any relation between dietary calcium intake and bone mass, although others have shown that the bone mass is lower and femoral neck fractures are more numerous when dietary calcium intake is low. With aging, dietary calcium intake decreases and there is a decrease in intestinal absorption of calcium and the ability to adapt to a low-calcium diet.

Caffeine, alcohol, aluminum-containing antacids, some medication (including glucocorticoids and anticonvulsants), and smoking may have a detrimental effect on calcium metabolism and lead to bone loss. Numerous hormonal factors, including parathyroid hormone (PTH), vitamin D and its metabolites, calcitonin, gonadal steroids, insulin, adrenocorticosteroids, growth hormone, thyroid hormones, and prolactin are important in maintaining skeletal integrity.

Postmenopausal and senile osteoporosis are the most common types of osteoporosis. Hypogonadism, hyperthyroidism, hyperparathyroidism, and adrenocortical hormone excess (endogenous or exogenous) are endocrine causes of osteoporosis. Chronic heparin administration, chemotherapeutic agents, and alcohol cause osteoporosis, as do immobilization, multiple myeloma, systemic mastocytosis, and perhaps rheumatoid arthritis and diabetes mellitus.

Symptoms

Symptomatic osteoporosis affects millions of older Americans, and fractures of the vertebrae, hip, and forearm are common complications of bone loss. For example, fractures of the proximal femur are uncommon before age 50, but the incidence approximately doubles with each 5-year increment after 60, and by the ninth decade the cumulative incidence of fractures of the proximal femur is about 30% for women and 17% for men.

Vertebral compression fractures are usually painful, although the severity is variable. Acute pain due to compression fractures usually disappears in 2 or 3 months. Chronic low-back pain, however, may arise from muscle spasm, microfractures, or the biomechanical effects of the skeletal deformity. Compression fractures usually occur first in the lower thoracic and upper lumbar vertebrae. Height loss progresses and sometimes amounts to as much as 8 inches, until the rib cage rests on the iliac crest. Dorsal kyphosis ("dowager's hump") develops with progressive vertebral compression fractures, and the abdominal creases are accentuated.

Diagnosis

The diagnosis of osteoporosis is based on roentgenographic evaluation and biochemical tests. The initial procedure should include laboratory tests for the various causative factors. There should be thoracic and lumbar spine x-rays for evaluation of any asymptomatic compression fractures. Because at least 30–40% of bone mineral must be lost before the diagnosis of osteopenia can be made on routine roentgenograms, additional quantitative information using photon absorptiometry and quantitative computed tomography is helpful, if available, and also establishes a baseline of reference on which to gauge the therapy. Bone biopsy of the iliac crest is sometimes needed in diagnosing osteomalacia and also in obtaining quantitative histomorphometric information. Tetracycline is taken up at new bone-forming surfaces. When tetracycline is administered on two occasions separated by approximately 10–14 days, and a biopsy specimen taken, estimates of the calcification rate can be made by viewing the specimen under a fluorescent microscope. In uncomplicated osteoporosis the biochemical parameters are usually normal; but after fractures, the alkaline phosphatase may be elevated. Some individuals with osteoporosis may have an increase in PTH levels indicating primary or secondary hyperparathyroidism. PTH secretion is pulsatile, however, and elevated PTH levels may also be seen with advancing age, making interpretation difficult. Low 25-hydroxyvitamin D (25-$[OH]_2$-D) levels in patients with osteoporosis indicate concomitant vitamin D deficiency.

Treatment

The therapy of osteoporosis is directed toward either the treatment of the acute episode of a fracture or the long-term use of agents to try to prevent further bone loss and increase bone strength. Adequate analgesics for pain relief after an acute compression fracture are important in keeping the patient comfortable and mobile, since immobilization accelerates bone resorption. Corsets and back braces may help mobility after a vertebral fracture. It is best that the patient avoid unnecessary lifting and exercise regularly, without stress on the back. Patients with vertebral collapse should avoid spinal flexion exercises. Precautions in the interest of home safety, such as removal of slippery rugs, will help prevent further fractures.

Estrogen. Estrogen administration to postmenopausal women increases serum levels of 1,25-dihydroxyvitamin D (1,25-$[OH]_2$-D) and PTH, increases intestinal calcium absorption, decreases urinary calcium excretion, reduces bone resorption and remodeling, decreases urinary hydroxyproline excretion, decreases serum calcium and inorganic phosphate concentration, and increases urinary phosphate clearance. There are many prospective, double-blind, randomized studies showing that chronic estrogen therapy in postmenopausal women prevents bone loss. It appears that a dose of conjugated estrogens of 0.6 mg daily or its equivalent is needed to obtain this beneficial effect on bone. When estrogen therapy is stopped, bone loss resumes. Chronic estrogen therapy also substantially reduces the likelihood of fractures of the vertebrae, hips, and forearms in postmenopausal women. Of course, estrogen should not be administered when there are contraindications to its use.

Chronic unopposed estrogen treatment increases the risk of endometrial carcinoma severalfold, but this risk appears to decline after discontinuation of the estrogen. Cystic hyperplasia of the endometrium is a premalignant condition, and the concurrent use of progestogens for several days of each estrogen cycle appears to decrease the occurrence of endometrial hyperplasia and the risk of endometrial cancer. A common therapeutic program for postmenopausal women with an intact uterus is the administration of estrogens on days 1–25 of each month and the addition of a progestogen on days 16–25. Women in the early stages of menopause will have a return of menses after the progestational agent is given. Although this may be bothersome to the patient initially, it will help diminish the risk of endometrial cancer. The incidence of gallbladder disease is increased with estrogen use, but the incidence of other problems with long-term hormonal use is still to be determined conclusively. It is not evident which women in the early menopausal period benefit from estrogen therapy nor if estrogen should be given to elderly women with osteoporosis. Estrogen administration to postmenopausal women should be individualized and should be carried out only after the patient understands the risks and benefits of this therapy.

Vitamin D and Calcium. The use of vitamin D and calcium for elderly persons with bone loss has gained widespread acceptance, although there are very few data to substantiate a specific role for the vitamin D endocrine system in the pathogenesis of age-related bone loss and osteoporosis. There are reports of abnormalities in circulating levels of the vitamin D metabolites (e.g., low 1,25-$[OH]_2$-D concentration) in elderly patients with osteoporosis and an impaired ability to make 1,25-$(OH)_2$-D in response to stimulation by human parathyroid hormone 1–34 fragment. The dose of vitamin D required to increase intestinal calcium absorption, which is low in elderly women, to premenopausal levels is of the order of 10,000–20,000 IU daily in many cases and may be higher in some. These high doses increase the risk of hypercalcemia and hypercalciuria. Lower doses of vitamin D, e.g., 400-800 IU daily, are useful in preventing vitamin D deficiency and subclinical osteomalacia. At this time, little information is available on the use of the vitamin D metabolites in osteoporosis.

Although there is evidence that calcium deficiency will produce osteoporosis in animals, there is no clear-cut evidence that this occurs in humans. The recommended dietary allowance of calcium is 800 mg daily, with no distinction between young healthy adults and the elderly; however, it appears that the calcium requirements of young healthy adults vary between 7.5 and 12.5 mg/kg/day or 200 and 810 mg/day, whereas elderly adults require much higher doses of calcium (approaching 1,500 mg/day) to attain calcium balance. No consistent improvement has been produced with intravenous calcium infusions to osteoporotic patients. Calcium supplementation that produces a total calcium intake of 1,500 mg/day seems to slow the rate of bone loss and decrease the vertebral fracture rate. Adequate calcium in the diet depends on the consumption of foods that have a high calcium content, such as milk, yogurt, cheese, and ice cream. Many elderly individuals have a low dietary calcium intake and therefore need calcium supplementation. The calcium content of calcium preparations varies depending on the calcium salt, e.g., 9% for calcium gluconate, 13% for calcium lactate, and 40% for calcium carbonate. Therefore, 1 gm of calcium gluconate contains only 90 mg of elemental calcium, 1 gm of calcium lactate contains 130 mg of elemental calcium, and 1 gm of calcium carbonate contains 400 mg of elemental calcium. Calcium supplements should be administered in divided doses.

Fluoride. Sodium fluoride is a potent stimulator of bone formation and increases the trabecular bone density in some patients with osteoporosis. Doses of sodium fluoride approaching 40–60 mg/day, however, are needed to stimulate bone formation. Dietary calcium supplements (1,000 mg in divided doses) should be added to fluoride therapy to prevent fluoride-induced osteomalacia. High doses of vitamin D were initially included with fluoride therapy but are probably unnecessary and cause hypercalcemia and hypercalcuria. Some of the adverse effects of chronic fluoride therapy are abdominal distress, nausea, vomiting, anemia, periarticular pain, bursitis, a painful plantar fascia syndrome, and fluorosis. The fluoridic bone is abnormal chemically and by crystallographic analysis. The long-term efficacy and safety of sodium fluoride have not been established, and fluoride is still considered experimental in the treatment of osteoporosis.

Other Agents. Synthetic anabolic steroids have been used in osteoporosis for years, but their efficacy is limited by side effects, which include hirsutism, liver abnormalities, and decreases in high-density lipoproteins. Salmon calcitonin has been tried in osteoporosis with some short-term prevention of bone loss, but little information is available on the long-term effects. Low doses of human PTH-(1–34) fragment increase bone accretion and trabecular bone volume, but this treatment is experimental.

The treatment of osteoporosis in the elderly is particularly difficult, since by the time many individuals seek help, they already have fractures and a very low bone mass. Older patients are best managed by prescribing an adequate supply of calcium (1000–1500 mg/day) and ensuring adequate vitamin D supplies, either through exposure to sunlight or with vitamin supplementation (e.g., 400–800 IU/day). The use of other agents should be based on the full assessment of the individual's status.

---

1. Albanese AA, Edelson AH, Lorenze EJ, Woodhull ML, Wein EH: Problems of bone health in the elderly: Ten year study. *NY State J Med* 75:326–336, 1975.
   A daily calcium intake of 1,200 mg increased bone density during 3 years in 12 elderly women with a mean age of 80 years.
2. Aloia JF: Fluoride: Will it have a place in the treatment of postmenopausal osteoporosis? *Geriatr Med Today* 2:58–64, 1983.
   Discussion of the effects of sodium fluoride on bone mass and fracture incidence, indicating a need for further long-term studies to determine efficacy.
3. Aloia JF: Exercise and skeletal health. *J Am Geriatr Soc* 29:104–107, 1981.
   Immobilization and weightlessness accelerate bone loss, and exercise can help preserve bone mass in elderly subjects.
4. Avioli LV: Aging, bone, and osteoporosis, in Korenman SG (ed): *Endocrine Aspects of Aging.* New York, Elsevier, 1982, pp 199–230.
   General review.
5. Chestnut CH III, Baylink DJ: The role of anabolic steroids in the treatment of osteoporosis. *Geriatr Med Today* 2:21–30, 1983.
   Anabolic steroids may be beneficial for some women, but complications including hirsutism, fluid retention, liver abnormalities, and lowering of HDL levels prevent its long-term use.
6. Daniell HW: Osteoporosis of the slender smoker: Vertebral compression fractures and

loss of metacarpal cortex in relation to postmenopausal cigarette smoking and lack of obesity. *Arch Intern Med* 136:298–304, 1976.
Smoking may be another risk factor in postmenopausal bone loss.

7. DeLuca HF, Frost HM, Jee WSS, Johnston CC Jr, Parfitt AM (eds): *Osteoporosis: Recent Advances in Pathogenesis and Treatment.* Baltimore, University Park Press, 1981.
Proceedings of the tenth Steenbock symposium devoted entirely to osteoporosis.
8. Gallagher JC, et al: 1,25-Dihydroxyvitamin D_3: Short- and long-term effects on bone and calcium metabolism in patients with postmenopausal osteoporosis. *Proc Natl Acad Sci USA* 79:3325–3329, 1982.
A significant increase in trabecular bone volume was found on bone biopsy at the end of 2 years' treatment with 1,25–$(OH)_2$–D_3.
9. Gallagher JC, et al: Intestinal calcium absorption and serum vitamin D metabolites in normal subjects and osteoporotic patients: Effect of age and dietary calcium. *J Clin Invest* 64:729–736, 1979.
In postmenopausal osteoporotic women calcium absorption was lower than normal, serum 25-OH-D was normal but 1,25–$(OH)_2$–D levels were low, and calcium absorption increased after 7 days of 1,25–$(OH)_2$–D_3 therapy.
10. Gambrell RD Jr: The menopause: Benefits and risks of estrogen-progestogen replacement therapy. *Fertil Steril* 37:457–474, 1982.
General discussion about the effects of estrogens and progestogens on vasomotor symptoms, urogenital atrophy, psychosomatic complaints, bone loss, cardiovascular disease, lipid metabolism, endometrial cancer, breast cancer, coagulation, and gallbladder disease.
11. Gusberg SB: The changing nature of endometrial cancer. *N Engl J Med* 302:729–731, 1980.
Close monitoring of all women on estrogens is necessary, especially in those who are at high risk for developing endometrial cancer as indicated by obesity, infertility, dysfunctional bleeding, failure of ovulation, and long-term estrogen use.
12. Heaney RP, et al: Calcium nutrition and bone health in the elderly. *Am J Clin Nutr* 36:986–1013, 1982.
Review of the role of calcium in the attainment of the peak bone mass, factors that affect calcium metabolism (e.g., diet and drugs), and calcium requirements in the elderly.
13. Horsman A, Gallagher JC, Simpson M, Nordin BEC: Prospective trial of oestrogen and calcium in postmenopausal women. *Br Med J* 2:789–792, 1977.
Estrogen-treated group did not lose bone during 2 years of therapy, while bone loss in the calcium-treated group was intermediate between placebo- and estrogen-treated groups.
14. Judd HL, Meldrum DR, Deftos LJ, Henderson BE: Estrogen replacement therapy: Indications and complications. *Ann Intern Med* 98:195–205, 1983.
General discussion of effects of estrogens on bone loss, genitourinary problems, endometrial cancer, breast cancer, hypertension, thromboembolic disease, and lipid metabolism.
15. Lee CJ, Lawler GS, Johnson GH: Effects of supplementation of the diets with calcium and calcium-rich foods on bone density of elderly females with osteoporosis. *Am J Clin Nutr* 34:819–823, 1981.
Some elderly persons can benefit from supplementary calcium and calcium-rich foods to improve bone density.
16. Libow LS, Ross F, Goldberg K: "One tablet per day" for osteoporosis: Hypercalcemia. *Ann Intern Med* 81:120–121, 1974.
Vitamin D, 50,000 units daily, can produce hypercalcemia, especially if an elderly patient is also on a thiazide diuretic.
17. Lindsay R, Hart DM, Forrest C, Baird C: Prevention of spinal osteoporosis in oophorectomized women. *Lancet* 2:1151–1154, 1980.
Prospective controlled trial of estrogen therapy with median follow-up of 9 years indicated that estrogen treatment prevents bone loss and reduces the incidence of vertebral compression fractures.
18. Parfitt AM, et al: Vitamin D and bone health in the elderly. *Am J Clin Nutr* 36:1014–1031, 1982.
Review including discussions of the factors that affect vitamin D metabolism, vitamin

D deficiency in elderly patients, and the need for a higher daily requirement for vitamin D in the elderly, which perhaps should approach 600–800 IV per day.
19. Raisz LG: Osteoporosis. *J Am Geriatr Soc* 30:127–138, 1982.
General review.
20. Recker RR, Saville PD, Heaney RP: Effect of estrogens and calcium carbonate on bone loss in postmenopausal osteoporosis. *Ann Intern Med* 87:649–655, 1977.
Postmenopausal treatment with estrogen-androgen combination decreased age-related bone loss, while a total calcium intake of 1,500 mg/day also prevented bone loss but was less effective than the hormones.
21. Reeve J, et al: Anabolic effect of human parathyroid hormone fragment on trabecular bone in involutional osteoporosis: A multicentre trial. *Br Med J* 280:1340–1344, 1980.
An increase in trabecular bone volume and bone accretion after 6–8 months of treatment with low doses of human PTH-(1–34).
22. Riggs BL, Seeman E, Hodgson SF, Taves DR, O'Fallon WM: Effect of the fluoride/calcium regimen on vertebral fracture occurrence in postmenopausal osteoporosis: Comparison with conventional therapy. *N Engl J Med* 306:446–450, 1982.
Fluoride, calcium, or estrogen therapy significantly reduces fractures, but a combination of the three is most effective.
23. Riggs BL, et al: Changes in bone mineral density of the proximal femur and spine with aging: Differences between the postmenopausal and senile osteoporosis syndromes. *J Clin Invest* 70:716–723, 1982.
The authors feel that postmenopausal osteoporosis is characterized by excessive and disproportionate trabecular bone loss and vertebral fractures, while senile osteoporosis is characterized by proportionate loss of both cortical and trabecular bone and hip and/or vertebral fractures.
24. Slovik DM: The vitamin D endocrine system, calcium metabolism and osteoporosis. *Spec Top Endocrinol Metab* 5:83, 1983.
Review of the role that the vitamin D endocrine system and calcium metabolism have on the development and maintenance of bone mass, and the use of vitamin D, or its metabolites, and calcium for the treatment of osteoporosis.
25. Slovik DM, Adams JS, Neer RM, Holick MF, Potts JT Jr: Deficient production of 1,25-dihydroxyvitamin D in elderly osteoporotic patients. *N Engl J Med* 305:372–374, 1982.
The deficient production of 1,25-$(OH)_2$-D in elderly osteoporotic patients may explain the decreased ability of older individuals to adapt to low-calcium diets and play some role in the pathogenesis of age-related bone loss.
26. Smith EL Jr, Reddan W, Smith PE: Physical activity and calcium modalities for bone mineral increase in aged women. *Med Sci Sports Exerc* 13:60–64, 1981.
Bone loss in elderly women (mean age $>$ 80 years) may be reversed by physical activity.
27. Thomson DL, Frame B: Involutional osteopenia: Current concepts. *Ann Intern Med* 85:789–803, 1976.
General review including diagnostic evaluation, pathogenesis, and therapy.
28. Zerwekh JE, Sakhaee K, Glass K, Pak CYC: Long term 25-hydroxyvitamin D_3 therapy in postmenopausal osteoporosis: Demonstration of responsive and non-responsive subgroups. *J Clin Endocrinol Metab* 56:410–413, 1983.
In 5 of 12 patients treated with 25-OH-D_3 in a daily dose of 50 μg, there was no change in intestinal calcium absorption or 1,25-$(OH)_2$-D levels, indicating that in some patients with postmenopausal osteoporosis there is an impairment in the renal alpha-1-hydroxylase enzyme.

80. OSTEOMALACIA

David M. Slovik

Causes

Osteomalacia is caused by a group of disorders that produce a defect in the mineralization of the newly formed organic matrix of bone. Its most common cause in the elderly is a deficiency of vitamin D due to inadequate dietary intake, lack of exposure to sunlight, or malabsorption of vitamin D in association with gastrointestinal disease or after operation, e.g., gastrectomy. Osteomalacia may be caused also by abnormalities in vitamin D metabolism due to impairment of 25-hydroxylase activity in the liver or of 1-hydroxylase activity in the kidney. Drugs (e.g., diphenylhydantoin) may cause alterations in the metabolism of vitamin D or its metabolites. Chronic acidosis, chronic renal failure, phosphate depletion and hypophosphatemia (e.g., mesenchymal tumors), generalized renal tubular disorders, inhibitors of mineralization (e.g., disodium etidronate), and defective mineral synthesis (e.g., fibrogenesis imperfecta ossium), are other underlying disorders that cause osteomalacia.

Clinical Features

The clinical picture of osteomalacia in the elderly varies. Although often without clinical symptoms or with vague, ill-defined skeletal pain, diffuse skeletal pain and bone tenderness, especially in the ribs, pelvis, vertebrae, and lower extremities may be present. The pain is worsened by weight bearing. Pain and weakness around the hips lead to an antalgic gait. Proximal muscle weakness of varying degrees also occurs, mimicking primary muscle disorders and contributing to the waddling gait.

Roentgenographic Findings

The roentgenographic features of osteomalacia may be indistinguishable from those of osteoporosis. There is a variable decrease of bone density, loss of trabeculae, and some thinning of the cortices. The trabecular pattern may be blurred, producing a homogeneous ground-glass appearance. Radiolucent bands, also called *pseudofractures* or *Looser's zones,* are the most characteristic roentgenographic finding in osteomalacia. These bands are symmetric, usually perpendicular to the surface of the bone, and located most commonly along the inner aspects of the femur near the femoral neck, pubic rami, and outer edge of the scapula. They are caused by stress from the pressure of major arteries crossing the bone. Subperiosteal resorption of the phalanges may be evident and is due to secondary hyperparathyroidism.

Laboratory Findings

Abnormalities in laboratory findings depend on the underlying cause of osteomalacia. In vitamin D deficiency the characteristic findings are low or low-normal calcium and inorganic phosphate levels and low 25-hydroxyvitamin D (25-OH-D) concentrations. Other findings that help to identify osteomalacia include high blood parathyroid hormone and alkaline phosphatase levels and low urinary calcium values. Patients with renal tubular disorders characteristically have low serum inorganic phosphate concentrations but normal serum calcium concentrations and may have aminoaciduria, glycosuria, acidosis, and hypouricemia. Chronic renal failure with renal osteodystrophy causes hypocalcemia, hyperphosphatemia, secondary hyperparathyroidism, and acidosis. In severe malabsorption, other findings, e.g., hypomagnesemia, may be present.

Histologic evidence of osteomalacia includes an increase in the amount of bone surface covered by incompletely mineralized osteoid (both an increase in osteoid volume and thickness) and a decrease in the calcification rate. Osteomalacia may be present in as many as 15–20% of elderly patients with femoral neck fractures, although the incidence of osteomalacia varies with the diagnostic criteria used. Low values of 25-OH-D may also be found in up to one-third of elderly patients with hip fractures.

Treatment

The therapeutic approach to osteomalacia depends on the underlying disorder. In elderly persons, bone pain and muscle weakness, if due to osteomalacia, often may be ameliorated, while bone mass remains low due to the concomitant presence of age-related bone loss and osteoporosis.

Vitamin D Deficiency. Approximately 400–500 IU of vitamin D (either ergocalciferol, vitamin D_2, or cholecalciferol, vitamin D_3) will increase or maintain 25-OH-D concentrations in the normal range; however, the vitamin D requirement includes all sources of vitamin D, part or all of which may be supplied by exposure to sunlight. Osteomalacia from inadequate exposure to sunlight or dietary deficiency of vitamin D should be treated with vitamin D_2 or D_3 given orally, in doses of 2,000–4,000 IU/day for 6–8 weeks, followed by supplements of 400 IU/day. Administration of lower doses only, such as 400–800 IU/day, will also promote healing of osteomalacia but will take longer than if higher doses are given initially. Generally, healing of pseudofractures will become evident within 3–4 weeks, although total healing will take approximately 6 months. Adequate calcium (1,000 mg/day) should be provided.

Malabsorption. Treatment of osteomalacia caused by malabsorption requires doses of vitamin D much larger than those needed in nutritional vitamin D deficiency. Patients with steatorrhea require oral doses of vitamin D of 40,000–100,000 IU/day in addition to large doses of oral calcium supplements. Small doses of 1,25-$(OH)_2$-D_3 (0.5–2.0μg/day) and, in some cases, ultraviolet irradiation of the skin in a controlled setting will cure the osteomalacia. If high doses of vitamin D are continued after bone healing has occurred, hypercalcemia and hypercalciuria become a risk; there should therefore be close monitoring of the blood calcium and the 24-hour urinary excretion of calcium. As roentgenographic healing becomes evident, the dose of vitamin D may have to be decreased.

Anticonvulsants. Patients with osteomalacia due to anticonvulsants may need high doses of vitamin D, varying from 4,000 to 40,000 IU/day, along with 1,000–1,500 mg/day of calcium. If anticonvulsants are necessary on a chronic basis, probably 800–2,000 IU of vitamin D daily along with calcium supplementation will be adequate to prevent osteomalacia.

Renal Tubular Disorders. Osteomalacia and severe hypophosphatemia can develop with renal tubular disorders and require oral supplementation with phosphate. The amount of phosphate must be individualized, but patients may eventually require 1–4 gm/day of elemental phosphorus, in divided doses q4–6h. The initial dose should be low, to avoid gastrointestinal distress and diarrhea, and may be gradually increased as tolerated. The addition of vitamin D or the more potent metabolites such as 1,25-$(OH)_2$-D_3 may be necessary for bone healing. If chronic acidosis is present, alkali is necessary.

Renal Failure and Other Disorders. In chronic renal failure, high doses of vitamin D are necessary to correct the abnormalities caused by its deficiency. Inasmuch as 1,25-$(OH)_2$-D_3 does not require the kidney for its activity and is the most potent agent to use to increase intestinal calcium absorption, it is the vitamin D preparation of choice for patients with chronic renal failure and renal osteodystrophy. It should be given in doses of 0.25–1.0 μg/day, with close monitoring of the serum calcium, as hypercalcemia can develop rapidly. Osteomalacia can develop with disodium etidronate (EHDP) therapy of Paget's disease, especially when high doses are administered. Low doses, e.g., 5 mg/kg BW/day, should be given; but even with this dosage mineralization defects may be seen. Osteomalacia can also develop during fluoride therapy for osteoporosis, and therefore calcium supplements of approximately 1,000–1,500 mg/day should be added to the fluoride regimen.

1. Aaron JE, et al: Frequency of osteomalacia and osteoporosis in fractures of the proximal femur. *Lancet* 1:229–233, 1974.
   Osteomalacia attributable to vitamin D deficiency is an important factor in the increase in femoral neck fractures with advancing age in the United Kingdom.
2. Anwar M: Nutritional hypovitaminosis-D and the genesis of osteomalacia in the elderly. *J Am Geriatr Soc* 26:309–317, 1978.
   Elderly individuals at high risk for developing nutritional vitamin D deficiency are those who have severe disabilities, mental illness, or dental problems; or are isolated, self-neglecting, or alcoholic.
3. Baker MR, McDonnell H, Peacock M, Nordin BEC: Plasma 25-hydroxyvitamin D concentrations in patients with fractures of the femoral neck. *Br Med J* 1:589, 1979.
   Of patients with fractures of the femoral neck, 40% had 25-OH-D levels below 10 ng/ml, the level below which most cases of histologic osteomalacia occur.
4. Corless D, et al: Response of plasma 25-hydroxyvitamin D to ultraviolet irradiation in long-stay geriatric patients. *Lancet* 2:649–651, 1978.
   Artificial UV irradiation increases plasma 25-OH-D levels in elderly female subjects.
5. Frame B, Parfitt AM: Osteomalacia: Current concepts. *Ann Intern Med* 89:966–982, 1978.
   General review.
6. Garry PJ, Goodwin JS, Hunt WC, Hooper EM, Leonard AG: Nutritional status in a healthy elderly population: Dietary and supplemental intakes. *Am J Clin Nutr* 36:319–331, 1982.

In a healthy, physically active population, vitamin D and calcium intakes were low, especially in women.

7. Justice CL, Howe JM, Clark HE: Dietary intakes and nutritional status of elderly patients. *J Am Diet Assoc* 65:639–646, 1974.
Most of these elderly patients consumed less calcium than any other nutrient.
8. Lips P, et al: Histomorphometric profile and vitamin D status in patients with femoral neck fracture. *Metab Bone Dis Relat Res* 4:85–93, 1982.
Serum concentrations of 25-OH-D, 24,25-$(OH)_2$-D, and 1,25-$(OH)_2$-D were lower in patients with femoral neck fractures than in age-matched controls, and there was a subgroup of patients with an increase in relative osteoid volume and surface.
9. MacLennan WJ, Hamilton JC: Vitamin D supplements and 25-hydroxy vitamin D concentrations in the elderly. *Br Med J* 2:859–861, 1977.
A daily dose of 500 IU of vitamin D produced a significant increase in 25-OH-D within 2 months, and is probably adequate in most elderly people to produce 25-OH-D levels sufficient to protect against osteomalacia.
10. Meredith SC, Rosenberg IH: Gastrointestinal-hepatic disorders and osteomalacia. *Clin Endocrinol Metab* 9:131–150, 1980.
Discussions of the roles that gastrointestinal disorders including gastric surgery, Crohn's disease, coeliac disease, pancreatic insufficiency, and jejunoileal bypass surgery, and liver diseases including cirrhosis and cholestatic liver disease have in the development of osteomalacia.
11. Omdahl JL, Garry PJ, Hunsaker LA, Hunt WC, Goodwin JS: Nutritional status in a healthy elderly population: Vitamin D. *Am J Clin Nutr* 36:1125–1133, 1982.
Greater than half of the subjects consumed less than the recommended dietary allowance for calcium and vitamin D.
12. Schlott GD, Wills MR: Muscle weakness in osteomalacia. *Lancet* 1:626–629, 1976.
Muscle weakness frequently accompanies osteomalacia, is predominantly proximal in nature, may be asymmetric, and leads to a waddling gait.
13. Snell AP, MacLennan WJ, Hamilton JC: Ultra-violet irradiation and 25-hydroxyvitamin D levels in sick old people. *Age Ageing* 7:225–228, 1978.
UV irradiation produced significant increases in plasma 25-OH-D levels by the end of the second week and can correct vitamin D deficiency in the elderly.
14. Stamp TCB: The clinical endocrinology of vitamin D, in Parsons JA, (ed): *Endocrinology of Calcium Metabolism.* New York, Raven Press, 1982, pp 363–422.
General review.
15. Toss G, Andersson R, Diffey BL, Fall PA, Larko O, Larsson L: Oral vitamin D and ultraviolet radiation for the prevention of vitamin D deficiency in the elderly. *Acta Med Scand* 212:157–161, 1982.
Although brief exposures to UV irradiation can prevent vitamin D deficiency, it is no more effective than oral vitamin D supplementation and is more time consuming.
16. Weisman Y, Salama R, Harell A, Edelstein S: Serum 24,25-dihydroxyvitamin D and 25-hydroxyvitamin D concentrations in femoral neck fractures. *Br Med J* 2:1196–1197, 1978.
No significant differences in the mean 25-OH-D and 24,25-$(OH)_2$-D levels of elderly patients with femoral neck fractures and elderly controls were found.
17. Barzel US: Vitamin D deficiency: A risk factor for osteomalacia in the aged. *J Am Geriatr Soc* 31:598–601, 1983.
In elderly persons who do not receive sunlight, drink milk, or take supplemental vitamins, vitamin D deficiency is common and physiologic replacement doses of vitamin D should be given.
18. Eddy RL: Metabolic bone disease after gastrectomy. *Am J Med* 50:442–449, 1971.
Osteomalacia may be present in 25% of postgastrectomy patients.

81. PAGET'S DISEASE OF BONE

David M. Slovik

Paget's disease of bone (osteitis deformans), rarely seen in individuals younger than 40 years of age, is a disorder characterized by excessive bone turnover in localized areas of the skeleton. It is estimated that 1–3% of the population over the age of 50 has the disease, even though it may be totally asymptomatic and detectable only with wide-scale screening techniques. The incidence increases with advancing age and is highest in western Europe, Australia, New Zealand, and the United States. The incidence is very low in Japan, the Middle East, India, and Scandinavia. Males appear to be affected slightly more often than females, and occasionally several family members are affected. Although the cause of Paget's disease is unclear, in recent years nuclear inclusion bodies have been found in osteoclasts from bone biopsies, suggesting a viral etiology.

Bone Involvement

The clinical features of Paget's disease are the result of a disorderly remodeling process. In the earliest phase of Paget's disease, bone resorption predominates, and osteoclastic activity produces focal areas of bone resorption. An increase in bone formation follows, as the osteoblasts lay down new bone in an irregular manner. During the second phase there is mixed osteoclastic and osteoblastic activity, and fibrous tissue and vascularity increase in the adjacent bone marrow. In the third *(sclerotic)* phase osteolytic activity decreases, and the bone becomes more dense and sclerotic. The disorderly remodeling process produces bone that is structurally weak, fractures easily, and causes physical deformities.

Paget's disease may involve one bone (monostotic) or multiple bones (polyostotic). The sites most commonly affected are the pelvis, sacrum, skull, spine, femur, and tibia. Approximately 25% of patients are symptomatic, although the clinical symptoms vary.

Skull. The osteolytic process in the skull is termed *osteoporosis circumscripta*. The subsequent osteoblastic reaction that causes thickening and enlargement of the skull is most prominent in the frontal and occipital areas. Cranial nerve encroachments occur with skull involvement, with the eighth cranial nerve most frequently affected. Up to 50% of patients with skull involvement have hearing loss; tinnitus and vertigo occur less frequently. Hearing loss may be mistaken for the expected decrease in hearing that occurs with advancing age, and the tinnitus and vertigo may be misinterpreted as arising from labyrinthine disorders. The other cranial nerves may be involved, and some patients have optic atrophy, extraocular muscle palsies, and diplopia. With extensive involvement there may be softening of the base of the skull, producing flattening known as *basilar impression,* or *platybasia*. Compression of the brainstem, spinal cord, cerebellum, and other contiguous structures produces neurologic findings. These include dysphagia, dysarthria, pharyngeal and lingual muscle weakness, ataxia, cerebellar signs, and pyramidal tract signs. Hydrocephalus can develop, and Valsalva maneuver–induced cranial pain from partial obstruction of the cerebrospinal fluid flow in the region of the medullary-cervical junction can occur. A pagetic "steal syndrome," in which blood is shunted from the internal carotid system into the highly vascular bone, may cause neurologic symptoms. Paget's disease can affect the spine, most frequently the lumbosacral area. Spinal cord and nerve root compression can develop slowly.

Pelvis and Extremities. Involvement of the pelvis and extremities leads to significant musculoskeletal abnormalities. Involvement of the acetabulum and femoral head narrows the joint space and limits motion. Protrusio acetabuli develops with more extensive disease. The femur is the most commonly affected of the long bones, although any long bone can be involved, especially with widespread disease. Involvement of the pelvis, proximal femur, and femoral head produces degenerative arthritis of the hip. Involvement of the distal portion of the femur produces degenerative arthritis of the knee. The arthritis causes pain, which is worse on weight bearing. Bowing of the femur and tibia can be seen grossly in some patients. Fewer symptoms are felt in the upper extremities, even with extensive disease, because there is no stress of weight bearing. The small bones of the hands and feet and the facial bones are usually spared, unless widespread disease is present. The mandible and maxilla are sometimes included in extensive facial bone involvement, causing an appearance known as *leontiasis ossea*.

Because the new bone is abnormal, patients with Paget's disease are susceptible to fractures involving both the long bones and the vertebrae. Patients have incomplete small fissure fractures as well as complete transverse fractures of the long bones. Fractures of the femur are most common.

Complications

Cardiovascular complications, including cardiomegaly and high-output congestive heart failure, occasionally occur but are not common, and congestive heart failure in patients with Paget's disease usually arises from coronary artery disease.

Hypercalciuria and urolithiasis develop during periods of increased bone resorptive activity and immobilization. Bone tumors also develop in patients with Paget's disease. The overall incidence of osteogenic sarcomas in patients with Paget's disease is probably about 1%; malignant changes are rare before age 50, but their likelihood increases with duration and extent of disease. However, Paget's disease is found in approximately 15–20% of patients with osteogenic sarcoma. The long bones, pelvis, and skull are most commonly involved, whereas vertebral involvement is rare. A sudden increase in bone pain is suggestive of malignant degeneration. The diagnosis is supported by a rapid rise in the serum alkaline phosphatase, roentgenographic evidence of destruction of the trabeculae, or a soft tissue tumor. The prognosis is very poor for these tumors. Benign giant cell tumors also develop in Paget's disease. Although the tumor is histologically benign, it can cause significant problems from local growth.

Diagnostic Evidence

Roentgenographic evidence of Paget's disease in the skull includes enlargement with thickening of the inner and outer table, chaotic deposition of bone (cotton-wool appearance), and basilar impression. Roentgenographic findings in other bones include coarsening of the trabeculae, thickening of the cortex in the long bones, and bone enlargement and deformity. Occasionally the roentgenogram shows osteolytic lesions characterized by osteoporosis circumscripta of the skull or a lytic wedge in the long bones. Osteoblastic or mixed osteoblastic-lytic metastases from prostatic or breast carcinoma may present a similar roentgenographic appearance, making the diagnosis difficult.

The diagnosis of Paget's disease in patients with the characteristic roentgenographic findings is confirmed by an elevation in serum alkaline phosphatase activity and urinary hydroxyproline excretion. Bone scans establish the extent of the disease but will give no information concerning the architecture of the lesions.

Treatment

Most patients (approximately 75%) with Paget's disease are asymptomatic and therefore require no specific therapy. Those who have mild or minimal disease require only analgesics and antiinflammatory agents. Patients with more extensive and symptomatic disease need specific therapy.

Indications. Indications for specific drug treatment are:

1. Moderate or severe disabling pain, corresponding to areas of known Paget's involvement, that is unrelieved by analgesics or antiinflammatory drugs
2. Progressive skeletal involvement with deformity and complications
3. Progressive hearing loss
4. Extensive resorptive disease
5. Neurologic complications
6. High-output cardiac failure
7. Preparation for a surgical procedure on pagetic bone
8. Prolonged immobilization
9. Hypercalcemia, renal stones, and hyperuricemia and gout, all due to Paget's disease

Drugs. Drug inhibitors of bone resorption that are used to treat Paget's disease are salmon calcitonin, disodium etidronate (EHDP), and mithramycin. Salmon calcitonin produces a decrease in the clinical and biochemical abnormalities of Paget's disease in 80% of cases treated. Clinical improvement is usually evident 2–8 weeks after initiation of treatment. Most patients reach a clinical and biochemical plateau, while some show a gradual drift upward in the biochemical parameters, despite continuation of calcitonin therapy. The dose of synthetic salmon calcitonin varies from 100 MRC units daily to 50 MRC units 3 times weekly. Many patients treated with calcitonin develop antibodies to calcitonin although only a small percentage of these patients will become clinically resistant.

EHDP, a diphosphonate, is administered in a dose of 5 mg/kg/day for up to 6 months. In responsive patients the clinical and biochemical improvement is usually complete within 6 months. EHDP also inhibits bone mineralization, and although this inhibition may occur at the 5 mg/kg/day dose, it is more likely to occur with higher doses. Since EHDP is excreted by the kidney, it should be administered with caution, if at all, to patients with renal failure because of possible excessive skeletal retention.

Mithramycin is usually administered in a dose of 25 μg/kg BW and infused over a period of 6–8 hours for 10 days. A rapid biochemical and clinical response is evident, even within a few days of the institution of therapy; however, gastrointestinal, hepatic, renal, and hematologic abnormalities, which are usually transient, limit its efficacy. Mithramycin is therefore reserved for patients with severe and symptomatic disease that is unresponsive to treatment with calcitonin and EHDP.

1. Altman RD, Singer F (eds): Proceedings of the Kroc Foundation Conference on Paget's disease of bone. *Arthritis Rheum* 23:1073–1240, 1980.
An entire issue devoted to Paget's disease, with several articles describing therapeutic agents including calcitonin, diphosphonates (EHDP, APD, and $C1_2MDP$), and mithramycin.
2. Bijvoet OLM, Hosking DJ, Frijlink WB, Te Velder J, Vellenga CJLR: Treatment of Paget's disease with combined calcitonin and diphosphonate (EHDP). *Metab Bone Dis Relat Res* 1:251–261, 1978.
A combination of EHDP and calcitonin produced complete biochemical remission in 25 of 30 patients treated for 6–12 months.
3. Chakravorty NK: Some unusual features of Paget's disease of bone. *Gerontology* 24:459–472, 1978.
Less common neurologic features include platybasia with neurologic deficit; involvement of second, fifth, and seventh cranial nerves; hydrocephalus; dementia; and dysphasia.
4. Feldman RG, Culebras A, Schmidek HH: Paget's disease and the nervous system. *J Am Geriatr Soc* 27:1–8, 1979.
Neurologic symptoms are related to skull, cranial nerve, spinal cord, and nerve root involvement.
5. Franck WA, Bress NM, Singer FR, Krane SM: Rheumatic manifestations of Paget's disease of bone. *Am J Med* 56:592–603, 1974.
Rheumatic problems not attributable to Paget's disease but frequently seen in patients with Paget's disease include gout, calcific periarthritis, and rheumatoid arthritis and its variant syndromes.
6. Henley JW, Croxson RS, Ibbertson HK: The cardiovascular system in Paget's disease of bone and the response to therapy with calcitonin and diphosphonate. *Aust NZ J Med* 9:390–397, 1979.
Before treatment, the cardiac index was elevated in 27 of 39 patients with Paget's disease of bone and there was a direct correlation between cardiac index, alkaline phosphatase, urine hydroxyproline and percentage skeletal uptake. After treatment with either diphosphonate or calcitonin, there was a fall in cardiac index in 17 of 18 patients.
7. Ibbertson HK, et al: Paget's disease of bone—clinical evaluation and treatment with diphosphonate. *Aust NZ J Med* 9:31–35, 1979.
Six-month treatment of Paget's disease with EHDP produced a mean reduction in serum alkaline phosphatase and urine hydroxyproline of 79% and 81%, respectively.
8. Krane SM: Etidronate disodium in the treatment of Paget's disease of bone. *Ann Intern Med* 96:619–625, 1982.
General discussion of the therapeutic uses and adverse effects of EHDP in Paget's disease.
9. MacIntyre I, Evans IMA, Hobitz HHG, Joplin GF, Stevenson JC: Chemistry, physiology, and therapeutic applications of calcitonin. *Arthritis Rheum* 23:1139–1147, 1980.
Review of chemistry, physiology, and therapeutic use of calcitonin.
10. Martin TJ: Treatment of Paget's disease with the calcitonins. *Aust NZ J Med* 9:36–43, 1979.
Discusses indications for calcitonin treatment in Paget's disease.

11. Ouslander JG, Beck JC: Paget's disease of bone. *J Am Geriatr Soc* 30:410–414, 1982.
General review.
12. Posen S, Clifton-Bligh P, Wilkinson M: Paget's disease of bone and hyperparathyroidism: Coincidence or causal relationship? *Calcif Tissue Int* 26:107–109, 1978.
Of 173 patients with Paget's disease and 105 patients with primary hyperparathyroidism, 9 patients were found to have both disorders.
13. Ryan WG, Schwartz TB: Mithramycin treatment of Paget's disease of bone. *Arthritis Rheum* 23:1155–1161, 1980.
During a 10-day course of mithramycin (15–25 μg/kg BW/day as a 12–24 hour infusion), there is typically a 60% reduction in serum alkaline phosphatase and usually a continued decline in the next month or two to a level approximately 25% of the pretreatment value.
14. Singer FR: *Paget's Disease of Bone*. New York, Plenum, 1977.
Book devoted entirely to Paget's disease.
15. Wallach S: Treatment of Paget's disease. *Adv Intern Med* 27:1–43, 1982.
Review with emphasis on clinical aspects and therapy.

XI. RENAL AND METABOLIC DISEASES

82. MINERAL-ION HOMEOSTASIS AND CALCIUM-REGULATING HORMONES

David M. Slovik

Abnormalities in mineral-ion metabolism and calcium-regulating hormones are common in the elderly and may have marked clinical effects.

Calcium

Over 99% of the total body calcium is located in the skeleton, and only about 1% of this is freely exchangeable with extracellular fluid. Approximately 46% of the total circulating calcium is protein-bound, primarily to albumin. About 48% circulates unbound in free or ionized form and is the fraction of calcium that is physiologically important. The remainder circulates complexed to other anions, e.g., citrate and phosphate. The normal range of serum calcium is about 8.5–10.4 mg/dl. Homeostatic calcium regulation involves changes in calcium fluxes in the intestine, bone, and urine and acts primarily through changes in parathyroid hormone (PTH) and 1,25-dihydroxycitamin D (1,25-$[OH]_2$-D). Intestinal calcium absorption is increased by PTH, which acts indirectly through 1,25-$(OH)_2$-D production; calcium mobilization from the skeleton is increased by both PTH and 1,25-$(OH)_2$-D, which act synergistically; and calcium resorption from the renal tubule is directly increased by PTH.

With advancing age, blood calcium levels decrease in normal males in parallel with a fall in serum albumin levels. In women, a slight rise in the serum calcium level occurs in the postmenopausal period, but the level then stabilizes or falls with advancing age. The ionized fraction of calcium changes little, if at all, up to age 60; it then may show a fall. Urinary calcium excretion is higher in postmenopausal women than in premenopausal women. The absolute increase in urinary calcium excretion may be slight and usually remains within the normal range; the difference is most obvious when expressed as a ratio of the fasting urinary calcium to creatinine. With advancing age there is a decrease in dietary calcium intake and intestinal calcium absorption in both sexes, which is most evident after the age 60. Normal individuals over age 60, unlike young normal individuals, are unable to adapt to a low-calcium diet by sufficiently increasing intestinal calcium absorption. The decreased intestinal absorption of calcium and the diminished adaptive ability of the elderly may be due to decreased production of 1,25-$(OH)_2$-D. Dietary calcium intakes approaching 1,500 mg/day may be necessary to maintain calcium balance in elderly women.

Phosphate

Approximately 85% of the total body content of phosphate is found in the mineral phase of bone, primarily as hydroxyapatite. The remaining 15% is found in muscle and soft tissue as an integral part of organic compounds. In contrast to calcium only 12% of phosphate is protein-bound; the remainder existing in the free state or complexed with other cations. Serum phosphate concentrations show a diurnal rhythm, with the nadir between 8:00 and 11:00 A.M. Carbohydrate ingestion lowers serum phosphate concentration by causing a shift of phosphate into cells. The intestinal absorption of phosphate is very efficient and averages 70% with a normal phosphate intake. The kidney regulates phosphate, and the daily urinary phosphate excretion approximates the net intestinal phosphate absorption. The tubular resorption of phosphate is normally between 85% and 95% of the filtered load. In normal males, phosphate concentrations decrease with advancing age. In women, serum phosphate levels rise after age 50 and are significantly higher in postmenopausal women than in premenopausal women. Dietary restriction of phosphate alone will not cause phosphate depletion, but depletion may occur in the elderly person with phosphate restriction who also ingests nonabsorbable antacids, which bind phosphate in the intestine. The daily urinary excretion of phosphate falls progressively with age, perhaps owing in part to decreased intake and absorption of phosphate. The TmP/GFR is higher in postmenopausal than in premenopausal women.

Magnesium

Of the total body magnesium content of 2,000 mEq, 50–65% is found in bone, with the remainder divided between muscle (15–20%) and other soft tissues. Approximately 55% of plasma magnesium circulates in the ionized form, whereas 33% is protein-bound, and the remainder usually complexes with various anions. Magnesium is primarily an intracellular ion that is important in many enzyme systems and cellular metabolic processes. Magnesium is absorbed primarily in the small intestine, although colonic absorption can occur. Its urinary excretion depends on dietary intake and intestinal absorption. Urinary magnesium losses fall to less than 1 mEq/day during magnesium deprevation, if renal function is normal. Little information is available concerning magnesium homeostasis in elderly individuals. Serum and urinary magnesium levels are higher in postmenopausal than in premenopausal women.

Parathyroid Hormone and Calcium Regulation

Parathyroid hormone is an 84-amino-acid single-chain polypeptide that is synthesized from precursors (Pre-ProPTH and ProPTH). The precursor forms are rapidly cleaved to produce the intact hormone, which is then secreted and undergoes peripheral metabolism, primarily in the liver and kidney. Decreases in the ionized fraction of the blood calcium stimulate the synthesis and secretion of PTH. At the target-tissue level, PTH acts by the stimulation of adenyl cyclase with subsequent generation of 3′5′ cyclic AMP. The principal actions of PTH are (1) acutely, to mobilize calcium from bone in response to decreases in serum calcium levels, and, chronically, to act on bone remodeling; (2) to stimulate intestinal calcium absorption, which is mediated through the production of 1,25-$(OH)_2$-D; and (3) to increase calcium and decrease phosphate resorption in the kidneys. With increasing age, immunoreactive PTH levels increase. This progressive rise has been assessed primarily by measurements of the biologically inactive carboxy-terminal fragment, and the small increase in PTH levels with aging may be partly due to a decrease in the glomerular filtration rate.

Vitamin D and Calcium Regulation

Vitamin D refers to a group of compounds with antirachitic properties. Previtamin D is formed from 7-dehydrocholesterol (7-DHC) in the epidermis, when it is exposed to ultraviolet radiation in the range of 290–320 nm, and is then converted to vitamin D_3. Ergocalciferol (vitamin D_2) is derived from the ultraviolet irradiation of the plant steroid, ergosterol, whereas cholecalciferol (vitamin D_3) is derived from 7-DHC in animal tissues. Vitamin D_3 synthesized in the skin, and vitamin D_2 or D_3 taken orally, are bound to a vitamin D–binding protein and transported to the liver, where 25-hydroxylation occurs and 25-hydroxyvitamin D (25-OH-D) is formed. The 25-OH-D is then transported to the kidney, where it is further hydroxylated to produce either 1,25-$(OH)_2$-D or 24,25-$(OH)_2$-D. The kidney enzyme, 25-hydroxyvitamin D_1–hydroxylase, is tightly regulated in comparison with the liver 25-hydroxylase. PTH and hypophosphatemia are the main factors that stimulate kidney 1-hydroxylase activity. The 25-OH-D is the major circulating vitamin D metabolite, and the 1,25-$(OH)_2$-D is the most active metabolite of vitamin D in stimulating intestinal calcium absorption and bone calcium mobilization.

Any reduction in the exposure of the skin to sunlight will diminish endogenous vitamin D_3 synthesis—including environmental and atmospheric factors such as cloud covering, ozone, pollutants, or even ordinary window glass. Circulating 25-OH-D concentrations show seasonal variations in normal individuals, who have the highest values in late summer through early autumn and the lowest values in winter. Plasma concentrations of 25-OH-D are significantly lower in elderly persons than in young, healthy persons, and especially in elderly persons who are chronically ill, house-bound, institutionalized, indigent, and poorly nourished. Even though there may be seasonal variation in 25-OH-D concentrations, the variation in the elderly is significantly less than it is in younger individuals. Increases in 25-OH-D concentration and intestinal calcium absorption can be produced in the elderly by administering ultraviolet radiation through artificial lighting. Interference with the intestinal absorption of vitamin D may also cause vitamin D deficiency, e.g., after a gastrectomy or a jejunoileal bypass or in medical conditions associated with malabsorption, steatorrhea, and liver disease, particularly in patients with bilary obstruction and bile salt abnormalities. Advanced renal insufficiency impairs the conversion of 25-OH-D to 1,25-$(OH)_2$-D. In addition, many elderly persons and patients with postmenopausal osteoporosis have low serum 1,25-$(OH)_2$-D levels and decreased production of 1,25-$(OH)_2$-D. Drugs may also adversely affect mineral-ion metabolism. Anticonvulsants can alter vitamin D metabolism, presumably by inducing hepatic microsomal enzymes that subsequently convert vitamin D and 25-OH-D to inactive polar metabolites. It now appears that these drugs also have direct effects on the bone and intestine. Glucocorticoids decrease intestinal calcium absorption and cause significant bone loss, but their relation to vitamin D and PTH is unclear.

Calcitonin

Calcitonin is a 32-amino-acid single-chain polypeptide hormone produced by the parafollicular cells of the thyroid gland. Its physiologic role in normal mineral homeostasis is uncertain. Its apparent major importance in humans lies in the detection of elevated levels characteristic of medullary carcinoma of the thyroid and in the treatment of Paget's disease and hypercalcemia. With advancing age, there is a progressive decrease in plasma calcitonin concentrations and the calcitonin response to intravenous calcium infusions.

---

1. Aitken JM, Gallagher MJD, Hart DM, Newton DAG, Craig A: Plasma growth hormone and serum phosphorus concentrations in relation to the menopause and to oestrogen therapy. *J Endocrinol* 59:593–598, 1973.
   An increase in serum inorganic phosphate was seen in postmenopausal women.
2. Allen LH: Calcium bioavailability and absorption: A review. *Am J Clin Nutr* 35:783–808, 1982.
   Good review, including discussion of (1) techniques used to measure calcium absorption, (2) physiology of calcium absorption, and (3) effects of dietary components, physiologic factors, and aging on calcium absorption.
3. Barragry JM, et al: Intestinal cholecalciferol absorption in the elderly and in younger adults. *Clin Sci* 55:213–220, 1978.
   Suggests that cholecalciferol absorption is reduced in the elderly.
4. Bulusu L, Hodgkinson A, Nordin BEC, Peacock M: Urinary excretion of calcium and creatinine in relation to age and body weight in normal subjects and patients with renal calculus. *Clin Sci* 38:601–612, 1970.
   The 24-hour urine calcium-creatinine ratio rose in women during the fifth and sixth decades.
5. Crilly RG, Francis RM, Nordin BEC: Steroid hormones, ageing and bone. *Clin Endocrinol Metab* 10:115–139, 1981.
   Discussion of hormonal changes and the effects of the menopause on bone and calcium metabolism.
6. Davie M, Lawson DEM: Assessment of plasma 25-hydroxyvitamin D response to ultraviolet irradiation over a controlled area in young and elderly subjects. *Clin Sci* 58:235–242, 1980.
   Young and elderly subjects respond similarly to artificial UV irradiation.
7. Deftos LJ, et al: Influence of age and sex on plasma calcitonin in human beings. *N Engl J Med* 302:1351–1353, 1980.
   There is a progressive decrease with age in basal calcitonin levels and the calcitonin response to an intravenous calcium infusion.
8. Epstein S, Van Mieghem W, Sagel J, Jackson WPU: Effect of single large doses of oral calcium on serum calcium levels in the young and the elderly. *Metabolism* 22:1163–1173, 1973.
   The rise in blood calcium levels after 4 gm of elemental calcium was lower in the elderly than that in younger subjects.
9. Gallagher JC, et al: Intestinal calcium absorption and serum vitamin D metabolites in normal subjects and osteoporotic patients: Effect of age and dietary calcium. *J Clin Invest* 64:729–736, 1979.
   Finds a decrease in 1,25–$(OH)_2$–D levels in elderly normal subjects.
10. Gallagher JC, Riggs BL, Jerpbak CM, Arnaud CD: The effect of age on serum immunoreactive parathyroid hormone in normal and osteoporotic women. *J Lab Clin Med* 95:373–385, 1980.
    Notes a significant increase in iPTH levels with age that was more pronounced with an antiserum that measured circulating carboxyl fragments rather than intact PTH.
11. Heaney RP, Recker RR, Saville PD: Menopausal changes in calcium balance performance. *J Lab Clin Med* 92:953–970, 1978.
    Estrogen-deficient postmenopausal women need 500 mg more dietary calcium (approximately 1,500 mg total calcium) to achieve zero balance than do premenopausal and estrogen-treated postmenopausal women.

12. Insongna KL, Lewis AM, Lipinski BA, Bryant C, Baran DT: Effect of age on serum immunoreactive parathyroid hormone and its biological effects. *J Clin Endocrinol Metab* 53:1072–1075, 1981.
The increased iPTH levels seen with aging also indicate biologically active PTH as nephrogenous cyclic AMP was increased and TmP/GFR was decreased in elderly healthy subjects.
13. Ireland PI, Fordtran JS: Effect of dietary calcium and age on jejunal calcium absorption in humans studied by intestinal perfusion. *J Clin Invest* 52:2672–2681, 1973.
Young subjects adapt better to a low calcium diet than do older subjects.
14. Keating FR Jr, Jones JD, Elveback LR, Randall RV: The relation of age and sex to distribution of values in healthy adults of serum calcium, inorganic phosphorus, magnesium, alkaline phosphatase, total proteins, albumin and blood urea. *J Lab Clin Med* 73:825–834, 1969.
Finds a decrease in serum calcium and phosphate but not magnesium levels with age in 298 healthy men.
15. Lester E, Skinner RK, Wills MR: Seasonal variation in serum 25-hydroxyvitamin-D in the elderly in Britain. *Lancet* 1:979–980, 1977.
Serum 25-OH-D levels were lower and showed less seasonal variation in elderly subjects compared to young adults.
16. Lindgarde F: Potentiometric determination of serum ionized calcium in a normal human population. *Clin Chim Acta* 40:477–484, 1972.
Notes a significant decrease in ionized calcium in both sexes and total calcium in men with advancing age.
17. Lindsay R, Hart DM, Forrest C: Effect of a natural and artificial menopause on serum, urinary and erythrocyte magnesium. *Clin Sci* 58:255–257, 1980.
Postmenopausal women have significantly higher serum and urinary magnesium levels than do premenopausal women, suggesting an increase in bone remodeling.
18. Neer RM, et al: Stimulation by artificial lighting of calcium absorption in elderly human subjects. *Nature* 229:255–257, 1971.
Ultraviolet light supplied from artificial lighting can significantly increase calcium absorption in elderly men.
19. Slovik DM: The vitamin D endocrine system, calcium metabolism and osteoporosis. *Spec Top Endocrinol Metab* 5:83–148, 1983.
Review of changes seen in vitamin D metabolism and calcium metabolism in elderly persons.
20. Slovik DM, Adams JS, Neer RM, Holick MF, Potts JT Jr: Deficient production of 1,25-dihydroxyvitamin D in elderly osteoporotic patients. *N Engl J Med* 305:372–374, 1981.
In response to a 24-hour intravenous infusion of human PTH–(1–34) fragment, elderly osteoporotic patients were unable to increase 1,25–$(OH)_2$–D secretion as well as younger normal subjects, and this deficient 1,25–$(OH)_2$–D production may explain the inability of elderly osteoporotic patients to adapt to low-calcium diets.
21. Weisman Y, Schen RJ, Eisenberg Z, Edelstein S, Harell A: Inadequate status and impaired metabolism of vitamin D in the elderly. *Isr J Med Sci* 17:19–21, 1981.
Serum 25-OH-D and 24,25–$(OH)_2$–D levels were lower in elderly subjects compared with younger subjects, and intestinal absorption of 25-OH-D is impaired in many old people.

83. AZOTEMIA IN THE ELDERLY

Leslie Fang

Symptoms

Azotemia or elevated blood urea nitrogen (BUN) in the elderly is associated with prominent systemic symptoms such as anorexia, easy fatigability, weakness, nausea, vomiting, diarrhea, and constipation. The most important clinical signs in the elderly are neurologic, however. Increasing lassitude, drowsiness, and disorientation, which are more severe in elderly patients than in younger patients, may be misconstrued as a primary neurologic illness.

Prerenal Azotemia

Prerenal azotemia occurs particularly in the elderly because of their marginal level of hydration and impaired cardiac function. Many elderly patients also receive medications that aggravate prerenal azotemia. The clinical presentation of prerenal azotemia falls into one of four major etiologic categories: hypovolemia, impaired cardiac output, peripheral vasodilatation, and increased renal vascular resistance. Prerenal azotemia is caused most frequently in the elderly by severe congestive heart failure, diuretic excess, gastrointestinal bleeding, gastrointestinal fluid losses, and high-protein tube feedings. Vasodilators also causes prerenal azotemia.

The physical examination in patients with azotemia should concentrate on the cardiac and volume status. Since blood in the gastrointestinal tract can accentuate prerenal azotemia, a positive finding on the stool guaiac test sometimes explains the azotemia.

Separating Prerenal from Renal Azotemia. It is important to differentiate between prerenal and renal disorders, because the management of the two disorders is quite different. In addition to the clinical clues, the ratio of BUN to creatinine and certain urinary indices is extremely helpful. In prerenal azotemia the BUN/Creat ratio is greater than 10 : 1, and the urinary sediment is normal: the urinary sodium concentration is usually less than 10 mEq/liter, and the urinary osmolality is usually greater than 350 mOsm/liter; the urine-to-plasma creatinine ratio (U/P_{Creat}) is usually greater than 40. Of the many parameters, the fractional excretion of sodium is the most sensitive index in the differentiation between prerenal azotemia and acute renal failure. The fractional excretion of sodium (FE_{Na}) is calculated by using plasma and urinary sodium and creatinine according to the formula

$$FE_{Na}(\%) = U_{Na}/P_{Na} \times P_{Creat}/U_{Creat} \times 100\%$$

In prerenal azotemia, the fractional excretion of sodium is consistently less than 1%, but in acute renal failure values of greater than 1% are usually obtained.

Complications

The major complications of azotemia arise from morbidity associated with alteration in mental status. Progressive lethargy and confusion increase the risk of aspiration pneumonia as well as complicating other medical and nursing care. Anorexia, nausea, and vomiting interfere with nutrition and can severely compromise an already debilitated patient.

Treatment

Therapy aims at determining the cause and optimizing cardiac and volume status. Azotemia in the elderly requires a search for reversible causes, but when irreversible azotemia is established, the physician attempts to optimize the metabolic parameters to minimize symptoms. Careful repletion of volume deficits and judicious use of diuretics, digoxin, or vasodilators help to maximize cardiac output and improve renal perfusion. Major complications arise from overvigorous therapy in any age group, but elderly patients with compromised cardiac reserve are particularly sensitive to even minor interventions. The most common problems arise from excessive fluid repletion or from toxicity from excessive use of digoxin. Moreover, prerenal azotemia can worsen following excessive or inappropriate use of diuretics or vasodilators.

1. Espinel CH: The FE_{Na} test: Use in the differential diagnosis of acute renal failure. *J Am Med Assoc* 236:579, 1976.
Indicates that the fractional excretion of sodium can be used to differentiate between prerenal azotemia and acute tubular necrosis. Patients with prerenal azotemia have FE_{Na} values less than 1% and patients with acute tubular necrosis have FE_{Na} values greater than 3%.
2. Perlmutter M, et al: Urine-serum urea nitrogen ratio: Simple test of renal function in acute azotemia and oliguria. *J Am Med Assoc* 170:1533, 1959.

Urine-serum urea nitrogen ratios were used to differentiate between prerenal azotemia and acute renal failure. A high ratio reflects prerenal azotemia.

3. Handa SP, Morrin PAF: Diagnostic indices in acute renal failure. *Can Med Assoc J* 96:78, 1967.
Review of uses of urinary osmolality, sodium, chloride, and urea in renal failure.
4. Miller TR, et al: Urinary diagnostic indices in acute renal failure. A prospective study. *Ann Intern Med* 89:47, 1978.
Prerenal azotemia is likely to be associated with urine osmolality greater than 500 mOsm/kg H_2O, urinary sodium concentration less than 20 mEq/liter, urine-to-plasma urea ratio greater than 8, and urine-to-plasma creatinine ratio greater than 40. Acute tubular necrosis is usually associated with urinary osmolality less than 350 mOsm/kg H_2O, urinary sodium greater than 40 mEq/liter, and urine-to-plasma creatinine ratio less than 20.
5. Schrier RW, Cronin RE: Acute renal failure, in Coggins CH, Cummings NB (eds): *Prevention of Kidney and Urinary Tract Diseases.* Washington DC, US Department of Health, Education and Welfare, 1978.
Excellent review of the diagnostic indices in acute renal failure.

84. PRIMARY RENAL DISORDERS

Leslie Fang

Metabolic derangements arising from renal failure often complicate the medical management of other disorders in the elderly. Significantly altered mental status can also be a symptom of renal disorder and signals a need for prompt intervention to minimize morbidity.

Acute Renal Failure

Elderly patients are particularly susceptible to acute renal failure because of their increased susceptibility to a wide variety of nephrotoxins and increased sensitivity to renal ischemia. The morbidity and mortality of acute renal failure are particularly high in the elderly, and the concurrent medical problems allow little margin for error in the management of the metabolic derangements associated with renal functional impairment.

Symptoms. While the etiologies of acute renal failure are diverse, the clinical presentation of the patient in acute renal failure is remarkably constant. Anorexia, hiccups, easy fatigability, and weakness are the common systemic symptoms. Dermatologic manifestations, such as pruritus and pale, sallow skin, accompany gastrointestinal manifestations of nausea, vomiting, mucosal ulceration, gastrointestinal bleeding, diarrhea and constipation. Cardiovascular abnormalities, including hypertension, biventricular failure, pericarditis, and arrhythmia, pose a serious threat to the patient's life. The neurologic abnormalities, especially prevalent in elderly patients, include lassitude, drowsiness, lethargy, disorientation, asterixis, seizure, and coma.

Causes. Although numerous etiologies have been known to cause acute renal failure in the elderly patient, the most common causes are ischemic disorders and nephrotoxins. Hemodynamic compromise during perioperative periods, periods of significant sepsis, and periods of volume depletion can result in reduction in renal perfusion sufficient to cause ischemic acute tubular necrosis. The nephrotoxins that most commonly cause acute tubular necrosis in the elderly patient are antibiotics and intravenous contrast media. Numerous antibiotics have been associated with nephrotoxicity, but the major culprits are aminoglycosides, semisynthetic penicillins, and, to a lesser degree, cephalosporins. The elderly patient with some preexisting renal disease is more susceptible to contrast media–induced acute renal failure. Many patients will have diabetes, multiple myeloma, or dehydration in addition to the contrast infection.

Management. Physical examination provides some clues to the degree of the azotemia. For instance, Kussmaul respiration denotes significant systemic acidosis, and the presence of a pericardial friction rub denotes significant uremia that warrants aggressive intervention. Volume status may be gauged on examination by measurement of changes in body weight and presence of edema. Moisture in mucous membranes may be indicative, but skin turgor may be misleading in elderly patients.

In about 80% of all cases of acute renal failure there is a period of transient oliguria, in which urine output is less than 400 ml/day. The duration of the oliguria is quite variable, ranging from hours to weeks, with a mean of about 10 days. Renal function gradually normalizes during this phase. Nonoliguric acute renal failure, occurring in 20% of cases, was initially observed in burn patients, but the most common etiology is nephrotoxicity.

Therapy of acute renal failure during the oliguric phase is directed at stabilization of the metabolic perturbation. Daily weights should be obtained whenever feasible, in order to monitor fluid overload. Patients should lose about ¼ pound each day during the oliguric phase. Careful recording of intake and output will provide data, so that fluid restriction can match urine output plus insensible fluid loss. Age should not be a contraindication when the fluid overload cannot be managed conservatively, making hemodialysis or peritoneal dialysis necessary. Acidosis can be managed with sodium bicarbonate in doses of 300–600 mg PO bid or qid, if the patient can tolerate the sodium load. Dialysis also may be needed, if the patient is already volume-overloaded and cannot tolerate the bicarbonate load. Hyperkalemia, perhaps the most threatening metabolic lesion, sometimes requires rapid lowering of the serum potassium. When there is some time to act, intravenous glucose, insulin, and bicarbonate and oral or rectal Kayexelate (25–50 gm in 50–100 ml of sorbitol) are effective. Dialysis for hyperkalemia may be necessary when other indications for it also exist.

Uremia itself responds to specific dietary controls that restrict dietary protein to 20–40 gm/day and ensure adequate caloric intake to minimize catabolism. The patient with acute renal failure requires about 2000 cal/day, which will usually prevent breakdown of body protein. It is best to use high-quality protein or essential amino acids whenever feasible.

Hyperphosphatemia and hypocalcemia also complicate the oliguric phase. Phosphate binders in the form of aluminum hydroxide, 30–120 ml PO 1 hour before each meal and at bedtime, help to reduce excess phosphate. If hypocalcemia persists after normalization of serum phosphate, elemental calcium can be supplemented either orally or via nasogastric tube. Drug toxicity during oliguria is a major source of danger. Careful monitoring of drug levels is a reasonable safeguard against drug toxicity.

Therapy during the diuretic or polyuric phase of acute renal failure aims at keeping the electrolyte and fluid balance by avoiding excessive losses. Of deaths due to acute renal failure, 15% occur during the polyuric phase. In general, it is reasonable to determine the electrolyte content of the urine and replace it with the same volume of fluid with the same content. Fluid replacement should continue until the patient's renal function improves (blood urea nitrogen [BUN] < 40 and creatinine < 2). Meticulous attention to the many metabolic perturbations in the patient with acute renal failure will minimize the morbidity and mortality of patients with acute renal failure.

Chronic Renal Failure

Chronic renal failure of various degrees is common in elderly patients, who have a high incidence of vascular disease and chronic obstructive renal disease. There is usually a slow but relentless deterioration of renal function over a period of years. Knowledge of an underlying condition such as poorly controlled or long-standing hypertension, diabetes, severe vascular disease, or collagen vascular disease, helps in delineation of the etiology of the renal impairment. The historical details associated with the separate diseases that contribute to renal dysfunction are obviously different for each disease and will not be listed in this chapter. Physical examination must be aimed at a careful assessment of the patient's volume status and cardiac function. Tests of renal function confirm the diagnosis. Markedly elevated BUN and creatinine with low creatinine clearance are the hallmarks, but normochromic, normocytic anemia, anion-gap metabolic acidosis, and hyperphosphatemia and hypocalcemia are frequent fellow travelers. A renal ultrasonogram can help to identify possible obstructive uropathy and can assess kidney size. Absence of caliceal dilatation in a patient with bilaterally small kidneys is a sign that further invasive investigation for obstructive uropathy is unnecessary.

Complications. The complications of chronic renal failure are similar to those of acute renal failure, only increased by their chronicity. Disorders of fluid balance occur with moderate renal insufficiency, causing hyposthenuria (dilute urine) and symptoms of polydipsia and polyuria. With further renal impairment, isosthenuria (isotonic urine) supervenes and then gives way to the oliguria of severe renal failure.

Moderate renal insufficiency causes an obligate urinary sodium loss, but as the damage progresses, sodium excretion becomes limited, and excessive sodium intake causes volume overload.

Hyperkalemia from the inability of the kidney to excrete a potassium load, muscle breakdown from abnormal catabolism, and systemic acidosis are the usual problems in the uremic patient. Hypokalemia occurs in patients with the rare type of potassium-losing nephropathy.

Disorders of acid-base balance follow failure to excrete organic acids formed from protein metabolism. The usual anion-gap metabolic acidosis comes from decreased excretion of ammonia and, in severe renal insufficiency, from reduced excretion of titratable acids. In instances of renal tubular acidosis, bicarbonate resorption or hydrogen ion excretion may also be reduced. Failure of waste product excretion also causes a wide variety of small- and middle-sized molecules to accumulate because of compromised renal function. Some of these retained molecules can produce uremic symptoms. Other systems also suffer in chronic renal failure. Uremic pericarditis develops in severely uremic patients and is believed to result from accumulation of a middle-sized molecule uremic toxin.

Hypertension, from volume overload and increased peripheral resistance, is an unwelcome complication, as is congestive heart failure, which threatens patients with volume overload and long-standing hypertension.

Metastatic calcification of vessels occasionally causes severe occlusive peripheral vascular disease. Hyperphosphatemia from inability of the kidneys to excrete phosphate contributes to hypocalcemia. Decreased calcium absorption from the gastrointestinal tract and decreased synthesis of 1,25-dihydroxycholecalciferol both contribute to hypocalcemia in patients with renal parenchymal diseases. Renal osteodystrophy, a bone disorder, accompanies chronic renal failure but also follows hyperthyroidism, abnormal vitamin D synthesis, and negative calcium balance from decreased gastrointestinal calcium absorption and decreased dietary intake. Acidosis and abnormal bone metabolism in uremic patients are also associated with renal osteodystrophy.

The anemia of renal failure is related to decreased red blood cell survival in uremic patients and in a few patients with hypersplenism. Bleeding because of impaired platelet adhesiveness in the uremic state and iron deficiency because of impaired gastrointestinal absorption both contribute to the anemia, as does inadequate production of red cells from decreased erythropoietin production. Hemolysis develops in some uremic patients with circulating inhibitors of hexose monophosphate shunt enzymes.

Management. Management of chronic renal failure is a complex endeavor that requires skill and patience. Patients with moderate renal insufficiency do not require fluid restriction, but patients with severe renal insufficiency and oliguria must have their fluid intake matched to output and insensible loss. With moderate renal insufficiency, enough dietary sodium should be given to balance the obligate urinary sodium losses. With further renal damage, sodium intake has to be restricted, usually with diets containing 1,000 mg sodium or less. Hypertension, when present at any stage, will also necessitate sodium restriction. Replacement of sodium bicarbonate should be undertaken with great care in the elderly, and starting doses (300–600 mg PO bid) should be titrated to maintain the serum bicarbonate level at 16–20 mEq/liter. Hyperkalemia can be prevented in part by minimizing endogenous potassium production, avoiding potassium in the diet, and avoiding potassium-retaining drugs. In the rare instances of potassium-losing nephropathy, careful potassium repletion may be necessary.

Management of waste product retention requires protein restriction to about 0.5 gm/kg BW/day. An adequate caloric intake (2000 cal/day) prevents muscle breakdown, and use of high-quality protein or essential amino acids reduces BUN.

Management of cardiovascular complications not only protects life but also makes the patient more comfortable. Blood pressure must be kept under control to prevent further renal damage and to prevent the other risks of hypertension. Maximizing hematocrit will help prevent high-output heart failure. The control of fluid overload and careful use of digoxin prevent congestive heart failure. Measurement of digoxin levels frequently avoids digoxin excess. Dialysis is needed in cases of intractable volume overload or uremic pericarditis. Phosphate binders are used to lower the serum phosphate level to less than 6 mg/100 ml. When the phosphate level is less than 6 mg/100 ml and hypocalcemia persists, one can add supplemental calcium or vitamin D. Renal osteodystrophy responds to improvement in calcium and phosphate balance and to correction of acidosis. Parathyroidectomy may be needed for patients with tertiary hyperparathyroidism. Iron and vitamin supplements help the anemia slightly. Judicious use of androgens may improve the hematocrit. Transfusions are indicated only if clinical symptoms are evident.

Chronic renal failure is usually characterized by inexorable progression. The rate of progression depends on the underlying diseases as well as on the mode of conservative management. After the serum creatinine level exceeds 10–15 mg/100 ml, the median survival time is usually less than 5 months, and dialysis and transplantation should be considered for appropriate candidates. Elderly patients who are otherwise healthy can be dialysed as needed. Transplant is also available to the active elderly patient.

Acute Renal Failure

1. Levinsky N: Pathophysiology of acute renal failure. *N Engl J Med* 296:1453, 1977.
   Pathogenetic mechanisms of acute renal failure are reviewed. Renal hemodynamic changes, tubular obstruction, and back-leak of glomerular filtrates are important mechanisms of acute renal failure.
2. Anderson RJ, et al: Nonoliguric acute renal failure. *N Engl J Med* 296:1134, 1977.
   Prospective examination of 92 patients with acute renal failure, 52 of whom had nonoliguric renal failure with urine output in excess of 600 cc/day. Nonoliguric patients had considerably less morbidity and mortality (2% vs. 17% mortality).
3. Baek SM, Makabali GG, Shoemaker WC: Clinical determinants of survival from postoperative renal failure. *Surg Gynecol Obstet* 140:685, 1975.
   Postoperative acute renal failure is associated with high mortality. The clinical determinants important in predicting outcome include oliguria, respiratory failure, cardiac failure, and infection.
4. Bhat JG, et al: Renal failure after open heart surgery. *Ann Intern Med* 84:677, 1976.
   Patients with significant acute renal failure after open heart surgery (serum creatinine > 5 mg/100 ml) have a mortality rate of nearly 60%. Duration of cardiopulmonary bypass, cardiac function, and sepsis determine outcome.
5. Ellenbogen PH, et al: Sensitivity of gray scale ultrasound in detecting urinary tract obstruction. *Am J Roentgenol* 130:731, 1978.
   A high degree of sensitivity and specificity in the detection of significant urinary tract obstruction is achieved by the use of gray scale renal ultrasonography.
6. Hall JW, et al: Immediate and longterm prognosis in acute renal failure. *Ann Intern Med* 73:515, 1970.
   The outcome of acute renal failure is described.
7. Kumar R, Hill CM, McGeown MG: Acute renal failure in the elderly. *Lancet* 1:90, 1973.
   Morbidity and mortality are significantly increased in elderly patients with acute renal failure.
8. Meyers C, Roxe DM, and Hans JE: The clinical course of nonoliguric acute renal failure. *Cardiovasc Med* 2:669, 1977.
   Nonoliguric renal failure is associated with less morbidity and mortality than is oliguric renal failure.
9. Linton AL, et al: Acute interstitial nephritis due to drugs. *Ann Intern Med* 93:735, 1980.
   Discussion of 9 cases of acute interstitial nephritis caused by drugs and a review of the literature.
10. Appel GB: A decade of penicillin-related acute interstitial nephritis—More questions than answers. *Clin Nephrol* 13:151, 1980.
    Review of the literature regarding acute interstitial nephritis secondary to penicillin and closely related antibiotics.
11. Galpin JE, et al: Acute interstitial nephritis due to methcillin. *Am J Med* 65:756, 1978.
    Clinical features of 14 patients with methcillin-induced acute interstitial nephritis. Hematuria and eosinophiluria are important features.
12. Cronin RE: Aminoglycoside nephrotoxicity: Pathogenesis and prevention. *Clin Nephrol* 11:251, 1979.
    Clinical features and possible pathogenetic mechanisms of aminoglycoside nephrotoxicity.

13. Gary NE, Buzzeo L, Salaki J, Eisenger RP: Gentamicin-associated acute renal failure. *Arch Intern Med* 136:1101, 1976.
Clinical features of aminoglycoside nephrotoxicity in 5 patients.
14. Byrd L, Sherman RL: Radiocontrast-induced acute renal failure: A clinical and pathophysiologic review. *Medicine* 58:270, 1979.
Clinical features of contrast-induced acute renal failure in 23 patients and the literature are reviewed. Diabetes mellitus, advanced age, and preexisting renal failure are major risk factors.

Chronic Renal Failure

1. Giovannetti S, Maggiore Q: A low nitrogen diet with proteins of high biological value for severe chronic uremia. *Lancet* 1:1000, 1964.
Beneficial effect of protein restriction in patients with chronic renal failure.
2. Berlyne GM: The place of dietary therapy in the treatment of chronic renal failure. *Clin Nephrol* 11:63, 1979.
Update of various aspects of dietary considerations in patients with chronic renal failure; protein, salt, potassium, and fluid restrictions; use of phosphate binders and calcium supplements; use of vitamins.
3. Yeh BPY, et al: Factors influencing sodium and water excretion in uremic man. *Kidney Int* 7:103, 1975.
Examination of sodium and fluid handling in patients with renal failure.
4. Maher JF, Nolph KD, Bryan CW: Prognosis of advanced chronic renal failure. *Ann Intern Med* 81:43, 1974.
Delineation of clinical course of patients with chronic renal failure.
5. Friedman EA, Giordano C: Uremia. *Kidney Int* (Suppl 8):1, 1978.
Entire issue discussing the many aspects of clinical manifestations and management of patients with chronic renal failure.
6. Massry SG, Goldstein DA, Malluche HH: Current status of use of 1,25 dihydroxycholecalciferol in the management of renal osteodystrophy. *Kidney Int* 18:409, 1980.
Discussion of the indications for and clinical use of vitamin D in patients with chronic renal failure.

85. OBSTRUCTIVE UROPATHY

Leslie Fang

Postrenal azotemia follows obstruction of the collecting system of the kidneys, ureters, or bladder outlet. Obstructive uropathy, potentially reversible, should be considered whenever an elderly patient presents with azotemia.

Causes

Obstructive uropathy clearly has to be considered in any case of an **anuric patient** with progressive azotemia. Since partial obstruction can result in progressive renal dysfunction, however, obstructive uropathy should not be overlooked even in the case of an azotemic patient with a reasonable urine output. Obstructive uropathy can occur as a result of obstruction at the urethra, bladder neck, or ureter. In the elderly male, benign prostatic hypertrophy constitutes the main cause of obstruction. In the elderly female, pelvic malignancy is the leading cause of obstructive uropathy.

Symptoms

Clinical presentation differs with the different etiologies of obstruction. Benign prostatic hypertrophy in the elderly male usually causes complaints of difficulty with initiation of urinary stream, hesitancy, dribbling, frequency, and nocturia. In cases of stone disease, a past history should raise suspicion of obstructive uropathy from renal calculi. The classic symptoms are severe colicky flank pain radiating to the groin and systemic symptoms of nausea and vomiting. Tumor generally causes progressive weight loss, anorexia, and painless hematuria in addition to obstructive azotemia. Some tumors may be asymptomatic except for the effects of the azotemia, or the azotemia may be discovered by chance.

The physical examination often helps focus the etiology. The presence of costovertebral angle tenderness heightens suspicion of possible obstructive uropathy. Its absence, however, does not preclude obstruction. Pelvic examination is mandatory in the elderly female in order to exclude the possibility of a pelvic mass causing bilateral ureteral obstruction. Rectal examination should be done routinely in the male to assess prostatic size. Palpation and percussion in the suprapubic area can identify a palpable bladder from either outlet obstruction or neurogenic cause, both of which can result in significant obstructive uropathy.

Diagnostic Tests

Renal function tests in early obstruction may show a blood urea nitrogen (BUN) elevation out of proportion to the elevation of creatinine. (The BUN/Creat ratio may be > 10.) Later in the course of obstructive uropathy, however, this disproportionate elevation is not present. Urinalysis may be normal in obstructive uropathy, or microscopic or macroscopic hematuria may provide clues to renal calculi, genitourinary tumors, or a pathologic condition of the prostate. Tissue debris in the urine may be the only clue to ongoing papillary necrosis. A urine cytologic specimen for tumor analysis should be obtained from the elderly patient with obstructive pathologic condition.

A number of diagnostic procedures are available to confirm the clinical suspicion of obstructive uropathy. If there is sufficient residual renal function for visualization of the caliceal system, the intravenous pyelogram (IVP) is an excellent diagnostic procedure. Two concerns limit the use of the IVP in elderly subjects. First, when there is significant renal dysfunction, it may not be possible to visualize the calyces. Second, contrast-induced acute renal failure is a danger, increasingly recognized, in patients with compromised renal function. Renal ultrasonography also has been increasingly useful in the work-up of obstructive uropathy. The gray scale ultrasonographic studies are quite sensitive and reliable in the diagnosis of caliceal and ureteral dilations that indicate obstruction. Cystoscopy and retrograde contrast studies also diagnose obstructive uropathy and in many instances can relieve the obstruction by the use of ureteral stints. The increasing sensitivity and reliability of the noninvasive studies, however, allow the invasive techniques to be reserved for instances in which the noninvasive studies or the clinical circumstances strongly suggest obstructive uropathy. Recently, percutaneous techniques have been devised to perform anterograde contrast studies in patients with dilated calyces. These studies permit manometric determination of pressure behind the obstructive lesion and allow delineation of the nature of the obstruction. Urologic consultation is necessary in cases of suspected obstructive uropathy.

Treatment

Obstructive uropathy is easily reversible when treated early but may cause irreversible renal damage if allowed to persist. Bacterial seeding of fluid behind an obstructive lesion in the genitourinary tract will result in significant infection, often with concomitant bacteremic urosepsis. The high-grade bacteremia in this setting mandates prompt decompression and constitutes a medical and urologic emergency. The method of treating the obstruction obviously depends on the site of the obstruction and the nature of the obstructing lesion. In bladder outlet obstruction, a Foley catheter, passed through the obstructing lesion, is certainly an easy and immediate solution. A suprapubic catheter may be necessary if a Foley catheter cannot be safely passed. Surgical correction of the bladder outlet obstruction is the ultimate goal but can be done when the patient is in the best possible health. For ureteral calculi, urologic intervention at the time of cystoscopy and retrograde pylography may remove obstructing stones. Ureteral stints also can be placed to relieve ureteral obstruction temporarily. Nephrostomy catheters, placed surgically or percutaneously, can be used to relieve obstructions as well. More extensive surgical intervention may be necessary to remove obstructing pelvic tumors or large renal calculi or to lyse retroperitoneal fibrosis.

Complications of therapy are common in the elderly. Obstruction of flow can occur in Foley catheters, ureteral stints, and suprapubic and nephrostomy catheters. Frequent irrigation with appropriate irrigating solutions is needed to prevent blockage of the catheters. Infection, the major difficulty of repeated instrumentation and indwelling catheters, demands frequent culturing and prompt antibiotic intervention. Definitive surgical correction ought to be carried out as soon as the patient's medical status is stable, in order to minimize the chances of infection. Bleeding is occasionally encountered because of irritation from the catheters but is seldom serious. Clots may obstruct the catheter and reinstate the obstruction. Postobstructive diuresis is usually short and can be managed by careful attention to the patient's intake, output, and overall volume status.

1. Ibraham A, Asha HA: Prediction of renal recovery in hydronephrotic kidneys. *Br J Urol* 50:222, 1978.
In 35 patients with obstructive uropathy, the pH of the urine of the obstructed kidneys in the absence of infection with urea-splitting organisms was a reliable indicator of the potential recovery of function after obstruction. Urinary pH less than 6 was associated with good recovery, whereas urinary pH greater than 7.3 was associated with poor recovery.
2. Torres VE, et al: The progression of vesicoureteral reflux nephropathy. *Ann Intern Med* 92:776, 1980.
Discusses 54 patients with reflux nephropathy. Patients with deteriorating renal functions were all found to have greater than 1 gm/day of proteinuria.
3. Guggenheim SJ, Schrier RW: Obstructive nephropathy: Pathophysiology and management, in Schrier RW (ed): *Renal and Electrolyte Disorders,* ed 2. Boston, Little, Brown, 1980.
Excellent review of obstructive uropathy, including clinical features and management.

86. HYPOCALCEMIC DISORDERS

David M. Slovik

Symptoms

Hypocalcemia is often mild and asymptomatic in elderly persons, although some patients have severe life-threatening problems. Patients with mild hypocalcemia may have nonspecific symptoms, such as fatigue and weakness. Other clinical features of hypocalcemia may be quite variable. Mental status changes include anxiety, lability of affect, agitation, depression, delirium, and psychoneurosis. Tetany and neuromuscular irritability are characterized by muscle contractions and cramps, carpopedal spasm, and paresthesias; the muscle contractions, depending upon the location, can produce dysphagia, pylorospasm, bronchospasm, laryngeal stridor, diplopia, and blepharospasm. CNS manifestations include seizures, electroencephalographic abnormalities, increased intracranial pressure with papilledema, and extrapyramidal disturbances. Cardiovascular abnormalities seen on ECG include a prolongation of the Q–T and S–T intervals. Abnormalities of teeth, hair, and fingernails may also occur, as well as lenticular cataracts and chronic dermatitis.

Causes

Hypoproteinemia is one of the most common causes of hypocalcemia in elderly subjects. It is not "true" hypocalcemia, because ionized calcium concentrations are normal, and the patients remain asymptomatic. Inasmuch as approximately 46% of calcium in the blood circulates bound to serum proteins, primarily albumin, a rough guide to follow to correct for changes in serum proteins is that the total serum calcium concentration decreases approximately 0.8 mg/dl for each decrease of 1.0 gm/dl in serum albumin. If the serum calcium concentration remains low after correction for hypoalbuminemia, then the presence of "true" hypocalcemia can be assumed, and further evaluation is necessary. Hypocalcemia in the elderly can be caused by abnormalities in parathyroid hormone (PTH) secretion or action. **Nonhypoparathyroid causes** of hypocalcemia include vitamin D deficiency, renal failure, malabsorption, pancreatitis, hyperphosphatemia, rapid deposition of calcium in bone (e.g., by osteoblastic metastases, or after surgical removal of a parathyroid adenoma), calcium-chelating agents (e.g., citrated whole blood), and hemodialysis with calcium-free dialysate.

Hypoparathyroidism in the elderly is most commonly seen after surgical removal of, or damage to, the parathyroid glands at the time of a thyroid or parathyroid surgical procedure, or with radical neck dissection. Less common causes of hypoparathyroidism in the elderly are radiation therapy to the neck, severe magnesium deficiency, and idiopathic hypoparathyroidism. The biochemical hallmarks of hypoparathyroidism are hypocalcemia, hyperphosphatemia, and inappropriately low or undetectable concentrations of immunoreactive PTH. **Pseudohypoparathyroidism,** an inherited disorder, is due to end-organ resistance to PTH due to an abnormality in the nucleotide regulatory protein and is characterized by short stature, round facies, short fourth and fifth metacarpals and metatarsals, mental retardation, ectopic calcification, and biochemical findings of hypocalcemia, hyperphosphatemia, and elevated circulating concentrations of immunoreactive PTH. Sometimes the intravenous administration of PTH is necessary to test the renal cyclic AMP and phosphaturic response and differentiate states of PTH deficiency from states of abnormal PTH responsiveness. In elderly persons, vitamin D deficiency is usually due to either lack of exposure to sunlight and insufficient oral vitamin D intake or intestinal malabsorption due to medical conditions or surgery.

Treatment

The acute treatment of hypocalcemic emergencies (e.g., tetany, seizures, and laryngeal stridor due to hypocalcemia) involves the intravenous administration of calcium with careful cardiac monitoring, especially of elderly patients taking digitalis. The rate and duration of intravenous calcium administration will vary depending on the severity of symptoms but is usually 30–100 mg/hr. The long-term treatment of the various disorders causing hypocalcemia depends on the chronic administration of calcium and vitamin D or its metabolites in various doses. The calcium content of different calcium preparations varies and is discussed in Chap. 79, and the treatment of vitamin D deficiency is discussed in Chap. 80. In other disorders, such as hypoparathyroidism and pseudohypoparathyroidism, high doses of vitamin D or smaller doses of dihydrotachysterol, 1,25-$(OH)_2$-D, or 1-alpha-OH-D are given. The aim of therapy is to prevent symptoms, restore the serum calcium to the low-normal range, and avoid hypercalciuria. In addition, oral calcium supplements (approximately 1,000–2,000 mg/day of elemental calcium) are needed. Thiazide diuretics may help by decreasing renal calcium clearance, but hypercalcemia may develop, especially with concomitant use of the potent vitamin D metabolites. Hyperphosphatemia, when present, should be controlled by reduction of the phosphate intake, the use of oral phosphate binders, and the substitution of oral calcium supplements for milk, since 8 ounces of milk contains approximately 250 mg of phosphorus. Treatment of the other causes of hypocalcemia should be directed to the underlying disorders, when necessary, calcium and vitamin D supplements should be used.

---

1. Avioli LV: The therapeutic approach to hypoparathyroidism. *Am J Med* 57:34–42, 1974.
   Dihydrotachysterol is more effective than vitamin D in the treatment of hypoparathyroidism.
2. Bunker JP, Stetson JB, Coe RC, Grillo HC, Murphy AJ: Citric acid intoxication. *JAMA* 157:1361–1367, 1955.
   In 130 patients, the transfusion of moderate to large volumes of citrated blood produced marked elevations in serum citrate levels sufficient to depress the ionized calcium level.
3. Chase LR, Melson GL, Aurbach GD: Pseudohypoparathyroidism: Defective excretion of 3′,5′-AMP in response to parathyroid hormone. *J Clin Invest* 48:1832–1844, 1969.
   Urinary excretion of 3′,5′-AMP in response to the exogenous administration of parathyroid hormone will distinguish between states of parathyroid hormone deficiency and parathyroid hormone unresponsiveness.
4. Coburn JW, Kurokawa K, Llach F: Altered divalent ion metabolism in renal disease and renal osteodystrophy, in Maxwell MH, Kleeman CR (eds): *Clinical Disorders of Fluid and Electrolyte Metabolism.* New York, McGraw-Hill, 1979, pp 1153–1250.
   General review of the multiple aspects of renal failure and renal osteodystrophy.
5. Kumar R, Riggs BL: Vitamin D in the therapy of disorders of calcium and phosphorus metabolism. *Mayo Clin Proc* 56:327–333, 1981.
   Review of the therapeutic use of vitamin D and its analogs.

6. Muldowney FP, McKenna TJ, Kyle LH, Freaney R, Swan M: Parathormone-life effect of magnesium replenishment in steatorrhea. *N Engl J Med* 282:61–68, 1970.
Of 9 patients with intestinal malabsorption, 5 had tetany associated with hypomagnesemia and hypocalcemia.
7. Nusynowitz ML, Frame B, Kolb FO: The spectrum of the hypoparathyroid states: A classification based on physiologic principles. *Medicine* 55:105–119, 1976.
Review. The authors classify the hypoparathyroid states into either (1) hormonopenic hypoparathyroidism (deficiency of hormone secretion) due to absence, damage, or insufficiency of parathyroid glands or suppression of PTH secretion, or (2) hormonoplethoric hypoparathyroidism (failure of hormone action) due to target tissue unresponsiveness to PTH or to the presence of ineffective circulating PTH.
8. Parfitt AM: Surgical, idiopathic, and other varieties of parathyroid hormone-deficient hypoparathyroidism, in DeGroot LJ, et al (eds): *Endocrinology.* New York, Grune & Stratton, 1979, pp 755–768.
General review of clinical features, diagnosis, and treatment of hypocalcemia.
9. Potts JT Jr: Pseudohypoparathyroidism, in DeGroot LJ, et al (eds): *Endocrinology.* New York, Grune & Stratton, 1979, pp 769–776.
General discussion of the pathophysiology, genetics, and clinical features of this syndrome.
10. Raskin P, McClain CJ, Medsger TA: Hypocalcemia associated with metastatic bone disease: A retrospective study. *Arch Intern Med* 132:539–543, 1973.
Hypocalcemia was present in 34% of patients with osteoblastic bone metastases from adenocarcinoma of the prostate.
11. Rude RK, Oldham SB, Sharp CF Jr, Singer FR: Parathyroid hormone secretion in magnesium deficiency. *J Clin Endocrinol Metab* 47:800–806, 1978.
Impaired PTH secretion is a significant factor contributing to the hypocalcemia of magnesium deficiency.
12. Schneider AB, Sherwood LM: Pathogenesis and management of hypoparathyroidism and other hypocalcemic disorders. *Metabolism* 24:871–898, 1975.
Good general review.

87. HYPERCALCEMIC DISORDERS

David M. Slovik

Mild hypercalcemia is often asymptomatic, especially when serum calcium concentrations are less than 11.5 mg/dl. The clinical features of hypercalcemia depend on the underlying etiology and duration of symptoms. The general symptoms caused by hypercalcemia include malaise, fatigue, lethargy, increased thirst, weakness, and pruritus. Other clinical features include:

Anorexia, nausea, vomiting, weight loss, constipation, dysphagia, vague abdominal pains, and pancreatitis
Polyuria, nocturia, defects in urinary concentrating ability, nephrosclerosis, nephrolithiasis, and renal failure
Cardiac arrhythmias, ECG changes (prolonged P–R interval and shortened Q–T interval), and increased sensitivity to digitalis
Depression, confusion, somnolence, decreased mental acuity, neuroses, psychoses, loss of consciousness, and coma
Proximal myopathy
Band keratopathy, when hypercalcemia is associated with hyperphosphatemia

Causes

Hypercalcemia in the elderly is caused by:

Endocrine disorders, including primary hyperparathyroidism, hyperthyroidism, and adrenal insufficiency

Malignant disorders, including osteolytic metastases, multiple myeloma, and hematologic malignancies, pseudohyperparathyroidism, and humoral hypercalcemia
Immobilization
Sarcoidosis, tuberculosis, and berylliosis
Vitamin D intoxication
Vitamin A intoxication
Milk-alkali syndrome
Drugs such as thiazide diuretics and lithium
Familial hypocalciuric hypercalcemia

It is important to determine the degree of the patient's vitamin ingestion and use of calcium supplements, dairy products, and antacids, because commercially available antacids, often not recognized as medications by the patient, have a high calcium content.

Diagnostic Pittfalls. In the evaluation of hypercalcemia, blood calcium and immunoreactive parathyroid hormone (iPTH) concentrations should be determined simultaneously. Because hypercalcemia should suppress iPTH activity in the parathyroid glands, hypercalcemic patients with elevated iPTH values or those with normal values that are inappropriate for the degree of hypercalcemia are manifesting evidence of hyperparathyroidism. Renal failure causes a decrease in the clearance of PTH and makes interpretation of the iPTH measurement difficult when a carboxyterminal assay is used.

Some pitfalls should be considered in the diagnosis of hypercalcemia in the elderly. A normal value of serum calcium in the presence of disorders known to lower serum calcium (e.g., vitamin D deficiency) should suggest a concomitant hypercalcemic disorder that will become obvious when the underlying disorder is successfully treated. Elevation of serum alkaline phosphatase or urinary hydroxyproline in a patient with primary hyperparathyroidism may be due to coexistent Paget's disease. Thiazide diuretics will produce sustained hypercalcemia in patients with other disorders that produce hypercalcemia. Palpable neck nodules in hypercalcemic patients are almost never parathyroid adenomas but coincidental thyroid nodules.

Primary Hyperparathyroidism. With increased use of multiphasic screening, asymptomatic hypercalcemia is being identified more frequently than in the past, and primary hyperparathyroidism may now be the most common cause of hypercalcemia. The peak incidence of primary hyperparathyroidism occurs in the third to fifth decade, but as many as 33% of patients are over the age of 60 years. It is estimated that the annual incidence of primary hyperparathyroidism is 1 in every 1,000 men over age 60, and 2 in every 1,000 woman over age 60.

Approximately 85% of all cases of primary hyperparathyroidism are caused by enlargement of a single gland, and 15% arise from hyperplasia of all four glands. Parathyroid carcinoma is a rare cause of hyperparathyroidism. Chronic symptoms of hypercalcemia favor the diagnosis of primary hyperparathyroidism, although there may not be any symptoms at all in many patients with primary hyperparathyroidism. Renal abnormalities include renal tubular defects, nephrolithiasis, nephrocalcinosis, a reduction in glomerular filtration rate, and renal failure. Bone disease, characterized by osteitis fibrosa cystica and generalized bone pain, is much less common now than in the past. Diffuse osteopenia from primary hyperparathyroidism is indistinguishable from senile or postmenopausal osteoporosis. Other complications caused by hyperparathyroidism are peptic ulcer disease, pancreatitis, chondrocalcinosis, pseudogout, calcific periarthritis, and hyperuricemia.

The biochemical findings of primary hyperparathyroidism are hypercalcemia (either sustained or intermittent), low or normal fasting serum inorganic phosphate concentrations, and a mild hyperchloremic acidosis. The iPTH concentration is usually elevated, although it may be in the high-normal range, which is inappropriately high in the setting of hypercalcemia.

Malignant Disorders. Malignant conditions are among the common causes of hypercalcemia in the elderly. Osteolytic metastases, primarily from carcinoma of the breast, lung, or kidney, and hematologic abnormalities such as multiple myeloma, lymphoma, and leukemia are high on the list. Pseudohyperparathyroidism is caused by the ectopic production of PTH or of a PTH-like substance by tumors, as in renal cell carcinoma and squamous cell carcinoma of the lung. Hypercalcemia may also be due to the production of other humoral substances ("tumor-humors," e.g., osteoclast-activating factor and prostaglandin). When hypercalcemia is caused by malignancy, it is severe (often $>$ 14 mg/dl) and causes rapid deterioration, elevated alkaline phosphatase, and bone pain. When hypercalcemia is caused by nonparathyroid factors, the patients have suppressed iPTH concentrations and normal serum inorganic phosphate concentrations. In addition, urinary calcium concentrations are higher in patients with malignancy than they are in patients with primary hyperparathyroidism and similar serum calcium values. In elderly patients, a known malignant condition is not always responsible for hypercalcemia, however, and other concomitant disorders, e.g., primary hyperparathyroidism, must be differentiated.

Vitamin D Intoxication. Vitamin D intoxication in the elderly may occur with the chronic ingestion of large doses of vitamin D—usually by inadvertent ingestion of 50,000–100,000 units of vitamin D daily, instead of once or twice a week, as is sometimes prescribed for osteoporosis; or by continued ingestion of high doses of vitamin D after the bones have healed in osteomalacia, or after parathyroidectomy. Hypercalcemia may develop rapidly after ingestion of one of the more potent vitamin D metabolites, e.g., 1,25-$(OH)_2$-D.

Immobilization and Thiazide. Immobilization of elderly patients who have increased bone turnover, e.g., from Paget's disease of bone or hyperparathyroidism, may produce marked hypercalcemia. Elderly patients who take thiazide diuretics and have abnormalities in calcium metabolism may become hypercalcemic due to decreased urinary calcium excretion.

Milk-Alkali Syndrome. The milk-alkali syndrome can occur in elderly patients who ingest very large quantities of calcium, commonly in the form of absorbable antacids containing calcium carbonate. When these patients are examined, they have hypercalcemia, normal or high serum inorganic phosphate concentrations, renal failure, and alkalosis (unless renal failure is severe).

Therapy

The therapy of hypercalcemia depends on the underlying disease and on the symptoms, severity, and rapidity of development of the hypercalcemia. Mobilization should be attempted if the clinical condition allows. Elderly patients may have marked dehyration because of nausea, vomiting, polyuria, and decreased fluid intake. The most important step in the treatment of hypercalcemia is to ensure adequate **hydration.** If intravenous fluids are required, physiologic saline solution is the fluid of choice, but saline solution must be administered cautiously to the elderly to avoid precipitation of congestive heart failure. Once adequate hydration has been established, **natriuresis** (and the coupled **calciuresis**) can be accomplished by administration of furosemide (40–160 mg/day) or ethacrynic acid (50–200 mg/day). Forced **diuresis** with vigorous administration of saline solution and furosemide or ethacrynic acid every 1 or 2 hours may be needed in severe hypercalcemia, in order to maintain a urine output of 200–500 ml/hr. Potassium and magnesium losses should be adequately replaced, especially if the patient is taking digitalis. Intestinal calcium absorption can be decreased by restriction of the dietary calcium.

Glucocorticoids are effective in treating hypercalcemia associated with certain disorders such as sarcoidosis, vitamin D intoxication, Addison's disease, hematologic malignant conditions, and certain tumors. Glucocorticoid therapy produces a decrease in intestinal calcium absorption, an increase in urinary calcium excretion, and an antitumor effect in susceptible malignant conditions. Prednisone, 40–100 mg, or its equivalent, given daily in divided doses, is often needed.

Mithramycin, a cytotoxic agent that inhibits bone resorption, is administered intravenously in a dose of 10–25 μg/kg BW. A beneficial response is evident by 12–24 hours, achieves its maximum effect in 72 hours, and sometimes lasts up to 7–10 days. Side effects vary from mild transient malaise, nausea, and vomiting to serious toxic effects, including thrombocytopenia, hepatocellular necrosis, proteinuria, and azotemia.

Calcitonin, in addition to inhibiting bone resorption, increases renal calcium clearance. In the elderly, especially those with cardiac disease, calcitonin may be useful for the short-term management of acute hypercalcemia. The usual initial dose of salmon calcitonin is 50–100 MRC (Medical Research Council, Great Britain) units q4–8h SC. After several days of therapy, tachyphylaxis develops, and the beneficial effect can disappear.

Indomethacin (25–50 mg PO q6h) can be given to those patients with suspected prostaglandin-mediated hypercalcemia.

The intravenous administration of **phosphate** will lower serum calcium concentrations rapidly but carries a high risk of ectopic calcification, e.g., in the heart, lung, and kidney.

Therefore phosphate should rarely, if ever, be administered intravenously and then only to treat acute life-threatening hypercalcemia. Oral phosphate therapy is useful in the treatment of chronic hypercalcemia in certain disorders associated with hypophosphatemia. Divided doses totalling 1–3 gm/day are usually prescribed. Low doses should be given initially, however, because diarrhea and gastrointestinal upset will occur. Phosphate supplements should not be given to elderly patients with hyperphosphatemia or renal failure. Patients with life-threatening hypercalcemia and severe renal failure may require dialysis with a calcium-free dialysate.

Patients with mild hypercalcemia (< 12 mg/dl) often do not require treatment except for the underlying disorder and for the maintenance of adequate hydration. The question of whether to remove the parathyroid glands in patients with mild or "asymptomatic" hyperparathyroidism is unresolved, but this issue is especially important in regard to elderly persons because of associated medical problems and the increased risk of anesthesia and surgical intervention.

---

1. Alveryd A, Boström H, Wengle B, Wester PO: Indications for surgery in the elderly patient with primary hyperparathyroidism. *Acta Chir Scand* 142:491–494, 1976.
   Seven of 8 elderly patients with neuromuscular symptoms, along with 2 of the 3 patients with extreme fatigue as the dominant symptom, improved after parathyroidectomy.
2. Baxter JD, Bondy PK: Hypercalcemia of thyrotoxicosis. *Ann Intern Med* 65:429–442, 1966.
   Approximately 15% of patients with hyperthyroidism had serum calcium levels over 10.6 mg/dl.
3. Binstock ML, Mundy GR: Effect of calcitonin and glucocorticoids in combination on the hypercalcemia of malignancy. *Ann Intern Med* 93:269–272, 1980.
   In patients with hypercalcemia of malignancy, the combination of calcitonin and glucocorticoids was more effective than calcitonin alone in lowering serum calcium concentrations.
4. Frame B, Jackson CE, Reynolds WA, Umphrey JE: Hypercalcemia and skeletal effects in chronic hypervitaminosis A. *Ann Intern Med* 80:44–48, 1974.
   Ingestion of excessive amounts of vitamin A should be considered in the differential diagnosis of hypercalcemia.
5. Habener JF, Potts JT Jr: Diagnosis and differential diagnosis of primary hyperparathyroidism, in DeGroot LJ, et al (eds): *Endocrinology.* New York, Grune & Stratton, 1979, pp 703–711.
   General review of differential diagnosis of hypercalcemia.
6. Habener JF, Potts JT Jr: Clinical features of primary hyperparathyroidism, in DeGroot LJ, et al (eds): *Endocrinology.* New York, Grune & Stratton, 1979, pp 693–701.
   Hypertension appears to occur more frequently in patients with hyperparathyroidism, particularly elderly patients, than in the general population.
7. Heath DA: The use of inorganic phosphate in the management of hypercalcemia. *Metab Bone Dis Relat Res* 2:213–215, 1980.
   Intravenous phosphate therapy has many serious side effects, including hypotension, heart failure, sudden death, hypocalcemia, acute renal failure, and extraskeletal calcification. The author feels intravenous phosphate should be reserved for the rare patient who is seriously ill and thought likely to die within the next 12–24 hours.
8. Heath DA, Wright AD, Barnes AD, Oates GD, Dorricott NJ: Surgical treatment of primary hyperparathyroidism in the elderly. *Br Med J* 1:1406–1408, 1980.
   The most common symptoms before surgery in 12 patients with primary hyperparathyroidism were muscle weakness, malaise, and mild to severe dementia. These were not related to the degree of hypercalcemia and showed some improvement after surgery.
9. Heath H III, Hodgson SF, Kennedy MA: Primary hyperparathyroidism: Incidence, morbidity, and potential economic impact in a community. *N Engl J Med* 302:189–193, 1980.
   Among women aged 60 years or older, primary hyperparathyroidism was diagnosed at an annual rate twice that of men of the same age.
10. Hosking DJ: Treatment of severe hypercalcemia with calcitonin. *Metab Bone Dis Relat Res* 2:207–212, 1980.

Calcitonin may be helpful in treating hypercalcemia in patients with renal and cardiac insufficiency.

11. Lafferty FW: Pseudohyperparathyroidism. *Medicine* 45:247–260, 1966.
Pseudohyperparathyroidism is favored over primary hyperparathyroidism when the illness is rapidly progressive; there is an absence of a history of renal calculi, peptic ulcer, or skeletal complaints; and the serum calcium is greater than 14 mg/dl.
12. Lee DBN, Zawada ET, Kleeman CN: The pathophysiology and clinical aspects of hypercalcemic disorders. *West J Med* 129:278–320, 1978.
General review of hypercalcemia, including a discussion of pathophysiology, causes, clinical manifestations, diagnostic consideration, and management.
13. McMillan DE, Freeman RB: The milk-alkali syndrome: A study of the acute disorder with comments on the development of the chronic condition. *Medicine* 44:485–501, 1965.
Patients with this syndrome present with hypercalcemia, elevated BUN and creatinine, and normal or elevated serum phosphorus.
14. Muller H: Sex, age, and hyperparathyroidism. *Lancet* 1:449–450, 1969.
An analysis of 200 consecutive cases of hyperparathyroidism showed that this disease was more common in menopausal and postmenopausal women.
15. Neer RM, Potts JR Jr: Medical management of hypercalcemia and hyperparathyroidism, in DeGroot LJ, et al (eds): *Endocrinology.* New York, Grune & Stratton, 1979, pp 725–734.
Review. Peritoneal dialysis and hemodialysis using calcium-free dialysate solutions may be necessary in patients with hypercalcemia and severe renal failure.
16. Patten BM, et al: Neuromuscular disease in primary hyperparathyroidism. *Ann Intern Med* 80:182–193, 1974.
Neuromuscular findings included weakness of proximal muscles, cranial nerve abnormalities, sensory changes, hyperreflexia, abnormal gait, and mental status changes.
17. Perlia CP, et al: Mithramycin treatment of hypercalcemia. *Cancer* 25:389–394, 1970.
Mithramycin, given as a single, intravenous injection (25 μg/kg) was effective in lowering serum calcium within 24–48 hours in patients with hypercalcemia caused by cancer.
18. Peskin GW, Greenburg AG, Salk RP: Expanding indications for early parathyroidectomy in the elderly female. *Am J Surg* 136:45–48, 1978.
The authors feel that, especially in the elderly female, the benefits in personality change, feeling of well-being, and lessened bone deterioration after parathyroidectomy warrant early operation.
19. Purnell DC, Smith LH, Scholz DA, Elveback LP, Arnaud CD: Primary hyperparathyroidism: A prospective clinical study. *Am J Med* 50:670–678, 1971.
Of 171 patients with proved primary hyperparathyroidism, 66 (39%) were over age 60 and 9% were over age 70, with a 2 : 1 female to male ratio.
20. Pyrah LN, Hodgkinson A, Anderson CK: Primary hyperparathyroidism. *Br J Surg* 53:245–316, 1966.
In reviewing 7 studies, only 18 of 890 patients with primary hyperparathyroidism were 70 years of age or more; and 92 were 60–69 years of age.
21. Roberts WC, Walter BF: Effect of chronic hypercalcemia on the heart. *Am J Med* 71:371–384, 1981.
Chronic hypercalcemia may be viewed as a risk factor to accelerated coronary atherosclerosis since it is associated with accelerated deposition of calcium in the cardiac annuli and valvular cusps, in the media and intima of the coronary arteries, and in individual myocardial fibers.
22. Roof BS, Gordan GS: Hyperparathyroid disease in the aged, in Greenblatt RB (ed): *Geriatric Endocrinology.* New York, Raven Press, 1978, Vol 5 in Aging Series, pp 33–79.
General review of hyperparathyroidism. Approximately 17% of the cases of hyperparathyroidism were in patients over the age of 60 years.
23. Shetty KR, Ajlouni K, Rosenfeld PS, Hagen TC: Protracted vitamin D intoxication. *Arch Intern Med* 135:986–988, 1975.
Vitamin D intoxication produces hypercalcemia, which may last for months.
24. Stenström G, Heedman P-A: Clinical findings in patients with hypercalcemia: A final investigation based on biochemical screening. *Acta Med Scand* 195:473–477, 1974.

The most common cause of hypercalcemia is hyperparathyroidism, closely followed by thiazides and malignant diseases.

25. Stewart AF, et al: Biochemical evaluation of patients with cancer-associated hypercalcemia: Evidence for humoral and nonhumoral groups. *N Engl J Med* 303:1377–1383, 1980.
   Nephrogenous cyclic AMP excretion was elevated in 41 patients and suppressed in 9 patients with cancer-associated hypercalcemia. Compared with patients with primary hyperparathyroidism, those patients with cancer-associated hypercalcemia had similar reductions in tubular phosphorus threshold, but higher fasting calcium excretion, reduced 1,25–(OH)$_2$–D levels and lower levels of immunoreactive PTH. Their findings suggested that the humoral factor responsible for this syndrome is not native 1-84 parathyroid hormone.
26. Suki WN: Effects of diuretics on calcium metabolism. *Miner Electrolyte Metab* 2:125–129, 1979.
   Significant elevations of serum calcium follow the administration of thiazide diuretics to patients (1) undergoing hemodialysis, (2) who have osteoporosis or hypoparathyroidism and are receiving vitamin D or its metabolites, or (3) who have hyperparathyroidism.

88. DISORDERS OF MAGNESIUM METABOLISM

David M. Slovik

Hypomagnesemia

Mild hypomagnesemia, often unsuspected in the elderly, may be present in various disorders and play a role in calcium and phosphate homeostasis. The clinical features of magnesium deficiency are:

Neuromuscular abnormalities, including lethargy, muscle weakness, neuromuscular irritability, fasciculations, athetoid movements, tremors, tetany, convulsions, and coma
Mental status changes, including disorientation, personality changes, anxiety, delirium, hallucinations, and psychoses
Cardiovascular abnormalities, including tachyarrhythmias, digitalis-toxicity arrhythmias, and low voltage on electrocardiograms

Severe magnesium deficiency ($<$ 1.0 mEq/liter) will lead to hypocalcemia, owing to inhibition of parathyroid hormone (PTH) secretion and end-organ resistance to PTH. Magnesium deficiency can exist without hypomagnesemia, but a substantial deficit is indicated by markedly low serum levels. In severe magnesium deficiency, urinary magnesium excretion will be very low if renal function is normal.

Causes. The causes of hypomagnesemia are:

Gastrointestinal disorders, including malabsorption due to bowel disease or resections, bowel and biliary fistulas, chronic pancreatitis, prolonged nasogastric suction, diarrhea, and the prolonged administration of magnesium-free fluids
Endocrine disorders, including hyperparathyroidism, hypoparathyroidism, primary hyperaldosteronism, and diabetic ketoacidosis
Renal diseases, including glomerulonephritis, pyelonephritis, nephrosclerosis, hydronephrosis, and renal tubular acidosis
Diuretic therapy with thiazides, mercurial diuretics, furosemide, ethacrynic acid, and osmotic diuretics
Alcoholism
The healing phase of osteitis fibrosa cystica

Treatment. The treatment of magnesium deficiency depends on the underlying disorder, the severity of the deficiency, and the clinical manifestations. When serum magnesium levels are below 1.0 mEq/liter and symptoms are present, parenteral magnesium is required. With serum magnesium levels of less than 1.0 mEq/liter there is usually a total body magnesium deficit of 150–200 mEq. Intravenous therapy has the potential of producing hypermagnesemia and should be given only when rapid correction is necessary. In such cases 40–60 mEq of magnesium can be given as 10–15 ml of 50% magnesium sulfate in 500 ml of D_5W over 4 hours. This will raise the serum magnesium concentration by several mEq/liter in patients with normal renal function. The infusion can be repeated daily for several days in cases of severe depletion, especially if the patient is unable to take oral preparations. After the severe depletion has been replenished, it is possible to use oral magnesium preparations, if they can be tolerated. Adequate replacement is established when daily urinary magnesium excretion approaches 90% of the daily intake. Magnesium may be administered intramuscularly when oral medication is not tolerated and when the intravenous route is not feasible. Intramuscular injections, however, are painful, and multiple injections are needed because of the low dose of magnesium in the solutions. Patients who have a continuous magnesium loss (e.g, malabsorption) need chronic oral magnesium supplementation. The optimal dose is difficult to judge, but the initial dose is usually in the range of 20–30 mEq/day in three or four divided doses. Increases in the dose should be made according to the serum magnesium values and the clinical status of the patient, inasmuch as the development of diarrhea is usually a limiting factor.

Hypermagnesemia

Hypermagnesemia occurs most frequently in patients with renal failure who take excessive amounts of magnesium-containing antacids. At concentrations of 3.0–5.0 mEq/liter, nausea, vomiting, and hypotension appear. Serum magnesium concentrations of 7.0–10.0 mEq/liter cause hyporeflexia, muscle weakness, drowsiness, and cardiac conduction disturbances (increases in P–R interval and QRS duration and heightened T wave). At concentrations approaching 15.0 mEq/liter, respiratory paralysis and coma occur; and as levels approach 25.0 mEq/liter, there is cardiac arrest in diastole.

Treatment of mild hypermagnesemia is directed primarily at removing the source of excess magnesium. If emergency treatment is required for patients with severe hypermagnesemia, intravenous calcium can be given, which will temporarily reverse the symptoms; however, because renal failure is a usual complication, therapy of severe hypermagnesemia with dialysis is sometimes necessary, especially in life-threatening situations.

---

1. Anast CS, Gardner DW: Magnesium metabolism, in Bronner F, Coburn JW (eds): *Disorders of Mineral Metabolism.* New York, Academic Press, 1981, vol 3, pp 423–506.
General review that includes sections on biochemistry, physiology, metabolism, hormonal interrelationships, and clinical manifestations.
2. Bellar GA, Hood WB Jr, Smith TW, Ablemann WH, Wacker WEC: Correlation of serum magnesium levels and cardiac digitalis intoxication. *Am J Cardiol* 33:225–228, 1974.
Hypomagnesemia was present in 21% of patients with digitalis toxicity.
3. Chipperfield B, Chipperfield JR: Magnesium and the heart. *Am Heart J* 93:679–682, 1977.
Decreased concentrations of magnesium in heart muscle may contribute to sudden death after myocardial infarction.
4. Fishman RA: Neurological aspects of magnesium metabolism. *Arch Neurol* 12:562–569, 1965.
The neurologic manifestations of hypomagnesemia include confusion, seizures, increased neuromuscular irritability, and a positive Chvostek's sign.
5. Iseri LT, Freed J, Bures AR: Magnesium deficiency and cardiac disorders. *Am J Med* 58:837–846, 1975.
Ventricular tachycardia and fibrillation may be associated with hypomagnesemia, and intravenous magnesium may be required to treat the arrhythmia.
6. Massry SG, Seelig MS: Hypomagnesemia and hypermagnesemia. *Clin Nephrol* 7:147–153, 1977.
Review. The main clinical manifestations of hypomagnesemia include neuromuscular disturbances and behavioral abnormalities.
7. Mordes JP, Wacker WEC: Excess magnesium. *Pharmacol Rev* 29:273–300, 1978.
Review. Hypermagnesemia most often occurs in patients with uremia who take mag-

nesium-containing antacids. In severe life-threatening hypermagnesemia, dialysis is capable of controlling hypermagnesemia.

8. Seelig MS, Heggtveit HA: Magnesium interrelationships in ischemic heart disease: A review. *Am J Clin Nutr* 27:59–79, 1974.
Magnesium is essential for maintenance of the functional and structural integrity of the myocardium.
9. Shils ME: Experimental human magnesium depletion. *Medicine* 48:61–85, 1969.
The occurrence of unexplained hypokalemia and hypocalcemia should suggest the possibility of significant magnesium depletion.
10. Wacker WEC, Parisi AF: Magnesium metabolism. *N Engl J Med* 278:658–663, 712–717, 772–776, 1968.
Review of magnesium metabolism that includes a discussion of clinical disorders.

89. DISORDERS OF PHOSPHATE METABOLISM

David M. Slovik

Hypophosphatemia in the elderly may result from chronic phosphate depletion, acute redistribution of phosphate from extracellular to intracellular spaces, or a combination of these two factors. Symptomatic hypophosphatemia, which is uncommon, can have marked consequences in elderly patients who already suffer from many chronic medical illnesses. Symptomatic hypophosphatemia usually begins to appear when the serum inorganic phosphate concentration decreases to a value between 1.8 and 2.0 mg/dl.

Clinical and Metabolic Features

The clinical and metabolic features of hypophosphatemia include:

1. Decreased erythrocyte ATP and 2,3-DPG levels, resulting in increased erythrocyte fragility and hemolytic anemia; and shifting of the oxyhemoglobin dissociation curve to the left, resulting in tissue hypoxia
2. Granulocyte dysfunction, resulting in increased susceptibility to infection
3. Platelet abnormalities, resulting in increased risk of bleeding
4. Bone pain, weakness, defective bone mineralization, and classic findings of osteomalacia
5. An increase in renal 1,25-$(OH)_2$-D production and an increase in intestinal calcium absorption
6. Renal bicarbonate-wasting, mild metabolic acidosis, and other tubular defects
7. Hypercalciuria, which may lead to renal stone formation
8. Generalized weakness, paresthesias, cranial nerve palsies, distal sensory defects, hyporeflexia, myalgias, and muscle weakness
9. Life-threatening serum phophate levels, usually below 0.8–1.0 mg/dl, flaccid paralysis, respiratory paralysis, acute muscle necrosis, confusion, EEG abnormalities, seizures, complete anesthesia, coma, and death

It is important to realize that large carbohydrate loads will produce transient hypophosphatemia and lower the serum phosphate level by as much as 1.0–1.5 mg/dl. This effect is maximal at approximately 2.0–2.5 hours after a meal and is proportional to the glucose load.

Causes

Chronic phosphate depletion arises from starvation and malnutrition, primary hyperparathyroidism, vitamin D deficiency, renal tubular defects, and mesenchymal and giant cell tumors. Acute phosphate redistribution occurs in association with carbohydrate ingestion, hyperalimentation, insulin treatment of diabetic ketoacidosis, acute respiratory alkalosis, refeeding of alcoholics, rapid bone mineralization, and the rapid correction of magnesium deficiency. Starvation and malnutrition can cause phosphate depletion but generally not clinical hypophosphatemia, owing to the efficiency of intestinal phosphate absorption and muscle catabolism. Elderly individuals with marginal phosphate intake, however, who ingest large quantities of phosphate-binding antacids, may develop severe hypophosphatemia.

Treatment

Treatment of hypophosphatemia is empiric and depends on the serum phosphate concentration, underlying disorder, and anticipated length of therapy. Serum inorganic phosphate values should be monitored closely. Phosphate salts should not be added directly to solutions containing calcium salts, because calcium phosphate will be precipitated. It is difficult to estimate total body deficits of phosphate, since under certain circumstances severe hypophosphatemia resulting from phosphate redistribution may occur in the presence of normal body phosphate stores. When the serum phosphate value is below 1.0 mg/dl, hypophosphatemia is severe and deserves prompt therapy. If intravenous phosphate is required, the initial dose should be 2.5–5.0 mg/kg BW, infused over a 4- to 6-hour period. Immediately after the infusion is completed, the serum phosphate value should be checked, and subsequent doses of phosphate should be adjusted according to the results and the clinical status of the patient. Even when treatment restores serum phosphate to normal, the patient may still have phosphate depletion and require close medical observation.

When serum phosphate values are 1.0–2.0 mg/dl, treatment depends on several factors. If the patient has significant symptoms, parenteral phosphate may be necessary, as just described. If symptoms are absent but the precipitating cause, e.g., hyperalimentation, is still present and the margin for developing symptoms narrow, parenteral therapy may again be necessary; otherwise, oral supplementation can be given. Large doses of oral phosphate supplements should generally not be given for acute therapy, because they are poorly tolerated, owing to severe gastrointestinal side effects that make absorption unreliable and diarrhea unacceptable.

Chronic treatment of hypophosphatemia depends on the underlying disorder and the degree of phosphate depletion. Therapy consists of the administration of oral phosphate salts, i.e., either sodium or potassium salts or a mixture of the two. Therapy is begun with low doses of phosphorus, e.g., 250 mg 3 times daily, and then increased. The amount of phosphate required must be individualized and ranges from 1.0–4.0 gm of elemental phosphorus daily in divided doses. The addition of vitamin D or its metabolites is sometimes necessary.

Hyperphosphatemia

Hyperphosphatemia is uncommon in the elderly and, if present, is most commonly due to chronic renal failure. The clinical features associated with hyperphosphatemia are due either to the underlying disorder or to the consequences of precipitating calcium-phosphate salts in extraskeletal tissues, if the calcium and phosphate product (CA $\times$ P) is too high. Other causes of hyperphosphatemia in the elderly include hypoparathyroidism, acute tissue necrosis (e.g., massive trauma and extensive burns), acute hemolytic reactions, cancer chemotherapy with massive cell death, acromegaly, and the ingestion of large quantities of phosphate, in either the diet or phosphate-containing medications.

Multiple other serious metabolic abnormalities usually accompany hyperphosphatemia, and any underlying disorder must be corrected. Treatment consists of correcting the underlying disorder and administering phosphate-binding antacids (e.g, aluminum hydroxide) to decrease intestinal absorption of phosphate.

---

1. Abrams DE, Silcott RB, Terry R, Berne TV, Barbour BH: Antacid induction of phosphate depletion syndrome in renal failure. *West J Med* 120:157–160, 1974.
   On two occasions, a patient on maintenance hemodialysis was found to have a serum phosphorus of less than 1.0 mg/dl, associated with symptoms of bone pain, weakness, and waddling gait. She had been ingesting large quantities of an antacid containing aluminum hydroxide. When this medication was stopped, her symptoms disappeared and the serum phosphorus returned to normal.
2. Betro MG, Pain RW: Hypophosphatemia and hyperphosphatemia in a hospital population. *Br Med J* 1:273–276, 1972.
   A low serum phosphorus concentration was most frequently due to the intravenous administration of carbohydrate, which accounted for 40% of cases.
3. Bringhurst FR, Potts JT Jr: Calcium and phosphate distribution, turnover, and met-

abolic actions, in DeGroot LJ, et al (eds): *Endocrinology.* New York, Grune & Stratton, 1979, pp 551–585.
Review that includes discussions on the distribution, absorption, excretion, metabolic effects, and clinical problems associated with phosphate.

4. Craddock PR, et al: Acquired phagocyte dysfunction: A complication of the hypophosphatemia of parenteral hyperalimentation. *N Engl J Med* 290:1403–1407, 1974.
Acquired granulocyte dysfunction induced by hypophosphatemia may explain the high rate of sepsis in patients undergoing hyperalimentation.
5. Daniels RA, Weisenfeld I: Tumorous phosphaturic osteomalacia. Report of a case associated with multiple hemangiomas of bone. *Am J Med* 67:155–159, 1979.
Tumorous phosphaturic osteomalacia is characterized by hypophosphatemia, decreased tubular reabsorption of phosphorus, hyperphosphaturia, and renal glycosuria with associated bone pain and weakness.
6. Fitzgerald FT: Hypophosphatemia. *Adv Intern Med* 23:137–157, 1978.
Review. Neuromuscular, hematologic, hepatic, and skeletal abnormalities are characteristic of hypophosphatemia.
7. Knochel JP: Hypophosphatemia. *Clin Nephrol* 7:131–137, 1977.
Review. A decline in red blood cell 2,3–DPG concentrations is seen in hypophosphatemia, and this may decrease the amount of oxygen released to peripheral tissues.
8. Knochel JP: The pathophysiology and clinical characteristics of severe hypophosphatemia. *Arch Intern Med* 137:203–220, 1977.
Review. Contraindications to the use of phosphate salts include hypercalcemia, hyperphosphatemia, oliguria, and tissue necrosis.
9. Lee DBN, Brautbar N, Kleeman CR: Disorders of phosphorus metabolism, in Bronner F, Coburn JW (eds): *Disorders of Mineral Metabolism.* New York, Academic Press, 1981, vol 3, pp 283–421.
Extensive review that covers phosphorus homeostasis and clinical disorders.
10. Lentz, RD, Brown DM, Kjellstrand CM: Treatment of severe hypophosphatemia. *Ann Intern Med* 89:941–944, 1978.
Severe hypophosphatemia may occur with normal or depleted body stores. Therapeutic guidelines are empiric, and serum inorganic phosphate concentrations should be monitored closely.
11. Lotz M, Zisman E, Bartter FC: Evidence for a phosphorus-depletion syndrome in man. *N Engl J Med* 278:409–415, 1968.
A syndrome of phosphorus depletion characterized by hypophosphatemia, hypophosphaturia, increased intestinal absorption of calcium, hypercalciuria, and increased skeletal resorption, as well as debility, anorexia, weakness, and bone pain, can be produced with prolonged administration of nonabsorbable antacids such as magnesium-aluminum hydroxides.
12. Newman JH, Neff TA, Ziporin P: Acute respiratory failure associated with hypophosphatemia. *N Engl J Med* 296:1101–1103, 1977.
In 2 alcoholic patients, the administration of intravenous 5% glucose produced a profound fall in serum inorganic phosphate concentration to 0.5 mg/dl; the ventilatory failure that ensued required tracheal intubation.
13. O'Connor LR, Klein KL, Bethune JE: Hyperphosphatemia in lactic acidosis. *N Engl J Med* 297:707–709, 1977.
Serum inorganic phosphate is increased in patients with lactic acidosis, and this is probably due to tissue ischemia.
14. O'Connor LR, Wheeler WS, Bethune JE: Effect of hypophosphatemia on myocardial performance in man. *N Engl J Med* 297:901–903, 1978.
The return of serum phosphate to normal levels in patients with hypophosphatemia improves myocardial contraction.
15. Silvis SE, Paragus PD Jr: Paresthesias, weakness, seizures, and hypophosphatemia in patients receiving hyperalimentation. *Gastroenterology* 62:513–520, 1972.
Severe life-threatening hypophosphatemia can be produced by hyperalimentation.
16. Slatopolsky E, Rutherford WE, Rosenbaum R, Martin K, Hruska K: Hyperphosphatemia. *Clin Nephrol* 7:138–146, 1977.
Review. The most common cause of hyperphosphatemia is a decrease in urinary phosphorus excretion secondary to renal failure. The most effective way to treat hyperphosphatemia is to decrease phosphorus absorption in the gut by the use of phosphate binders.

XII. DISEASES OF EYE AND EAR

90. GLAUCOMA

Don Bienfang

Glaucoma, largely a disease of the elderly, affects one million patients in the United States today, of whom 200,000 have already lost vision from the disease. A major cause of visual loss, glaucoma, like hypertension, causes few symptoms until its later stages, when vision is irrecoverably lost.

Screening

Measurement of Intraocular Pressure. Screening for glaucoma (usually done by an ophthalmologist) is the only way to prevent the complications of increased intraocular pressure. The first step is measurement of intraocular pressure, done with a device that measures the pressure required to indent the eyeball a given amount. This should be done routinely in elderly patients.

Gonioscopy. Gonioscopy, a more complicated technique, is a method of direct observation of the angle formed between the iris and the sclera of the eye. Within this angle is the filtering meshwork of the eye. The relationship between the iris and the filtering meshwork, as well as the appearance of the filtering meshwork, is important in the diagnosis of angle-closure glaucoma, potential angle-closure glaucoma, and the various types of open-angle glaucoma.

Tonography. Tonography, a test requiring considerable experience, is best left to the ophthalmologist. The test measures the increase in aqueous flow through the filtering meshwork that is caused by a standard weight placed upon the eye. The relationship between the weight and the rapidity of outflow serves as a measurement of resistance.

Provocative Testing. Provocative testing is most useful in patients thought to be at risk for an attack of angle-closure glaucoma. Through gonioscopy, the appearance of the angle is determined and then the intraocular pressure is measured; the patient is put in a dark room in the brow-down position for 1 hour. The intraocular pressure is remeasured, and if there is an elevation of 6 mm Hg or more, the patient is then examined by gonioscopy to see if the anterior chamber angle has closed significantly. This procedure separates patients who have shallow anterior chambers and are at risk for angle closure from those patients who have shallow anterior chambers that will not close. The provoked angle closure is readily reversible, so that an acute attack is rarely precipitated.

In all cases of glaucoma it is necessary to map the visual fields for loss of peripheral vision, especially in the Bjerrum portion of the field.

Possible Misleading Results. Although usually reliable, the tests for glaucoma have some pitfalls. Low pressure with pathologic cupping of the optic disc may be measured because the random intraocular pressure taken in the office may not reflect the true state of the patient's eye pressure at other times of the day. Certain patients, even with what might be considered normal intraocular pressures, may have such susceptible nerve heads that they will develop pathologic cupping even at "normal" pressures.

Apparent high intraocular pressure without cupping may be found in patients who become so tense during measurement of intraocular pressure that they falsely elevate their eye pressure by contracting the extraocular muscles. A high initial reading will be obtained from such patients, but if several readings are taken, the pressure will be seen to decrease gradually as the aqueous humor is squeezed out of the eye. (In effect, these patients are performing their own tonography.) Confusion of cupping and atrophy may occur when the examining physician is unable to separate a pale optic nerve head from true loss of the substance of the optic nerve head, as is seen in chronically elevated intraocular pressure.

Chronic Open-Angle Glaucoma

Symptoms. Chronic open-angle glaucoma has very few symptoms except loss of central vision and visual field changes associated with gradual excavation of the optic nerve head, which is caused by chronically elevated intraocular pressure. There may be a family history of glaucoma, in either parents or siblings. Use of systemic corticosteroids or topical corticosteroids may precipitate open-angle glaucoma, as may prior injuries or inflammations of the eye. On physical examination the most important sign of chronic open-angle glaucoma is elevation of the intraocular pressure. The normal levels for intraocular pressure have indistinct upper and lower limits, but in glaucoma the upper limit is of importance. Most patients without pathologic cupping from glaucoma have an intraocular pressure lower than 22 mm Hg. Some people who have intraocular pressures chronically elevated between 22 and 30 mm Hg without evidence of damage to the optic nerve head. Such patients, without evidence of damage, have *ocular hypertension*. Just as many patients with the same relatively modest elevation of intraocular pressure do sustain optic nerve damage, however. Patients with intraocular pressures above 30 mm Hg, with or without damage to the optic nerve head, are at risk for damage to the optic nerve head and usually should be treated. The peripheral field is usually lost first, as the visual fields become progressively constricted later, only a small central island of vision remains and then disappears, causing loss of central visual acuity.

Differential Diagnosis. The ultimate effect of elevated intraocular pressure in most cases is progressive pathologic cupping of the optic nerve head. Recognition of the difference between cupping and atrophy of the optic disc is essential to diagnosis. Atrophy indicates a loss of nerve fibers without a loss of supporting structures of the optic nerve head. The atrophic disc is the pale, chalk-white nerve head that one associates with compressive lesions of the nerve or demyelination. In glaucomatous cupping there is true loss of the substance of the optic nerve head, so that it becomes carved out and excavated. Ultimately the excavation may reach the rim of the optic nerve head, at which point an arclike scotoma always can be detected in the visual field. When the cupping reaches the papillomacular bundle in the central temporal portion of the optic nerve head, central vision is lost. Pathologic cupping usually begins in the upper or lower temporal quadrant of the optic nerve head.

With markedly elevated intraocular pressures, patients may experience pain and corneal edema, but pathologic cupping is usually found alone. With severe loss of optic nerve head substance, one may see a defective afferent pupillary response to light (Marcus Gunn pupil), in which the pupil dilates when a light is shifted from the normal eye into the affected eye.

Treatment. The decision to treat in cases of elevated intraocular pressure must be an individual one, based on prior family history, degree of intraocular pressure, visual loss, and susceptibility of discs, e.g., myopia. Extreme sensitivity of an eye to small doses of medication, allowing pressure to be lowered significantly with simple and inexpensive therapy, is an encouragement to treat.

Pilocarpine and Epinephrine. Drugs used in the treatment of glaucoma follow a standard progression. First attempts are made with low doses of pilocarpine, 1% or 2%, 4 times daily. Relatively weak doses of pilocarpine seldom cause ocular side effects, although stronger doses certainly cause ocular side effects related to induced myopia and a small pupil. Epinephrine may be a good choice for a younger patient whose eyes are responsive to the drug, although the chronic ocular inflammation caused by the drug is undesirable. Epinephrine may be added to pilocarpine in lieu of a stronger dose of pilocarpine, or it may be added to the maximum dosage of pilocarpine, which is almost always pilocarpine 4%. The systemic side effects of pilocarpine and epinephrine are so uncommon as to be hardly worth mentioning. Occasionally one sees a patient who suffers from the cardiostimulatory effects of epinephrine.

Timolol Maleate. Timolol maleate has proved to be remarkably effective in many cases of open-angle glaucoma. This drug is used only twice daily and in responsive patients may be extremely effective. Cautious ophthalmologists are wary of using timolol maleate as the only treatment for open-angle glaucoma, since long-term experience with it is lacking, and since pilocarpine is usually so well tolerated. It is, however, a valuable adjunct when used with pilocarpine and epinephrine or in those cases in which the intraocular pressure is not sensitive to either pilocarpine or epinephrine. Timolol maleate, a beta-adrenergic blocker, can precipitate asthmatic attacks, bradycardia, or congestive heart failure. Phospholine Iodide (echothiophate iodide) and carbachol are drugs that act similarly to pilocarpine. They are used less frequently, although they may be effective in certain cases. Phospholine Iodide, which depletes serum pseudocholinesterase, can cause prolonged apnea if succinylcholine is used concurrently as part of general anesthesia.

Acetazolamide. If the other drugs are ineffective, oral doses of acetazolamide (Diamox), an oral carbonic anhydrase inhibitor used to reduce aqueous production in the ciliary body, may lower the intraocular pressure; but this drug is usually used last because of its side effects. The systemic side effects of acetozolamide are caused by acidosis created by the drug. The acidosis is necessary, however, for the drug to be effective. Lethargy, loss of appetite, numbness and tingling in the extremities, and potassium loss are the most common problems with acetozolamide. In most patients the adverse effects pass in a few days or weeks. All patients who are using acetozolamide are given potassium supplements.

Operation. Operation for open-angle glaucoma is usually done when maximum medical therapy is insufficient to control the intraocular pressure and prevent further loss of visual fields. Surgical intervention is always carried out late in the course of glaucoma because of the potential postoperative complications to the eye. Operation for glaucoma may result in cataract formation, corneal damage, or intraocular infection.

The operation for open-angle glaucoma creates a fistula between the anterior chamber and the subconjunctival space, allowing an exit for the aqueous humor, which is then absorbed by the vessels of the conjunctiva.

Angle-Closure Glaucoma

Diagnosis. In contrast to chronic open-angle glaucoma, acute angle-closure glaucoma is marked by striking and prominent symptoms. The abrupt onset of blurred vision and halos around lights results from corneal edema caused by high intraocular pressure. Pain in the eye is precipitated by the relatively rapid increase of intraocular pressure from normal to very high levels but is unusual except when the intraocular pressure is markedly elevated, usually to 50 mm Hg or more. The patient may have, in addition to ocular pain, nausea, vomiting, and abdominal pain, which may be misdiagnosed as an attack of acute cholecystitis. As with chronic open-angle glaucoma, there may be a family history of a similar problem, and the patient may also have a history of previous, less severe attacks. Topical dilators of the pupil and systemic use of atropine can precipitate attacks of angle-closure glaucoma.

All patients with angle-closure glaucoma have a shallow anterior chamber with the iris already close to the filtering meshwork of the eye. The iris need move only a small amount before it covers the filtering meshwork. The observant physician will identify the problem on seeing a globe with deep dilated vessels on its surface, radiating from the edge of the cornea. The cornea will be cloudy, the pupil semidilated, and the intraocular pressure high when tested.

Treatment. Angle-closure glaucoma is caused by a blockage of the normal flow of aqueous humor from the posterior chamber of the eye (i.e., the area behind the iris) through the pupil into the anterior chamber. A peripheral iridectomy creates an alternative access to the anterior chamber, lowers the pressure gradient between the posterior and anterior chambers, and allows the iris to fall back away from the filtering meshwork. Therefore, angle-closure glaucoma is treated by surgical creation of a second pupil, but the first step is to lower the intraocular pressure, using pilocarpine to constrict the pupil, which pulls the iris away from the filtering meshwork. Acetazolamide also can be used to reduce aqueous humor production, and glycerol to shrink the vitreous body. Medical treatment almost always precedes surgical treatment, because it is much safer to perform a peripheral iridectomy on an eye in which the attack is already halted. Such an eye is not inflamed and is a better target for surgery. Unfortunately, in some cases of angle-closure glaucoma, particularly those in which the attack has been prolonged, there is irreversible damage to the filtering meshwork. In such cases further lowering of the intraocular pressure, with topical medications, may be required after operation.

Although the acute attack may occur in only one eye, anatomic predisposition is almost always present in both eyes, so that peripheral iridectomies should be done in both eyes.

Visual Field Loss

The most common complication of any type of glaucoma is the loss of peripheral visual fields. The pathologic cupping from glaucoma extends largely into the upper and lower temporal quadrants of the optic disc; therefore, the characteristic field loss from chronically raised intraocular pressure, in either angle-closure or open-angle glaucoma, is a semicircle extending from the upper or lower poles of the blind spot. Bjerrum scotoma is characteristic of glaucoma and other diseases of the anterior portion of the optic nerve head. This scotoma advances toward the macula and out toward the periphery as the disorder progresses. In severe cases the entire upper or lower half of the visual field may be lost, or even both the upper and the lower half, at which point the patient is effectively blind. Central vision is usually lost late in eyes with chronically elevated intraocular pressure, but if progressive cupping is not managed by dramatic lowering of the intraocular pressure, loss is almost certain.

1. Blackwell B: Drug therapy, patient compliance. *N Engl J Med* 289:249–252, 1973.
The most important contribution to compliance is the patient's understanding of the illness and the need for treatment.
2. Vincent PA: Patients' viewpoint of glaucoma therapy. *Sight-Saving Rev* (Winter):213–221, 1972–73.
The prescription was not followed by 58% of clinic patients.
3. Richardson KT: Diagnostic evaluation and therapeutic decision in the glaucomas. *Br J Ophthalmol* 56:216–222, 1972.
Suggests a method for organizing diagnostic data so that therapy can be monitored more easily.
4. Duke-Elder S: *System of Ophthalmology, Diseases of the Lens and Vitreous: Glaucoma and Hypotony.* St Louis, Mosby, 1969, vol 11.
A major reference work.
5. Chandler PA, Grant WM: *Lectures on Glaucoma.* Philadelphia, Lea & Febiger, 1965.
General reference source.
6. Grant WM: Antiglaucoma drugs. Problems with carbonic anhydrase inhibitors, in Leopold IH (ed): *Symposium on Ocular Therapy.* St Louis, Mosby, 1973, pp 19–38.

91. CATARACT

Don Bienfang

One and one-half million Americans have decreased vision from cataracts (lens opacification), and approximately 300,000 cataract operations are performed every year. Cataract, probably the most widely encountered eye problem in the elderly, continues to engender a considerable amount of fear among older patients.

Symptomatology

Cataract patients generally present with a rather typical set of complaints. Visual loss is usually gradual, although occasionally a patient first notices a monocular cataract when the better eye is covered and may interpret this as visual loss of sudden onset. The visual loss is always painless, and the patient may describe the obscuration of vision as a veil in front of the eye.

Cataracts that affect the posterior surface of the lens, such as a posterior subcapsular cataract, may cause the vision to be much worse for close objects and in bright light than for distance, because when the pupil is small, all the light must pass through the area of the cataract. Occasionally there is a history of injury to the eye, prior operation on the eye, or use of topical or systemic corticosteroids.

Diagnosis

With the slit lamp one can see the details of the cataractous changes in the lens, but, curiously, the slit lamp is probably the least valuable method of diagnosing the severity of cataracts. Using the +10 lens on the direct ophthalmoscope, the physician may identify a cataract by looking at the opacity against the red reflex. To an experienced physician, this is the best method of assessing a cataract: to observe the macula of the patient's eye, wih the ophthalmoscope, through the undilated pupil. The amount of difficulty that the examiner has in looking through the cataract to see the macula is an indication of the degree of visual obscuration caused by the cataract. The depth of the anterior chamber should be checked, since in some cataracts the lens may swell and reduce the anterior chamber. Likewise, checking the intraocular pressures may identify glaucoma as a complication or cause of the cataract. The pupillary response to light is normally preserved in even the densest cataract. Failure of the pupillary response to light strongly suggests a concomitant pathologic condition in the optic nerve or in the retina behind the cataract. Color perception also is preserved except in the most opaque cataract.

After the visual assessment has been made, the pupil should be dilated and the fundus examined as thoroughly as possible, to exclude a coexisting retinal pathologic condition that may preclude a successful surgical outcome. The major diagnostic pitfall in assessment of cataracts is failure to recognize the coexistence of macular disease. The ability of the examiner to see the macula more easily than would be indicated by the patient's visual acuity suggests that the cataract is not the cause of the patient's poor vision. Optic nerve disease usually produces an afferent pupillary defect (Marcus Gunn pupil), in which the pupil dilates when a light is shone first in the good eye and then in the suspect eye.

Finally, the state of the fellow eye is extremely important, since the visual capacity of a patient turns on the visual acuity of the better eye.

Cataract Surgical Procedure

It is extremely important to assess both visual acuity and the amount of functional difficulty that a cataract patient seems to be experiencing. The decision to perform a cataract operation depends almost entirely on the patient's needs, and there are no hard and fast rules for the timing of the procedure. The major complaint of patients with cataracts is inability to see well enough to lead a normal life. People with certain lifestyles may find that they are very little disabled by what would be a severely disabling cataract in more active persons. A few patients are unable to ignore the cataract; but most people, if they have a dense cataract in one eye and a relatively normal lens in the other, will ignore the eye with the cataract. Certain types of cataract cause a significant amount of glare, which may disturb the patient enough to warrant a surgical procedure. A swollen mature cataract may close the anterior chamber angle and cause an acute attack of glaucoma, or it may leak lens proteins and cause an inflammatory response in front of the eye. Such lenses should be removed. A cataract that obscures the retina also may interfere with a diagnosis of tumor or retinal detachment, or with observation of the course of optic nerve cupping or other changes in the retina and disc.

Intracapsular cataract extraction can be carried out safely in patients over 40 years old, when the attachments between the lens and the vitreous body have loosened. It has the advantage of being a complete cataract extraction, so that no membranes are left behind for secondary opacification. Although it requires a large incision and the removal of the natural barrier between the anterior chamber, the posterior chamber, and the vitreous body, intracapsular cataract surgery is undoubtedly the method preferred by most ophthalmic surgeons.

Postoperative Management

When a patient has had a binocular cataract surgical procedure, or has had a monocular procedure and has very poor vision in the other eye, he or she experiences the optical problems of vision without an intraocular lens (aphakic vision). The elderly have more difficulty with aphakic vision than younger patients. The patient with aphakic vision notices enhanced movement of the environment and peripheral distortion of the visual field. Usually a period of adjustment is necessary to learn to perform tasks that involve movement, and the patient with aphakic vision who has recently begun to wear a spectacle correction will complain of difficulty in managing stairs and sidewalks and even in getting around at home.

The patient who has had a cataract operation on one eye and has a relatively normal fellow eye must regain the ocular balance between the two eyes. In most cases this cannot be accomplished by a spectacle correction for the eye that was operated on, because of the image size disparity between the two eyes. The best solution is often a contact lens, which elderly people may find difficult to handle. The alternative to an external lens is an intraocular lens, placed at the time of operation. Lens insertion, however, is associated with complications that make the surgeon choose patients with great care. Intraocular lenses are nonetheless gaining popularity in the United States. They are an additional step at the time of operation and therefore add an additional set of intraoperative complications. The postoperative management of patients with intraocular lenses is far more complicated than that of patients who have had only a standard cataract operation. Prolonged use of steroids and careful management of pupillary size is needed, and if a retinal detachment occurs, the surgical management is complicated. Postoperative care of the cataract patient includes protecting the eye with a hard shield or glasses to prevent injury and prescribing medication to quiet the inflammation and prevent infection. Depending on the type of surgical procedure patients are able to resume a normal active life within a few weeks or at least in 2 months. With modern techniques, most activities can be resumed a few weeks after operation.

Aphakia is the greatest complication of cataract surgical procedures and must be anticipated by the surgeon. Careful assessment of the patient's acceptance of aphakia is crucial to success. Newer spectacle glass designs have reduced some of the problems of aphakia. Glaucoma and retinal detachments are unusual complications that are managed as in nonaphakic patients.

The drooping of the upper lid usually goes away within a year, and fortunately so does most of the macular edema. Surgical complications include corneal damage, postoperative glaucoma, rare instances of intraocular infection, vitreous loss and consequent retinal detachment, ptosis of the upper lid, and transient macular edema with loss of central vision. Diabetic retinopathy may be worsened by a cataract operation.

1. Duke-Elder S: *System of Ophthalmology*. St Louis, Mosby, 1969, vol 11.
   A major reference source.
2. Jaffe NS: *Cataract Surgery and Its Complications*. St Louis, Mosby, 1972.
   A complete reference to the subject.
3. Chandler PA: Symposium: Cataract extraction: Complications after cataract extraction: Clinical aspects. *Trans Am Acad Ophthalmol Otolaryngol* 58:382–395, 1954.
   Details the problems and their treatments.
4. Kornzweig AL, Feldstein M, Schneider J: The eye in old age. *Am J Ophthalmol* 44:29–37, 1957.
   Ocular survey of over 1,000 aged persons showed cataracts in 61%. In those over 80 years the incidence was 76%.

92. SENILE MACULAR DEGENERATION

Don Bienfang

Senile macular degeneration, a disease with no clearly effective treatment, is diagnosed in 165,000 new cases every year. It is a major problem for the elderly, but fortunately the vision is not so severely impaired as to preclude self-sufficiency.

Clinical Features

A slow onset is characteristic of senile macular degeneration, although the disease causes acute retinal hemorrhage in some cases. A painless, progressive loss of central vision over many months or years, with relative preservation of peripheral vision, is the usual course. Senile macular degeneration affects fine discrimination and not coarse peripheral vision, so the chief complaint regards close reading, since this requires the finest discrimination. Drugs such as chloroquine (which is used little today), hydroxychloroquine, and thioridazine hydrochloride (Mellaril) cause a type of macular degeneration similar to that seen in older patients. Macular degeneration is also a problem among severely myopic patients.

When central visual acuity is profoundly affected, a disturbance of the normal pigmentation of the macular region is expected. In most cases a disturbance in the smooth retinal pigment epithelial layer causes clumps of black pigment in the macular area. In more subtle cases the normal foveal dimple may be absent and be replaced by an irregular roughened foveal area.

The visual fields show a relative central scotoma with the peripheral fields intact. The central scotoma reflects the loss of visual acuity from damage to the fine receptor elements in the macular area. Pupillary response to light is normal except in the grossest cases of macular degeneration.

Assessment

The major problem in assessing macular degeneration is relating ophthalmoscopic findings to the patient's visual acuity. There is a gross correlation between the amount of macular damage that is visible and the degree of visual loss. However, patients with ophthalmoscopically severe macular degeneration may have relatively good visual acuity, and patients with minor-appearing macular changes may have poor visual acuity. If the patient's visual acuity is better than 20/200, a simple test may identify the macula as the cause. The patient looks at a bright light for a fixed time, the light is removed, and the time for the glare to disappear is measured. Patients with sick maculae have a prolonged recovery time. A more complicated method, fluorescein angiography, uses an intravenous injection of fluorescein dye, which is photographed as it passes through the retinal vasculature to show leakage from the blood vessels in macular degeneration. The incongruity of signs and symptoms makes the macular photostress test and fluorescein angiography very useful.

Since senile macular degeneration is a disease of the elderly, it is routine to find a cataract complicating the problem. It is extremely difficult to assess the relative contributions of the cataract and the macular change to visual loss. In most cases the macular degeneration precedes the cataract, so it is possible to have a good idea of how much the cataract has added to the visual loss. A cataract operation does pose a particular problem to patients with macular degeneration, however. Spectacle aphakic correction makes the patient particularly dependent on central vision at the cost of peripheral vision. In macular degeneration the patient's peripheral vision is the primary visual function remaining, so to reduce peripheral vision by a cataract operation often worsens overall function. Patients faced with such a dilemma, however, may be good candidates for intraocular lenses.

There are no complications from senile macular degeneration other than the loss of central visual acuity. It should be emphasized to the patient that central visual acuity is all that is usually lost in senile macular degeneration, that total blindness will not ensue, and that peripheral vision will likely remain intact.

Management

The principle for the management of senile macular degeneration is magnification of the visual image, so that it falls upon seeing retina. This is most easily accomplished for near vision by the use of stronger reading glasses or a magnifying glass. Magnifying the image with telescopes may cause an apparent increase in visual acuity for distance, but telescopes also magnify the movement of objects when the head is turned and sacrifice peripheral field, so that such devices are of limited use. Moreover, telescopes provided to patients to allow them to pass driving tests are rarely successful in actual driving. The patient with senile macualr degeneration will benefit, however, from a strong bright light on his reading material.

Ocular devices are most useful in the more active, younger patients with macular degeneration and become less useful as the patients grow older.

1. Friedman ES, Smith TR: Senile changes of the chorio-capillaris of the posterior pole. *Trans Am Acad Ophthalmol Otolaryngol* 69:652–661, 1965.
   The changes were mild and consisted of a decrease in cellularity and an increase in periodic acid Schiff staining of the capillary wall.
2. Hogan MJ: Role of pigment epithelium in macular disease. *Trans Am Acad Ophthalmol Otolaryngol* 76:64–79, 1972.
   Discusses the ultrastructural pathology.
3. Maumenee AE, Emery JM: An anatomic classification of diseases of the macula. *Am J Ophthalmol* 74:594–597, 1971.
   A comprehensive anatomic classification of macular disease.
4. Kornzweig A: The eye in old age. *Am J Ophthalmol* 44:29–37, 1957.
   A survey of 1,068 aged persons, 86% of whom had good vision. Macular disease occurred in 29%.
5. Sarks SH: Aging and degeneration in the macular region. *Br J Ophthalmol* 60:324–340, 1976.
   A total of 378 eyes were examined clinically and pathologically.

93. RETINAL DETACHMENT

Don Bienfang

There are 25,000 new cases of retinal detachment annually. Many occur in elderly patients. Although there is a modestly increased incidence of retinal detachment in patients who have a family history of the disorder, the higher incidence is eliminated when one removes the hereditary diseases known to predispose to retinal detachment. Therefore, the risk to patients who have relatives with retinal detachment should not be a concern.

Causes

Most cases of retinal detachment are idiopathic, but some detachments are associated with ocular conditions that create a retinal hole by vitreous traction on the retina. Anything that irritates the vitreous or manipulates its shape or position can lead to retinal holes and detachment. For example, cataract operations cause vitreous traction and the development of retinal holes, either from movement of the vitreous into the anterior chamber because of the absence of the lens or from loss of vitreous at the time of surgical procedure. Another example is inflammation of the vitreous body following inflammation of the uvea, so-called *iridocyclitis* or *uveitis,* which creates scars and bands within the vitreous body. Injuries can cause similar disturbances to the vitreous, and the myopic eye is vulnerable to retinal detachment because the retina is stretched out. Formation of vitreous bands is more common in the myopic eye, and the vitreous body becomes liquefied, allowing the vitreous bands to move more easily.

Diabetic proliferative retinopathy is also associated with retinal detachment. The new vessels frequently grow on the surface of the retina and into the vitreous body. In so doing, they drag the retina up into the vitreous and lead to a traction detachment. In SC hemoglobinopathy a proliferation of new blood vessels can lead to retinal detachment. The use of miotics for treatment of glaucoma also may be associated with retinal detachment, although the mechanism is not well understood.

Signs and Symptoms

A warning sign of a developing retinal hole is a flashing light, usually in the periphery of the visual field, since most retinal holes occur in the periphery of the retina. Associated with the flash of light, which is a sign of vitreous traction upon the retina, the patient may have a prominent new floater from a small piece of retina torn loose. The onset of a new symptomatic floater may appear as a black spot, often described as a worm or a fly appearing before the eye. Floaters are very common ocular symptoms, and only a few of them are from retinal breaks. A new floater ($<$ 1 yr old) that causes prominent symptoms for the patient requires an ophthalmologic examination of the entire retina out to its edges, by indirect ophthalmoscopy, usually with scleral depression.

All myopes, all patients who are aphakic, all diabetics, all patients with SC and SS hemoglobinopathies, and patients with a prior history of uveitis should have a dilated fundus examination at intervals, even without symptoms. Not all retinal holes need to be treated, but high myopia, a prior history of retinal detachment, evidence of vitreous traction, and superior location of the hole are indications for treatment.

When the retina actually detaches, the patient usually experiences a slowly moving shade that passes from below upwards, gradually obscuring the vision. In contrast to amaurosis fugax, this visual loss is permanent.

If the macula is still attached, the central visual acuity remains but is limited by the presence of vitreous blood, which is a consequence of the retinal hole. Visual field examination will usually show a relative loss of visual field in the area of the detachment. There is not absolute loss of vision, since the freshly detached retina functions to some degree, having retained some of its anatomic integrity, but the close attachment has been lost between the receptor elements of the retina and the retinal pigment epithelium that nourishes the rods and cones.

Funduscopic examination in the areas of detachment reveals a billowing retina that resembles a collection of adjacent gray hills just touching one another. There may be a small amount of blood in the vitreous, and the ophthalmologist, using the indirect ophthalmoscope, will be able to detect one or more retinal holes.

In an ordinary case of retinal detachment, laboratory studies are useful mainly preoperatively. Blood sugar and blood count may detect patients who have diabetic retinopathy or sickle cell disease, but these cases usually are detectable from examination of the retina itself. The electroretinogram is useful in determining the prognosis for vision.

For the experienced ophthalmologist the diagnosis of retinal detachment should present little difficulty. Intraocular tumor may cause retinal detachment, and therefore when a retinal hole is not found, tumor should be seriously considered. Another cause of retinal detachment without hole formation is eclampsia of pregnancy, but other clinical features make this diagnosis obvious.

Treatment

The principle of therapy for retinal detachment is reattachment of the receptor elements of the retina to the underlying nutritive retinal pigment epithelium. The chance of successful treatment of retinal detachment depends on the duration of the detachment. At operation the eye is indented in the area of the retinal break, so the retinal pigment epithelium comes nearer to the rods and cones and the element of vitreous traction on the retina is reduced. A variety of artificial elements may be sewn or pressed into the wall of the eye to indent it. The surgeon scars the retinal pigment epithelium directly in the vicinity of the area of the holes with a freezing probe or by diathermy. The scars reduce visual acuity, but in most cases they are so far on the periphery that there is no problem. The surgeon usually drains the subretinal fluid that has leaked under the retina from the vitreous body through the retinal hole, but in certain cases the retinal fluid may not be drained, but the indentation of the eye used to cause spontaneous resorption.

Surgical reattachment is successful in almost 95% of all cases. The retina in a few cases does not respond to initial attempts at attachment or redetaches in a short period of time. A macula that has been detached for a period of time, however, may not recover sufficiently for normal visual acuity. Moreover, the reattachment process itself may lead to distortion of the macula, preventing it from lying flat on the eye and causing distortion of the patient's central vision.

The usual surgical technique involves manipulation and even frank removal of the extraocular muscles, which are then reattached to the globe at the end of the procedure. Muscle detachment and the placement of an indenting band as part of the procedure may result in disturbances of extraocular motility, which may be permanent. If necessary, the muscular imbalance induced by the surgical procedure may be corrected later. Another complication follows, in which the placement of a plastic band around the eye and removal of a number of muscles reduces the circulation to the front part of the eye, leading to a vascular hypoperfusion of the front of the eye known as *anterior segment ischemia*. The ischemia may lead to cataract formation and corneal opacities.

Retinal detachment surgical intervention usually takes several hours and is performed on elderly patients under general anesthesia. The procedure may, under certain circumstances, be done under local anesthesia, using a long-acting local anesthetic such as bupivacaine hydrochloride (Marcaine). This method is safer for elderly patients who are poor risks for general anesthesia.

The key to prevention of complications is the rapid detection and treatment of the detachment. The use of surgical techniques that spare the vasculature to the front of the eye is also important for long-term success.

1. Goldmann H: Senile changes of the lens and the vitreous: The Arthur J. Bedell Lecture. *Am J Ophthalmol* 57:1–12, 1964.
   Aging in the lens and vitreous helps explain the observed pathologies.
2. Norton EWD: Retinal detachment in aphakia. *Trans Am Ophthalmol Soc* 61:770, 1963.
   A summary of the problem that complicates lens removal.
3. Ashrafzadeh MT, et al: Aphakic and phakic retinal detachment. *Arch Ophthalmol* 89:476–483, 1973.
   A comparison of nearly 5,000 cases.
4. Byer NE: The natural history of the retinopathies of retinal detachment and preventive treatment. *Isr J Med Sci* 8:1417–1423, 1972.
   Explains the causes and types of retinal breaks.
5. Schepens CL, Marden D: Data on the natural history of retinal detachment: I. Age and sex relationship. *Arch Ophthalmol* 66:631–642, 1961.
   A statistical survey of 3,821 patients reviewed retrospectively shows older males have highest risk.
6. Schepens CL, Marden D: Data on the natural history of retinal detachment: Further characterization of certain unilateral nontraumatic cases. *Am J Ophthalmol* 61:213–226, 1966.
   Discusses the detachments in terms of the morphologic types.

94. OTOLOGIC PROBLEMS IN THE ELDERLY

William R. Wilson

Hearing loss is a common problem of the elderly. Almost all individuals who live in a noisy, industrialized society will gradually experience some hearing loss due to a life-time of noise exposure. Older patients may lose hearing as the result of exposure to ototoxic medications, disease, or both. Certain families have a strong genetic predisposition to progressive presbycusis usually beginning in the fifth and sixth decades. It has been estimated that approximately ten million elderly patients in the United States have impaired hearing; therefore hearing loss represents a major national health problem as well as a common complaint among the elderly.

Sensorineural Hearing Loss

The clinical history of sensorineural hearing loss should specify the time of onset and rate of progression and establish the loss as unilateral or bilateral, constant or fluctuating. These data, once obtained, greatly facilitate identification of the causes of sensorineural hearing loss.

Presbycusis is the most common etiology for bilateral symmetrically decreased hearing in the elderly. Other causes are acoustic or head trauma, ototoxic drugs (aminoglycosides, ethacrynic acid, quinine, or aspirin), acquired syphilis, and, rarely, psychogenic deafness.

Unilateral sensorineural hearing loss is less common than the bilateral type and follows a separate set of causes. The most common are viral cochleitis, intracochlear membrane rupture, and possible obstruction of microvasculature of the inner ear. Acoustic neurinoma or other cerebellopontile angle tumors can present as unilateral hearing loss at any age.

Tinnitus

Subjective tinnitus, which is heard only by the patient, may accompany either sensorineural or conductive hearing loss. In general, it does not respond to therapeutic measures, other than those that restore hearing to normal. Tinnitus is an annoying, but rarely debilitating, symptom that is best handled by a sympathetic explanation. Tinnitus presents little trouble to active persons during the day. At night, a clock radio or mild sedative is helpful.

Objective tinnitus can be heard by the examiner as well as by the patient. Pulsatile objective tinnitus may represent partial vascular occlusion such as seen with carotid artery obstruction, or a vascular tumor, such as glomus tympanicum or jugulare. Clicking sounds can be caused by myoclonic spasms of the palatal musculature. Breath sounds in the ear are secondary to a patent eustachian tube and may occur following marked weight loss.

Conductive Hearing Loss

Conductive hearing loss is far less common in the elderly than sensorineural loss. Otosclerosis is most commonly a disorder of young adults that, if untreated, may persist in the elderly.

Frequently, unilateral or bilateral conductive hearing loss in the elderly represents long-neglected impacted cerumen. In addition, serous otitis secondary to nasopharyngeal carcinoma may occur. Rarely, myxedema results in a mixed conductive and sensorineural hearing loss. Other causes that a physician must consider are foreign bodies in the ear canal, chronic otitis externa, chronic otitis media, and occasionally tumors involving the canal or middle ear.

Otologic Examination

Several features of the otologic examination should be emphasized when the patient is elderly. The auricle should be examined briefly for evidence of tophi, pressure sores, and basal or squamous cell carcinoma. The posterior auricular sulcus may bear the scar or depression of a forgotten childhood mastoid operation. A preauricular tragal crease indicates advanced atherosclerotic cardiovascular disease. Often, impacted cerumen among the elderly is too hard to free with a curette or syringe, and is best removed with twice-daily applications of 10 drops of hydrogen peroxide–glycerin ear drops (Debrox). After a week it is loosened sufficiently for easy removal with a syringe and warm water.

Other than increased opacity of the tympanic membrane, there are no features of the external canal or middle ear that are the direct result of aging. The best gauge of hearing is simply how well the patient hears and understands a conversational speaking voice. The examiner should make certain that the patient has bilateral hearing by whispering in each ear separately, and, if a hearing loss is suspected, should test the hearing with a 512-Hz tuning fork. Patients with normal hearing, perceive air conduction as louder than bone conduction (positive Rinne test). This is also true, however, if the patient has a sensorineural hearing loss. With a conductive hearing loss of 15 db or greater, the patient will perceive bone conduction as louder (negative Rinne test); bone conduction is also greater in the case of a unilateral complete sensorineural loss (false-negative Rinne test). A 512-Hz fork placed in the center of the forehead will lateralize to the ear with the greatest conductive hearing loss (Weber test).

Presbycusis

Features. The pathologic features of presbycusis includes hair cell loss, first-order neuron degeneration, and deterioration of the auditory centers in the central nervous system. Early in the course, many older persons either deny or fail to recognize their hearing loss until it is pointed out by others, usually family members. They often blame their problems on mumbling or on background noise. Like other forms of hearing loss, early presbycusis is accompanied by tinnitus, which may be the first symptom. Other indications of mild hearing loss are increased inability to hear at meetings, a need to turn up the television, and difficulty in speaking to someone in the next room. Patients complain that the higher-pitched voices of women and children are difficult to hear. Some patients with presbycusis find sounds so loud as to be irritating yet have poor word comprehension. Loss of speech discrimination is a common feature. Presbycusis may progress relatively rapidly over several years or slowly over a decade or more.

As presbycusis progresses the patient experiences increased failure to hear on the telephone and complains of missed door and phone bells. The hearing loss may gradually become very handicapping and a source of irritation to the patient and his or her family. Communication may begin to require a loud voice or a shout. Some patients learn to rely on visual clues and acquire self-taught lipreading skills, others become frustrated and angry. The most common complication of hearing loss in the elderly is depression and withdrawal. The embarrassment of not hearing well all too often results in the patient's avoiding social contacts. The hard-of-hearing lose interest in social gatherings, church, and at times their families. Conversely, friends fail to call because of the difficulty of communicating with the patient, thus reinforcing feelings of isolation.

Management. The treatment of patients with hearing deficits incorporates several aspects of medical care. Family and friends must seek out the hard-of-hearing in spite of the difficulty. Communication is best accomplished in quiet surroundings with a minimum of auditory distraction. Most elderly hear better when spoken to directly. Speaking slowly and clearly is more helpful than shouting, as patients with loss of discrimination may have to think about words and derive their meaning from the context of sentences, lip movements, or facial expressions. For the hard-of-hearing the act of listening alone requires concentration, and in some, cognitive function may be impaired, compounding the deficit.

Patients with presbycusis must be encouraged to seek professional assistance for their hearing problem. Medical treatment begins with an ear examination by an otolaryngologist and a thorough hearing evaluation, usually by an associated audiologist. (Unless personal and religious reasons forbid it, recent FDA regulations require a medical evaluation prior to the fitting of a hearing aid.) If amplification is recommended, a hearing aid evaluation is necessary. At that time the proper hearing instrument is selected for the patient, and the patient is given a prescription for it. A qualified hearing aid salesperson will fit the aid to the patient and teach him or her how to use it. The process requires several visits for adjustments and fittings. Many elderly are stymied by this time-consuming, expensive procedure and are clearly unable to accomplish it without the enthusiastic assistance of family or friends.

Hearing aids are very helpful for well-motivated patients, particularly those with good speech discrimination. Among the drawbacks are the initial cost and the cost of battery replacements. Hearing aids are small and difficult to handle for patients with poor eyesight, arthritis, or neurologic disease. Hearing aids amplify ambient noises (wind, traffic, kitchen noises) as well as useful sounds and require frequent adjustment because of changing noise levels. In all, they help, but do not overcome the problem of speech discrimination and therefore are of only partial benefit to many patients with presbycusis. As a result, many hearing aids go unused.

Vestibular Disorders

As presbycusis affects the hearing, progressive degeneration both centrally and peripherally affects the vestibular system. Loss of vestibular function does not necessarily accompany or parallel the degree of hearing loss.

Patients with chronic vestibular disorders suffer from a constant sense of imbalance and fear of falling, rather than vertigo. Their gait is characterized by short, brisk, shuffling steps but is not wide-based. A cane, walker, or handrail and good lighting are helpful. Ataxia is a most discouraging and confining debility for those patients with active minds and spirits. Medications used in the treatment of vertigo are of no benefit.

Otalgia

Otalgia is a complaint that requires careful evaluation in the elderly. Among the causes are carcinoma of the tonsil, base of tongue, hypopharynx, epiglottis, and larynx. Also, dental disease, temporomandibular joint disorders, cervical spine arthritis, and occasionally thyroiditis and angina are found. Ear pain from serous otitis media or otitis media should be followed up by an examination for nasopharyngeal carcinoma in the elderly.

Malignant Otitis Externa

Malignant otitis externa is a life-threatening infection found mostly in the elderly diabetic. It begins, often after swimming as routine otitis externa, but, despite adequate antibiotic drop therapy, fails to improve. The presence of granulations in the ear canal represent the onset of *Pseudomonas* chondritis of the external canal, and, despite what appears to be only a small, localized infection, the patient must be hospitalized and otologic consultation obtained. Prior to the availability of effective antibiotics, *Pseudomonas* chondritis and osteitis were usually fatal in spite of aggressive otologic surgical drainage procedures. Serum creatinine, blood urea nitrogen, and an audiogram must be included among the studies at admission. In addition, the patient's gait and state of balance should be carefully noted.

Treatment consists of combined antibiotic therapy, using either gentamycin or tobramycin in combination with carbenicillin, debridement, and control of the diabetes. In malignant otitis externa, the dosages of gentamycin or tobramycin for patients with normal blood urea nitrogen and creatinine levels are 3–5 mg/kg/day, divided into 3 doses given q8h either slowly IV over 1 hour (by means of a heparin lock) or IM. Peak therapeutic serum levels for gentamycin (4–11 μg/ml) or tobramycin (6–8 μg/ml), measured 15 minutes after IV injection or 1 hour after IM injection, can be monitored and are usually below toxic levels at the doses given here.

Ototoxicity from the drugs is first manifested by balance disturbances. Audiograms are obtained once weekly or as needed to evaluate the clinical symptoms. Full resolution of the infection may require several months of hospitalization.

Indications for Surgical Treatment of Otologic Disorders

The decision to perform an otologic operation on an elderly patient must be made on an individual basis, but several rules are applicable. Stapedectomy for the correction of a conductive hearing loss that will provide the patient with good useful hearing should be performed regardless of age. The procedure is short, can be performed under monitored local anesthesia, and has a very high success rate. The return of hearing to an elderly deafened patient will often result in marked emotional, and possibly physical, improvement. However, other middle ear disorders, such as chronic otitis media with and without drainage, and cholesteatoma, should be treated medically in patients over 65 years of age. The main reason for avoiding a surgical procedure is that reduced vascularity in this age group hampers healing of repaired tympanic membranes and makes poor surgical results likely. Surgical intervention is reserved for patients in whom ear infection or cholesteatoma has led to the onset of attacks of vertigo, facial weakness, or threat of acute bacterial labyrinthitis or meningitis. Because of the potential complications, chronic ear disease should be treated by an otolaryngologist.

1. Butler RN, Gastel B: Hearing and age. *Ann Otol Rhinol Laryngol* 88:676–683, 1979.
Describes research and activities of the National Institute on Aging relevant to hearing in the elderly.
2. Chandler JR: Malignant external otitis. *Laryngoscope* 78:1257–1294, 1968.
Description of this life-threatening disorder, which occurs most commonly among elderly diabetics.
3. Cohn AM: Progressive necrotizing otitis: Malignant external otitis. *Arch Otolaryngol* 99:136–140, 1974.
Describes the progressive course and treatment of pseudomonas infections of the external and middle ear and mastoid in elderly diabetic patients.
4. Hansen C, Reske-Nielsen E: Pathological studies in presbycusis. *Arch Otolaryngol* 82:115–131, 1965.
In 10 of 12 patients the basal cochlear coils were histologically abnormal.
5. Lowell SH, Paparella MM: Presbycusis: What is it? *Laryngoscope* 87:1710–1717, 1977.
A comprehensive discussion of audiological and clinical findings in presbycusis.
6. Lowry LD, Isaacson SR: Study of 100 patients with bilateral sensorineural hearing loss for lipid abnormalities. *Ann Otol Rhinol Laryngol* 87:404–408, 1978.
Finds a lesser incidence of lipoprotein abnormalities than expected from the general population.
7. Makishima K: Arteriolar sclerosis as a cause of presbycusis. *Otolaryngology* 86:322–326, 1978.
Presbycusis is caused in part by the pathologic changes of angiosclerosis.
8. Nadol JB Jr: Electron microscopic findings in presbycusis degeneration of the basal turn of the human cochlea. *Otolaryngol Head Neck Surg* 87:818–836, 1979.
Notes changes indicative of primary neural, hair cell, and supporting cell degeneration.
9. Sanders JW: The successful hearing aid user. *Otolaryngol Clin North Am* 11:187–193, 1978.
Improvements in design, construction, and evaluation procedures have increased the number of successful hearing aid users.
10. Schukenecht HF: *Pathology of the Ear.* Cambridge, Mass, Harvard University Press, 1974, pp 388–403.
Details changes with age.
11. Schuknecht H: Further observations on the pathology of presbycusis. *Arch Otolaryngol* 80:369–382, 1964.
Sensory, neural, metabolic, and mechanical lesions underlie the loss of hearing with age.
12. Stephens SDG: Rehabilitation of the hearing impaired adult in Denmark. *Clin Otolaryngol* 4:95–98, 1977.
The overall success of the Danish system of rehabilitation services is the result of its comprehensiveness.
13. Stephens SDG: Hearing aid use by adults: A survey of surveys. *Clin Otolaryngol* 2:385–402, 1977.
Summary and analysis of investigative studies on the use of hearing aids.
14. Suga F, Lindsay JR: Histopathological observations of presbycusis. *Ann Otol Rhinol Laryngol* 85:169–184, 1976.
Audiometric curve does not necessarily indicate a lesion in a specific cochlear element.
15. Weber HJ, Pirkey WP: Selection of hearing aids. *Otolaryngol Clin North Am* 11:173–186, 1978.
Discourages the use of a hearing aid with excessive power output.
16. Alpiner JG (ed): *Handbook of Adult Rehabilitative Audiology.* Baltimore, Williams & Wilkins, 1978.
17. Glorig A, Hearing aids and the otolaryngologist. *J Cont Ed Otol Rhinol Laryngol Allergy* 41:15, 1979.
18. Katz J: *Handbook of Clinical Audiology.* Baltimore, Williams & Wilkins, 1978, pp 426–441.
19. Radcliffe D: The aging of America: Impact on hearing health. *Hearing Aid J* 8:1, 1978.
20. Rintelmann W: *Hearing Assessment.* Baltimore, University Park Press, 1979.
These references discuss the role of audiology and use of hearing aids.

XIII. NEUROLOGIC DISEASES

95. PARKINSON'S DISEASE

Thomas M. Walshe

Symptoms

Parkinson's disease usually begins insidiously in patients who are older than 50 years and has its onset after age 60 in about 20% of cases. It is a chronic disorder in which the pigmented neurons of the substantia nigra and other nuclei degenerate, to be replaced by a reactive gliosis. Intracytoplasmic hyaline inclusions, called *Lewy bodies,* are found in the pigmented neurons of the substantia nigra and the locus ceruleus. Cell loss also occurs in the globus pallidus, putamen, and caudate nucleus. The primary lesion, however, is in the dopaminergic tract, which connects the cells of the substantia nigra with the corpus striatum. There are also losses in cholinergic neuronal groups in the caudate and in the deep diencephalic nuclei, such as the nucleus basalis.

The diagnostic finding of most importance in Parkinson's disease is slowness of movement, or *bradykinesia.* The diagnosis is suggested by a gradual onset of bradykinesia, rigidity, and tremor. Aging causes slower reaction time, but the changes in Parkinson's disease are much more marked than those seen in usual aging.

Although tremor is the most obvious finding, it is not essential to the diagnosis. Most Parkinson's patients have a typical resting tremor at one time or another but also have bradykinesia and rigidity, which confirm the diagnosis. Parkinsonian patients have a slow response time, and each movement seems as if it is done in "slow motion." In addition, patients have an abnormality of tone that causes the limbs to feel rigid on passive movement. Many Parkinson patients have an essential tremor superimposed upon the rigidity, which causes the well-known "cogwheel" phenomenon elicited by passively moving the limb.

When a patient develops a slowly progressive motor disorder in which bradykinesia, rigidity, and resting tremor coexist, the diagnosis is usually Parkinson's disease. The deficits are frequently bilateral, but one side or one extremity may be involved alone, early in the course. The facial expression becomes "starched," with little spontaneous blinking; gait is usually abnormal because of the slowness and loss of the usual associated movements. Small steps, stooped posture, and a tendency to shuffle are also characteristic.

Patients with Parkinson's disease seldom have disorders of language, praxis, vision, or sensation. It is distinctly unusual for them to have hemiparesis or Babinski signs, although some may develop such pyramidal signs late in the disease from concomitant diseases. Late in the disease, dysphonia causes the patient's speech to be nearly inaudible. Motor power is good, although tasks are performed slowly.

Although most physicians can diagnose Parkinson's disease by history and examination alone, most obtain an EEG and CT scan to ensure that there is no unsuspected lesion. In Parkinson's disease the EEG and CT are usually normal, although there may be signs of mild brain atrophy on the CT scan.

Mild or moderate dementia occurs in over one-third of advanced cases of Parkinson's disease, usually well after the motor abnormality is clearly established. Patients who experience an early decline in memory, and develop the findings of Parkinson's disease later, usually become severely demented, and at autopsy some have the neuropathologic changes of both Parkinson's and Alzheimer's disease. Treatment of the movement disorder is less successful in patients with early dementia than in patients whose dementia follows the movement disorder.

Diagnosis

The diagnosis of Parkinson's disease is difficult in older patients because neurologic changes that accompany aging superficially imitate the signs of parkinsonism. Elderly persons develop slowness of response, become unsteady on their feet, do not respond quickly on tests, and may develop mild rigidity. The bradykinesia seen in normal elderly patients is almost always symmetric and is much less marked than in patients with Parkinson's disease. The typical extrapyramidal tremor does not occur in normal aging, but a misdiagnosed essential tremor, along with the extrapyramidal changes of aging, might lead an unwary physician into making an erroneous diagnosis of Parkinson's disease.

Very few disorders resemble the clinical syndrome of Parkinson's disease. The most important, because it is reversible, is the neuroleptic drug–induced parkinsonian syndrome. The differentiation is made by getting the drug history. The parkinsonian symptoms usually disappear when the neuroleptic drugs are removed. When patients need neuroleptics and have severe parkinsonism, benztropine (Cogentin), 2–4 mg bid, or Trihexyphenidyl (Artane), 1–5 mg tid, may reduce the severity of bradykinesia. Tardive dyskinesia, another complication of neuroleptics, is not prevented with anticholinergic drugs.

System degenerations with prominent extrapyramidal signs superficially resemble Parkinson's disease but can usually be separated by a careful history and physical examination. Progressive supranuclear palsy and striatonigral degeneration have neurologic signs not found in Parkinson's disease.

Treatment

The treatment of Parkinson's disease requires careful titration of anticholinergic and dopaminergic drugs. The goal of therapy is to allow as much normal activity as possible. When the disease is mild and does not impede the patient's daily routine, no therapy is required. When treatment is needed, an anticholinergic drug, benztropine (Cogentin), 2–4 mg bid or tid, may keep the patient functional for years. The side effects even in the elderly are minor, although acute glaucoma and bladder retention become a problem in a few. The initial blurred vision and dry mouth usually disappear with prolonged use of the medicine or a reduced dose. In some elderly persons, anticholinergics produce a confusional state. The medicine is stopped or the dose reduced to reverse the confusion.

Dopaminergic Drugs. The most important and successful drug in Parkinson's disease is a combination of L-dopa and carbidopa (Sinemet). Most combinations come as 100 mg or 250 mg of L-dopa and 10 or 25 mg of carbidopa. Carbidopa, which inhibits decarboxylation of the peripheral L-dopa, allows a higher dose to be used without gastrointestinal and other systemic side effects. For older patients it is best to initiate therapy with 100/25 (L-dopa–carbidopa) tablets bid. The dose can be increased weekly until maximal improvement or the first signs of toxicity. A total of 2,000 mg of L-dopa is the limit in most patients. The dose needed to improve symptoms varies widely, and patients should be allowed to time their doses to suit their activities.

Complications of L-Dopa. The major problem with elderly patients receiving L-dopa is a drug-induced confusional state or acute psychotic reaction. Involuntary movements that resemble chorea or myoclonus are side effects of excess L-dopa, and orthostatic hypotension develops in some patients. When side effects become intolerable, the dose must be reduced. When a patient has a toxic reaction from L-dopa, the dose must be reduced but not stopped altogether. It is usually sufficient to reduce the daily dose by one or two pills. The toxic effects will usually abate in several days.

Although many patients with Parkinson's disease are improved by L-dopa with relative ease, some patients have a great deal of difficulty arriving at a dose that is effective without causing excessive toxicity. Very gradual increases in the dose help to avoid the problem in some cases. Another problem is end-of-dose akinesia, in which the patient becomes stiff toward the end of the dose interval. This can usually be relieved by shortening the dose interval and increasing the total dose of drug. More difficult to treat is the on-off phenomenon, in which the patient suddenly becomes bradykinetic not in association with the end of dose. On-off patients may have fluctuating blood levels of L-dopa or other absorption problems. Reducing the dose interval may help, but not always. Longer-acting drugs are sometimes useful for on-off patients, and Bromocriptine, a dopamine agonist, is the one currently available. The Bromocriptine dose is 10–20 mg qd but may be increased to 40–50 mg qd.

Other Treatments. Amantadine hydrochloride (100 mg bid) is sometimes useful, either alone as initial therapy or in addition to the other medicine. Amantadine acts by preventing neuronal uptake of dopamine, so it may augment the effect of L-dopa.

Although the movement disorder is the most disabling feature of Parkinson's disease, other symptoms need specific treatment also. Proper nutrition and hydration are sometimes difficult because the patient is so slow. Awareness of the difficulty will allow family or nursing staff to give the patient enough time to finish his meals. Adequate hydration and exercise go a long way in reducing constipation, which is a frequent complaint in Parkinson's disease. Most parkinsonian patients require a laxative or suppository, at least occasionally. Parkinsonian patients who develop bowel obstruction need a thorough evaluation, because there is almost always a cause in addition to the Parkinson's disease.

1. Bianchine JR: Drug therapy for parkinsonism. *N Engl J Med* 295:814–818, 1976.
A brief, accessible review.
2. Bosches B: Sinemet and the treatment of parkinsonism. *Ann Intern Med* 94:364–370, 1981.
A discussion of the long-term use of Sinemet.
3. Calne DB, Kebabian J, Silbergeld E, Evarts E: Advances in the neuropharmacology of parkinsonism. *Ann Intern Med* 90:219–229, 1979.
A discussion of basic pharmacology.
4. Carman JB: Anatomic basis of surgical treatment of Parkinson's disease. *N Engl J Med* 279:919–930, 1968.
Extensive review with clear illustrations.
5. Fann S: On-off phenomenon with levodopa therapy in parkinsonism. *Neurology* 24:431–441, 1974.
Discussion of the pharmacology behind the phenomenon.
6. Fann WE, Whelan JC: Therapeutic principles in the management of movement disorders in elderly patients. *Interdiscipl Top Gerontol* 15:194–210, 1979.
Includes tardive dyskinesia, Huntington disease, and Parkinson's disease.
7. Hakim AM, Mathieson G: Dementia in parkinson disease: A neuropathologic study. *Neurology* 29:1209–1214, 1979.
Plaques, neurofibrillary tangles, granulovacuolar degeneration, and cortical cell loss were present in 33 of 34 brains.
8. Klawans HL, Topel JL: Parkinsonism as a falling sickness. *JAMA* 230:1555–1557, 1974.
Subtle changes in postural reflex may cause falling even with mild parkinsonism.
9. Lesser RP, et al: Analysis of the clinical problems in parkinsonism and the complications of long-term levodopa therapy. *Neurology* 29:1253–1260, 1979.
A discussion of 131 patients and their progressive course. Others do not agree that L-*dopa contributes to the more rapid decline.*
10. Lieberman A, et al: Dementia in Parkinson disease. *Ann Neurol* 6:355–359, 1978.
Demented patients were older, developed Parkinson's disease later, had a more severe course, and responded to L-*dopa poorly.*
11. Lieberman A, Kupersmith M, Estey E, Goldstein M: Treatment of Parkinson's disease with bromocriptine. *N Engl J Med* 295:1400–1404, 1976.
Notes early success using high doses. At present, lower doses are used.
12. Martin WE, Lowenson RB, Resch JA, Baker AB: Parkinson's disease: Clinical analysis of 100 patients. *Neurology* 23:783–790, 1973.
Discusses a series of patients who were not treated with L-*dopa.*
13. Presthus J: Diagnostic problems in extrapyramidal disorders. *Acta Neurol Scand* 57 (supp 67):123–137, 1978.
A well-conceived view that stresses the importance of the neurologic examination.
14. Richardson EP: Remarks on the pathology of Parkinson's disease. *Monographs in Biology and Medicine.* New York, Grune & Stratton, 1965, pp 63–68.
The lesions are invariably in the substantia nigra in both postencephalitic and idiopathic Parkinson's disease.
15. Teravainen H, Calne DB: Action tremor in Parkinson's disease. *J Neurol Neurosurg Psychiatry* 43:257–263, 1980.
A discussion of the occasional finding of essential tremor in Parkinson's disease.
16. Young RR: The differential diagnosis of Parkinson's disease. *Int J Neurol* 12:210–235, 1977.
A good review of the clinical problem.
17. Forno LS, Barbour PJ, Norville RL: Presenile dementia with Lewy bodies and neurofibrillary tangles. *Arch Neurol* 35:818–822, 1978.
The overlap of degenerative diseases pathologically is illustrated by this case.
18. Davison AN: Neurochemical observations in pathological forms of central nervous system aging. *Interdiscipl Top Gerontol* 15:1–12, 1979.
Summary of aspects of the degenerative disorders.
19. Marttila RJ, Rinne UK: Dementia in Parkinson's disease. *Acta Neurol Scand* 54:431–441, 1976.
Prevalence of dementia was 29% in 444 parkinsonism patients. The frequency of dementia increases with age.

20. Kosaka K, Mehraein P: Dementia-parkinsonism syndrome with numerous Lewy bodies and senile plaques in cerebral cortex. *Arch Psychiatr Nervenkr* 226:241–250, 1979.
Five cases with progressive dementia and rigidity had both Parkinson's and Alzheimer's disease at autopsy.
21. Ikeda K, Hori A, Bode G: Progressive dementia with "diffuse Lewy-type inclusions" in cerebral cortex. *Arch Psychiatr Nervenkr* 228:243–248, 1980.
A 69-year-old man with dementia preceding the motor disorder had both Parkinson's and Alzheimer's disease.
22. Forno LS, Barbour PJ, Norville RL: Presenile dementia with Lewy bodies and neurofibrillary tangles. *Arch Neurol* 35:818–822, 1978.
This case lies between Parkinson's and Alzheimer's disease, both clinically and pathologically.
23. Loranger AW, Goodell H, McDowell FH, Lee JH, Sweet RD: Intellectual impairment in Parkinson's syndrome. *Brain* 95:405, 1972.
A slight degree of intellectual impairment is almost the rule; about half the 63 patients were subnormal on the WAIS.
24. Pollack M, Hornabrook RW: The prevalence, natural history and dementia of Parkinson's disease. *Brain* 89:429–448, 1966.
The diagnostic groups leave some doubt about the findings. The "atherosclerotic" cases were more often demented.
25. Pearce J: The extrapyramidal disorder of Alzheimer disease. *Eur Neurol* 12:94–103, 1974.
Points out that the features of Parkinson's disease are frequent in patients with Alzheimer's disease. No mention of drug treatment or pathology.

96. SEPARATING DEMENTIA FROM CONFUSIONAL STATES

Thomas M. Walshe

There is nothing more devastating in an aged individual than diminished mental function. Several disorders cause altered mental function in elderly patients, but the clinician is often required to separate two interrelated syndromes, dementia and confusion. Each has a separate set of pathologic features that requires a specific evaluation.

Definition of Dementia and Confusion

Dementia describes a chronic symptom complex in which memory fails but the patient remains alert. The term was introduced in 1806 by Pinel, when he described the state of "demency" as "a peculiar debility of the understanding and the acts of the will." Maudsley refined the definition in 1874, describing the demented patient as one whose "memory is impaired, feelings quenched, and intelligence is enfeebled or extinct." Since then, dementia has been used to describe the symptoms of cognitive failure associated with many causes.

Dementia usually occurs with well-established intracranial lesions, whereas *confusional states* in elderly patients are most commonly caused by systemic disease outside the central nervous system. Intracranial lesions, such as meningitis or right hemisphere stroke, may cause the acute confusional state, but for the most part other signs make the diagnosis clear. The separation of dementia and the confusional state is not always complete, especially when patients with chronic dementia have acute episodes of confusion. The confusional state in chronic dementia often appears at night and improves during the day. There is usually no underlying illness, although when the acute confusional state persists, an underlying illness is often the cause. When patients are in an acute confusional state, the memory cannot be properly tested; so the diagnosis of dementia or assessment of the degree of dementia should be postponed until the acute phase is over. Because of the interrelationship between dementia and the acute confusional state, usage of the terms has become vague; unless clearly defined, they will not help to distinguish different etiologic categories.

Features and Types of Dementia

Modern practice separates several types of memory disorder. **Memory loss** is the common feature of all dementias. Memory loss may be progressive over months or years, as in senile dementia of the Alzheimer type (SDAT); or, in disorders such as stroke or trauma, it may remain unchanged after the initial damage. The amnestic state is easily separated from other dementias because it is characterized by isolated loss of memory with preserved language and personality. In Huntington's disease, progressive supranuclear palsy, and Parkinson's disease, memories associated with incidental experience or with projection of information (planning) are most affected, and language is usually intact. The degree of the dementia depends on the stage of the illness or the size and location of the cerebral lesions.

The character of the memory deficit is related to the underlying pathologic state. Patients with SDAT fail in memory, personality, language, praxis, and ability to process information. Korsakoff's psychosis from thiamine deficiency or other lesions in the medial temporal lobe or dorsal medial thalamic regions causes a failure in access of memories, but personality, language, and other cognitive functions are usually spared. Dementia (or the amnestic state, which is a specific type of dementia) implies a lesion in the brain itself. There are patients, however, with early Alzheimer's disease or with Korsakoff's psychosis that exhibit no obvious changes on gross examination of the brain. The psychoses are marked by changes in affect, attention, or thought content but, in almost all cases, can be separated from the dementias because the memory remains clear. Depression sometimes prevents adequate memory testing, making it hard to separate it from dementia.

Features and Types of Confusional States

The confusional state differs from the syndrome of dementia because of its acute onset, changing character, attention deficit, and obtundation. Patients in an acute confusional state have a reduced, erratically shifting attention span—a condition that usually comes on over several hours. Patients are unable to maintain a coherent stream of thought or action. When tested, confusional patients seem to know a number of correct facts, but they fail to associate them in the usual order. The ability to answer test questions correctly varies from time to time. Some patients are somnolent and fall asleep unless stimulated, others are hyperalert. The patient fails to attend to the examination and is easily distracted by extraneous stimuli. Memory may not be affected, or the patient may confabulate. The confusional state remits and relapses over several days; in elderly patients the mental abnormality may not clear for days after the underlying illness is resolved.

Acute confusional states are often reversible, and it is axiomatic that the elderly patient with acute confusion requires a general medical evaluation along with a neurologic one. Elderly patients develop acute confusion and stupor more easily than normal young persons, and elderly patients with existing neurologic disease, either dementing or not, are quite likely to become confused when ill from any cause.

Patients with head trauma, stroke, or other lesions affecting the right hemisphere sometimes develop a chronic confusional state that resembles the acute state in some ways. The chronic confusional state is stable over months or years and usually does not include somnolence; but it does produce inattentiveness, apathy, and incoherent thinking, in which fragments of information are available but poorly associated. Patients with Parkinson's or Huntington's disease may have a confusional state early in the course of their disease but gradually develop a memory loss that is more profound than that seen in the confusional state. Small infarctions in the nondominant hemisphere also may cause such a state.

Other Syndromes of Mental Deficiency

There are other syndromes in which there is alteration of the mental state but memory is not defective. Patients with frontal lobe lesions develop a state of apathy, in which the personality is blunted and spontaneity lost. Such listless states, called *abulia,* are not always associated with impairment of intellect, memory, or reasoning. The prototype frontal lesions are surgical frontal lobotomies, which cause personality changes but do not affect memory per se. In late stages of degenerative dementias and in other disorders that do not affect the frontal lobes alone, abulia may coexist with dementia.

Mental retardation is another abnormality of cognition, in which the patient cannot learn and reason effectively. Mental retardation is usually evident in childhood, but chronic mental institutions house retarded patients who are erroneously thought to suffer a degenerative dementia. The diagnosis is made when the history of developmental delay is available, and when it is evident that the condition is not progressing. Some patients with Down's syndrome develop dementia at an early age, superimposed on their retardation. Pathologic examination usually shows changes similar to those found in SDAT.

Sometimes patients with aphasia may be erroneously diagnosed as being demented. When given non verbal tests, however, the aphasic patient can respond adequately. When a history is obtained, the speech disorder can usually be recognized as a result of a specific event. Aphasia is a regular feature of Alzheimer dementia but is seldom seen in confusional states. Agraphia without aphasia occurs, however, in the confusional state.

1. Chedru F, Geschwind N: Disorders of higher cortical function in acute confusional states. *Cortex* 8:395–411, 1972.
   Acute onset of inattention, disturbance of mood, lack of concern for the illness, mild word-finding difficulty, constructional apraxia, and memory deficit were reported in 24 patients.
2. Flint FJ, Richards SM: Organic basis of confusional states in the elderly. *Br Med J* 2:1537–1539, 1956.
   Even without modern technology, 188 of 242 patients had diagnosable disease, most of which was extracranial.
3. Mesulam MM, Geschwind N: Disordered mental states in the postoperative period. *Urol Clin North Am* 3:199–215, 1976.
   Describes the clinical picture of acute confusion.
4. Mesulam MM, Waxman SG, Geschwind N, Sabin TD: Acute confusional states with right middle cerebral artery infarctions. *J Neurol Neurosurg Psychiatry* 39:84–89, 1976.
   The role of the right hemisphere in maintainence of attention is emphasized as a feature of acute confusion.
5. Seymour DG, Henschke PJ, Cape RDT, Campbell AJ: Acute confusional states and dementia in the elderly: The role of dehydration/volume depletion, physical illness and age. *Age Ageing* 9:137–146, 1980.
   One-fourth of the confused elderly were also demented.
6. Rabins PV, Folstein MF: Delirium and dementia: Diagnostic criteria and fatality rates. *Br J Psychiatry* 140:149–153, 1982.
   An altered level of consciousness was the most important feature in separating the delirious from the demented patients. The delirious patients had a higher mortality.
7. Engle G, Romano J: Delirium: A syndrome of cerebral insufficiency. *J Chronic Dis* 9:260–277, 1959.
   Defines the confusional state and points out its relationship to systemic disorders.
8. Lipowski JZ: Delirium, clouding of consciousness and confusion. *Nerv Ment Dis* 145:227–255, 1967.
   A review with 139 references.
9. Wolff HG, Curran D: Nature of delirium and allied states: The dysergastic reaction. *Arch Neurol Psychiatry* 33:1175–1215, 1935.
   Describes 106 cases in which poor memory and concentration, fear, anxiety, suspicion, misinterpretation, hallucinations, and restlessness were major features.
10. Romano J, Engle GL: Delirium I and II. *Arch Neurol Psychiatry* 51:356–392, 1944.
    A two-part treatise points out the many medical causes and the EEG features.

97. SENILE DEMENTIA OF THE ALZHEIMER TYPE

Thomas M. Walshe and Cheri Leonard

Senile dementia of the Alzheimer type (SDAT), a progressive neuronal degeneration manifested clinically by an unremitting deterioration of memory, learning, and personality, is the most common cause of dementia in elderly patients. The symptom of dementia occurs in 5% of individuals over age 65, and in nearly 20% of patients over age 80. Two-thirds of all demented patients have SDAT, usually sporadic, which is a dominant trait in certain families. Furthermore, the incidence of all degenerative disorders is four times greater in the families of patients who have SDAT. Mortality in SDAT is higher by 30% than in age-matched controls, making SDAT fifth in the leading causes of death in the United States. The chronic morbidity it causes, however, is one of the greatest health problems in the country.

Pathologic Features

The clinical course and neurologic features are suggestive, but only the pathologic findings in Alzheimer's disease are diagnostic. The cerebral cortex and the subcortical nuclei become grossly atrophic. Cell loss occurs in the basal nucleus of Meynert, a primarily cholinergic nucleus with extensive cortical projections. On microscopic examination neurofibrillary tangles are seen in the neurons and senile plaques in the gray matter. The number of plaques and tangles has been found to have a correlation with the degree of dementia. The neurofibrillary tangles are composed of abnormal paired helical filaments, and the plaques consist of degenerating neurons surrounding an amyloid core. Biochemical analysis of postmortem brain tissue has identified a 90% reduction in the level of the enzyme choline acetyltransferase, indicating a selective loss of cholinergic activity.

Clinical Course

Differences Between Age Groups. The clinical features of SDAT begin insidiously and progress over a period of several years. Memory and intellect are always impaired. The clinical syndrome differs slightly between patients in whom the disease begins at a young age and those with the onset in the senium. Patients with early age of onset are more likely to develop language difficulties and to be left-handed. Furthermore, a more rapid and malignant course is the rule in the presenile group. Older patients develop gait disturbances that are greater in severity than would be expected from the degree of other impairment. Older patients also have less language deficit, so that they maintain a circumlocutory stream of speech despite their severe dementia. Longevity is reduced in both groups, but patients with early onset have a more rapid course.

Benign Senescent Forgetfulness. Elderly patients who have minimal memory loss are sometimes described as having *benign senescent forgetfulness*. Benign forgetfulness is not progressive, does not interfere with daily activity, and does not seriously limit the patient. Benign forgetfulness is manifested by the singular intermittent failure to remember relatively unimportant pieces of information—a name, a date, a place. The memory disturbance waxes and wanes, and the patient is usually not disabled by the loss of memory. Mild SDAT in elderly patients may be indistinguishable from benign senescent forgetfulness, but the clinical diagnosis of SDAT becomes evident as patients progress to a more severe state of dementia without other medical or neurologic disease.

Difficulty in Diagnosis. During the early phases of SDAT, the diagnosis is not always clear, and the physician must evaluate the patient for curable disorders. Clinical features of depression may be prominent early in SDAT, so that the two disorders are hard to separate. A trial of antidepressants will improve patients with depression and is useful in diagnosis in some cases. The CT scan in SDAT usually shows enlarged ventricles but is not diagnostic. Likewise, the EEG is often abnormal but may be normal. Spinal fluid is normal even in advanced cases. The major diagnostic clue in SDAT is the clinical history and neurologic examination.

First Stage. The initial stage of SDAT lasts 2–4 years and is characterized by gradually increasing memory loss (names, appointments, daily events, possessions). Carelessness in work and appearance, loss of spatial perception, and disturbance in planning and judgment add to the subtle changes in behavior and personality (apathy, irritability, hyperactivity). There are generally no other neurologic signs. Usually the patient is unaware of the deficits, even when others point them out. When symptoms exist for several years the diagnosis of SDAT becomes more obvious. The insidious progression, memory loss, aphasia, loss of interest in usual pursuits, and lack of motor and/or sensory findings can point to almost nothing else.

Second Stage. In the second stage of the disease the dementia becomes more profound. The patient is unable to comprehend simple instructions and fails to carry out even simple tasks. Complete visual and/or spatial disorientation and aimless wandering also mark this stage. Extrapyramidal signs become manifest, and other focal symptoms, including aphasia, apraxia, and agnosia, are the rule. Language may be fluent but devoid of any information. Patients have echolalia and palilalia; and, as language fails, verbal utterances may be reduced to nonsensical jargon—logoclonia (the repetition of nonsense), klatzomania (repeated loud utterances), or other noises (humming, moaning). Dressing, grooming, and the use of even the most rudimentary implements becomes impossible. Patients sometimes have voracious appetites, and some develop a peculiar behavior called the *Klüver-Bucy syndrome,* in which the person compulsively puts things into his or her mouth and persistently reaches for and handles objects. A few patients become sexually uninhibited. The behavioral aberrations, often coupled with aggressive, agitated, restless activity, wandering, and incontinence, eventually lead to institutionalization.

Final Stage. In the final stages the patient becomes bedridden, contracted, and mute. Neurologic signs are generally symmetric, although in a few cases there are unilateral dystonic postures or other asymmetries of tone. Pyramidal tract signs are absent, unless the course has been complicated by other neurologic disease. Marked rigidity causes the patient to lie motionless and become contracted in flexion. Myoclonus and seizures occur in the late stages in about one-third of patients. Patients have grasping, sucking, and rooting reflexes, and they become difficult to feed because of choking and aspiration of food. Even those who eat well lose weight, so that the end stage is marked by severe cachexia.

SDAT patients survive on the average for 7 years following diagnosis. Some may live 10–12 years or longer when institutionalized in a facility with staff adept at preventing the usual complications. Aspiration pneumonia and bacterial infections account for most of the deaths.

Differential Diagnosis

Pick's Disease. In an established case of dementia there are a few diseases to consider other than SDAT. Pick's disease resembles SDAT over the whole course of the illness. Pick's disease usually has its onset before age 65. Language is affected equally in SDAT and Pick's disease. Subtle and not necessarily diagnostic clinical differences have been described to differentiate Pick's from Alzheimer's disease. Patients with Pick's disease seem to retain their spontaneity and their spatial orientation later than those with SDAT. Even after many years they are better at interaction and attention and are able to find their way about their environment in a way that belies their otherwise severe dementia. They fail early in the social graces and often exhibit inappropriate or unacceptable behavior. In addition, patients with Pick's disease seem to have less extrapyramidal involvement, gait disturbance, and seizures, except in the very late stages. Their EEG is often normal. The CT scan may be helpful by showing predominant frontotemporal atrophy in early cases, but patients with SDAT may have nearly the same gross appearance on CT. Separation of the two disorders is, however, usually difficult, and no clinical criteria have yet been shown to be specific for one or the other. Pathologically, Pick's disease is quite distinct from SDAT and shows marked frontal, temporal, and insular atrophy on gross examination. Microscopically, there are no neurofibrillary changes or senile plaques diagnostic of SDAT; instead there are abnormal, ballooned, eosinophilic neurons with inclusions, called *Pick bodies,* found mostly in the hippocampus, subiculum, amygdala, and anterior temporal cortex.

Stroke. When a patient has both SDAT and stroke, it is sometimes difficult to know which condition is responsible for the clinical features. Vascular cases usually have a more abrupt onset, stepwise progression, fluctuating course, and focal signs. There is often a history of previous stroke, hypertension, or other vascular disease. The dementia is usually less severe than in patients with SDAT, unless there is extensive infarction (see Chap. 20). No doubt the mixture of lesions produces a hybrid syndrome that takes its clinical form from the entity that predominates.

Sudden Mental Decline in Established SDAT

Sudden decline in the mental status of a patient with SDAT usually indicates a systemic disorder. Although SDAT patients occasionally have stroke or subdural hematoma, an extracranial cause is generally responsible for an acute change. At times elderly SDAT patients with confusion of subacute onset have no measurable metabolic abnormality and no identifiable infection or primary neurologic event. After several days in hospital the patient returns to the baseline, and the true cause of the episode remains obscure, the only therapeutic event having been use of IV fluid to reverse dehydration. Another important cause of acute or subacute failure in the clinical condition of patients with SDAT is the overuse of neuroleptic drugs. Neuroleptic drugs in small doses are useful but tend to accumulate over time and reduce the level of function in the patient. Short-acting benzodiazepine drugs (lorazepam or oxazepam) do not accumulate and are usually as effective as the neuroleptic drugs. Almost any drug, however, can worsen the mental status in an elderly demented patient.

---

1. Brinkman SD, Sarwar M, Levin HS, Morris HH: Quantitative indexes of computed tomography in dementia and normal aging. *Radiology* 138:89–92, 1981.
Compared to 30 normal patients, 28 Alzheimer's patients showed increased atrophy as measured between the third ventricle and the sylvian fissure.
2. Cassel CK, Jameton AL: Dementia in the elderly: An analysis of medical responsibility. *Ann Intern Med* 94:802–807, 1981.
Management of symptoms is helpful even though a cure is impossible.
3. Colblentz JM, et al: Presenile dementia. *Arch Neurol* 29:299–308, 1973.
Discusses the differentiation of SDAT and hydrocephalus.
4. Davison AN: Neurochemical observations in pathological forms of central nervous system aging. *Interdiscipl Top Gerontol* 15:1–12, 1979.
Summary of aspects in the degenerative disorders.
5. DeBoni U, Crapper DR, McLachlan DR: Senile dementia and Alzheimer's disease: A current view. *Life Sci* 27:1–14, 1980.
Reviews the cellular changes and experimental models so far concocted in SDAT.
6. Drachman DA, Glosser G, Fleming P, Longnecker G: Memory decline in the aged: Treatment with lecithin and physostigmine. *Neurology* 32:944–950, 1982.
Normal aged persons given lecithin did not improve on memory tests. Addition of physostigmine did not improve their memory either.
7. Forno LS, Barbour PJ, Norville RL: Presenile dementia with Lewy bodies and neurofibrillary tangles. *Arch Neurol* 35:818–822, 1978.
Case illustrates the pathologic overlap of degenerative diseases.
8. Forno LS, Barbour PJ, Norville RL: Presenile dementia with Lewy bodies and neurofibrillary tangles. *Arch Neurol* 35:818–822, 1978.
This case lies between Parkinson's and Alzheimer's disease, both clinically and pathologically.
9. Frackowiak RSJ, et al: Regional cerebral oxygen supply and utilization in dementia. *Brain* 104:753–778, 1981.
Positron tomography shows no increase in oxygen extraction, which is evidence against chronic ischemia as a cause of dementia.
10. Fuld PA, Katzman R, Davies P, Terry RD: Intrusions as a sign of Alzheimer dementia: Chemical and pathological verification. *Ann Neurol* 11:155–159, 1981.
The substitution of a word that was previously used as the response to a new stimulus was a frequent finding in SDAT.
11. Gaspar D: Hollymoor Hospital Dementia Service. *Lancet* 1:1402–1405, 1980.
Of the patients studied, 76.1% had behavioral problems. This group favored neuroleptics to control behavior; complications were not studied.
12. Huckman MS, Fox JH, Ramsy RG: Computed tomography in the diagnosis of degenerative diseases of the brain. *Semin Roentgenol* 12:63–75, 1977.
This article has no pathological verification and attempts to replace pathology with radiology. Bibliography is the high point.
13. Hughes CP, Mohktar G: Computed tomography and aging brain. *Radiology* 130:391–396, 1981.
A survey of 100 patients older than 65 years showed that ventricular size was related to age and not to mental status.
14. Jacoby RJ, Levy R: Computed tomography in the elderly: II. Senile dementia: Diagnosis and functional impairment. *Br J Psychiatry* 136:256–269, 1980.
Compared with normals, demented patients showed more tissue loss on CT scans, but there was a lot of overlap between abnormal and normal.
15. Katzman R: Dementia, in Tyler HR, Dawson DM (eds): *Current Neurology.* Boston, Houghton Mifflin, 1979, pp 138–158.
General discussion of all types of dementia.
16. Katzman R: Early detection of senile dementia. *Hosp Pract* 16:61–76, 1981.

Of nursing home residents, 60% have dementia; most have Alzheimer's disease or strokes.

17. Katzman R: The prevalence and malignancy of Alzheimer's disease. *Arch Neurol* 33:217–218, 1976.
A brief comment containing the most often quoted statistics.
18. Marsden DC, Harrison MJG: Outcome of patients with presenile dementia. *Br Med J* 2:249–252, 1972.
Points out the importance of looking for treatable disease that causes dementia. In this group 15% had treatable dementia.
19. McMenemy WH: Alzheimer's disease. *J Neurol Neurosurg Psychiatry* 3:211–240, 1940.
A review of 6 cases with clinical and pathological data.
20. Nakano I, Hirano A: Neuron loss in the nucleus basalis of Meynert in parkinsonism-dementia complex of Guam. *Ann Neurol* 13:87–91, 1983.
Presents more evidence to suggest a relationship between SDAT and other degenerative disorders.
21. Newton RD: The identity of Alzheimer's disease and senile dementia and their relationship to senility. *J Ment Sci* 94:225–249, 1948.
The brains from 150 consecutive autopsies at a mental hospital were examined.
22. Pear BL: The radiographic morphology of cerebral atrophy, in Smith LW, Kinsbourn M (eds): *Aging and Dementia.* New York, Spectrum Publications, 1977, pp 57–75.
The most useful linear measurement in determining ventricular enlargement in CT or pneumoencephalography is the width of the ventricular floor between the caudate nuclei. Most patients with a third ventricle width greater than 9 mm were too demented to work.
23. Pearce J: The extrapyramidal disorder of Alzheimer disease. *Eur Neurol* 12:94–103, 1974.
Points out that the features of Parkinson's disease are frequent in patients with SDAT. No mention of drug treatment or pathology here.
24. Pearce J: The extrapyramidal disorder of Alzheimer's disease. *Eur Neurol* 12:94–103, 1974.
Of 65 demented patients, 40 had features of parkinsonism.
25. Pearce J, Miller E: *Clinical Aspects of Dementia.* London, Bailliere-Tindal, 1973.
This monograph is one of the best clinical sources, despite its age.
26. Rothchild D: Alzheimer's disease. *Am J Psychiatry* 91:485–519, 1934.
Discusses 5 cases with extensive detail of the pathology and clinical features.
27. Sanford JR: Tolerance of debility in elderly dependents by supporters at home: Its significance for hospital practice. *Br Med J* 3:471–473, 1975.
A good general discussion with emphasis on the caretaker's role.
28. Seltzer B, Sherwin I: "Organic brain syndromes": An empirical study and critical review. *Am J Psychiatry* 135:13–21, 1978.
Organic brain syndrome can usually be diagnosed as a specific neurologic disease.
29. Sim M, Sussman I: Alzheimer's disease: Its natural history and differential diagnosis. *J Nerv Ment Dis* 135:489–499, 1962.
A study of 22 cases of Alzheimer's disease.
30. Sjögren H: Presenile brain atrophic syndromes related to the micro and macroscopical analyses and to weight of the brain. *Acta Psychiatr Scand* 41:446–461, 1965.
In a study of 400 brains, those from demented patients had a lower weight than those from patients with psychiatric disease.
31. Sjögren T, Sjögren H, Lindgren AG: Morbus Alzheimer and Morbus Pick. *Acta Psychiatr Scand* [Suppl] 82:1–152, 1952.
A very large study with a detailed description of the clinical features. There were 18 Alzheimer's and 18 Pick's cases diagnosed pathologically. Others were clinically diagnosed.
32. Sourander P, Sjögren H: The concept of Alzheimer's disease and its clinical implications, in Walstenholme GEW, O'Connor M (eds): *Alzheimer's Disease and Related Conditions.* London, Churchill Livingstone, 1970, pp 11–32.
A discussion of clinical and pathological features. The volume contains other monographs on dementia.
33. Squire LR, Moore RY: Dorsal thalamic lesion in a noted case of human memory dysfunction. *Ann Neurol* 6:503–506, 1979.

CT scans show the lesion. A good bibliography.
34. Thompson EG, Eastwood MR: Survivorship and senile dementia. *Age Ageing* 10:29–32, 1981.
About 50% of patients with senile dementia who live in institutions die within 2 years; 70% die within 4 years.
35. Tomlinson BE: Morphological changes and dementia in old age, in Smith LW, Kinsbourn M (eds): *Aging and Dementia.* New York, Spectrum Publications, 1977, pp 25–55.
Summarizes the data previously collected by the author.
36. Tomlinson BE, Blessed G, Roth M: Observations on the brain of non-demented old people. *J Neurol Sci* 7:331–356, 1968.
Mean age was 75 years. Patients had a few neurofibrillary tangles and senile plaques. Some had strokes.
37. Tomlinson BE, Blessed G, Roth M: Observations on the brains of demented old people. *J Neurol Sci* 11:205–242, 1970.
Brain weight did not indicate whether patients were demented. The numbers of pathological changes were related to the dementia. Many patients also had strokes.
38. Tomlinson BE, Irving D, Blessed G: Cell loss in the locus ceruleus in senile dementia of Alzheimer type. *J Neurol Sci* 49:419–428, 1981.
39. Wang HS: Dementia of old age, in Smith LW, Kinsbourn M (eds): *Aging and Dementia.* New York, Spectrum Publications, 1977, pp 1–4.
Epidemiologic data.
40. Wells CE, Duncan GW: Dangers of over reliance on computerized axial tomography. *Am J Psychiatry* 134:811–813, 1977.
There is no substitute for history and physical exam.
41. Whitehouse PJ, Hedreen JC, White CL, Price DL: Basal forebrain neurons in the dementia of Parkinson disease. *Ann Neurol* 3:243, 1983.
References to the cholinergic depletion in SDAT as well as in Parkinson's disease.
42. Whitehouse PJ, Price DL, Clark AW, Coyle JT, DeLong MR: Alzheimer disease: Evidence for selective loss of cholinergic neurons in the nucleus basalis. *Ann Neurol* 10:122–125, 1981.
Other nuclei are also affected, including the amygdala.
43. Willanger R, Thygesen P, Nielsen R, Peterson O: Intellectual impairment and cerebral atrophy. A psychological, neurological and radiological investigation. *Dan Med Bull* 15:65–93, 1968.
In this pneumoencephalographic study, the 4% of patients with the most atrophy had no intellectual impairment while 18% had doubtful impairment.

98. MANAGEMENT OF SENILE DEMENTIA OF THE ALZHEIMER TYPE

Thomas M. Walshe

Senile dementia of the Alzheimer type (SDAT) is a devastating illness that affects almost 600,000 middle-aged and elderly persons. Because of the total helplessness inflicted by the progressive course of SDAT, the emotional and financial cost to the patient and society is enormous. The disorder has been recognized since 1906, when Alois Alzheimer reported the initial neuropathologic findings, but its etiology and pathophysiology have yet to become clear. The disease is common, malignant, and poorly understood, so there have been many attempts at treatment. At present there is no drug or other therapy to alter or reverse the memory loss or halt the deteriorating course of SDAT.

Dememtia is a neurologic sign associated with several illnesses its management therefore must be adapted to each cause. When there is a treatable underlying disease, the dementia is accompanied by other signs and symptoms, and treatment is aimed at the specific etiolgy. When there is no treatment, as in the degenerative disorders, cure is not possible, but management of the symptoms is of great benefit to the patient and his or her family. Attempts at treatment of senile dementia of the Alzheimer type focus on two aspects of the disorder: the cognitive deficit itself and the complications caused by the cognitive deficit. Neither approach provides a completely satisfactory solution, but at least the complications can be controlled in many cases without increasing the deficits.

Caretaking

The litany of failure to improve cognitive function with pharmacologic treatment leaves a false impression that there is nothing a physician can do for the demented patient. Although cure is impossible, management of unacceptable behavior provides a real service to both patient and his providers. The major management problems in demented patients concern failure to control behavior. Most nursing home staffs and well-equipped families can manage the physical nursing care required for a demented patient, but the caretakers balk when assaultive and threatening behavior develops. Other problems which make home care difficult are nocturnal wandering, reversed sleep-wake cycle, yelling, and failure to respond to directions. Bowel and bladder incontinence, although major nursing problems, are not as destructive to continued home care as is assaultive behavior. Control of behavior requires special care, since overtreatment lowers the patient's limited functional ability, and undertreatment precludes remaining at home.

At the beginning of care the physician, family, and caretaking staff must realize that much of the unacceptable behavior is beyond control with medicines. The first requirement in management of the dement is an understanding caretaker who can tend to the patient's needs and tolerate the uncivilized behavior. In the home or chronic ward the caretaker must accept the pacing, aimless handling of objects, muttering, following, and other nuisance behaviors. The dement requires total effort and has little personality or other emotional output with which to reward the caretaker. The physical and emotional strain is felt in short order, and either at home or on the chronic ward there must be provision for adequate help. Families, no longer able to tolerate the burden without help, insist upon institutionalization. When the hospital caretakers are exhausted with the task, they demand that the patient be sedated. The patient then sinks even lower on the functional scale. Part of the solution for the family is day care and home health workers, and for the professional caretakers, adequate staff to care for the demented patient. Short stays in hospital give the families needed rest and delay the patient's institutionalization. When a patient regularly awakens during the night, night care several days a week may offer needed relief for the family.

Just as one does not sedate a child to prevent him from wandering into the street, one is loath to stupefy a demented patient in order to control unwanted behavior. Modifications of the home (adding fences, locking doors, roping off certain areas) are sometimes enough to contain the patient safely.

Drug Therapy

When the problem is more than nuisance behavior, drugs are needed. Drug therapy helps to make the patient sleep at night and reduces assaultive, aggressive, and unacceptable behavior. Drugs are not very useful in the control of wandering, yelling, and other nuisance behaviors, unless the patient is made stuporous or akinetic. The goal of drug therapy in SDAT is to reduce or eliminate aberrant behavior without reducing the patient's overall functional ability.

Sedatives. The short-acting benzodiazepines (oxazepam, lorazepam) are useful drugs that calm aggressive patients, help to reduce nocturnal mischief, and reduce unwanted behavior without making the patient stuporous. When the benzodiazepines are used in small doses, the patient can often function at home or on the ward without excess sedation. Drugs with a short half-life do not accumulate and are fast-acting. Patients who develop an unacceptable behavior, such as assaultiveness, can be treated acutely with high sedative doses. The patient then sleeps for 8–12 hours, and the crisis is over. Recurrent behavioral problems can be handled with lower doses given chronically. Use of the short-acting drugs at night will allow patient and family to avoid the unpleasant nocturnal wandering that often appears. If benzodiazepines or barbiturates are given, the patient is spared the disfiguring movement disorders that interfere with all aspects of care. Other hypnotics are also effective in acute control of serious unacceptable behavior. Chloral hydrate in doses of 1,000 mg bid or tid for 1 or 2 days will slow up the most ardent dement. The longer-acting sedative drugs (diazepam) are also useful, as long as the physician remembers that the peak levels do not occur for days and that the drug, after it is stopped, will linger for days or longer in elderly patients. The sedative drugs may increase agitation in some demented patients. If the drug is to be used for a short time, it may help to increase the dose until a hypnotic effect is produced. Most patients who become agitated when treated with minor tranquilizers require neuroleptics to control their behavior.

Antidepressants. For patients with minimal dementia who develop a depressed affect and who withdraw from their surroundings, a trial of tricyclic antidepressants may be helpful. In most cases of SDAT, however, tricyclics cause minimal if any improvement. When they are used, those with a minimal anticholinergic effect (Norpramin [desipramine], 25–100 mg) are best tolerated. Other drugs that may help the apathetic, demented patient include amphetamines and methylphenidate. Improvement is usually limited to more alertness without betterment in the activities of daily living. Both amphetamine and methylphenidate may produce an acute confusional state. In the occasional SDAT patient who has marked extrapyramidal signs, a trial of L-dopa may help rigidity. Most patients with SDAT do not improve when given L-dopa.

Neuroleptics. When the sedative drugs fail to control behavior in doses that are not hypnotic, the next stage of management is use of the neuroleptics (Haldol, Mellaril, Thorazine, and others). The neuroleptics are very effective against problem behavior. Their side effects, however, especially in the demented patient, make them a second choice under most circumstances. The neuroleptics are not very effective acutely except in huge parenteral doses, and then they linger for weeks in some cases. They seldom change nuisance behavior unless given in large enough amounts to cause a severe parkinsonian syndrome, which interferes with ambulation. The parkinsonian syndrome sometimes interferes with speech and swallowing. Severe tardive movement disorders are also produced in demented patients by neuroleptics. It seems most reasonable to save the neuroleptic medications for patients who can be controlled in no other way.

It is futile to place early well-mannered demented patients, early in the disease, on neuroleptics, and it may well lead to decline in the patients' level of activity. The favorite neuroleptic drug for patients with dementia, haloperidol, even in small doses, induces devastating movement disorders in SDAT patients. The patient overtreated with haloperidol becomes rigid, fails to eat (most demented patients eat well because of their vigorous sucking reflex), and becomes obtunded and ill. In addition to rigidity, the patient may develop dyskinesia, dystonia, or akathisia. Often the restlessness that is being treated is far less severe than the movement disorder induced. Patients with extrapyramidal features are especially vulnerable to life-threatening rigidity. The malignant neuroleptic syndrome (increased confusion, coma, hyperthermia) and hypotension, are risks in patients treated with neuroleptics, unless the goal is to induce rigidity (as in Huntington's disease). Other neuroleptics have the same unneeded effects as haloperidol. Even the minimal dopamine-blockers induce movement disorders in the demented patient. Because of the sedative effects, Chlorpromazine (Thorazine) is most effective in reducing dangerous behavior. Thorazine need only be used, however, after other, safer drugs have failed.

There are no absolute rules in the management of SDAT. The prognosis for useful life is nil, and death in a state of subhuman existence inevitable. Management must focus on helping the patient stay as well as possible for as long as possible. Help is also needed for those who take care of the patient. Drugs are best avoided, unless there is no other choice. Selection of benign, short-acting drugs usually avoids many complications and solves all but the most severe behavior problems.

---

1. Bowen DM, Smith CB, White P, Davison AN: Neurotransmitter-related enzymes and indices of hypoxia in senile dementia and other abiotrophies. *Brain* 99:459–496, 1976.
   The original finding of decreased choline acetyl transferase in SDAT.
2. Boyd WD, et al: Clinical effects of choline in alzheimer senile dementia. *Lancet* 2:711, 1977.
   Finds "behavior" but not memory improved.
3. Branconnier RJ, Cole JO: The therapeutic role of methylphenidate in senile organic brain syndrome, in Cole JO, Barrett JE (eds): *Psychopathology in the Aged.* New York, Raven Press, 1980, pp 183–196.
   Depression, confusion, vigor, and fatigue all showed improvement, but no objective parameter improved.
4. Burian E: An ergot alkaloid preparation (hydergine) in the treatment of presenile brain atrophy (Alzheimer's disease): Case report. *J Am Geriatr Soc* 22:126–128, 1974.
   Of patients with biopsy-proved SDAT, 1 of 4 had improvement.
5. Cowley LM, Glen RS: Double-blind study of thioridazine and haloperidol in geriatric

patients with a psychosis associated with organic brain syndrome. *J Clin Psychiatry* 40:411–419, 1979.
In 12 weeks 3 patients developed movement disorders that required intervention; no mention was made of less dramatic movement disorders.
6. Davies P, Maloney AJF: Selective loss of central cholinergic neurons in Alzheimer's disease. *Lancet* 2:1403, 1976.
A brief and early revelation of the importance of the cholinergic lesion in SDAT.
7. Davis KL, et al: Physostigmine: Improvement of long-term memory process in normal humans. *Science* 201:272–274, 1978.
Slow intravenous injection enhanced the storage of information into long-term memory.
8. DeWied D, et al: Vasopressin and memory consolidation. *Prog Brain Res* 45:181–191, 1976.
In rats, the drug facilitates consolidation of learned behavior, improves acquisition of avoidance behavior, and impedes extinction behavior.
9. Drachman DA, Glosser G, Fleming P, Longnecker G: Memory decline in the aged: Treatment with lecithin and physostigmine. *Neurology* 32:944–950, 1982.
Normal aged persons given lecithin did not improve on memory tests. Addition of physostigmine did not improve the memory either.
10. Drachman DA, Leavitt J: Human memory and the cholinergic system. *Arch Neurol* 30:113–121, 1974.
Scopolamine caused changes in memory similar to those seen in aging.
11. Etienne P, Gauthier S, Dastoor D, Collier B: Lecithin in Alzheimer's disease. *Lancet* 2:1206, 1978.
Of 7 patients with mild Alzheimer's disease, 3 improved subjectively.
12. Etienne P, et al: Clinical effects of choline in Alzheimer's disease. *Lancet* 1:508–509, 1978.
"No clinical or laboratory signs of improvement were found."
13. Growdon JH, Corkin S: Neurochemical approaches to the treatment of senile dementia, in Cole JO, Barretts JE (eds): *Psychopathology in the Aged.* New York, Raven Press, 1980, pp 281–296.
A review holding that choline treats tardive dyskinesia and may benefit dementia. Good literature review.
14. Havens WW, Cole JO: Successful treatment of dementia with lithium. *J Clin Psychopharmacol* 2:71–72, 1982.
Less wandering, agitation, and hostility in an 87-year-old patient with SDAT on clinical exam.
15. Haycox JA: Late care of the demented patient. *N Engl J Med* 303:165–166, 1980.
An insightful, brief commentary on the time when patients need to be institutionalized.
16. Hier DB, Caplan LR: Drugs for senile dementia. *Drugs* 20:74–80, 1980.
A practical rendition of the available treatments by reliable clinicians.
17. Kristensen V, Olsen M, Theilgaard A: Levodopa treatment of presenile dementia. *Acta Psychiatr Scand* 55:41–51, 1977.
The patients tested were of "normal intelligence"; no effect was measured.
18. Legros JJ, et al: Influence of vasopressin on learning and memory. *Lancet* 1:41, 1978.
In 11 patients given placebo and 12 given vasopressin, the treated group showed improvement in attention, concentration, and motor rapidity.
19. McDonald RJ: Hydergine: A review of 26 clinical studies. *Pharmacopsychiatria* 12:407–422, 1979.
Most of the studies are less than satisfactory.
20. Messing RB, et al: Naloxone enhancement of memory. *Behav Neural Biol* 27:266–275, 1979.
21. Meyer JS, et al: Neurotransmitter precursor amino acids in the treatment of multi-infarct dementia and Alzheimer's disease. *J Am Geriatr Soc* 25:289–298, 1977.
Improvement was seen in 2 of 10 patients with multiple infarcts and/or SDAT.
22. Perry EK, Perry RH, Tomlinson BE: Dietary lecithin supplements in dementia of Alzheimer type? *Lancet* 2:242–243, 1977.
Suggests that lecithin is more convenient to give than choline.
23. Peters BH, Levin HS: Memory enhancement after physostigmine treatment in the amnestic syndrome. *Arch Neurol* 34:215–219, 1977.

Improvement of retrieval and storage after subcutaneous treatment with 0.8 mg occurred in a case of encephalitis.

24. Pritchard JG, Mykyta LJ: Use of a combination of methylphenidate and oxyprenolol in the management of physically disabled, apathetic, elderly patients: A pilot study. *Curr Med Res Opin* 3:26–29, 1975.
Half of the institutionalized patients treated were able to be discharged from the chronic ward.
25. Rabins PV: Management of irreversible dementia. *Psychosomatics* 22:591–597, 1981.
Restraint in the use of neuroleptics is one wise suggestion in this review.
26. Reisberg B, et al: Effects of naloxone in senile dementia: A double blind trial. *N Engl J Med* 308:721–722, 1983.
This letter describes 7 patients with minimal improvement.
27. Reisberg B, Ferris SH, Gershon S: An overview of pharmacologic treatment of cognitive decline in the aged. *Am J Psychiatry* 138:593–598, 1981.
Places more emphasis on vasodilators than is warranted.
28. Reisberg B, Ferris SH, Gershon S: Pharmacotherapy of senile dementia, in Cole JO, Barrett JE (eds): *Psychopathology in the Aged.* New York, Raven Press, 1980, pp 233–264.
A review with 204 references.
29. Shimamoto T, Murase H, Numano F: Treatment of senile dementia and cerebellar disorders with phthalazinol. Cyclic AMP increasing agent, pthhalazinol, in therapeutic trials, in hitherto incurable morbid conditions. *Mech Ageing Dev* 5:241–250, 1976.
Some improvement occurred in 5 cases of SDAT and 7 cases of cerebellar degeneration.
30. Signoret JL, Whiteley A, Lhermitte F: Influence of choline on amnesia in early Alzheimer's disease. *Lancet* 2:837, 1978.
Minimally demented patients had better recall after 9 gm of choline daily for 21 days.
31. Sitaram N, Weingartner H, Gillin JC: Human serial learning: Enhancement with arecholine and choline and impairment with scopolamine. *Science* 201:274–276, 1978.
Normal human subjects were used.
32. Smith CM, Swash M: Physostigmine in Alzheimer's disease. *Lancet* 1:42, 1979.
A single patient improved on the drug.
33. Spillane JA, et al: Selective vulnerability of neurones in organic dementia. *Nature* 266:558–559, 1977.
Reduced choline acetyl transferase was found in patients with SDAT. Glutamic acid decarboxylase reduction is thought to result from postmortem changes.
34. Thal LJ, Fuld PA: Memory enhancement with oral physostigmine in Alzheimer's disease. *N Engl J Med* 308:720–721, 1983.
Oral physostigmine is absorbed. The best dose is 2.5 mg 6 times daily.
35. Williams KH, Goldstein G: Cognitive and affective responses to lithium in patients with organic brain syndrome. *Am J Psychiatry* 136:800–803, 1979.
The diagnosis was not made with accuracy.
36. Vasodilators in senile dementia, editorial. *Br Med J* 2:511–512, 1979.
This editorial expresses a negative impression of vasodilators.

99. VASCULAR DEMENTIAS

Thomas M. Walshe

Stroke, either single or multiple, is the underlying cause of vascular dementia. Chronic ischemia from carotid, vertebral, or intracerebral atherosclerosis is not the cause of vascular dementia. Dementia is a prominent feature of several distinct vascular states: (1) multiple infarctions involving the larger vessels, (2) multiple infarctions involving the smaller penetrating vessels (lacunar infarcts), (3) infarction from low blood flow and hypoxic states, e.g, after cardiac arrest, and (4) single infarctions that affect specific memory structures.

Characteristics of Vascular Dementia

Cerebrovascular disease, the most common neurologic malady in the elderly, comprises several disorders, each having specific clinical and pathologic characteristics that separate it from primary degenerative disease. Dementia is only one sign associated with cerebrovascular disease. An abrupt onset, focal signs, and a fluctuating course point to a vascular etiology. In vascular disease, the memory deficit waxes and wanes between examinations, and the patients have poor attention. Patients usually have only moderate dementia and retain much correct information, but they fail to integrate the information into coherent answers. The course of vascular dementia is usually intermittent, with fluctuations and stable periods. Hypertension, congestive heart disease, valvular heart disease, atrial fibrillation, and other arrhythmias are commonly associated with but not always found in vascular dementias caused by multiple emboli.

The EEG shows an asymmetric slowing when the infarcts involve the cortex but may be normal when the damage lies in the deep nuclei or white matter. The CT scan shows enlarged ventricles similar to those found in degenerative dementias and may show the areas of infarction. The lumbar puncture is usually normal, with a normal pressure.

A few patients with vascular dementia fail insidiously over months or years and have few other obvious neurologic signs. Such patients resemble clinically those with dementia of the Alzheimer type, but at autopsy, they have many small areas of cerebral infarction. In such cases the CT scan may help by showing discrete areas of infarction, and often a careful neurologic examination reveals telltale focal signs of past stroke.

Single Cerebral Infarctions

Single cerebral infarctions caused by large vessel thrombosis (carotid or vertebral artery) or by embolism to their distal branches almost always cause motor, sensory, visual, or other focal signs. Cerebral infarctions usually affect functions such as speech or praxis more than memory. When a patient is aphasic, memory testing is sometimes difficult, but in most cases it is clear that a language disturbance is the major problem. Patients with fluent aphasia, however, are sometimes erroneously identified as being demented.

Cerebral infarctions in the right hemisphere, especially in elderly patients, may produce a confusional state that is different from the dementia found in degenerative diseases (see Chap. 96). The confusional state usually clears, but in some patients it becomes fixed, leaving the patient with a deficit of attention and difficulty in developing a coherent line of thought.

Another single-stroke syndrome that produces dementia is occlusion of the posterior cerebral artery by thrombosis or embolism. The memory disorder is almost always associated with bilateral medial temporal lesions, although memory deficits occur with left posterior cerebral artery occlusion alone. A contralateral hemianopia and an acute memory loss may be the only signs. There is usually no hemiplegia, and there are usually no signs of brainstem dysfunction, which one expects in more proximal posterior cerebral artery occlusions. The memory deficit resembles Korsakoff's syndrome (similar to that seen in thiamine deficiency), where the major memory deficit is failure of recent memory, with less obvious failure of remote memory. There is usually preservation of personality and language. In posterior cerebral artery occlusions the memory usually improves after several weeks or sooner.

Amnestic Syndrome

Patients who suffer cardiac arrest or hypoxia and hypotension from other reasons can develop Korsakoff's syndrome without other signs. Like patients with posterior cerebral artery lesions, they retain language and personality but have a chronic, fixed memory loss that can be quite severe. Bilateral ischemic lesions in the medial temporal regions, hippocampus, and thalamus are found postmortem. There is usually no hemianopia in the anoxic-hypotensive cases, but some patients are left with motor and other focal deficits that make the diagnosis much simpler.

Multiple Cerebral Infarctions

Small cerebral infarctions clear completely and are sometimes forgotten by the patient. Small lesions away from the motor cortex may go completely unrecognized clinically, even by a physician. Such lesions are often caused by emboli but also occur from thrombotic vascular disease of the deep penetrating vessels as seen in hypertension. Elderly patients may have had many such small infarctions, with only the slimmest remembrance of them.

Some patients with hypertension develop thickening of the media and degenerative changes in the subcortical arteries, which occlude, causing small, discrete infarcts in the basal ganglia and patchy areas of infarction in the periventricular and subcortical white matter. The patients may not have had clear strokes but have a stepwise or fluctuating course marked by progressive dementia. This disorder, known as *Binswanger's disease,* is a variant of the syndrome associated with multiple small lacunar infarcts. The diagnosis can be made if a history of past stroke is obtained from the medical record or if the neurologic examination shows signs indicative of old lesions. In such cases the neurologist finds brisk tendon reflexes, brisk jaw jerk, dysarthria, dysphagia, upgoing toes, or a mild hemiparesis. A labile affect is more common in vascular dementia but also occurs in the late stages of Alzheimer's disease.

Multiple infarction dementia can be stabilized by reducing the risk of further stroke. Reduction of hypertension in the lacunar state can prevent futher decline. Anticoagulation to avoid recurrent emboli may prevent deterioration in cases of multiple embolism. Once the dementia is established, however, there is usually no reversal, and the purpose of treatment is prevention of new lesions.

Combined Degenerative and Vascular Dementia

In about 20% of elderly demented patients, degenerative changes (SDAT) and vascular changes coexist. Both disorders are common in the senium, so it would be expected to find both in some cases. When an adequate history and neurologic examination are available, the two syndromes can be separated clinically in most cases. Treatment is usually determined by the degree of the dementia. Patients who are severely and hopelessly demented do not require treatment of vascular risk factors to prevent further deterioration. Patients with early disease generally are evaluated for sources of emboli and treated vigorously if they have hypertension.

The separation of vascular dementia from primary degenerative dementia is clinically useful, since the prognosis and overall management differ in each. The vascular dement may go years without becoming worse, especially if the sources of stroke are under control. On the other hand, the patient with senile dementia of the Alzheimer type will progress steadily, no matter what is done. There is little to gain by treating cerebrovascular disease in a patient who also has progressive degenerative dementia.

1. Pearce J, Miller E: *Clinical Aspects of Dementia.* London, Bailliere-Tindal, 1973.
This monograph is one of the best clinical sources, despite its age.
2. Tomlinson BE, Blessed G, Roth M: Observations on the brains of non-demented old people. *J Neurol Sci* 7:331–356, 1968.
Mean age was 75 years. Patients had a few neurofibrillary tangles and senile plaques. Some had strokes.
3. Tomlinson BE, Blessed G, Roth M: Observations on the brains of demented old people. *J Neurol Sci* 11:205–242, 1970.
Brain weight did not indicate which patients were demented. The numbers of pathological changes were related to the dementia. Many patients also had strokes.
4. DeReuck J, Sieben G, DeCoster W, Van der Ecken H: Stroke pattern and topography of cerebral infarcts. *Eur Neurol* 20:411–415, 1981.
Clinically silent strokes occurred in 22% of patients. Reversible strokes occur mostly in PCA and PICA territories.
5. O'Brien MD: Vascular diseases and dementia in the elderly, in Smith LW, Kinsbourn M (eds): *Aging and Dementia.* New York, Spectrum Publications, 1977, pp 77–90.
This review suggests that there are populations of ischemic brain cells that are still viable but hypoactive following stroke; such cells may benefit from increased cerebral blood flow.
6. Rossor MN, et al: A postmortem study of the cholinergic and GABA systems in senile dementia. *Brain* 105:313–330, 1982.
Choline acetyl transferase was reduced in all cortical areas examined in patients dying before age 79. GABA was reduced only in the temporal cortex (areas 20,21,28). The patients with vascular dementia had much less loss of cholinergic activity.

7. Alvarez WC: *Little Strokes*. Philadelphia, Lippincott, 1966.
An early identification of the results of multiple strokes.
8. Caplan L: Chronic vascular dementia. *Primary Care* 5:843–848, 1979.
A brief review of the subject with 3 cases.
9. Caplan LR, Schoene WC: Clinical features of subcortical arteriosclerotic encephalopathy (Binswanger disease). *Neurology* 28:1206–1215, 1978.
Clinicopathological study of 5 cases and clinical study of 6.
10. De Reuck J, Crevits L, De Coster W, Sieben G, Van der Ecken H: Pathogenesis of Binswanger chronic progressive subcortical encephalopathy. *Neurology* 30:920–928, 1980.
Only 1 patient in 4 postmortem cases had been demented. The pathology is the same as multi-infact cases and the clinical syndrome is not a distinct entity.
11. Fisher CM: Dementia in cerebral vascular disease, in Siekert R, Whishant J (eds): *Cerebral Vascular Diseases, Sixth Conference*. New York, Grune & Stratton, 1968, pp 232–236.
A review of the causes of vascular dementia and a warning about overdiagnosis of little strokes.
12. Frackowiak RSJ, et al: Regional cerebral oxygen supply and utilization in dementia. *Brain* 104:753–778, 1981.
Positron tomography shows no increase in oxygen extraction, evidence against chronic ischemia as a cause of dementia.
13. Gerin J: Symptomatic treatment of cerebrovascular insufficiency with hydergine. *Curr Therapeutic Res* 11:539–546, 1969.
Few use this drug and expect improvement.
14. Hachinski VC, Lassen NA, Marshall J: Multi-infarct dementia: A cause of mental deterioration in the elderly. *Lancet* 2:207–209, 1974.
A new name for small strokes.
15. Paulson GW, Perrine G: Cerebral vascular disease in mental hospitals, in Siekert R, Whisnant J (eds): *Cerebral Vascular Diseases, Sixth Conference*. New York, Grune & Stratton, 1968, pp 237–241.
Angiograms of demented inpatients in a state hospital indicated that vascular disease was a rare cause of dementia in that group.
16. Rosen WG, Terry RD, Fuld PA, Katzman R, Peck A: Pathological verification of ischemic score in differentiation of dementias. *Ann Neurol* 7:486–488, 1980.
Although not infallible, it is the best test available. The score is a summary of a good neurologic history and exam.
17. Tomlinson BE, Blessed G, Roth M: Observations on the brains of demented old people. *J Neurol Sci* 11:205–242, 1970.
Pathological study shows many demented old people have both stroke and Alzheimer's disease.
18. Wells CE: Role of stroke in dementia. *Stroke* 9:1–3, 1978.
Editorial that puts vascular disease in perspective.
19. Yarnell PR: Neurological outcome of prolonged coma survivors of out of hospital cardiac arrest. *Stroke* 7:279–282, 1976.
Describes the dementia that occurs with anoxia in 2 of 9 patients.
20. Marie P: Desfoyers lacunaires de desintegration et des differents autres états cavitaires du cerneau. *Rev Med de Nancy* 21:281–298, 1901.
The original description of the lacunar state.
21. Bousser MG: Les conceptions actuelles des demences arteriopathiques. *Encephale* 3:357–372, 1977.
Describes the five types of vascular dementia.
22. Cook P, James I: Cerebral vasodilators (two parts). *N Engl J Med* 305:1508–1513, 1560–1564, 1981.
Many references and general review. Short discussion of cerebral blood flow changes with aging.
23. Gustafson L, Nilsson L: Differential diagnosis of presenile dementia on clinical grounds. *Acta Psychiatr Scand* 65:194–209, 1982.
In 57 patients, scales to differentiate Alzheimer's, Pick's, and vascular dementia were applied; 26 postmortems showed 12 SDAT, 6 atrophies other than SDAT, 4 multiple strokes, 3 Creutzfeld-Jacob disease, 1 bilateral encephalitis. This is a confusing paper.

24. Hachinski VC, et al: Cerebral blood flow in dementia. *Arch Neurol* 32:632–637, 1975.
Multiple-stroke patients had decrease in blood flow proportional to the severity of their dementia.
25. Olzewski J: Subcortical arteriosclerotic encephalopathy: Review of the literature on the so-called Benswanger's disease and presentation of two cases. *World Neurol* 3:559–575, 1962.
Includes scant clinical detail but detailed pathology.
26. Sourander P, Walinder J: Hereditary multi-infarct dementia. *Acta Neuropathol* (Berl) 39:247–254, 1977.
Discusses three generations of multiple strokes.
27. White JC: Periodic EEG activity in subcortical arteriosclerotic encephalopathy (Binswanger's type). *Arch Neurol* 36:485–489, 1979.
A report of an autopsy-proved case.
28. Vasodilators in senile dementia, editorial. *Br Med J* 2:511–512, 1979.
This editorial expresses a negative impression of vasodilators.
29. Benson DF, Marsden CD, Meadows JC: The amnestic stroke. *Neurology* 23:400, 1973.
An abstract that describes 9 patients with amnesia and hemianopia.
30. Perez FI, et al: Analysis of intellectual and cognitive performance in patients with multi-infarct dementia, vertebrobasilar insufficience with dementia and Alzheimer's disease. *J Neurol Neurosurg Psychiatry* 38:533–540, 1975.
The patients with Alzheimer's disease were more demented than those with vascular dementia.
31. Arnold KG: Cerebral blood flow in geriatrics—a review. *Age Ageing* 10:5–9, 1981.
Brief discussion but many references.
32. Tomonaga M: Cerebral amyloid angiopathy in the elderly. *J Am Geriatr Soc* 29:151–163, 1981.
The lesion occurred in 58% of patients over 90 years. Cerebral hemorrhage is a complication.
33. von Cramon D, Kuhnlein J, Wolfram A: Die Thalamische Demenz. *Fortschr Neurol Psychiatr* 49:129–135, 1981.
Discusses a syndrome reminiscent of bifrontal lesions.

100. CURABLE DEMENTIAS

Thomas M. Walshe

The majority of elderly patients whose major complaint is dementia have an incurable degenerative or vascular dementia. There are many treatable illnesses that cause impairment of mental ability, but in most cases the mental deficiency is a secondary part of the whole illness and seldom is confused with primary dementing illnesses. Patients with toxic, metabolic, and other acute illness usually develop an acute change in mental state, a confusional state distinct from the chronic dementias.

The overall incidence of curable disease as the basis for chronic, well-established dementia is below 1% but in cases of confusional state of brief duration or of short-term, mild dementia, the incidence of curable causes may be as high as 15%. Moreover, there are scattered cases of curable diseases that cause a syndrome similar to senile dementia of the Alzheimer type (SDAT). The chance of identifying a curable disorder makes careful clinical assessment necessary, even in chronic dementia.

Identification of Curable Dementia

The curable dementias can be separated clinically in most cases from degenerative disorders by the initial history, physical examination, and routine laboratory tests. Most demented patients can be evaluated as outpatients, although hospitalization may be useful when there is a suspicion of chronic drug intoxication.

A major discriminating feature of the curable disorders is the character of the dementia. Patients with altered attention, lethargy, or remissions in the dementia seldom have degenerative disease as the only problem. The elderly patient must be in the best medical condition possible before the characteristics and severity of the dementia are evaluated;

otherwise a false impression of the dementia may lead the physician to conclude that the patient has severe, hopeless, degenerative disease. In curable dementia the memory disorder is often mild, without language abnormality. Early degenerative disease causes mild dementia but usually affects language and praxis. In the curable dementias, personality and emotional life may remain complex and in fact be a major source of complaint. There may be specific psychiatric signs such as paranoia, hallucinations, mania, and depression. In SDAT there is a bland, lusterless affect, even early. Curable dementias usually occur over weeks or months and the patient is brought in early by the family. The curable disorders sometimes progress to severe dementia, but usually they stabilize at a mild or moderate level of dysfunction. Most patients with Alzheimer's disease decline noticeably over 6–18 months, so the progression of the dementia becomes obvious.

Causes of Curable Dementias

Systemic Illness. A number of specific medical disorders produce memory loss. Dementia seldom is the presenting sign or symptom, and, when it is, other signs are usually abundant when sought. Chronic metabolic imbalance may cause mild dementia, but usually there is the telltale addition of lethargy. Patients with chronic hypoxia and hypercarbia develop a mild dementia, papilledema, headache, and myoclonus. Elderly patients with hypocalcemia from parathyroid failure may develop a syndrome almost identical to SDAT.

Endocrinopathies. Endocrinopathies, especially hypothyroidism, may precipitate dementia in older persons. Hyperthyroidism, hyperadrenalism, hypoadrenalism, and panhypopituitarism also have been associated with dementia. It is usually not difficult to identify the cause after a thorough medical examination. Hyperthyroid patients can develop an agitated, hyperactive state with emotional lability, mood changes, and loosely associated thoughts. Hallucinations and delusions occur in some patients. Hyperthyroidism in the older patient causes a state of listless inertia, in which mood and energy levels are depressed. The patient may complain of fuzzy thinking and may have diarrhea. The hypothyroid patient has impoverished thinking, lethargy, and a slow EEG. Somnolence, which affects some hypothyroid patients, is not found in SDAT. Thyroid function tests are diagnostic.

Chronic Renal Failure. Chronic renal failure and uremia may cause dementia, but more often a confusional state or stupor is the major neurologic sign. Patients on hemodialysis develop a dementia that superficially resembles the degenerative dementias. The dialysis encephalopathy syndrome is found only in patients on chronic hemodialysis and is marked by a progressive mental decline despite good metabolic control. Attacks of dysarthria, stuttering, seizures, psychotic episodes, and myoclonus progress to death, usually in less than 18 months. Some cases are associated with elevated aluminum in the dialysate, but the true pathophysiology is not clear.

Chronic Hepatic Failure. Chronic liver failure is associated with stupor and coma and only occasionally with a dementing illness known as *hepatocerebral degeneration.* Once the degeneration occurs there is no treatment, but it can be prevented by treating the liver failure and avoiding a hepatosystemic shunt.

Dehydration. Elderly patients are especially subject to dehydration, either from poor intake or from chronic diuretic use. Dehydration may cause mild dementia with few other signs. The electrolytes are usually abnormal, but not always. Dehydration that occurs over a few days generally causes a confusional state.

Cancer. The remote effects of cancer have been associated with a progressive decline in memory, usually developing over several months. When the tumor is removed, the neurologic symptoms may abate.

Hypoglycemia. Acute hypoglycemia usually causes stupor and coma but, when chronic or repeated, may cause a dementia, which, when recognized, can be prevented from worsening, if not improved. When hypoglycemia is severe and prolonged, it causes amnesia similar to that seen in Korsakoff's syndrome. Multiple hypoglycemic episodes produce a chronic stable dementia similar to that seen in multiple strokes.

Intoxication. Toxins usually cause an acute confusional state rather than chronic dementia, but there are several toxins that cause dementia. Chronic intoxication with barbiturates, bromides, and heavy metals such as mercury, thallium, and lead causes dementia. Other sedative and neuroleptic drugs, when used chronically, may cause an elderly patient to appear demented. Chronic use of alcohol may produce a syndrome easily mistaken for degenerative dementia. A careful history from the family is crucial to identifying drug toxicity. Cimetidine and propranolol are both associated with confusion and dementia in older patients.

Chronic Systemic Illness. In elderly patients who have mild senescent mental impairment, an underlying chronic systemic illness may produce signs of dementia rather than the acute confusional syndrome usually associated with acute illness. Similarly, degenerative dementia may worsen with a systemic illness, so that a patient with established dementia seems to deteriorate suddenly. When the underlying acute illness is treated, the patient improves to his or her previous state. In both cases it is valuable to identify the underlying illness, so that the degree of dementia can be ascertained. The patient with an acute confusional condition is not reliably testable for memory function and should not be diagnosed as having chronic dementia until the acute illness is over. Drugs that cause sedation are notorious for reducing mental acumen in elderly patients.

Neurosyphilis. Neurosyphilis is a rare cause of dementia, and the dementia, once established, is not curable. The disease usually occurs in patients under 60. The diagnosis is made by a positive FTA-ABS in serum, a positive FTA-ABS in the cerebrospinal fluid, and cells in the CSF. If there are no cells in the CSF, the neurosyphilis is not active. The dementia may occur alone or with signs of tabes dorsalis. Psychiatric and behavioral signs, such as delusions, aggressive behavior and paranoid ideas, are also part of the syndrome.

Meningitis. Chronic meningitis occasionally causes dementia, usually as a late complication. In TB or fungal meningitis, the patient is usually acutely ill, lethargic, and has fever. It is unusual for patients with TB meningitis to develop dementia if they survive, unless they have hydrocephalus or another complication. Sarcoid meningitis is a rare cause of dementia, and its diagnosis requires a biopsy.

Hydrocephalus. One of the major concerns of physicians who detect dementia is the possibility of occult hydrocephalus. About two-thirds of patients with occult hydrocephalus have a predisposition for it, such as previous intracerebral bleeding or infection. Hydrocephalus is usually associated with an elevated pressure in the CSF, but hydrocephalus with normal lumbar pressure has been known since the mid-1960s. Patients who have hydrocephalus sometimes have an elevated CSF pressure if it is checked several times; the "normal" pressure is almost always over 100, and usually at the high-normal range (180–190). There are a few cases of idiopathic hydrocephalus in near-normal pressure is maintained. About half the patients are younger than 60, and hydrocephalus is seldom the cause for enlarged ventricles on the CT scan in elderly patients.

The clinical syndrome of chronic hydrocephalus develops gradually over several months. Key findings are a decline in mental acuity with memory loss, poor attention, and somnolence. The patient may also lack spontaneity and develop primitive reflex signs, such as a grasp reflex. The mental changes precede a gait disorder that is not easily characterized but that causes the patient to become clumsy, fall, and remain in a chair or bed most of the time. There is usually no paresis of the legs, although tendon reflexes may be more active than expected. Later, the patient's social awareness fails, and he becomes incontinent of urine. The signs are not specific, since the same complaints can be found in patients who have early SDAT or Creutzfeld-Jakob disease. In hydrocephalus the CSF pressure is usually high or high-normal, but there are no other changes in the CSF. The CT scan shows ballooned, enlarged ventricles with little space between skull and brain. The EEG is almost always slower than normal. Ventricular radionucleotide scans are not of great use, since patients with enlarged ventricles from degenerative dementia may also have abnormal CSF flow dynamics. When the isotope remains in the ventricles after 48 hours without any activity over the convexity, the correlation with hydrocephalus is good.

Patients who have hydrocephalus as the cause of their dementia improve with a ventricular shunt. Periventricular hypodensity on the CT scan has been identified as a predictor of good results from shunt. There is usually no sure way to predict the efficacy of a shunt, unless the patient has the clinical syndrome and the expected findings on CT scan.

Tumor of the third ventricle, fungal or other chronic meningitis, head trauma, intracranial bleeding, and other primary disorders may produce hydrocephalus and dementia. The clinical and laboratory evaluation will separate these disorders from idiopathic hydrocephalus.

Chronic Subdural Hematoma. Another curable syndrome that must be sought in elderly patients who present with memory problems is chronic subdural hematoma. Chronic subdural hematoma causes lethargy in almost all elderly patients who have it.

Rarely does dementia occur alone; there is usually a confusional state with inattention, lethargy, and mild motor signs. The problem generally develops over a few days or weeks, often causing a progressive change in mental status that ultimately ends in stupor or coma. Other signs that suggest subdural hematoma in an elderly patient are headache, personality change, and seizures. The CSF is normal in about half of cases. When CSF is abnormal, the most common findings are xanthochromia, pleocytosis, and elevated opening pressure. The EEG is usually abnormal, with slowing or diminished amplitude on the side of the lesion. The CT scan may not show a chronic subdural hematoma if it is isodense with brain; however, there may be a shift of the midline with unilateral lesions, or contrast may separate vascularized brain from the hematoma. The technetium brain scan also shows the hematoma in most cases, but the definitive test is cerebral angiography, which is diagnostic. The treatment is surgical evacuation of the subdural collection when the patient is symptomatic and is a surgical candidate. Some elderly patients do not improve following the removal of the clot, when the hematoma has been present for a long time and the deficit is severe. Small subdural collections can be treated medically with dexamethasone.

Brain Tumors. Other space-occupying lesions also cause a disturbance of memory under some circumstances. About 1% of the patients in geriatric wards have brain tumors. The majority of tumors begin with clear focal signs and, in elderly patients, most are metastatic. Meningioma is a benign tumor whose earliest sign may be a simple progressive dementia. Most meningioma patients have seizures, which may be focal, and gradual mental impairment with progressive appearance of neurologic signs. The CT scan with contrast enhancement diagnoses most meningiomas. Technetium brain scan and EEG are also abnormal in most cases. Glioma, unusual in patients over 70 years old, may cause dementia, but the course is rapidly progressive, and there are almost always clear focal signs. When the lesion is bifrontal, the abulic state is most common. A diffusely infiltrating glioma (gliomatosis cerebri) or a temporal lobe tumor sometimes causes a progressive neurologic syndrome with dementia as a major feature. The course is usually over months, but a few patients who are treated with radiation may live with the dementia for several years. The dementia is generally not so profound as in the usual case of Alzheimer's disease.

Thiamine Deficiency. Thiamine deficiency causes a specific memory disorder in which new memories are not formed. The condition called *amnesic,* or *Korsakoff's dementia* is characteristic, because the patient cannot learn new material but can recollect previously learned information. On careful testing there is a deficit of both recent and remote memory, but recent memory is more greatly affected. In most patients with Korsakoff's psychosis, immediate recall is preserved. The amnesic state usually spares the personality, and language is normal. An apathetic, global, confusional state usually is associated with it, and at onset the memory deficit may not be testable. The confusional state and memory disorder blend into a mixed syndrome that is often not easily separable. Korsakoff's psychosis develops in alcoholics but also in elderly patients with poor nutrition. It may arise suddenly in older persons who enter the hospital for a surgical procedure (fractured hip) and receive infusions of glucose. The treatment is thiamine, 50–100 mg IV initially and 50 mg PO later. The syndrome is usually reversible to some degree, but in alcoholics with severe impairment it may not be curable. Other signs associated with thiamine deficiency may be absent, but usually nystagmus, ocular palsy, and ataxia appear.

Vitamin B_{12} and Niacin Deficiencies. Other deficiency diseases occasionally cause dementia. Vitamin B_{12} deficiency is rare and almost always accompanies hematologic abnormality. The dementia is mild and seldom is confused with degenerative disease. When the posterior columns or corticospinal tracts are also affected, diagnosis becomes easier. A loss of vibratory sense in the feet is invariable, the hematocrit is usually low, the red blood cell indices are high, and there are hypersegmented polymorphonuclear leukocytes. Serum B_{12} and the Schilling test are diagnostic. Many patients with chronic later-stage Alzheimer's disease also have anemia, but few show megaloblastic changes on smear or marrow. Niacin deficiency causes pellagra, which is a syndrome of rough, red, vesicular rash; sore mouth; red tongue; diarrhea; and dementia. A confusional state is more common than dementia.

Transient Global Amnesia. Transient global amnesia is an acute state of memory loss in which the patient fails to remember recent events. Although the patient is agitated, there is little change in personality, and language is normal. Remote memory is usually better then recent memory. The syndrome is not associated with other neurologic signs, except when it is a part of a basilar artery stroke. The idiopathic form, which is not associated with lesions in the basilar artery, may be a seizure disorder. There is no treatment for transient global amnesia, which usually lasts for a few hours, is seldom recurrent, and is benign. Patients should be watched, however, for signs of brainstem ischemia, indicating an evolving stroke.

Depression. Depressed elderly patients perform poorly on clinical and neuropsychiatric tests. Attention is poor and they give up easily. Often the patient complains bitterly of memory loss, an unusual finding in other dementias. Severe depression may resemble SDAT occasionally when the patient is mute and refuses to cooperate with tests. In milder cases memory can be shown to be spared and with persistent questioning the patient will answer questions correctly. There are usually no language or praxis deficits in depression. A therapeutic trial of antidepressants will improve the depression in most patients. EEG and CT scan are normal.

Evaluation

The evaluation of a demented patient begins with a careful assessment of the severity and character of the dementia. A history focused to search for clues of the common treatable disorders often makes the diagnosis easy. Blood chemistry, VDRL, thyroid function tests, complete blood count, ECG, and chest x-ray should be performed on all patients evaluated for dementia. Special chemistries need to be done only when there is an indication on history or examination. EEG and CT scan are most helpful and are required in all dementia evaluations. Lumbar puncture is needed to measure CSF pressure and to identify infection, if the history or examination is suggestive. When it is not possible to distinguish depression from primary dementia, the patient should be treated for depression and followed for improvement. The most useful test in difficult cases of dementia is a reexamination in several months to assess the progression of the dementia and to search for new signs that might indicate the underlying disorder.

1. Adams RD, Rosman NP: Emotions and mentation, in Werner SC, Ingbar SH (eds): *The Thyroid*, ed 3. New York, Harper and Row, 1978, pp 775–776.
   In hypothyroidism, somnolence is more apparent than in hydrocephalus, chronic subdural hematoma, or SDAT.
2. Bennett R, Hughes GRU, Bywaters EGL, Holt PJL: Neuropsychiatric problems in systemic lupus erythematosus. *Br Med J* 4:342–345, 1972.
   Five patients had anxiety and depression but none were demented.
3. Bergin JD: Rapidly progressing dementia in disseminated sclerosis. *J Neurol Neurosurg Psychiatry* 20:285–292, 1957.
   Two patients had irritability and mild dementia that progressed along with other signs to a severe dementia. EEGs, were abnormal.
4. Black PM: Idiopathic normal pressure hydrocephalus. Results of shunting in 62 patients. *J Neurosurg* 52:371–377, 1980.
   The patients' mean age was 67 2/3 years; large ventricles with little atrophy on CT predicted improvement after shunting.
5. Borgesen SE, Gjerris F: The predictive value of conductance to outflow of CSF in normal pressure hydrocephalus. *Brain* 105:65–86, 1982.
   Two CT findings were related to improvement after shunting: periventricular hypodensity and cortical sulci below 1.9 mm.
6. Brain R, Henson RA: Neurological syndromes associated with carcinoma. *Lancet* 2:971–975, 1958.
   Progressive dementia was reported in 14 patients. Mood was euphoric. Onset was in months. It may be associated with cerebellar or neuropathic changes.
7. Bulens C: Neurological complications of hyperthyroidism. *Arch Neurol* 38:669–670, 1981.
   Spastic paraplegia, dementia, and optic neuropathy improved in a 72-year-old patient treated for excess thyroid hormone.
8. Campbell ACP, Biggart JH: Wernike's encephalopathy (polioencephalitis hemorrhagica superior): Its alcoholic and non-alcoholic incidence. *J Pathol Bacteriol* 48:245–262, 1939.
   This study supports the then-novel notion that nutrition was the cause of the syndrome. The emphasis is on the pathology.
9. Carney MW: Five cases of bromism. *Lancet* 2:523–524, 1971.
   Confusion and psychiatric changes were noted.

10. Carroll BJ: The dexamethasone suppression test for melancholia. *Br J Psychiatr* 140:292–304, 1982.
A review that describes the method and rationale for the test.
11. Clarke EC, Yoss RE: Nervous system findings associated with systemic lupus erythematosus. *Minn Med* 39:517–520, 1956.
A case of personality changes, memory loss, and multiple temporary focal signs is reported in a 46-year-old woman.
12. Eraut D: Idiopathic hypoparathyroidism presenting as dementia. *Br Med J* 1:429–430, 1974.
Case report.
13. Fisher CM: The clinical picture in occult hydrocephalus. *Clin Neurosurg* 24:270–284, 1976.
The inside story of occult symptomatic hydrocephalus and the clinical details of 30 cases.
14. Fisher CM, Adams RD: Transient global amnesia. *Acta Neurol Scand* 40 (suppl 9):7–83, 1964.
Careful clinical description that established the disorder as a clinical entity.
15. Gilbert DN, Johnson MT, Luby JP, Sanford JP: Herpes virus hominis type I encephalitis treated with cytarabine, an unresolved problem in encephalitis. *Medicine* 52:331–338, 1973.
In 8 patients, confusion, personality change, and aphasia were prominent presenting complaints; 2 reported survivors had fixed deficits, including dementia in 1.
16. Graham K, Williams BO, Rowe MJ: Idiopathic hypoparathyroidism: A cause of fits in the elderly. *Br Med J* 1:1460–1461, 1979.
A collection of case reports.
17. Greenberg JO, Sherikin HA, Adam R: Idiopathic normal pressure hydrocephalus—a report of 73 patients. *J Neurol Neurosurg Psychiatry* 40:336–341, 1977.
Gait disorder and large ventricles were signs predicting best result of shunt in patients thought to have hydrocephalus.
18. Green R: The thyroid gland: Its relationship to neurology, in Vinken PJ, Bruyn GW (eds): *Handbook of Clinical Neurology.* Amsterdam, North Holland Publishing, 1976, pp 255–278.
A major review.
19. Heilman KM, Fisher WR: Hyperlipidemic dementia. *Arch Neurol* 31:61–63, 1974.
Diabetes, stroke, and possible thyroid disease make this case suspect.
20. Hooshmand H, Escobar MR, Kopf SW: Neurosyphilis. *JAMA* 219:726–729, 1972.
Reviews 241 patients, 12 of whom had general paresis.
21. Hunter R, Blackwood M, Bull J: Three cases of frontal meningoma presenting psychiatrically. *Br Med J* 3:9–16, 1968.
Apathy, incontinence, and seizures were the major signs; 1 patient was symptomatic for 43 years before diagnosis.
22. Hyldstrup L, Ladefoged SD: Reversible dementia in idiopathic hypoparathyroidism. *Dan Med Bull* 28:74–75, 1981.
Describes a 71-year-old man with dementia and seizures, which disappeared with treatment.
23. Isbell H, et al: Chronic barbiturate intoxication. *Arch Neurol Psychiatr* 64:1–28, 1950.
The study done on young prisoners showed slowness of thought, poor judgment, and failures on psychometric tests but no dementia. This study would not be allowed today.
24. Johnson KP, Rosenthal MS, Lerner PI: Herpes simplex encephalitis: The course in five virologically proven cases. *Arch Neurol* 27:103–108, 1972.
Headaches and acute onset of confusional states, which led to unresponsiveness, were manifested in 5 patients.
25. Johnson RT, Richardson EP: The neurological manifestations of systemic lupus erythematosus. *Medicine* 47:337–369, 1968.
A definitive description in 24 cases with 222 references.
26. Kimble ST, Stieglitz EJ: Hypothyroidism: A geriatric problem. *Geriatrics* 7:20–31, 1952.
This study is dated, but it gives some clinical and historical information that is still of use.
27. Koenig IT: Dementia associated with the benign form of multiple sclerosis. *Trans Am Neurol Assoc* 93:227–228, 1968.

Seven patients had memory loss with multiple neurologic signs. There was no pathology and little to rule out more than one etiology.

28. Kurland ML: Organic brain syndrome with propranolol. *N Engl J Med* 300:366, 1979.
A letter reporting 3 cases (ages 60, 49, 56) using daily doses between 160 mg and 320 mg.
29. Langworthy OR: Lesions of the central nervous system characteristic of pellagra. *Brain* 54:291–302, 1931.
A detailed pathologic study of a simple case in which the patient developed nervousness, irritability, and defects in memory after the onset of diarrhea and dermatitis.
30. Lederman RJ, Henry CE: Progressive dialysis encephalopathy. *Ann Neurol* 4:199–204, 1978.
Sudden onset of hesitant, nonfluent speech was the most characteristic early sign in this group of 42 patients.
31. Lehrich JR, Kleinman GM: Case 44–1979. *N Engl J Med* 301:987–994, 1979.
A clinical description of herpes simplex encephalitis. "Her thoughts wandered, and her information was imprecise." The patient was oriented to month and year. Onset, beginning with headache, was over in about 5 days.
32. Lidz T: Emotions and mentation, in Werner SC, Ingbar SH (eds): *The Thyroid,* ed 3. New York, Harper & Row, 1978, pp 627–629.
Brief description of the mental state in hyperthyroidism; no mention of dementia.
33. Luxon L, Lees AJ, Greenwood RJ: Neurosyphilis today. *Lancet* 1:90–93, 1979.
Reviews 17 cases; 3 patients had dementia.
34. Mahurkar DD, et al: Dialysis dementia. *Lancet* 1:1412–1415, 1973.
Describes a progressive course with dysarthria leading to mutism. A confusional state with fluctuating attention, misarticulation, dysprosady, and dysgraphia.
35. Mair WGP, Warrington EK, Weiskrantz L: Memory disorder in Korsakoff's psychosis: A neuropathological and neuropsychological investigation of two cases. *Brain* 102:749–783, 1979.
Both patients had a pure long-term memory impairment without a short-term loss. The minimal lesion was thought to be in the mamillary bodies and dorsal medial thalamus.
36. Marsden DC, Harrison MJG: Outcome of patients with presenile dementia. *Br Med J* 2:249–252, 1972.
Points out the importance of looking for treatable disease causing dementia. In this group 15% had treatable dementia.
37. McGovern GP, Miller MG, Robertson EE: A mental syndrome associated with lung carcinoma. *Arch Neurol Psychiatry* 81:341–347, 1959.
Two patients developed psychotic depression in which the intellectual deficits were too severe to be attributable to the depression.
38. Morgan M, Jakobovits A, Elithorn A, James IM, Sherlock S: Successful use of bromocriptine in the treatment of a patient with chronic protosystemic encephalopathy. *N Engl J Med* 296:793–794, 1977.
Describes the use of 15 mg/day for 3 months.
39. Olivarius B, Roder E: Reversible psychosis and dementia in myxedemia. *Acta Psychiatr Scand* 46:1–13, 1970.
Review of 3 cases and the literature.
40. Perlmutter I: Subdural hematoma in older patients. *JAMA* 176:212–214, 1961.
In 2 cases drowsiness was a major clue.
41. Robinson KC, Kallberg MH, Crowley MF: Idiopathic hypoparathyroidism presenting as dementia. *Br Med J* 2:1203, 1954.
Case report.
42. Rowan AJ, Protass LM: Transient global amnesia: Clinical and electroencephalographic findings in 10 cases. *Neurology* 29:869–872, 1979.
Abnormal routine EEGs were found in 4 patients. Nasopharyngeal leads show abnormality in 5 of 7 tested.
43. Sanders HI, Warrington EK: Memory for remote events in amnestic patients. *Brain* 94:661–668, 1971.
There was no evidence of sparing of remote memory.
44. Slyter H, Idiopathic hypoparathyroidism presenting as dementia. *Neurology* 29:393–394, 1979.
Case report.
45. Sparling PF: Diagnosis and treatment of syphilis. *N Engl J Med* 284:642–653, 1971.

Large review with 136 references.

46. Steinberg H, Waldron BR: Idiopathic hypoparathyroidism: Analysis of fifty-two cases, including the report of a new case. *Medicine* 31:133–154, 1953.
Extensive review.
47. Strachan RW, Henderson JG: Psychiatric syndromes due to avitaminosis B_{12} with normal blood and marrow. *Q J Med* 34:303–317, 1965.
This is a unique report of neurologic disease without blood findings in B_{12} deficiency.
48. Stuteville P, Welch K: Subdural hematoma in the elderly person. *JAMA* 168:1445–1449, 1958.
The chief complaint was mental status change or personality change in 12 of 75 cases. CSF was normal in three-fourths of the patients.
49. Thomas RB, Mazzaferri EL, Skillman TG: Apathetic thyrotoxicosis: A distinctive clinical and laboratory entity. *Ann Intern Med* 72:679–685, 1970.
The patients were older than typical hyperthyroid patients and seemed to have depression. The 2 case reports illustrate somnolence and confusion rather than dementia.
50. Tsai FY, Huprich JE, Segall HD, Teal JS: The contrast enhanced CT scan in the diagnosis of isodense subdural hematoma. *J Neurosurg* 50:64–69, 1979.
With newer scans there are fewer problems, but an occasional case may be overlooked if the technical quality is poor. The patients in this study were young.
51. Twomey C: Brain tumors in the elderly. *Age Ageing* 7:138–145, 1978.
Mental impairment with motor signs was the most common finding in malignant tumors. Headache was common in the benign cases.
52. Victor M, Yakovlev PI: S.S. Korsakoff's psychic disorder in conjunction with peripheral neuritis. *Neurology* 5:394–406, 1955.
Subtitle: A translation of Korsakoff's original article with brief comments on the author and his contribution to clinical medicine.
53. Wells CE: Pseudodementia. *Am J Psychiatry* 136:895–900, 1979.
Depression was not the only cause: conversion reaction, hysteria, and other neuroses were at fault.
54. Whybrow PC, Prange AJ, Treadway CR: Mental changes accompanying thyroid gland function. *Arch Gen Psychiatry* 20:48–63, 1969.
A good review and reference source that reports 17 cases. The hypothyroid patients were inattentive and poor at abstraction and in memory. Long-standing hypothyroidism may cause irreversible memory loss. Hyperthyroid patients had less deficit, and their memory loss was completely reversible.
55. Williams M, Smith HV: Mental disturbances in tuberculous meningitis. *J Neurol Neurosurg Psychiatry* 17:173–182, 1954.
In 19 cases only 4 patients had minimal residual memory loss, but all had amnesia for the period of illness. The acute syndrome was confusion and amnesia.
56. Wintzen AR: The clinical course of subdural hematoma. *Brain* 103:855–867, 1980.
Chronic subdurals occur without trauma and have a better prognosis than acute subdurals. Age was not mentioned.

101. APPROACH TO CEREBROVASCULAR DISEASE

Thomas M. Walshe

The cerebrovascular diseases include a number of syndromes in which the diagnosis depends on recognition of the vascular and neural pathologic features. Management and prognosis then depend on the type of lesion and its severity. There is no known therapy to regenerate brain tissue once it is infarcted; therefore a major concern in cerebrovascular disease is anticipation of stroke, so that it can be prevented before infarction is complete.

Etiology

The primary pathologic condition of stroke lies in the blood vessel, and the brain lesion results from hemorrhage or ischemia caused by the vascular abnormality. The chief types of vascular pathologic conditions are large or small vessel thrombosis, embolism, aneurysmal change, and rupture of arteries. Malformations of arteries also may cause stroke but are usually considered as a separate disease, because they are associated with other syndromes. Another group of cerebral ischemic syndromes occur when the vessels are normal but either the total blood flow or the oxygen content of the blood is reduced, so that the brain undergoes diffuse ischemia and infarction. Disorders of the veins are much less common than disorders of the arteries. Venous thrombosis occurs occasionally in infants, the elderly, and women in the puerperium.

Incidence

Approximately 275,000 persons die each year from all types of stroke. Three hundred thousand are disabled, of whom 10% are required to live in chronic care facilities. Over 80% of the patients who suffer a stroke are older than 65 years. The prevalence of stroke in persons over 65 is about 60 in every 1,000; in persons over 75 the prevalence is 95 in every 1,000 persons. The incidence of stroke is hard to determine from mortality statistics because of changes in diagnostic fashions and coding practices, low accuracy of diagnosis, and variability in death certificate reporting. Morbidity statistics are more accurate, but comparison between different study groups is difficult.

The incidence of ischemic and hemorrhagic stroke has declined by about one-half, as measured by computer record index methods at the Mayo Clinic. Patients older than 80 years had a 60% reduction in stroke rate. Stroke nonetheless remains six times more common in older age groups. There has been no change, however, in the incidence of subarachnoid hemorrhage. The reasons for the declining rate of stroke are not known. Epidemiologic studies estimate the incidence of infarction to be about 80% of all strokes, and of hemorrhage, about 20%.

Prognosis

Following the first 24–48 hours after a stroke, the prognosis for survival can generally be made. Most patients who survive the first 3 or 4 days live through their strokes. Patients who develop coma, no matter from which type of stroke, have the worst prognosis. The prognosis for active ability to perform in society depends on the size of the lesion and the area of brain involved. It is generally better to reserve the prognosis for activity until well into the rehabilitation phase. In general, patients with hemiparetic strokes improve rapidly in the first month and then gradually for up to 6 months. Overall ability to function depends on the patient's personality, the size of the infarct, and the quality of the rehabilitation.

The degree of disability from stroke depends on the size and location of the lesion. About 16% of stroke patients require institutionalization, 31% require help with self-care, and 20% are not ambulatory without help. Seventy-one percent of patients have decreased ability to work at their jobs. These percentages have not been broken down according to type of stroke. Of stroke patients able to go to rehabilitation, 80% return home after an average stay of 43 days. Of these, 85% are ambulatory, and 56% are able to carry out their own activities of daily living. Bad signs for recovery are "severe" weakness, cognitive or perceptual deficits, or the combination of hemianopia with motor weaknesses. Unrelated to the rehabilitation prognosis are age, dysphagia, hemisensory deficit, diabetes mellitus, hypertension, and atherosclerosis in other parts of the body.

Survival rate is higher after infarction than after hemorrhage. Subarachnoid hemorrhage has a better survival prognosis than intracerebral hemorrhage. Young persons survive better than old persons.

It is difficult to assess the large studies that predict incidence and prognosis in stroke because the diagnosis is often not clearly established. The prognosis and severity of stroke depends entirely on the size and location of the cerebral lesion. Certainly the larger the lesion, the worse the prognosis. Each case must be understood on its own merits, and although the statistics may provide trends, they have very little to do with day-to-day management of stroke patients.

Death from stroke is generally delayed. In about 20% of cases it occurs within 24 hours. Most early deaths are caused by intracerebral hemorrhages, and only a few by infarctions. Often an infarction that causes death is in the pons or is associated with intractable seizures.

Diagnosis

The recognition of an event as cerebrovascular is usually simple. The rapid onset of a neurologic deficit is the hallmark by which even laymen can recognize a stroke. Through the history and, to a lesser extent, the neurologic findings, the physician can then distinguish a specific vascular syndrome.

Diagnosis becomes more difficult in the case of patients with small cerebral lesions or lesions of the brainstem that are not accompanied by a gross motor deficit. Sometimes patients complain of signs or symptoms that may go misunderstood without careful and specialized effort. Analysis of a stroke includes separating it into the general types of thrombosis, embolism, intraparenchymal hemorrhage, or subarachnoid hemorrhage. The specific subtype usually can be discerned by looking at the history carefully, doing a complete neurologic examination, and then selecting proper tests.

Angiography. Angiography and computerized tomography have become indispensable in confirming the clinical diagnosis. Cerebral and neck angiograms identify and localize the vascular lesion precisely. Angiography should be used when carotid lesions are suspected and in many cases of suspected basilar artery or vertebral artery lesions. The cerebral angiogram not only shows lesions of the artery, it also reveals the available collaterals that come into play after complete occlusions or with tight stenosis. Embolic lesions may not appear on angiograms or may show only subtle changes in the distal branches. The angiogram is less helpful in embolic disease than in thrombotic disease, although it may show the embolic source to be an ulcerated plaque in one of the extracranial vessels.

Digital subtraction angiography (DSA) uses intravenous contrast material for imaging of the large extracranial and intracranial vessels. The technique requires computer subtraction to enhance the dilute contrast material, so that the large extracranial arteries are easily seen. DSA is much safer, cheaper, and easier than conventional angiography and will identify plaques and stenosis in the carotid artery. DSA is not adequate for aneurysms, arteriovenous malformation or carotid-cavernous fistulas, because its small vessel resolution is not as good as that of conventional angiography. DSA is also useful in diagnosing venous occlusion or assessing the patency of temporal artery–middle cerebral artery bypass grafts. Patient motion and other technical problems, however, prevent adequate imaging in 10–15% of patients studied with DSA.

Patients who are not candidates for any medical or surgical intervention do not require angiography. Patients in this group are demented, suffer from massive medical or neurologic disease, or are unwilling to undergo therapy.

Computerized Tomography. The computerized tomogram (CT) will show brain infarcts reliably but is most helpful in diagnosing brain hemorrhages. A contrast-enhanced CT scan may show the area of infarction in ischemic lesions. When hemorrhage is suspected, an unenhanced scan should be used to search for a high-density lesion. CT scan has replaced lumbar puncture as the initial diagnostic procedure of choice in intraparenchymal hemorrhages. CT is not so useful in subarachnoid hemorrhage, although it may show cisternal blood, which identifies the site of the aneurysm. In very large aneurysms, contrast enhancement may identify the aneurysm itself on CT scan.

Lumbar puncture remains the diagnostic procedure of choice if subarachnoid hemorrhage is suspected, but it is generally of limited value in the overall assessment of an ischemic stroke. With thrombotic infarction there may be a few white cells in the CSF; in embolic cases the CSF occasionally has some white cells and sometimes up to 10,000–15,000 red cells. It is usually wise to check the spinal fluid before putting an embolic stroke patient on anticoagulation. It is, however, very rare for a hemorrhagic infarct to develop a hematoma, even with anticoagulation.

Electroencephalography. The electroencephalogram has little place in the diagnosis of acute stroke. There may be a nonspecific lateralizing focus of slow-wave activity in patients whose cortex is involved. The EEG of patients with lacunar infarction is normal. Patients who have seizures and postictal paralysis may be identified occasionally with electroencephalography. In stroke, the clinical history usually is more enlightening than the EEG. Seizure disorders are often a long-term complication of cerebrovascular disease, and an EEG is indicated later in the course if the patient has intermittent symptoms, to ensure that no paroxysmal activity is present.

Technetium Brain Scan. The CT scan has virtually eliminated the use of a technetium brain scan in the evaluation of acute stroke. When used, the technetium brain scan is often negative early in the course and then becomes positive several days to a week later, when the infarct is well established.

Management

General medical measures that are important in the care of stroke patients include taking the usual precautions to protect the patient from aspiration and to prevent other respiratory complications. Excess hydration, particularly with hypotonic fluid such as D_5W, should be avoided, because it increases brain swelling. Some neurologists prefer to use saline or half normal saline, if an intravenous fluid is necessary. Patients with stroke who are able to swallow can be hydrated orally. Careful observation of the neurologic syndrome with an eye to further progression is necessary, since patients who begin with a partial deficit may progress to a more severe problem. In addition, later complications such as hydrocephalus and seizures can be reduced when recognized early. Myocardial infarction and arrhythmias are common in stroke patients, so ECG monitoring is helpful during the acute phase.

It is quite important to reassure stroke patients that the problem is under control. Patients with strokes are among the most anxious and frustrated of all patients encountered in medicine, and their psychological care is often quite difficult. Patients who are aphasic are particularly difficult, because they cannot express their feelings. Frequent reassurance and explanations often help tremendously.

1. Leonberg SC, Elliott FA: Prevention of recurrent stroke. *Stroke* 12:731–735, 1981.
The 5-year mortality was 17% and the stroke rate was 16% in 88 survivors of ischemic stroke when risk factors were "controlled." Endarterectomy, anticoagulants, and aspirin were used in some cases.
2. Siekert RG (ed): *Cerebrovascular Survey Report.* Bethesda, Maryland, NINCDS, National Institutes of Health, January 1980 (revised).
A comprehensive collection of essays on stroke with many references.
3. Britton M, DeGaire U, Helmers C, Miah K: Prognostication in acute cerebrovascular disease. *Acta Med Scand* 207:37–42, 1980.
The degree of neurologic deficit rather than the type of stroke was important in prognosis.
4. Garraway W, et al: The declining incidence of stroke. *N Engl J Med* 300:449–452, 1979.
For every 100 strokes that occurred from 1945–1949, only 55 occurred from 1970–1975.
5. Kannel W, Pawber T, Sorlie P, Wolf P: Components of blood pressure and risk of atherothrombotic brain infarction: The Framingham Study. *Stroke* 7:327, 1976.
The 18-year follow-up of 5,209 patients showed hypertension to be the main risk factor in ischemic stroke; the incidence was 7 times higher in hypertensive patients.
6. Shekelle R, Ostfeld A, Klawans H: Hypertension and risk of stroke in an elderly population. *Stroke* 5:71–75, 1974.
Suggests that more than 25% of strokes in persons aged 65–74 years are caused by hypertension.
7. Terent A, Anderson B: The prognosis for patients with cerebrovascular stroke and transient ischemic attacks. *Ups J Med Sci* 86:63–74, 1981.
Of 281 patients with stroke and 44 with TIA, 30% of the stroke patients died in 3 months; in 4 years 70% of the stroke patients died and 40% of TIA patients died.
8. Torvik A, Stenwig JT: Changes in frequency of cerebrovascular diseases in Oslo, Norway, 1968–1977. *Stroke* 12:816–823, 1981.
Autopsy study showed an overall fall of 14% in a 20-year survey, but for patients over 70 years only a small drop was noted. For patients aged 40–60 years, the drop was 25%.
9. Wolf PA, et al: Epidemiology of stroke, in Thompson RA, Green JR (eds): *Advances in Neurology: Stroke.* New York, Raven Press, 1977.
Summary of the Framingham study.
10. Furlan AJ, Whisnant JP, Elveback LR: The decreasing incidence of primary intracerebral hemorrhage: A population study. *Ann Neurol* 5:367–373, 1979.
Hemorrhage accounts for about 10% of strokes.
11. National Heart and Lung Institute Task Force on Arteriosclerosis: Arteriosclerosis: A report. Washington, DC, US Department of Health, Education, and Welfare, Pub No. (NIH) 72–219, 1971, vol 2.
Describes the epidemiology of stroke.
12. Thompson RA, Green JR: *Stroke.* New York, Raven Press, 1977.
A complete review of the clinical aspects.
13. Vitek JJ: Femoro-cerebral angiography: Analysis of 2000 consecutive examinations, special emphasis on carotid arteries catheterization in older patients. *Am J Roentgenol* 118:633–647, 1973.

Reports 2 deaths, 5 permanent complications, and 25 transient complications in 2,000 studies.

14. de Reuck J, et al: Epilepsy in patients with cerebral infarcts. *J Neurol* 224:101–109, 1980.
An autopsy study that showed seizure that preceded stroke came from causes other than cerebral ischemia.
15. Hinshaw DB, Thompson JR, Hasso AN, Casselman ES: Infarctions of the brainsteim and cerebellum: A correlation of computed tomography and angiography. *Radiology* 137:105–112, 1980.
The CT scan was better at showing more rostral lesions in the brainsteim. The bone artifact at the skull base probably obscures lower lesions.
16. McHenry LC, Toole JF, Miller HS: Long-term EKG monitoring in patients with cerebrovascular insufficiency. *Stroke* 7:264–269, 1976.
Of these patients, 10 had syndromes and arrhythmia but only 1 had arrhythmia that seemed to be the cause of the TIA. Another patient had the expected syncopal attack with the arrhythmia.
17. Simonsen N, et al: Long-term prognosis after transient ischemic attacks. *Acta Neurol Scand* 63:156–168, 1981.
Death from stroke occurred in 20% and from MI in 38% of patients over a 10-year period. The diagnosis was from medical records, and treatment was not controlled.

102. TRANSIENT NEUROLOGIC SYMPTOMS AND SIGNS

Thomas M. Walshe

Differential Diagnosis

All transient neurological symptoms and signs are not transient ischemic attacks. The physician confronted with a transient neurologic deficit must make a differential diagnosis. By careful analysis of the history of the spell, one can usually determine if it is transient ischemia or one of the many other causes of transient signs. Deficits commonly confused with transient ischemic attacks include focal seizures, syncopal attacks, labyrinthine disorders, migrainous accompaniments, multiple sclerosis with transient symptoms, hypoglycemia, hyperventilation, cervical discopathy, and carpal tunnel syndrome.

As a general rule, transient ischemic attacks can be identified as coming from a specific vascular territory. Transient ischemic attacks (TIAs) are episodes of temporary and focal cerebral dysfunction of vascular origin that have their onset within minutes and usually last 2–15 minutes. TIAs that fit this description usually indicate thrombotic stenosis of a large vessel in the neck or of a proximal intracranial vessel.

Carotid Artery Obstruction. Pure transient hemispheric symptoms such as arm weakness or numbness affect about half of patients with carotid artery disease, and isolated monocular blindness occurs in about one-third. In transient hemispheric attacks that last 1 hour or longer, the carotid arteries often reveal no notable stenosis. Hemispheric and ocular attacks occurring at different times in the same vascular distribution have a high correlation with tight carotid stenosis.

A typical hemispheric attack includes numbness, tingling, or weakness of an extremity and face or, when the lesion is on the left, a transient episode of aphasia. The importance of a transient ischemic attack lies in its warning of an impending stroke. Approximately 60% of carotid stenosis patients may have transient ischemic symptoms before their stroke. The mechanism of transient ischemia relating to stenosis of the carotid artery is not known. Emboli that form in and around the narrowing are not the major cause, but whether changes in hemodynamics through the stenosis play a role has not yet been proved, either.

Once the physician identifies a patient as having transient ischemic attacks related to the carotid artery, a cerebral angiogram should be obtained, and further therapeutic considerations can follow it. Overall, about 25–40% of patients with transient ischemic attacks have a stroke within 5 years. When the attacks are frequent, close together, and in the carotid territory, the incidence is probably higher. Moreover, when the attacks conform to the definition of *short* (< 4 hrs), the incidence of stroke is probably higher. Transient ischemic attacks that last as long as 24 hours are often embolic strokes. Because *long* transient ischemic attacks are often embolic, it seems best to separate those cases from the ischemic attacks lasting less than 4 hours.

In general, the angiogram reveals a 1- to 1½-mm opening when a transient ischemic attack is associated with carotid stenosis. Rarely are larger openings associated with short transient ischemic attacks. Longer TIAs may be caused by small emboli from any source, including a thrombus on an ulcerated nonstenotic plaque in the carotid artery. Transient ischemic attacks can occur even when the internal carotid artery is occluded. Amaurosis fugax, hemispheric signs, or both, have been found in patients who have occluded carotid arteries and ipsilateral external carotid stenosis; following endarterectomy of the external carotid, the transient ischemic attacks stop. The exact mechanism of this rare clinical situation is unclear, but in most cases the external carotid supplies the internal carotid territory. Carotid artery lesions have been known to cause vertebrobasilar transient ischemic syndromes. Usually there is an anomalous vascularization; for instance, through the trigeminal artery or through the hypoglossal artery feeding the basilar artery.

Transient monocular blindness occuring in isolation, without other symptoms or signs, is infrequently associated with carotid artery stenosis. Young patients who have transient monocular blindness, and patients who do not have other symptoms, need not be examined by angiography; however, patients with transient monocular blindness who have cholesterol emboli in the retina may have a carotid plaque as revealed by the angiogram. Patients with bruits in the neck or other physical findings indicative of carotid artery disease should be studied also.

Vertebrobasilar TIA. Vertebrobasilar transient ischemic attacks are often subtle and difficult to diagnose. The most common features are numbness and decreased sensation or weakness in one or both sides of the face, arm, or leg. Complete or partial loss of vision in both eyes, with or without vertigo or dizziness, may be a clue. Homonymous hemianopia, ataxia, imbalance, or staggering of gait, diplopia, dysphagia, dysarthria, transient global amnesia, and drop attacks have all been identified with vertebrobasilar stenosis. These symptoms generally last only a few minutes, and the patient may have many transient attacks before the stroke. In most cases, however, the patient has only a few or a single TIA before acquiring a fixed deficit.

The overall incidence of transient ischemic attacks in stroke is only 10%. Of that 10%, however, most are patients who have large vessel disease and are therefore therapeutic targets for stroke prevention.

Treatment

Therapy of TIA remains controversial. Several options are open to the clinician.

Endarterectomy. When stenotic carotid artery disease causes TIA, endarterectomy is the best treatment for many patients. The success of carotid endarterectomy, as found in the major studies, depends mainly on the skill of the surgeon. Patients who have stable (incomplete or unchanging) neurologic deficits, no medical complications, and relatively uncomplicated atherosclerotic lesions have a very low morbidity and mortality from endarterectomy in experienced hands. Patients with symptomatic coronary artery disease, congestive heart failure, severe hypertension, or extreme obesity do much worse following operation. Patients who are older than 70 years have a much higher risk of stroke and death also. Roentgenographic signs help to assess the risks. When the angiogram shows occlusion of the carotid artery opposite to the one being operated on, or extensive plaque extending above into the siphon, or loose thrombus on the ulcerated plaque, there is a slightly greater operative risk. The highest risk of postoperative death or stroke is in patients who have major unstable neurologic deficits. Such patients may have complication rates of 10% or more.

Some surgeons have tried to treat the unstable neurologic cases with endarterectomy. Patients with smaller lesions appear to do well, but those with large lesions do not benefit from the procedure. When a surgical team can offer patients a postoperative stroke risk of less than 3%, carotid endarterectomy is useful in management of TIA in carotid territory.

Acute Stage Anticoagulation. Heparin is given acutely to patients who have angiographically proved carotid stenosis with transient symptoms related to the lesion. Heparin is also used for angiographically defined basilar or middle cerebral artery stenosis, and the patients are usually put on chronic anticoagulation with sodium warfarin (Coumadin). When patients have inoperable carotid stenosis, that is, narrowing in the carotid siphon or above, chronic anticoagulation is also used. Patients with complete occlusions of the carotid or other arteries are not given anticoagulants, unless there is some other indication. Some patients who have a complete carotid occlusion and stenotic disease in other vessels may develop symptoms in the territory of the nonoccluded vessel; such patients are treated like others with stenosis. Patients who have embolism, presumably from thrombus associated with a carotid occlusion, are treated for the embolism (see Chap. 105).

Long-Term Anticoagulation. Anticoagulation with Coumadin has been studied in nine trials. A 1958 study by Fisher, in which 23 patients were untreated and 29 patients treated, showed a 34% stroke rate in the untreated, and a 3% stroke rate in the treated group. The 1961 Cooperative VA Study tested 15 untreated and 22 treated patients, with a 53% stroke rate in the untreated group and a 4.5% stroke rate in the treated group. The follow-up time, however, was less than a year in the treated group. Neurologists at the Mayo Clinic studied 160 controls and 175 anticoagulant-treated patients for 5 years. The stroke rate was 32% in the untreated TIA group and only 4% in the treated. Cerebral hemorrhage occurred in 4% of the untreated and in 7% of the treated patients. A recent study of anticoagulation compared 124 controls to 163 treated TIA cases. The study lasted less than 2 years, and the stroke rate for controls was 15% and for treated patients was zero. In a study that showed no improvement, 29% of treated patients had stroke, but only 13% of the untreated had stroke. Follow-up of the treated group was almost 5 years, and of the untreated, 4 years. Using this information, one can say that anticoagulation reduces the stroke rate in TIA cases, despite the flaws inherent in each study. In addition, anticoagulation seems to reduce the number of TIAs. The risks of heparin and Coumadin are usually minimal when the patient is monitored closely, but even with care the complications are greater in the elderly than in younger patients.

Antiplatelet Therapy. Data from the U.S. Aspirin TIA Study showed that the fewest strokes developed in patients who had endarterectomy and were then treated with aspirin. Other studies of antiplatelet treatment in TIA are not clear-cut. Dipyridamole (Persantin) was used in a controlled double-blind study and was no better than the placebo.

There are two major antiplatelet studies from which physicians must try to derive clinical guidance. The U.S. study used 308 selected patients, of whom 130 were treated surgically and 178 nonsurgically. The separation was not random but was determined by the clinicians. In each of the groups, half received aspirin and half placebo. Among those who did not undergo an operation there were fewer recurrent TIAs in the aspirin-treated group. The stroke rate in the ASA-treated group was 12%, in the placebo group 15%. Of patients who underwent a carotid surgical procedure, 13% of the operation-placebo group had a stroke, but only 3% of the operation-aspirin group had stroke.

The Canadian study used aspirin and sulfinpyrazone in patients with "threatened stroke." Among the symptoms were drowsiness, seizures, hearing loss, hoarseness and mental changes. Over half the 585 patients selected for inclusion had neurologic signs on admission to the study. The groups were given placebo alone, aspirin alone, sulfinpyrazone alone, and aspirin plus sulfinpyrazone. Among the 406 males in the study, the stroke rate for the aspirin group was about 16%. The rate for the placebo group was 17%. The stroke rate for aspirin and sulfinpyrazone was about 6%.

These data do not make one confident that aspirin alone will reduce stroke. The limits of the patient selection make the study difficult to use in more narrowly defined TIA cases.

Although treatment of TIA remains controversial, it seems an acceptable approach to perform endarterectomy on patients with carotid stenosis and to handle inoperable carotid and basilar lesions with anticoagulants.

1. Baker RN, et al: Anticoagulant therapy in cerebral infarction. *Neurology* 12:823–835, 1962.

   This 2-year follow-up study reports a 25% stroke rate in untreated TIA and 4% stroke rate in the treated group.

2. Baker RN, Schwartz W, Rose AS: Transient ischemic attacks—A report of a study of anticoagulant treatment. *Neurology* 16:841–847, 1966.

   Follows up 60 patients after about 3 years of anticoagulant treatment; reports one-third fewer strokes in the treated group.

3. DeWeese JA, et al: Results of carotid endarterectomies for transient ischemic attacks—5 years later. *Ann Surg* 178:258–264, 1973.

Of these patients, 46% were in the 60- to 70-year age group; 34% died in 5 years and 84% had relief of symptoms after their operation.

4. DeWeese JA, et al: Endarterectomy for atherosclerotic lesions of the carotid artery. *Gen Cardiovasc Surg* 12:299–308, 1971.
Reviews 349 operations. Most patients had warning signs before stroke.
5. Fields WS, et al: Joint study of extracranial arterial occlusion: V. Progress report of prognosis following surgical or non-surgical treatment for transient cerebral ischemic attacks and cervical carotid artery lesions. *JAMA* 211:1993–2003, 1970.
For 169 patients, there were 3% operative deaths; 41% were normal in 42-month follow-up.
6. Friedman GD, et al: Transient ischemic attacks in a community. *JAMA* 210:1428–1431, 1969.
Discusses 2-year follow-up of 44 patients; none of the treated group had stroke.
7. Jonas S, Hass WK: An approach to the maximum acceptable stroke complication rate after surgery for transient cerebral ischemia (TIA). *Stroke* 10:104, 1979.
Suggest that surgical risk must be less than 3%.
8. Ollson JE, Muller R, Berneli S: Long-term anticoagulant therapy for TIAs and minor stroke with minimum residuum. *Stroke* 7:444–451, 1976.
Discusses the follow-up of 287 patients for 2 years; there was a 15% stroke rate in the untreated group and a 0% rate in the treated group.
9. Pearce JMS, Gribby SS, Walton JM: Long-term anticoagulant therapy in transient cerebral attacks. *Lancet* 1:6–9, 1965.
Only a few patients were included with less than 1-year follow-up.
10. Toole JF, et al: Transient ischemic attacks due to atherosclerosis: Prospective study of 160 patients. *Arch Neurol* 32:5–13, 1975.
Finds more strokes in the anticoagulated group.
11. Barnett HJM: Delayed cerebral ischemic episodes distal to occlusion of major cerebral arteries. *Neurology* 28:769–774, 1978.
In 237 patients with occluded carotid arteries, 27 had TIA or stroke in distribution of the occlusion.
12. Harrison MJG, Marshall J, Thomas DJ: Relevance of duration of transient ischemic attacks in carotid territory. *Br Med J* 1:1578–1579, 1978.
Carotid stenosis was more likely in patients with attacks lasting less than 1 hour.
13. Humphrey PRD, Marshall J: Transient ischemic attacks and strokes with recovery prognosis and investigation. *Stroke* 12:765–769, 1981.
Of these TIA patients, 51% of those whose attacks lasted less than 5 minutes had subsequent stroke, 30% with short TIAs had operable lesions, but 10% with longer TIAs had operable lesions. Age over 50 years was more common in patients with stenosis.
14. Pessin MS, et al: Clinical and angiographic features of carotid transient ischemic attacks. *N Engl J Med* 296:358–362, 1977.
Hemisphere attack and monocular blindness at separate times on the appropriate side are indications of tight carotid stenosis.
15. Fisher CM: in Scheinberg P (ed): *Cerebrovascular Diseases*. New York, Raven Press, 1976, pp 50–53.
Dr. Fisher gives 37 reasons for TIA not being caused by embolism.
16. Toole JF, et al: Transient ischemic attacks: A study of 225 patients. *Neurology* 28:746–753, 1978.
The series closed in 1973. Subsequent surgical mortality declined. Selected patients had stenosis but not occlusion and only the most skilled surgeons were used; regional anesthesia has improved results.
17. Torvik A, Skullerud K: How often are brain infarcts caused by hypotensive episodes? *Stroke* 7:255–257, 1976.
Very seldom.
18. Walter PF, Reid SD, Wenger NK: Transient cerebral ischemia due to arrhythmia. *Ann Intern Med* 72:471–474, 1970.
Of 28 patients with blackouts, 8 had arrhythmia. Of 11 with focal deficits, 2 had arrhythmia, but no conclusion could be drawn as to the role of the arrhythmia.
19. McAllen PM, Marshall J: Cardiac dysrhythmia and transient cerebral ischaemic attacks. *Lancet* 1:1212–1215, 1973.
The cases illustrate that dysrhythmia causes nonfocal complaints rather than the usual unilateral signs associated with thrombosis.

20. Brust JC, Plank CR, Healton EB, Sanchez GF: The pathology of drop attacks: A case report. *Neurology* 29:786–790, 1979.
Finds a basilar artery stenosis and infarction of the lower basis pontis.
21. Eisenberg RL, Nemzek WR, Moore WS, Mani RL: Relationship of transient ischemic attacks and angiographically demonstrable lesions of carotid artery. *Stroke* 8:483–486, 1977.
Reports carotid lesions in 89% of patients with amaurosis fugax, a higher percentage than usually seen.
22. Millikan CH, McDowell FH: Treatment of transient ischemic attacks. *Stroke* 9:299–308, 1978.
Emphasizes the importance of TIA as a risk factor for stroke. The answer is not absolute.
23. Mohr JP: Transient ischemic attacks and the prevention of strokes. *N Engl J Med* 299:93–95, 1978.
Editorial that reviews the Canadian Study of aspirin in TIA.
24. Reed RL, Siekert RG, Meridith J: Rarity of transient focal cerebral ischemia in cardiac dysrhythmia. *JAMA* 223:893–895, 1973.
About 1% of patients with cardiac arrhythmia have an associated focal neurologic symptom.
25. Sandok BA, Furlan AJ, Whisnant JP, Sundt TM: Guidelines for the management of transient ischemic attacks. *Mayo Clin Proc* 53:665–674, 1978.
A clear plan calling for medical treatment of vertebrobasilar TIA and endarterectomy for carotid lesions.
26. Stewart MR, Samson D, Diehl J, Hinton RC, Ditmore QM: Unruptured cerebral aneurysms presenting as recurrent transient neurologic deficits. *Neurology* 30:47–51, 1980.
In 4 patients, focal signs lasted less than 30 minutes.
27. Ueda K, Toole JF, McHenry LC: Carotid and vertebrobasilar transient ischemic attacks: Clinical and angiographic correlation. *Neurology* 29:1094–1101, 1979.
In 30% of carotid cases and 48% of vertebral cases the arteries were not stenosed or occluded. The duration of the attacks was not recorded.
28. Whisnant JP, Niall EF, Cartlidge MB, Elveback LR: Carotid and vertebral-basilar transient ischemic attacks: Effect of anticoagulants, hypertension, and cardiac disorders on survival and stroke occurrence—a population study. *Neurology* 3:107–113, 1978.
Discusses a follow-up of 199 patients after TIA who showed no difference in survival from those treated with anticoagulants. Risk of hemorrhage on anticoagulants was highest after 1 year of treatment and in patients older than 65 years.
29. Jonas S, Klein I, Dimant J: Importance of Holter monitoring in patients with periodic cerebral symptoms. *Ann Neurol* 1:470–474, 1977.
Arrhythmia does not cause focal signs or symptoms but may cause dizziness, lightheadedness, and blackout spells.
30. Simonsen N, et al: Long-term prognosis after transient ischemic attacks. *Acta Neurol Scand* 63:156–168, 1981.
Death from stroke occurred in 20% of patients and from MI in 38% over a 10-year period. The diagnosis was from medical records, and treatment was not controlled.
31. Olsson JE, et al: Anticoagulant vs. antiplatelet therapy as prophylactic against cerebral infarction in transient ischemic attacks. *Stroke* 11:4–9, 1980.
Suggests an acute treatment with anticoagulants followed by chronic treatment with antiplatelet drugs.

103. THROMBOTIC STROKES

Thomas M. Walshe

Thrombosis, almost always associated with atherosclerosis, occurs in the common and internal carotid arteries. Less frequently, thrombotic stenosis or occlusion reduces flow in the vertebral or basilar arteries. Middle cerebral and other cerebral arteries are uncommonly affected by thrombosis, and, when they are, the lesions are almost always in the most proximal parts. Small vessel thrombosis occurs in hypertensive patients, causing small deep infarcts known as *lacunes*.

The major clinical clue to the diagnosis of thrombotic stroke is a history of transient ischemic attack (TIA). In addition to TIA, which affects about two-thirds of patients with thrombotic cerebrovascular disease, the past history may indicate intermittent claudication in the legs, hyperlipidemia, or diabetes mellitus. A history of coronary artery disease is a common finding. Indeed, one of the major complications of transient ischemic attack is death by coronary artery disease.

The temporal course in about 20% of cases of thrombotic stroke is stepwise, with waxing and waning focal signs. The course is usually uneven rather than smoothly progressive. The thrombotic stroke may occur early in the morning or during sleep.

Carotid Artery Thrombosis

In nearly 80% of carotid artery thrombosis there is transient ischemic attack or a stepwise course, therefore there is often time for preventive action before the completed infarction. In the other 20% of cases, carotid stroke occurs as a single sudden event with no warning.

The neurologic syndrome of carotid stenosis is variable, but classically a syndrome develops in the area of the middle cerebral artery. At times there is a combined middle and anterior cerebral artery deficit, or an ischemic attack of the border zone, causing numbness, tingling, or weakness at the corner of the mouth and hand. Headache is present in some cases of carotid occlusion but not in most. The severity of the deficit following carotid artery occlusion depends on the collateral circulation. About 15% of carotid artery occlusions are asymptomatic. Mild deficits appear in 25%, and severe motor and other deficits in the rest. There is no way to predict the result of occlusion before the incident.

Basilar Artery Thrombosis

Basilar artery stenosis is less common than carotid artery stenosis. The basilar artery and its branches supply the brainstem, the contents of the posterior fossa, and the occipital lobes. The basilar artery arises from the union of the two vertebral arteries, a unique anatomic feature. Atherothrombosis may occur in the vertebral or basilar arteries, but most basilar occlusions arise in the lower one-third of the artery. Transient brainstem signs are common in basilar artery thrombosis. Almost 80% of patients with basilar strokes have preceding TIA. Only half the patients who have transient ischemic attacks in the basilar distribution have a subsequent basilar occlusion. About 20% experience a partial syndrome, and 8–10% have transient ischemic attacks only, without stroke. In a minority of cases (10–12%) the stroke is a progressive deficit, without preceding TIA. In basilar thrombosis the time from onset of TIA to full stroke is usually within 7–8 weeks. Dizziness is a prominent symptom in 80% of basilar cases, but dizziness alone rarely indicates vertebrobasilar disease. Pallor, sweating, diplopia, weakness, slumping to the ground, numbness bilaterally or unilaterally, dysarthria, or headache almost always accompanies the dizziness in basilar artery lesions. Transient global amnesia, with other symptoms, may provide warning of a basilar artery stroke.

Basilar artery occlusion, described in 1946 by Kubik and Adams, causes the progressive development of bilateral long tract signs, segmental brainstem signs, and cerebellar signs with coma. In half the cases the syndrome progresses within 24 hours to a complete stroke; by day 6 in almost all cases the maximum deficit has been reached. At this stage there is little to be done, so the aim of the physician is to anticipate the problem at the earliest stage. The history is generally the best clue to the diagnosis, especially when transient ischemic attacks are present. Patients with dizziness and fleeting brainstem signs, especially diplopia, are suspect.

Anticoagulants seem to provide a better chance of survival in basilar thrombosis. Patients with progressing basilar thrombosis are treated with heparin and then with Coumadin for chronic anticoagulation. There are no reliable data to indicate how long a patient will need to be anticoagulated for a thrombotic lesion. Anticoagulation is not given to patients with completed strokes and unchanging deficits following large vessel occlusion.

Angiography is important in the diagnosis of basilar artery disease, because some basilar syndromes are not related to large vessel thrombosis but, rather, to basilar branch thrombosis. Patients with basilar branch occlusion have a more benign course and usually do well when treated with only short-term anticoagulation or left untreated. The basilar branch syndromes vary and are usually discrete brainstem syndromes that improve rapidly. Angiography shows no arterial lesion when the problem is a basilar branch occlusion, since the branches are too small to appear on conventional angiography.

Treatment

A stroke must be defined as thrombotic or embolic, so that suitable therapy may be chosen. In carotid artery stenosis angiography is usually needed; if large vessel stenosis is found, heparinization and early endarterectomy may reduce the final deficit. Strokes from carotid thrombosis usually do not progress after the first 12–24 hours. Progressive carotid artery strokes seem to stop with anticoagulation more often than without.

Basilar artery occlusion progress over 8–12 hours and is often lethal. The usual treatment for basilar thrombosis is anticoagulation, although there is no definite evidence that it prevents the stroke from progressing. There is no proved operative therapy as yet for vertebrobasilar stroke, although some centers are doing bypass operations between posterior cerebral and occipital arteries.

Middle Cerebral Artery Thrombosis

Thrombosis of the middle cerebral artery is distinctly uncommon. Although the middle cerebral artery syndrome is the most common stroke syndrome in neurology, the etiology is almost always embolus rather than thrombosis. Thrombosis of the middle cerebral artery occurs at the most proximal branches, usually in the middle cerebral stem. It is more common in women treated with birth control pills, in pregnant women, or in the puerperium. Middle cerebral artery occlusion is never asymptomatic. Only a minority of patients have minor strokes, the vast majority having severe disabling deficits. In most cases there are prodromal transient ischemic attacks, and in many a stepwise, progressive deficit. Most patients managed before the infarction with anticoagulation follow a benign course.

---

1. Ackerman RH: A perspective on non-invasive diagnosis of carotid disease. *Neurology* 29:615–622, 1979.
   A balanced view of the limits of the available tests.
2. Barnett HJM: Delayed cerebral ischemic episodes distal to occlusion of major cerebral arteries. *Neurology* 28:769–774, 1978.
   Of 237 patients with occluded carotid arteries, 27 had TIA or stroke in distribution of the occlusion.
3. Berguer R, McCaffrey JF, Bauer RB: Bilateral internal carotid artery occlusion. Its surgical management. *Arch Surg* 115:840–843, 1980.
   Of these 7 patients, 5 had basilar symptoms. Operations were performed on 2 patients with acute carotid occlusion.
4. Bogousslavsky J, Regli F: Delayed TIAs distal to bilateral occlusion of carotid arteries—evidence for embolic and hemodynamic mechanisms. *Stroke* 14:58–61, 1983.
   Of 4 patients, 2 had emboli and 2 had signs with head turning or orthostatic hypotension.
5. Caplan LR: "Top of the basilar" syndrome. *Neurology* 30:72–79, 198.
   A good description of the clinical features.
6. Caplan LR: Vertebrobasilar disease: Time for a new strategy. *Stroke* 12:111–114, 1981.
   A brief review of the syndromes and thoughts on management.
7. Castaigne P, et al: Internal carotid artery occlusion. *Brain* 93:231–258, 1970.
   Discusses the arterial pathology of the carotid in detail and indicates that artery-to-artery embolism may cause stroke.
8. Cooperman M, Martin EW, Evans WE: Significance of asymptomatic bruits. *Arch Surg* 113:1339–1440, 1978.
   Stroke rate was 15% over 2–7 years with a bruit; 5% without bruit.
9. Countee RW, Vijayanathan T: External carotid artery in internal carotid artery occlusion. Angiographic, therapeutic, and prognostic considerations. *Stroke* 10:450–460, 1979.
   Of 22 patients, 12 had later problems that were solved by external carotid endarterectomy.

10. Ferguson GG: Intraoperative monitoring and internal shunts: Are they necessary in carotid endarterectomy? *Stroke* 13:287–289, 1982.
Author believes not and stirred up a controversy.
11. Fisher CM: Occlusion of carotid arteries: Further experiences. *Arch Neurol Psychiatry* 72:187–204, 1954.
The sequel to earlier work and a careful clinicopathologic correlation.
12. Fisher CM: Use of anticoagulants in cerebral thrombosis. *Neurology* 8:311–332, 1958.
Small personal series with 34% stroke rate in the untreated group and 3% in the treated group.
13. Fisher CM: Occlusion of the internal carotid artery. *Arch Neurol Psychiatry* 65:346–377, 1951.
The modern realization that lesions of extracranial vessels caused stroke.
14. Fisher CM, Ojemann RG, Roberson GH: Spontaneous dissection of cervicocerebral arteries. *Can J Neurol Sci* 5:9–19, 1978.
The 16 patients had headache, facial pain, subjective bruit, oculosympathetic palsy, and monocular blindness.
15. Goldstone J, Moore WS: Emergency carotid artery surgery in neurologically unstable patients. *Arch Surg* 111:1284–1291, 1976.
An aggressive approach is sometimes of benefit.
16. Harrison MJG, Marshall J, Thomas DJ: Relevance of duration of transient ischemic attacks in carotid territory. *Br Med J (Clin Res)* 1:1578–1579, 1978.
Carotid stenosis was more likely in patients with attacks lasting less than 1 hour.
17. Humphrey PRD, Marshall J: Transient ischemic attacks and strokes with recovery prognosis and investigation. *Stroke* 12:765–769, 1981.
Of these TIA patients, 51% of those whose attacks lasted less than 5 minutes had subsequent stroke, 30% with short TIAs had operable lesions, but 10% of longer TIAs had operable lesions. Age over 50 years was more common in stenosis.
18. Jones HR, Millikan CH: Temporal profile (clinical course) of acute carotid system cerebral infarction. *Stroke* 7:64–71, 1976.
When hemiplegia develops in 3 hours and lasts for 36 hours, it usually remains a major deficit; altered consciousness predicts high mortality.
19. Kubik CS, Adams RD: Occlusion of the basilar artery—A clinical and pathological study. *Brain* 69:73–121, 1946.
The classic description, still worth reading.
20. Marshall J, Wilkinson IMS: The prognosis of carotid transient ischemic attacks in patients with normal angiograms. *Brain* 94:395–402, 1971.
Of these patients, 20% continued to have TIA, while 13% had completed stroke. Hypertension and abnormal ECG were bad prognostic signs. Are these lacunar strokes?
21. McAllen PM, Marshall J: Cardiac dysrhythmia and transient cerebral ischaemic attacks. *Lancet* 1:1212–1215, 1973.
The cases illustrate that dysrhythmia causes nonfocal complaints rather than the usual unilateral signs associated with thrombosis.
22. Mohr JP, et al: The Harvard Cooperative Stroke Registry: A prospective registry. *Neurology* 28:754–762, 1978.
A prospective study of 694 patients showed 53% had thrombosis either of a large vessel (34%) or as lacunar infarct (19%).
23. Nunn DB: Carotid endarterectomy: Analysis of 234 operative cases. *Ann Surg* 182:733–738, 1975.
Mean age was 64. Of the 69 late deaths, 58% were caused by heart disease, 16% by stroke.
24. Pessin MS, et al: Clinical and angiographic features of carotid transient ischemic attacks. *N Engl J Med* 296:358–362, 1977.
Hemisphere attack and monocular blindness at separate times on the appropriate side are indications of tight carotid stenosis.
25. Pessin MS, et al: Mechanisms of acute carotid stroke. *Ann Neurol* 6:245–252, 1979.
Embolism from carotid stenosis or occlusion caused moderate or severe deficit with transient attacks.
26. Romanul FC, Abramovicz A: Changes in brain and pial vessels in arterial border zones: A study of 13 cases. *Arch Neurol* 11:40–65, 1964.
Only 5 of 13 patients had occlusion of the carotid artery.

27. Sanford JR, Lubow M, Vasko JS: Prevention of stroke by carotid endarterectomy. *Surgery* 83:259–263, 1978.
Discusses 154 patients who had 187 carotid endarterectomies. In 6 months to 6 years, 4.7% had strokes and 7% had recurrence of their symptoms.
28. Siekert RG, Whisnant JP, Millikan CH: Surgical and anticoagulant therapy of occlusive cerebral vascular disease. *Ann Intern Med* 48:637–641, 1963.
This 5-year follow-up showed 32% incidence of stroke in the TIA-untreated group and 4% in the treated group.
29. Sundt TM: The ischemic tolerance of neural tissue and the need for monitoring and selective shunting during carotid endarterectomy. *Stroke* 14:93–98, 1983.
An experienced review of carotid endarterectomy, which author believes is best done with selective shunting and intraoperative monitoring. Good bibliography.
30. Thompson JE, Austin DJ, Patman RD: Carotid endarterectomy for cerebrovascular insufficiency: Long-term results in 592 patients followed up to 13 years. *Ann Surg* 172:663–679, 1970.
TIAs occurred in 293 patients; operative deaths were 1.4%.

104. LACUNAR STROKES

Thomas M. Walshe

Lacunes are thrombotic infarcts of restricted size that usually occur in the deeper parts of the brain in the presence of hypertension. The arterial lesions underlying lacunes involve vessels less than 200 μ in diameter and thus cause small infarcts, usually measuring less than 10–12 mm. The involved arteries have *lipohyalinosis,* a vasculopathy that narrows the lumen and causes thinning of the vessel wall, which becomes infiltrated with macrophages. Some lacunar infarcts are up to 2 cm across. The larger lesions are associated with atheromatous lesions in the distal portions without the vasculopathy; the stroke may be from embolism.

Clinical Course

In general, the clinical course of a lacune consists of the stepwise onset of a stereotyped syndrome. In 30% of cases there are transient ischemic attacks, sometimes as many as 50 isolated ones. There is never aphasia, apraxia, hemianopia, or stupor in lacunar syndromes. Patients with lacunar infarcts often have multiple lesions. When the lesions are diffuse and numerous, the clinical picture is one of dementia.

Syndromes

Pure motor hemiplegia was the first lacunar syndrome described. The lesions have been identified pathologically in the upper part of the internal capsule. The motor deficit is greater proximally than distally; the arm and leg are equally affected. There is no mental change, but up to two-thirds of patients have slurred speech. There is no gaze palsy; in most cases, however, a pontine gaze preference has been reported (eyes toward the strong side), which is usually gone in 24 hours. Sensation is normal, and there is often an upgoing toe on the side of the hemiparesis. The EEG, CSF, angiogram, and CT scan are all normal.

Another well-described lacunar syndrome is **pure sensory stroke** in which the patient presents with a hemianesthesia. The posterolateral nucleus of the thalamus was identified as the site of the lacune in one autopsied case. **Ataxic hemiparesis** causes a mild weakness and an ipsilateral cerebellar ataxia. The lesions identified at postmortem have been in the upper basis pontis contralateral to the deficit. In **dysarthria, clumsy hand, and facial weakness syndrome** the patient presents with a leisurely progression of dysarthria and a clumsy hand. There is often an upgoing toe on the same side, and the lesion, when found at postmortem, is in the basis pontis. In the **lacunar state** the patient presents with pseudobulbar palsy, dementia, and motor signs. There are usually at least four to six isolated, small infarcts at postmortem. Sites commonly involved are the caudate, the lenticular nuclei, the thalamus, pons, and the deep white matter of the hemisphere.

Treatment

The approach to a patient with lacunar infarct aims at treatment of the hypertension with observation for expected improvement. Most patients improve in 6–8 weeks, although some patients are left with a moderate to severe deficit. Some neurologists treat with heparin if the patient is seen within the first hours of onset. There are no data to suggest that anticoagulants are efficacious in altering the course of these thrombotic lesions.

1. Caplan LR, Schoene WC: Clinical features of subcortical arteriosclerotic encephalopathy (Binswanger disease). *Neurology* 28:1206–1215, 1978.
   Clinicopathological study of 5 cases and clinical study of 6.
2. Fisher CM, Curry HB: Pure motor hemiplegia of vascular origin. *Arch Neurol* 13:30–44, 1965.
   Case report and pathology.
3. Fisher CM: Lacunar strokes and infarcts: A review. *Neurology* 32:871–877, 1982.
   There are 20 recognizable lacunar syndromes. The lacunar state may be a result of hydrocephalus rather than the few infarcts.
4. Fisher CM: Capsular infarcts: The underlying vascular lesions. *Arch Neurol* 36:65–73, 1979.
   Serial sections show the type of pathology in lacunar stroke.
5. Fisher CM: Pure sensory stroke and allied conditions. *Stroke* 13:434–447, 1982.
   A review of 134 cases with case reports and a discussion of migrainous accompaniments.
6. Fisher CM: Ataxic hemiparesis. *Arch Neurol* 35:126–128, 1978.
   The pathologic lesions were in the mid-basis pons, contralateral to the clinical findings.
7. Fisher CM: The arterial lesions underlying lacunes. *Acta Neuropathol (Berl)* 12:1–15, 1969.
   Pathological description of types of thrombosis involved in lacunes.
8. Fisher CM: The dysarthria—clumsy hand syndrome. *Neurology* 17:614–617, 1967.
   Reports 2 clinical cases, 1 postmortem. The lesion was in the basis pontis, but there were 2 lesions in the brain.
9. Fisher CM: Lacunes: Small, deep cerebral infarcts. *Neurology* 15:774–784, 1965.
   Among 1,042 postmortem cases, 376 lacunes were found in 114 patients.
10. Fisher CM: Pure sensory stroke involving face, arm, and leg. *Neurology* 15:76–80, 1965.
    Some patients had transient sensory symptoms alone or before the stroke.
11. Fisher CM, Cole M: Homolateral ataxia and crural paresis: A vascular syndrome. *J Neurol Neurosurg Psychiatry* 28:48–55, 1965.
    This syndrome is renamed ataxic hemiparesis.
12. Marie P: Desfoyers lacunaires de desintegration et des differents autres états cavitaires du cerneau. *Rev Med de Nancy* 21:281–298, 1901.
    The original description of the lacunar state.
13. Mohr JP: Lacunes. *Stroke* 13:3–11, 1982.
    A complete, enlightened review of the subject.
14. Rascol A, et al: Pure motor hemiplegia: CT study of 30 cases. *Stroke* 13:11–16, 1982.
    The lesion was seen in 29 patients; 2 had small hemorrhages; only 16 were known hypertensives.
15. Weisberg LA: Computed tomography and pure motor hemiparesis. *Neurology* 29:490–495, 1979.
    One case had a small hemorrhage.

105. EMBOLIC STROKES

Thomas M. Walshe

Etiology

Cerebral embolism occurs when an intraarterial object passes from a large proximal artery or from the heart and lodges in one of the more distal cerebral vessels. The embolus may be a fragment of calcium, bacterial vegetation, or other material dislodged from a heart valve; cholesterol from an atherosclerotic plaque; or platelet material. In trauma, fat from fractures of the large bones may be introduced into the circulation and act as an embolus. The size of the embolus determines its position in the arterial tree. Large calcium fragments from a heart valve may lodge in the carotid, but most emboli are very small and pass up to the distal cerebral vessels.

Atrial fibrillation, with or without valvular heart disease, constitutes a major risk, as high as 35% for cerebral embolism. Of patients with embolic stroke and atrial fibrillation, 70% develop a severe deficit or die. The majority of the patients are over 70 years old and in good health before the stroke. Atrial fibrillation is persistent in most patients but may occur paroxysmally in some. The presence of valvular heart disease increases the risk, but patients with atrial fibrillation alone are at as high a risk for embolism. A second episode of embolism occurs in about 10% of patients, and some have reembolization within 10 days of the initial stroke.

Clinical Syndromes

Middle Cerebral Artery Embolism. The artery of embolism is the middle cerebral artery (MCA), the site of occlusion in about three-quarters of embolic strokes. Contralateral hemiparesis, hemianesthesia, and hemianopia appear in the classic case, along with aphasia (dominant side) or constructional apraxia (nondominant side). In smaller emboli, only one division of the MCA may be involved. The superior-division MCA syndrome comprises loss of motor and sensory function (hemiparesis and hemisensory syndrome) and motor (expressive) aphasia. The inferior MCA syndrome may not include hemiparesis but produces hemianopia or an inferior quadrantanopsia and a fluent aphasia, if on the dominant side. The severity and exact detail of the lesion depend on the severity and size of the infarct. Although embolism is most commonly the cause of middle cerebral artery occlusion, a carotid artery thrombosis may also present with a neurologic syndrome very similar to one produced by an embolus. The embolic deficit is usually fixed but may clear in several hours or days.

Anterior Cerebral Artery Embolism. Embolization occurs to other arteries less commonly than to the MCA. In the case of an anterior cerebral artery syndrome, one must consider thrombosis, since only 3% of embolic lesions occur in that territory. The signs of anterior cerebral artery occlusion are not particularly well worked out because of the rarity of the lesion. There are usually excellent collaterals in the anterior system, and the areas of brain served by the anterior cerebral artery are relatively silent. The syndrome occurs when both anterior cerebral arteries are derived from the same carotid source. The signs are generally bilateral pyramidal and sensory, with the foot being affected more than the hands and arms. Dementia may occur, along with lack of spontaneity and what has been called *abulia*. Frontal release reflexes, such as a grasp or snout reflex, may appear. There may be graphesthesia, poor two-point discrimination, and other cortical sensory loss. In pure anterior cerebral artery occlusion, aphasia and hemianopia do not occur. Some patients are unable to name an object held in the left hand without looking at it because the fibers crossing from the right side of the brain to the left speech area are interrupted.

Posterior Cerebral Artery Embolism. The posterior cerebral artery (PCA) is a branch of the basilar system and is subject to embolic occlusion. Thrombotic occlusion also occurs, but embolus is more likely. The key sign in PCA occlusion is hemianopia. Often the upper quadrant deficit is denser than the lower quadrant, and in some cases there is a slight headache over the brow on the ipsilateral side. In pure cases there is lack of paralysis, aphasia, cortical sensory signs, and apraxia.

Treatment

Once an embolus is identified as the cause of a neurologic syndrome, the usual procedure is to observe the patient and to seek sources for the embolus. Embolism may arise from ulcerated plaques in the carotid and from other arterial sources. A large atrial clot or myxoma can be identified by echocardiography; an arrhythmia may be seen with cardiac monitoring. Elderly patients have a higher risk of nonbacterial thrombotic endocarditis, which may be the source of single and multiple emboli. Patients with nonbacterial thrombotic endocarditis often have a malignancy and may also show signs of venous thrombosis, disseminated intravascular coagulation, or other systemic disease before the embolism occurs.

Patients with cerebral embolism pose a different therapeutic problem than those with large vessel thrombosis. Anticoagulation does not alter the stroke and serves only to reduce the chances of future embolization. If the patient has a embolic source, chronic anticoagulation using Coumadin is necessary. Otherwise heparin is continued for several days and followed by several months of Coumadin. Patients selected for chronic anticoagulation are those at high risk of further emboli, such as patients with atrial fibrillation, recent myocardial infarction, or valvular lesions. Patients with very large strokes, especially in the left hemisphere, are not treated with anticoagulants, mainly because the maximum deficit has occurred, and the next stroke may not alter their marginal lifestyle. Acute heparin therapy is very rarely complicated by an intracerebral hematoma, but minor bleeding is common, especially in older patients. Minor bleeding can usually be handled without stopping the anticoagulation. Anticoagulation with heparin is generally instituted once the possibility of a hemorrhage is excluded by lumbar puncture or CT scan.

Patients with bacterial endocarditis do not receive heparin routinely. In rheumatic heart disease, anticoagulation reduces the likelihood of stroke and is used chronically for patients who have had an embolus to any part of the body. Chronic anticoagulation is generally recommended for patients with a prosthetic valve, except when the valve is a homograft.

Patients with atrial fibrillation should be cardioverted or treated chronically with anticoagulants. Patients who have a cerebral embolism following myocardial infarction require 6–8 months of anticoagulation; then the drugs can be stopped. Patients with mitral valve prolapse are at increased risk for cerebral embolism, but most physicians do not put such patients on anticoagulation treatment unless they have had an embolism.

---

1. Biller J, Challa VR, Toole JF, Howard VJ: Nonbacterial thrombotic endocarditis. *Arch Neurol* 39:95–98, 1982.
   Of these 99 patients, 57 were older than 60 years.
2. Easton JD, Sherman DG: Management of cerebral embolism of cardiac origin. *Stroke* 11:433–442, 1980.
   An updated summery of acute and preventive treatment.
3. Fisher CM, Pearlman A: The non-sudden onset of cerebral embolism. *Neurology* 17:1025–1032, 1967.
   Makes the point with 16 cases in detail.
4. Furlan AJ, Cavalier SJ, Hobbs RE, Weinstein MA, Modic MT: Hemorrhage and anticoagulation after nonseptic embolic brain infarction. *Neurology* 32:280–282, 1982.
   One patient had CT scan evidence of hemorrhagic infarct; none had hemorrhage even with immediate anticoagulation; 13% had recurrent embolism in 7 days.
5. Hinton RC, et al: Influence of the etiology of atrial fibrillation on the incidence of systemic embolism. *Am J Cardiol* 40:509–513, 1977.
   In 333 autopsy cases with AF, symptomatic, systemic embolism occurred in 41% that also had mitral valve disease, 35% that also had ischemic heart disease, and 35% that also had both. Of the controls, 7% had embolism.
6. Mohr JP, et al: The Harvard Cooperative Stroke Registry: A prospective registry. *Neurology* 28:754–762, 1978.
   Many embolic strokes have no source; about one-fifth of emboli are non-sudden in onset.
7. Pessin MS, et al: Mechanisms of acute carotid stroke. *Ann Neurol* 6:245–252, 1979.
   Embolism from carotid stenosis or occlusion caused moderate or severe deficit with transient attacks.
8. Wood EH, Correll JW: Atheromatous ulceration in major neck vessels as a cause of cerebral embolism. *Acta Radiol* 9:520–536, 1969.
   Ulcers that were potential sources of emboli were found in 54% of endarterectomy specimins. This paper introduces the idea of artery-to-artery embolism.
9. Castaigne P, et al: Internal carotid artery occlusion. *Brain* 93:231–258, 1970.
   Discusses the arterial pathology of the carotid in detail and indicates that artery-to-artery embolism may cause stroke.
10. Marshall J, Wilkinson IMS: The prognosis of carotid transient ischemic attacks in patients with normal angiograms. *Brain* 94:395–402, 1971.
    Of these patients, 20% continued to have TIA, 13% had completed stroke. Hypertension and abnormal ECG were bad prognostic signs. Are these lacunar strokes?

11. Koller RL: Recurrent embolic cerebral infarction and anticoagulation. *Neurol* 32:283–285, 1982.
Of 44 untreated patients, 2 reembolized in 48 hours, another in 6 days. In all, 11% reembolized within a year.

106. CEREBELLAR INFARCTION

Thomas M. Walshe

Clinical Syndrome

One of the most difficult strokes to diagnose is cerebellar infarction, since there is usually no hemiparesis. The syndrome begins with the sudden onset of vomiting, dizziness, vertigo, cerebellar ataxia, and dysarthria. Most patients with cerebellar infarction are past middle age, many have other evidence of atherosclerosis, and acute vertebral artery occlusion is the most frequent finding on cerebral angiography. The malignancy of the syndrome arises from the swelling that follows the infarction; death may follow progressive brainstem compression when cerebellar swelling reaches its peak in 3–6 days. In large cerebellar infarcts, the mass effect may cause death within 6 hours. Usually the stroke begins without warning, and there are seldom signs of transient ischemia. The patient complains of falling down and being unable to stand up again, and only rarely complains of a headache. Gait ataxia and dysarthria may develop between 12 and 96 hours after the ictus. A progressive decline in mental status and signs of brainstem compression foreshadow death, if osmotic agents and steroids are not given. A small cerebellar infarction may cause only a gait disorder that is difficult to recognize as a sign of cerebellar dysfunction. Patients who have small cerebellar infarctions often recover full neurologic function and may go undiagnosed.

The best single sign of cerebellar infarct is a sudden disorder of gait without weakness. About two-thirds of the patients have decreased alertness early in the illness. Some become comatose rapidly because of brainstem compression or hydrocephalus. An ipsilateral gaze palsy or sixth nerve palsy is also a frequent early sign and probably represents brainstem dysfunction. Upward gaze disorders are not so common but occur occasionally.

Cerebellar Infarction and Brainstem Findings. Facial nerve (VII) deficit and deficits of the trigeminal (V), vagus (X), and glossopharyngeal (IX) nerves, when they occur at the onset of the stroke, usually indicate that the brainstem as well as the cerebellum is infarcted. The vessels that provide blood to the cerebellum are important in supplying the pons, therefore in many cases cerebellar infarcts occur with pontine or medullary infarcts. On the other hand, strokes of the brainstem that destroy the cerebellar connections cause cerebellar signs without a lesion in the cerebellum itself. Infarcts in the brainstem alone do not carry a risk of herniation. Cases of brainstem infarction can be identified by the early segmental brainstem signs and by the absence of a cerebellar lesion on CT scan.

Hemorrhage vs. Infarct. The CT scan also will distinguish hemorrhage from infarct and is safer than the lumbar puncture. Surgical evacuation of the hematoma to protect the brainstem is often necessary, but in some cases of cerebellar infarction there is also enough brain swelling to warrant surgical removal of the infarct. Generally, however, osmotic agents and steroids will control brain swelling through the critical phase in cerebellar infarcts. Anticoagulation is not used unless there is angiographic evidence of large vessel thrombosis. Angiography may be needed acutely when basilar artery thrombosis is suspected, but usually it is delayed until after the acute syndrome is over.

Specific Vascular Lesions. Cerebellar infarction may be associated with occlusion of the posterior inferior cerebellar (PICA), anterior inferior cerebellar (AICA), or superior cerebellar arteries. The PICA syndrome, in addition to ipsilateral cerebellar ataxia, causes pain and numbness over half the face; vertigo and nausea; nystagmus; Horner's syndrome; dysphagia; and numbness of the arm, trunk, and leg. On the opposite side of the lesion one finds impaired pain and thermal sensation. In many cases of the PICA syndrome the vertebral artery from which the PICA arises is occluded. When the AICA is occluded, deafness and facial paralysis are added to the signs of the PICA syndrome. The superior cerebellar artery causes chorea on the side of the lesion and a contralateral sensory deficit of face and body. The amount of cerebellar involvement depends on the availability of collateral flow.

Labyrinthine Disorders. Cerebellar infarction must be considered in cases of acute vertigo and imbalance, a common syndrome usually caused by labyrinthine disorders. Separating the benign labyrinthine diseases from the cerebellar cases is sometimes difficult at onset, but patients with labyrinthine disorders do not have brainstem findings, do not have nystagmus when there is no dizziness, do not have cerebellar ataxia, and often have a past history of hearing loss or tinnitus. The best approach is to observe the patient carefully over 24–48 hours to identify progressing signs that indicate a central nervous system lesion.

1. Scotti G, Spinnler H, Sterzi R, Vallar G: Cerebellar softening. *Ann Neurol* 8:133–140, 1980.
   Study emphasizes the risks of swelling in the posteria fossa. CT scan showed the size of the lesion.
2. Adams RD: Occlusion of the anterior inferior cerebellar artery. *Arch Neurol Psychiatry* 35:765–770, 1936.
   A discussion of the PICA and superior cerebellar syndromes in addition to AICA.
3. Duncan GW, Parker SW, Fisher CM: Acute cerebellar infarction in the PICA territory. *Arch Neurol* 32:364–368, 1975.
   Clinicopathological correlation of cerebellar infarcts without brainstem involvement.
4. Sypert GW, Alvord EC: Cerebellar infarction. *Arch Neurol* 32:357–363, 1975.
   Discusses 28 cases in which the brainstem was compressed.
5. Feely MP: Cerebellar infarction. *Neurosurgery* 4:7–11, 1979.
   The infarct acted as a mass lesion in 55 of 75 cases.
6. Greenberg J, Skubick D, Shenkin H: Acute hydrocephalus in cerebellar infarct and hemorrhage. *Neurology* 29:409–413, 1979.
   Three cases were treated with ventricular drainage alone.
7. Heros RC: Cerebellar infarction resulting from traumatic occlusion of a vertebral artery. *J Neurosurg* 51:111–113, 1979.
   The syndrome is described in a patient following a gunshot wound to the neck.
8. Hinshaw DB, Thompson JR, Hasso AN, Casselman ES: Infarctions of the brainstem and cerebellum: A correlation of computed tomography and angiography. *Radiology* 137:105–112, 1980.
   The CT scan was better at showing rostral lesions in the brainstem. The bone artifact at the skull base probably obscures lower lesions.
9. Brouckaert L, Sieben G, DeReuck J, Vander Eecken H: The syndrome of the anterior inferior cerebellar artery. *Acta Neurol Belg* 81:65–73, 1981.
   Two cases: 1 with a small lesion in the basis pontis showed a pure motor hemiplegia. The other case had bilateral opthalmoplegia, facial numbness, hemiplegia, and bilateral upgoing toes. A review of 52 autopsy specimens shows the artery to be variable in its distribution.
10. Ho SU, Kim KS, Berenberg RA, Ho HT: Cerebellar infarction: A clinical and CT study. *Surg Neurol* 16:350–352, 1981.
    Of 7 patients reported, 4 were over 65 years; all but 1 over 60 years.
11. Lehrich JR, Winkler GF, Ojemann RG: Cerebellar infarctions with brain stem compression: Diagnosis and surgical treatment. *Arch Neurol* 22:490–498, 1970.
    Four cases illustrate the syndrome.
12. Woodhurst WB: Cerebellar infarction—Review of recent experiences. *Can J Neurol Sci* 7:97–99, 1980.
    Describes 6 patients. The average age was 59 years.

107. INTRACEREBRAL HEMORRHAGE

Thomas M. Walshe

About 10% of all strokes are caused by hemorrhage into the brain parenchyma. Intraparenchymal brain hemorrhage is a disorder separate from a bleeding aneurysm or arteriovenous malformation that bleeds into the subarachnoid space. About half the cases of intraparenchymal hemorrhage occur in patients older than 70 years. The hemorrhage can occur anywhere in the brain, but there are several common sites that produce clinically recognizable syndromes. The vessels involved in hemorrhage are usually the small deep penetrating branches that supply the basal ganglia, thalamus, brainstem, and cerebellum. Chronic hypertension is associated with intraparenchymal hemorrhage, and the vascular pathologic picture seems to be related to fibrinoid necrosis induced by hypertension in the small penetrating arteries. Because of this close association with high blood pressure, the term *hypertensive hemorrhage* is used interchangeably with *intraparenchymal hemorrhage*.

Clinical Findings and Diagnosis

The clinical findings of hypertensive hemorrhage vary with the site and size of the lesion. The neurologic deficit develops gradually over several hours, unless the pons is the site of bleeding, when the onset may be in minutes. Improvement and decline of the neurologic signs does not occur as in thrombotic stroke; rather, the hemorrhage causes a smoothly increasing deficit with declining alertness. Patients seldom have a severe headache but frequently vomit at the beginning of the neurologic deficit. Almost all patients with hypertensive hemorrhage have an altered level of consciousness. Even small hemorrhages cause listlessness and somnolence; the larger hemorrhages are associated with stupor and coma. At the time of hemorrhage the blood pressure is usually elevated, but more important to the diagnosis is a past history of chronic hypertension.

The temporal profile and the general characteristics associated with hemorrhage, added to the neurologic signs of hemorrhage specific to each site, allow a clinical diagnosis to be made in most cases. Confirmation of the clinical suspicion is made reliably by non-contrast CT scanning. The only hemorrhages that may not appear on CT scan are small pontine hemorrhages, and with high-resolution machines, even these are usually identifiable. In patients who have a low hemoglobin (< 9 gm/dl) the hemorrhage may appear as a low-density mass rather than the usual high-density lesion. Lumbar puncture shows blood in all but the smallest putaminal hemorrhages and is a useful diagnostic test if CT scan is not available.

Common Sites of Hemorrhage

There are five sites frequently involved in hemorrhage that each produce an identifiable neurologic syndrome. The majority of hypertensive hemorrhages (47%) occur in the putamen, 29% occur in the thalamus, 9% in the pons, 8% in the cerebellum, and 7% in the subcortical white matter.

Putaminal Hemorrhage. A putaminal hemorrhage causes a neurologic picture similar to that of middle cerebral artery occlusion: contralateral hemiplegia, hemisensory loss, and hemianopia. Vomiting, obtundation, and an ipsilateral gaze preference suggest that the lesion is hemorrhage rather than infarct. The hemiplegia or hemiparesis usually involves the foot equally with the hand, suggesting a capsular lesion in hemorrhage. Aphasia and apraxia occur in both ischemic and hemorrhagic lesions. The CT scan identifies the putaminal hemorrhage in all cases, and the size of the lesion helps to predict the overall prognosis. Most patients with small lesions do well, and many return to near their previous lifestyles. The larger hemorrhages create increased intracranial pressure, coma, and marked neurological deficits; the patients usually die or, if they live, suffer total disability.

Thalamic Hemorrhage. The syndrome of thalamic hemorrhage often begins with a sensory complaint. Examination shows a dense deficit to pin, touch, and position sense, along with a variable hemiparesis. The corneal reflex is often absent on the side affected. Patients are usually obtunded and some, in whom the hematoma extends caudally, are comatose even at onset. A diagnostic clue is a downward and inward deviation of the eyes, as if the patient were looking down at the tip of the nose. In most cases the sign is more subtle and the eyes are slightly deviated downward and will not elevate. A very small thalamic hemorrhage has been associated with an amnesic (Korsakoff) dementia as the only sign. In thalamic hemorrhage the pupils are small (3 mm) and do not react well to light. The CT scan accurately identifies the lesion and helps predict the outcome, as in putaminal hemorrhage. The prognosis in thalamic hemorrhage is the same as in putaminal hemorrhage.

Pontine Hemorrhage. The pontine hemorrhage has its onset in several minutes or over an hour. Initial complaints vary, but patients commonly arrive at the hospital stuporous or comatose, with neurologic signs related to brainstem dysfunction. Bilateral extensor plantar responses, quadriplegia, skew deviation of the eyes, and absent oculovestibular (ice-water calorics) or oculocephalic (doll's head) reflexes localize the lesion to the brainstem. The pupils are often small (1–2 mm) but react to strong light. The spinal fluid is bloody, and CT scan usually shows the leison. The prognosis is poor, and even the few who survive are severely disabled and totally dependent on others for their care.

Cerebellar Hemorrhage. Cerebellar hemorrhage constitutes a relative emergency, because the hematoma causes death from compression of the brainstem. If the hematoma is removed, the patient can recover to a relatively normal state. The clinical diagnosis of cerebellar hemorrhage is sometimes subtle early in the course, but the CT scan has made it easier to identify. The onset is usually abrupt over several minutes or hours and consists of headache, nausea, vomiting, dizzy feeling, and difficulty in walking. After the initial complaints, the patient gradually becomes stuporous and then comatose. Ataxia of the arms and legs, ipsilateral gaze palsy, and a peripheral seventh nerve palsy are also found in patients with cerebellar hemorrhage. Nystagmus, dysarthria, and upgoing toes are present in some cases. There is usually no hemiplegia. Even alert patients who have cerebellar hemorrhage are at great risk, because they can develop brainstem compression with coma very rapidly. Cerebellar hemorrhage is usually suspected clinically and confirmed by CT scan, and the patient is sent at once for surgical removal of the hematoma. Once the patient becomes comatose, with signs of brainstem damage, there is little hope of resolution even with surgical intervention. Mortality is very high, especially in patients who develop coma, reaching 75% in some groups studied.

Lobar Hemorrhage. Lobar hemorrhages occur most frequently at the white matter-gray matter interface. Vomiting, headache, a smoothly progressive deficit, and obtundation occurs with signs that depend on the lobe in which the lesion occurs. Small lobar hemorrhages may have few specific signs and go undiagnosed, unless a CT scan is done.

Treatment

There is no specific treatment for hypertensive hemorrhage except for the cerebellar hematoma, which requires prompt surgical removal. Surgical removal of a hematoma in other locations does not alter the prognosis except to maintain life, usually, with unacceptable disability. Communicating hydrocephalus occurs early in the course in some cases and usually resolves without placement of an intraventricular drain. Hydrocephalus also occurs as a late complication and then requires a ventricular shunt.

With good medical support, prevention of respiratory complications, and careful nursing, patients who have small or medium-sized supratentorial lesions improve without other treatment. It is usually of no value to use corticosteroid or osmotic diuretics. Blood pressure should not be lowered rapidly after an acute hemorrhage because of the increased intracranial pressure. Chronic blood pressure control, however, is important in preventing hypertensive hemorrhage, and even acute slight lowering of blood pressure may be needed when the systolic pressure is above 180 mm Hg.

After the acute stage, vigorous physical therapy to prevent contracture and to educate the patient to use his remaining function is helpful in getting the patient to an acceptable lifestyle.

---

1. Boudouresques G, Hauw JJ, Escourolle R: Etude anatomique de 318 hémorragies intra-parenchymateuses de l'adulte. *Rev Neurol (Paris)* 135:845–865, 1979.
English abstract. Parietal lobe hematoma was more common in elderly patients; cerebellar hematoma is found in younger patients. Average age for all patients was 62 years.
2. Collomb H, Dumas M, Girard PL, Lemercier G, Tap D: Hémorragies primitives du tronc cérébral. Etude anatomique et clinique de 36 cas. *Rev Neurol (Paris)* 129:185–210, 1973.
The best study of the clinical and pathologic aspects of pontine hemorrhage.
3. Crowell RM, Ojemann RG: Surgery for brain hemorrhage, in Moossy J, Reinmuth OM (eds): *Cerebrovascular Diseases, Twelfth Research (Princeton) Conference.* New York, Raven Press, 1981, pp 233–254.
An extensive review.

4. Dinsdale NB: Spontaneous hemorrhage in the posterior fossa: A study of primary cerebellar and pontine hemorrhage with observations on the pathogenesis. *Arch Neurol* 10:200–217, 1964.
Discusses 82 cases studied pathologically, with clinical comments. Sixty percent of the patients with cerebellar hemorrhages were between 60 and 80 years old.
5. Epstein AW: Primary massive pontine hemorrhage. *J Neuropathol Exp Neurol* 10:426–448, 1951.
Finds a 9% incidence in postmortem material.
6. Fisher CM, et al: Acute hypertensive cerebellar hemorrhage. *J Nerv Ment Dis* 140:38, 1965.
Good clinical description.
7. Fisher CM: Clinical syndromes in cerebral thrombosis, hypertensive hemorrhage, and ruptured aneurysm. *Clin Neurosurg* 22:117–147, 1975.
The details of the clinical syndromes based on the author's personal observations illustrate the variability of each disorder.
8. Furlan AJ, Cavalier SJ, Hobbs RE, Weinstein MA, Modic MT: Hemorrhage and anticoagulation after nonseptic embolic brain infarction. *Neurology* 32:280–282, 1982.
One patient had CT scan evidence of hemorrhagic infarct; none had hemorrhage even with immediate anticoagulation. In 13%, embolism recurred within 7 days.
9. Furlan AJ, Whisnant JP, Elveback LR: The decreasing incidence of primary intracerebral hemorrhage: A population study. *Ann Neurol* 5:367–373, 1979.
Hemorrhage accounts for about 10% of stroke patients.
10. Greenberg J, Skubick D, Shenkin H: Acute hydrocephalus in cerebellar infarct and hemorrhage. *Neurology* 29:409–413, 1979.
Three cases were treated with ventricular shunts.
11. Herbstein DJ, Schaumberg HH: Hypertensive intracerebral hematoma: An investigation of the initial hemorrhage and rebleeding using Cr-51 labeled erythrocytes. *Arch Neurol* 30:412–414, 1974.
Finds no evidence of rebleeding.
12. Heros RC: Cerebellar hemorrhage and infarction. *Stroke* 13:106–109, 1982.
This review emphasizes the need for prompt removal of the mass effect.
13. Hier DB, Davis KR, Richardson EP, Mohr JP: Hypertensive putaminal hemorrhage. *Ann Neurol* 1:152–159, 1977.
Summary of the clinical and CT scan features of putaminal hemorrhage.
14. Kase CS, Williams JP, Wyatt DA, Mohr JP: Lobar intracerebral hematomas: Clinical and CT analysis of 22 cases. *Neurology* 32:1146–1150, 1982.
Most lesions were in the parietotemporal lobes. Large lesions had a bad prognosis and should be considered for surgical removal.
15. Kelley RE, Berger JR, Scheinberg P, Stokes N: Active bleeding in hypertensive intracerebral hemorrhage: Computed tomography. *Neurology* 32:852–856, 1982.
Hematomas were enlarged after contrast; the supposition is that there was rebleeding.
16. Kowada M, Yamaguchi K, Matsuoka S, Ito S: Extravasation of angiographic contrast material in hypertensive intracerebral hemorrhage. *J Neurosurg* 36:471–473, 1972.
Rebleeding is rare but occurs in some patients.
17. Kwak R, Kadoya S, Suzuki T: Factors affecting the prognosis in thalamic hemorrhage. *Stroke* 14:493–500, 1983.
Level of consciousness, bilateral Babinski's signs, large hematoma, and ventricular dilatation were bad signs.
18. Moscow NP, Margolis MT: Angiography of pontine hemorrhage. *Neuroradiology* 7:125–127, 1974.
Of historic interest now that CT scanning is available.
19. Muller HR, Wuthrich R, Wiggli U, Hurrig R, Ecke M: The contribution of computerized axial tomography to the diagnosis of cerebellar and pontine hematomas. *Stroke* 6:467–475, 1975.
CT is reliable in identifying posterior fossa hematoma; hydrocephalus with blood in tips of the posterior ventricular horns points to a posterior fossa hematoma with fourth ventricular rupture.
20. Nakajima K: Clinical pathological study of pontine hemorrhage. *Stroke* 14:485–492, 1983.
Discusses 60 patients, of whom 17 survived.
21. Ojemann RG: Spontaneous brain hemorrhage: What treatment should we recom-

mend? *Stroke* 14:467, 1983.
The conclusion is, no one knows.

22. Ojemann RG, Heros RC: Spontaneous brain hemorrhage. *Stroke* 14:468–474, 1983.
A review of each type of lesion with suggestions for management.
23. Ott KH, Kase CS, Ojemann RG, Mohr JP: Cerebellar hemorrhage: Diagnosis and treatment. *Arch Neurol* 31:160–167, 1974.
Discusses clinical findings in 56 cases.
24. Ropper AH, Davis KR: Lobar cerebral hemorrhages: Acute clinical syndromes in 26 cases. *Ann Neurol* 8:141–147, 1980.
Headache was a prevalent symptom and hypertension was unusual.
25. Rosenberg GA, Kaufman DM: Cerebellar hemorrhage: Reliability of clinical evaluation. *Stroke* 7:332–336, 1976.
Correct diagnosis was made in only 13 of 33 patients using clinical parameters; 10 cases were unsuspected and 10 cases were suspected but proved to be something else.
26. Scott WR, New PFG, Davis KR, Schnur JA: Computerized axial tomography of intracerebral and intraventricular hemorrhage. *Radiology* 112:73–80, 1974.
An early description of the usefulness of CT scanning.
27. Waga S, Yamamoto Y: Hypertensive putaminal hemorrhage: Treatment and results. Is surgical treatment superior to a conservative one? *Stroke* 14:480–484, 1983.
There is little difference in the mortality in the large hemorrhage.
28. Walshe TM, Davis KR, Fisher CM: Thalamic hemorrhage. Computed tomographic-clinical correlation. *Neurology* 27:217–222, 1977.
Discusses clinical and CT scan observations in thalamic hemorrhage.
29. Weisberg LA: Computed tomography and pure motor hemiparesis. *Neurology* 29:490–495, 1979.
One case had a small hemorrhage.

APPENDIXES

A. DRUG TABLES

Table A-1. Factors affecting drug therapy in the aged

Changes in elderly	Clinical effect on drug therapy
Reduced gastric acidity	None
Reduced mesenteric blood flow	None
Reduced GI motility	None
Reduced first pass effect	Elevated serum drug levels
Reduced protein binding	Elevated free drug fraction
Reduced total body water	No consistent change
Increased percent body fat	No consistent change
Reduced hepatic blood flow and metabolism	Slower biotransformation, longer drug half-life
Reduced renal function	Slower excretion, longer drug half-life
Altered drug receptors	Variable clinical responses
Altered homeostatic function	Increased sensitivity to drug
Drug-drug interaction	Variable clinical response
Poor memory, inadequate income	Failure to comply with therapy

Table A-2. Comparative pharmacokinetics in young and elderly patients

	Half-life (hr)	
Drug	Young	Elderly
Acetaminophen	1.8	2.2
Antipyrine	12	17
Benzylpenicillin	24	55
Doxycycline	12	18
Kanamycin	1.8	4.7
Penicillin	0.5	1.0
Digoxin	51	73
Lidocaine	1.3	2.3
Quinidine	7	10
Chlordiazepoxide	10	37
Desipramine	34	76
Diazepam	20	90
Imipramine	19	24
Oxazepam	~5	~5
Phenobarbital	71	107
Phenytoin	NC	NC
Phenylbutazone	87	110
Ampicillin	1	1.2
Warfarin	37	44
ASA	NC	NC

NC = no change.

Table A-3. Desired peak and trough serum concentrations for aminoglycosides[a] and vancomycin[b]

Antibiotic	Peak (μg/ml)	Trough (μg/ml)
Amikacin	20–30	5–10
Gentamicin	6–8	1–2
Streptomycin	20–30	<5
Tobramycin	6–8	1–2
Vancomycin	30–40	5–10

[a]In patients with normal renal function, peak value is determined by obtaining blood 30 min after intravenous administration or 45–60 min after intramuscular injection. In patients with renal insufficiency or changing renal function, peak value blood is drawn 1 hr after administration. Blood for trough values is obtained 15–30 min prior to administration of the next dose.
[b]Blood for peak value is obtained 1 hr after intravenous infusion.
Source: Adapted from Barza M, Scheife RT: *Am J Hosp Pharm* 34:723, 1977.

Table A-4. Guidelines for antibiotic therapy in the elderly

Antimicrobial	Usual dosage	Route	Maintenance dose intervals (hr) based on creatinine clearance (cc/min)[a] 100	80–50	50–10	<10
Amikacin[b,c]	10 mg/kg (loading dose); then, 7.5 mg/kg q12h	IM or IV	12	12–18	24–36	36–48
Ampicillin	0.5–2.0 gm q6h	PO or IV	6	6	8	12
Azlocillin	2–3 gm q4–6h	IV	6	6	6–8	8–12
Carbenicillin	4–5 gm q4h	IV	4	4	6–12	12–24
Cefamandole	0.5–2.0 gm q6h	IM or IV	6	6	8	12
Cefazolin	0.25–1.0 gm q6h	IM or IV	6	6	8–12	12–24
Cefoperazone[d]j	2–3 gm q8h	IV		Unchanged		
Cefotaxime	1–2 gm q4–6h	IM or IV	6	6	6–8	8–12
Cefoxitin	1–2 gm q4–6h	IM or IV	6	6	8	12
Cephalothin	1–2 gm q4–6h	IV	4	4	6–8	8–12
Chloramphenicol[d]	0.5–1.0 gm q6h	IV		Unchanged		
Clindamycin[d]	0.6–1.2 gm q6h	IV		Unchanged		
Dicloxacillin	0.125–0.5 gm q6h	PO		Unchanged		
Doxycycline	0.1–0.2 gm q12h	PO or IV		Unchanged		
Erythromycin	0.25–1.0 gm q6h	PO or IV		Unchanged		
Ethambutol	15 mg/kg/day as single dose	PO or IV	24	24	24–36	48–72
Gentamicin[b,c]	2 mg/kg (loading dose); then, 1.75 mg/kg q8h	IM or IV	8	8–12	12–24	24–48
Isoniazid	300 mg/day as single dose	PO or IM		Unchanged		
Methicillin	1–2 gm q4–6h	IM or IV	4	4	4–6	6–8
Mezlocillin	2–3 gm q4–6h	IV	6	6	6–8	8–12
Moxalactum	1–2 gm q8h	IM or IV	8	8	8–12	8–12
Nafcillin	0.5–2.0 gm q4–6h	PO, IM, or IV		Unchanged		
Oxacillin	0.5–2.0 gm q4–6h	PO, IM, or IV		Unchanged		

A-4. Continued

Antimicrobial	Usual dosage	Route	Maintenance dose intervals (hr) based on creatinine clearance (cc/min)[a]			
			100	80–50	50–10	<10
Penicillin G	600,000–1,200,000 units q6h	PO or IV	6	6	6–8	8–12
	10,000,000–12,000,000 units/day (serious infections)	IV	6	6	6–8	8–12
Piperacillin	2–3 gm q4–6h	IV	6	6	6	6–8
Rifampin	600 mg/day as single dose	PO	Unchanged			
Streptomycin[b,c]	7.5 mg/kg q12h	IM	12	12–24	24–72	72–96
Tetracycline[e,f]	0.25–0.5 gm q6h	PO or IV	6	Not Recommended		
Ticarcillin	2–3 gm q4h	IV	4	4	6–8	12
Trimethoprim-sulfamethoxazole	2 tablets (80 mg TMP and 400 mg SMZ/tablet) q12h	PO	12	12	18	24
Tobramycin	2 mg/kg (loading dose); then, 1.7 mg/kg q8h	IM or IV	8	8–12	12–24	48
Vancomycin[c]	0.5 mg q6–8h	IV	12	24–72	72–240	240

IM = intramuscular; IV = intravenous; PO = oral; U = units.

[a]Creatinine clearance (C_{cr}) for males can be estimated with the following formula: $C_{cr}\ (\text{ml/min}) = \frac{(140 - \text{age}) \times \text{kg body weight}}{72 \times \text{serum creatinine (mg/dl)}}$. For females, C_{cr} is multiplied by 0.85.

[b]Doses of aminoglycosides based on ideal body weight.
[c]Dosage best monitored by frequent measurements of serum concentrations (Table A-3). Loading dose employed only in presence of life-threatening infection.
[d]Dosage should be decreased in presence of hepatic failure.
[e]Tetracycline should be avoided in presence of renal insufficiency.
[f]Intravenous administration must not exceed 1.5 gm/day.
Source: Maintenance dose intervals (hr) based on creatinine clearance (cc/min) adapted from Bennett WM, et al: Drug therapy in renal failure: Dosing guidelines for adults. *Ann Intern Med* 93:62, 1980.

Table A-5. Antibiotic toxicities of special significance in the elderly

Antimicrobial	Adverse reaction	Precaution
Aminoglycosides (amikacin, gentamicin, tobramycin)[a]	Nephrotoxicity	Measure serum blood urea nitrogen (BUN), creatinine, and creatinine clearance before therapy; monitor serum BUN or creatinine 2–3 times weekly, more frequently in presence of changing renal function; avoid intravascular volume depletion, concomitant use of methoxyflurane, and other potentially nephrotoxic drugs (e.g., vancomycin, cephalosporins)
	Ototoxicity	Monitor audiograms if aminoglycoside administered for longer than 10 days; avoid simultaneous use of drugs that can mask symptoms of ototoxicity (e.g., Benadryl)
Ampicillin	Diarrhea, pseudomembranous colitis	Monitor for appearance of gastrointestinal tract symptoms; daily stool counts
Carbenicillin, ticarcillin, and newer derivatives (e.g., azlocillin, mezlocillin, piperacillin)	Volume overload	Monitor fluid status by physical examination, daily weights, and measurements of daily fluid intake and output
	Hypokalemic alkalosis	Measure serum electrolytes 2–3 times/week; obtain frequent ECGs
	Coagulopathy	Monitor for occult bleeding (e.g., stool for guaiac); avoid use of other drugs that interfere with hemostasis (e.g., aspirin)
Cephalosporins	Nephrotoxicity	Measure serum BUN and creatinine 2–3 times/week; avoid volume depletion and the simultaneous use of other potential nephrotoxins (e.g., aminoglycosides)

A-5. Continued

Antimicrobial	Adverse reaction	Precaution
	Coagulopathy	Patients receiving moxalactum, cefamandole, or cefoperazone should be monitored for occult bleeding, avoid the use of other drugs that interfere with hemostasis, and have a prothrombin time (PT) measured 2–3 times/wk. Patients receiving moxalactum or cefoperazone can be given vitamin K 5–10 mg 1–2 times/wk
	Ethanol intolerance	Patients given cefoperazone, cefamandole, or moxalactum should not receive alcohol or alcohol-containing products (e.g., some cough syrup preparations) because of possibility of disulfiramlike reactions (i.e., nausea, vomiting, flushing, hyypotension)
Chloramphenicol	Bone marrow suppression	Perform complete blood count (CBC) before therapy and 2–3 times/week during treatment
	Aplastic anemia	Avoid oral administration
Clindamycin	Diarrhea, pseudomembranous colitis	Monitor for appearance of gastrointestinal symptoms and perform daily stool counts
Ethambutol	Optic neuritis	Monthly ophthalmologic examination for red-green color perception and visual acuity
Isoniazid	Peripheral neuropathy	Administer pyridoxine 100 mg/day
	Hepatitis	Obtain liver function tests before initiating therapy; monitor monthly for symptoms suggestive of hepatitis (e.g., "flulike illness"—fever, malaise, anorexia, fatigue, nausea, vomiting); avoid concomitant use of potential hepatotoxins (e.g., ethyl alcohol)

Penicillin G (high dose)	Hyperkalemia Hypokalemia	Measure serum BUN, creatinine, and electrolytes before treatment and 2–3 times/week during therapy
	Hemolytic anemia	Obtain CBC before treatment and 2–3 times/week during therapy and a Coombs' test if anemia occurs
	Volume overload	Monitor fluid status by physical examination, daily weights, and daily measurements of fluid intake and output
Rifampin	Hepatitis	As described for isoniazid
Tetracycline	Azotemia	Measure serum BUN and creatinine before treatment and 2–3 times/week during therapy; avoid in the presence of moderate to severe renal insufficiency
	Hepatic failure	Avoid intravenous administration (when necessary, maximum dose in presence of normal renal function is 1.5 gm/day); monitor liver function tests 2–3 times/week
Vancomycin	Nephrotoxicity, ototoxicity	As described for aminoglycosides

Note: See also Table A-6, Drug-antibiotic interactions.

[a]Dosing intervals of aminoglycosides are best determined by level of creatinine clearance, not serum creatinine (see Table A-4). Peak and trough serum levels should be monitored frequently (Table A-3).

Table A-6. Drug antibiotic interactions

Antibiotic	Interacting drugs	Effect
Amantadine	Anticholinergics, L-dopa	Agitation, confusion, hallucinations
Aminoglycosides	Carbenicillin, ticarcillin	Inactivation of aminoglycoside in patients with renal insufficiency
	Cephalosporins, vancomycin, methoxyflurane, *cis*-platinum	Enhanced potential for nephrotoxicity
	Neuromuscular blocking agents	Enhanced possibility of neuromuscular blockade
Ampicillin	Allopurinol	Enhanced potential for rash
Cephalosporins	Aminoglycosides	Enhanced potential for nephrotoxicity
	Probenecid, phenylbutazone, sulfinpyrazone	Increased serum levels and decreased urine levels of cephalosporins
	Ethanol	Antabaselike reaction (i.e., nausea, flushing, diarrhea, tachycardia)
Chloramphenicol	Diphenylhydantoin	Diphenylhydantoin toxicity
	Oral anticoagulants	Enhanced anticoagulation
	Barbiturates	Barbiturate toxicity
	Sulfonylureas	Hypoglycemia
Clindamycin	Neuromuscular blocking agents	Enhanced neuromuscular blockade
Doxycycline	Phenobarbital, phenytoin, carbamazepine	Shortened half-life of doxycycline
	Preparations (e.g., antacids) containing calcium, aluminum, iron, magnesium, or zinc salts	Impaired absorption of doxycycline
Erythromycin	Theophylline	Increased serum levels of theophylline
Isoniazid	Aluminum hydroxide	Impaired absorption of isoniazid
	Diphenylhydantoin	Diphenylhydantoin toxicity
	Disulfiram	Alterations in effect and behavior
	Ethanol, rifampin	Enhanced potential for hepatotoxicity
Penicillins	Acetylsalicylic acid (3–4 gm/day), probenecid, phenylbutazone, sulfinpyrazone	Increased serum levels and decreased urine levels of penicillin

A-6. Continued

Antibiotic	Interacting drugs	Effect
Rifampin	Methadone	Increased metabolism of methadone
	Glucocorticoids	Enhanced catabolism of glucocorticoids
	Quinidine	Decreased quinidine effect
	Halothane, isoniazid	Enhanced potential for hepatotoxicity
	Digitoxin, digoxin	Decreased cardiac glycoside effect
	Oral anticoagulants	Inhibition of anticoagulation
	Oral hypoglycemics	Decreased effect of hypoglycemics
	Probenecid	Increased serum levels of rifampin
Sulfonamides	Diphenylhydantoin	Enhanced potential for diphenylhydantoin toxicity
	Methotrexate	Enhanced antifolate activity
	Oral anticoagulants	Enhanced anticoagulation
	Oral hypoglycemics	Hypoglycemia
Tetracycline	Antacids containing calcium, aluminum, or magnesium; ferrous sulfate, zinc sulfate, sodium bicarbonate; milk products	Impaired absorption of tetracycline
	Methoxyflurane	Enhanced potential for nephrotoxicity
	Oral anticoagulants	Enhanced anticoagulation

Table A-7. Antimicrobial therapy for bacterial endocarditis

Organism	Antibiotic	Dose	Alternate
Streptococcus viridans	Penicillin G[a]	2–4 million units IV q4h	Vancomycin[b] 500 mg IV q6–8h
Staphylococcus aureus			
Penicillin-sensitive	Penicillin G[a]	2–4 million units q4h	Vancomycin[b] 500 mg IV q6–8h
Penicillin-resistant	Oxacillin or nafcillin	2 gm IV q4h	Vancomycin[b] 500 mg IV q6–8h
Enterococcus	Penicillin G[a]	2–4 million units q4h	Vancomycin[b] 500 mg IV q6–8h
	or		
	Ampicillin	2 gm IV q4h	
	plus		**plus**
	Gentamicin[b]	1.75 mg/kg q8h	Gentamicin[b] 1.75 mg/kg IV q8h
Unknown (presumptive diagnosis)[c]			
ABE	Ampicillin	2 gm IV q4h	Vancomycin[b] 500 mg IV q6–8h
	plus		**plus**
	Oxacillin	2 gm IV q4h	Gentamicin[b] 1.75 mg/kg IV q8h
	plus		
	Gentamicin[b]	1.75 mg/kg IV q8h	
SBE	Penicillin G[a]	2–4 million units IV q4h	Vancomycin[b] 500 mg IV q6–8h
	or		
	Ampicillin	2 gm IV q4h	
	plus		**plus**
	Gentamicin[b]	1.75 mg/kg IV q8h	Gentamicin[b] 1.75 mg/kg IV q8h

Note: All antibiotic regimens to be administered for 4–6 weeks without interruption. Alternate therapies, particularly those that employ both vancomycin and gentamicin, possess a high potential for toxicity; they should be employed only for elderly patients with a prior history of a significant adverse reaction to penicillin. Scrupulous monitoring of therapy is mandatory (see Tables A-3, A-4, A-5).

[a]Adjust dose of penicillin G to achieve serum-cidal levels of 1 : 8 or greater.

[b]See Table A-5 for toxicities and precautions.

[c]These regimens are to be employed while awaiting results of blood cultures or in the setting of sterile cultures; these treatments should be modified when offending pathogen has been isolated.

IV = intravenous; IM = intramuscular; ABE = acute bacterial endocarditis; SBE = subacute bacterial endocarditis.

Table A-8. Community-acquired bacteremia in patients age 65 and older

Urinary tract (34%)	Biliary tract (16%)	Pulmonary (14%)	Cutaneous (10%)	Endocarditis (8%)	Unknown (8%)	Abdominal (5%)
E. coli	*E. coli*	*S. pneumoniae*	*Streptococcus*	*Streptococcus*	*E. coli*	*E. coli*
Klebsiella	*Klebsiella*	*Klebsiella*	*S. aureus*	*S. aureus*	*Pseudomonas*	*Bacteroides*
Proteus	*Enterococcus*	*S. aureus*	*Proteus*		*Streptococcus*	*Klebsiella*
Enterococcus	*Bacteroides*	*E. coli*	*E. coli*		*Bacteroides*	*Pseudomonas*
Pseudomonas	*Streptococcus*	*H. influenzae*				*Streptococcus*

Note: Percentages refer to total number of community-acquired bacteremias. Miscellaneous foci generate 5% of total bacteremias. Bacteria are listed in order of frequency of isolation.
Source: From Esposito AL, Gleckman RA: Community-acquired bacteremia in the elderly: An analysis of one-hundred consecutive episodes. *J Am Geriatr Soc* 28:315, 1980.

Table A-9. Nosocomial bacteremia in patients over age 65

Urinary tract (35%)	Surgical wound (16%)	catheter (15%)	Pulmonary (14%)	Abdominal (12%)	Cutaneous (5%)	Unknown (3%)
E. coli	*S. aureus*	*S. aureus*	*S. aureus*	*E. coli*	*Proteus*	*E. coli*
Proteus	*Proteus*	*S. epidermidis*	*E. coli*	*Bacteroides*	*S. aureus*	*S. aureus*
Pseudomonas	*Bacteroides*	*Serratia*	*Klebsiella*	*Proteus*	*E. coli*	*Proteus*
Enterococcus	*Klebsiella*	*E. coli*	*S. pneumoniae*	*Pseudomonas*	*Enterococcus*	*Pseudomonas*
Klebsiella	*S. epidermidis*	*Entercoccus*	*Pseudomonas*	*Klebsiella*		
Serratia	*E. coli*	*Acinetobacter*	*Serratia*	*Clostridia*		

Note: Percentages refer to total number of nosocomial bacteremias. Bacteria are listed in order of frequency of isolation.
Source: From Esposito AL, Gleckman RA: Unpublished data, 1979.

Table A-10. Fever of unknown origin in patients 65 yr of age or older

Category	Percent total cases
Infection	36
Abscess	
Abdominal	11
Hepatic	6
Endocarditis	8
Tuberculosis	8
Brucellosis	1
Other	2
Neoplasm	24
Lymphoma	
Non-Hodgkin's	8
Hodgkin's disease	6
Carcinoma	
Renal	4
Hepatobiliary	3
Pancreatic	1
Unknown primary	2
Connective tissue disorder	25
Giant cell arteritis	17
Polyarteritis nodosa	5
Other	3
Miscellaneous	10
Pulmonary emboli	5
Periodic fever	3
Drugs	2
Undiagnosed	5

Source: Adapted from Esposito AL, Gleckman RA: Fever of unknown origin in the elderly. *J Am Geriatr Soc* 26:498, 1978.

Table A-11. Drugs used in the treatment of obstructive airway disease

Type	Dose	Toxicity	Comment
Methylxanthines (e.g., aminophylline, theophylline)	Loading dose for IV use = 5.6 mg/kg Maintenance dose (IV or PO) for young normal = 0.9 mg/kg/hr, 22 mg/kg/day; for elderly = 0.7 mg/kg/hr, 16.5 mg/kg/day Liver disease and CHF = 0.45 mg/kg/hr, 11 mg/kg/day	Anorexia, nausea, dysrhythmias, seizures (at high levels)	Therapeutic level usually 10–20 μg/ml; most oral compounds contain methylxanthine as the efficacious agent; dosing should be based on methylxanthine content; following drug levels may be helpful
Beta-adrenergic agents			
Nonselective ($B_1 + B_2$)		Tachycardia, tachyarrhythmias, benign tremor, angina pectoris (in the presence of coronary artery disease)	Not recommended for use when relatively B_2 selective agents are available
Isoproterenol	Inhaled = 0.5 –1.0 mg q6–8h		
Epinephrine	Subcutaneously = 0.25–0.5 mg q2–6h		
Relatively selective (B_2)			
Salbutamol	Inhaled = 0.5–1.0 mg q2–6h IV = 1–4 mg/min infused Subcutaneously = 0.25 –0.5 mg q2–6h Oral = 2–4 mg 4 times/day	Occasional tachyarrhythmia	Most B_2 selective agent available
Isoetharine mesylate	Inhaled = 0.5–1.0 mg q2–6h	Occasional tachyarrhythmias	
Terbutaline	Subcutaneously = 0.25–0.5 mg every 4–6 hours Oral = 2.5–5.0 mg 4 times/day	Benign tremor, tachycardia, tachyarrhythmias (especially subcutaneously, which have effects similar to epinephrine)	Oral administration is useful when patients cannot use inhaled medication

A-11. Continued

Type	Dose	Toxicity	Comment
Metaproterenol	Oral = 30 mg 4 times/day	Tachycardia	
Ephedrine			Found in many proprietary preparations (not particularly useful)
Corticosteriods	IV = 250–1,000 mg hydrocortisone equivalent dose q2–12h for first 24–48 hr with transfer to oral dose after	Little acute toxicity	Use in status asthmaticus; frequently difficult to document benefit in groups of patients treated for COPD

B. GOVERNMENT AGENCIES SERVING THE ELDERLY

Alabama
Alabama Commission on Aging
502 Washington Avenue, Floor 2
Montgomery, Alabama 36130

Alaska
Older Alaskans Commission
Department of Administration
Pouch C, Millstop. 209
Juneau, Alaska 99811

Arizona
Aging and Adult Administration
1400 West Washington Street
P.O. Box 6123
Phoenix, Arizona 85007

Arkansas
Office on Aging and Adult Services
Department of Human Services
1428 Donaghey Building
7th and Main Streets
Little Rock, Arkansas 72201

California
Health and Welfare Agency
1600 9th Street, Room 443
Sacramento, California 95814

California Department of Aging
Health and Welfare Agency
1020 19th Street
Sacramento, California 95814

Colorado
Division of Services for the Aging
Department of Social Services
1575 Sherman Street, Room 803
Denver, Colorado 80203

Connecticut
State Department on Aging
80 Washington Street
Hartford, Connecticut 06106

Delaware
Department of Health and Social Services
Delaware State Hospital
Office of the Secretary Administration Building, Floor 3
New Castle, Delaware 19720

Division of Aging
Department of Health and Social Services
1901 North Dupont Highway, Floor 2
New Castle, Delaware 19720

District of Columbia
D.C. Office of Aging
1424 K Street, Northwest, Floor 7
Washington, D.C. 20005

Florida
Department of Health and Rehabilitation Services
1323 Winewood Boulevard
Tallahassee, Florida 32301

Aging and Adult Services
Department of Health and Rehabilitative Services
1323 Winewood Boulevard
Tallahassee, Florida 32301

Georgia
Office of Aging
Department of Human Resources
878 Peachtree Street, Northeast, Room 682
Atlanta, Georgia 30309

Guam
Department of Public Health and Social Services
Government of Guam
P.O. Box 2816
Agana, Guam 96910

Division of Senior Citizens
Department of Public Health and Social Services
Government of Guam
P.O. Box 2816
Agana, Guam 96910

Hawaii
Executive Office on Aging
Office of the Governor
State of Hawaii
1149 Bethel Street, Room 307
Honolulu, Hawaii 96813

Idaho
Idaho Office on Aging
Statehouse, Room 104
Boise, Idaho 83720

Illinois
Department on Aging
421 East Capitol Avenue
Springfield, Illinois 62701

Indiana
Indiana Department on Aging and Community Services
115 North Pennsylvania Street, Suite 1350
Indianapolis, Indiana 46204

Iowa
Commission on Aging
914 Grand Avenue
Jewett Building, Suite 236
Des Moines, Iowa 50319

Kansas
Kansas Department on Aging
610 West 10th Street
Topeka, Kansas 66612

Kentucky
Department of Human Resources
Capital Annex, Room 201
Frankfort, Kentucky 40601

Division of Aging Services
Department of Social Services
275 East Main Street
Frankfort, Kentucky 40621

Louisiana
Office of Elderly Affairs
P.O. Box 80374
Baton Rouge, Louisiana 70898

Maine
Department of Human Services
State House
Augusta, Maine 04333

Bureau of Maine's Elderly
Department of Human Services
State House, Station 11
Augusta, Maine 04333

Maryland
Office on Aging
State Office Building
301 West Preston Street
Baltimore, Maryland 21201

Massachusetts
Department of Elder Affairs
38 Chauncey Street
Boston, Massachusetts 02111

Michigan
Office of Services to the Aging
300 East Michigan
P.O. Box 30026
Lansing, Michigan 48909

Minnesota
Minnesota Board on Aging
204 Metro Square Building
121 East Seventh Street
St. Paul, Minnesota 55101

Mississippi
Council on Aging
Executive Building, Suite 301
802 North State Street
Jackson, Mississippi 39201

Missouri
Department of Social Services
Broadway State Office Building
P.O. Box 1527
Jefferson City, Missouri 65102

Division of Aging
Department of Social Services
Broadway State Office Building
P.O. Box 1337
Jefferson City, Missouri 65102

Montana
Department of Social and Rehabilitation Services
P.O. Box 4210
Helena, Montana 59601

Aging Services Bureau
Department of Social and Rehabilitation Services
P.O. Box 4210
Helena, Montana 59601
(406) 8-587-5650

Nebraska
Department of Aging
State House Station 95044
Lincoln, Nebraska 68509

Nevada
Division for Aging Services
Department of Human Resources
505 East King Street
Kinkead Building, Room 101
Carson City, Nevada 89710

New Hampshire
New Hampshire State Council on Aging
14 Depot Street
Concord, New Hampshire 03301

New Jersey
Division on Aging
Department of Community Affairs
CN807
363 West State Street
Trenton, New Jersey 08625

New Mexico
State Agency on Aging
La Villa Riviera Building, Floor 4
224 East Palace Avenue
Santa Fe, New Mexico 87501

New York
Office for the Aging
Agency Building 2
Empire State Plaza
Albany, New York 12223

North Carolina
Department of Human Resources
Albermarle Building
325 North Salisbury Street
Raleigh, North Carolina 27611

Division of Aging
Department of Human Resources
708 Hillsborough Street, Suite 200
Raleigh, North Carolina 27603

North Dakota
North Dakota Department of Human Services
State Capitol Building
Bismarck, North Dakota 58505

Aging Services
Social Services Board of North Dakota
State Capitol Building
Bismarck, North Dakota 58505

Northern Mariana Islands
Department of Community and Cultural Affairs
Commonwealth of the Northern Mariana Islands
Civic Center, Susupe
Saipan, Mariana Islands 96950

Ohio
Commission on Aging
50 West Broad Street, Floor 9
Columbus, Ohio 43215

Oklahoma
Department of Human Services
P.O. Box 25352
Oklahoma City, Oklahoma 73125

Special Unit on Aging
Department of Human Services
P.O. Box 25352
Oklahoma City, Oklahoma 73125

Oregon
Human Resources Department
318 Public Service Building
Salem, Oregon 97310

Senior Services Division
Human Resources Department
313 Public Services Building
Salem, Oregon 97310

Pennsylvania
Department of Aging
231 State Street
Barto Building
Harrisburg, Pennsylvania 17101

Puerto Rico
Department of Social Services
P.O. Box 11398
Santurce, Puerto Rico 00910

Gericulture Commission
Department of Social Services
P.O. Box 11389
Santurce, Puerto Rico 00910

Rhode Island
Department of Elderly Affairs
79 Washington Street
Providence, Rhode Island 02903

Samoa
Territorial Administration on Aging
Government of American Samoa
Pago Pago, American Samoa 96799

South Carolina
Commission on Aging
915 Main Street
Columbia, South Carolina 29201

South Dakota
Department of Social Services
Office of the Secretary
Richard F. Kneip Building
Illinois Street
Pierre, South Dakota 57501

Office of Adult Services and Aging
Division of Human Development
Department of Social Services
Richard F. Kneip Building
Illinois Street
Pierre, South Dakota 57501

Tennessee
Commission on Aging
703 Tennessee Building
535 Church Street
Nashville, Tennessee 37219

Texas
Governor's Committee on Aging
Capitol Station
P.O. Box 12786
Austin, Texas 78711

Trust Territory of the Pacific
Office of Elderly Affairs
Grants Management Division
Government of the Trust Territory of the Pacific Islands
Saipan, Mariana Islands 96950

Utah
Department of Social Services
221 State Capitol Building
Salt Lake City, Utah 84102

Division of Aging
Department of Social Services
150 West North Temple, Suite 326
Salt Lake City, Utah 84103

Vermont
Agency of Human Services
103 South Main Street
Waterbury, Vermont 05676

Office on Aging
103 South Main Street
Waterbury, Vermont 05676

Virginia
Office on Aging
830 East Main Street
Suite 950
Richmond, Virginia 23219

Virgin Islands
Commission on Aging
P.O. Box 539
Charlotte Amalie
St. Thomas, Virgin Islands 00801

Washington
Department of Social and Health Services
Mailstop OB-44-M
Olympia, Washington 98504

Bureau of Aging
Department of Social and Health Services
Mailstop OB-43-G
Olympia, Washington 98504

West Virginia
Commission on Aging
State Capitol
Charleston, West Virginia 25305

Wisconsin
Department of Health and Social Services
1 West Wilson Street, Room 686
P.O. Box 7850
Madison, Wisconsin 53707

Office on Aging
Department of Health and Social Services
1 West Wilson Street, Room 480
Madison, Wisconsin 53702

Wyoming
Wyoming Office on Aging
140 Hathaway Building
Cheyenne, Wyoming 82002

INDEX

INDEX